Financial Management for Nurse Managers and Executives

Financial Management
for Nurse Managers
and Executives

Steven A. Finkler, Ph.D., C.P.A.

Program in Health Policy
and Management
New York University

Christine T. Kovner, Ph.D., R.N., FAAN

Division of Nursing
New York University

W.B. SAUNDERS COMPANY
A Division of Harcourt Brace & Company
Philadelphia   London   Toronto   Montreal   Sydney   Tokyo

W.B. SAUNDERS COMPANY
A Division of
Harcourt Brace & Company

The Curtis Center
Independence Square West
Philadelphia, Pennsylvania 19106

> **Library of Congress Cataloging-in-Publication Data**
> Finkler, Steven A.
>   Financial management for nurse managers and executives / Steven A. Finkler,
> Christine T. Kovner.
>   p.   cm.
>   Includes bibliographical references and index.
>   ISBN 0-7216-3285-8
> 1. Nursing services—Business management.   2. Health facilities—Business
> management.   I. Kovner, Christine Tassone.   II. Title. [DNLM: 1. Delivery of
> Health Care—economics—United States—nurses' instruction.   2. Financial
> Management—methods—nurses' instruction.   W 74 F499f]
> RT86.7F46   1993
> 362.1'73'0681—dc20
> DNLM/DLC   92-49444

FINANCIAL MANAGEMENT FOR NURSE MANAGERS
AND EXECUTIVES   ISBN 0–7216–3285–8

Printed in the United States of America

Last digit is the print number: 9   8   7   6   5   4   3   2

To Our Parents,
With love and appreciation for all you taught us.

S.A.F. and C.T.K.

Preface

A book on financial management for nurses. "For whom? To what end?" our peers might ask. Our finance colleagues could tell us that there are already numerous books on financial management. Our nursing colleagues could argue that financial management is for finance people. "If nurses want to know the material, send them to business school." We do not agree that such an approach is optimal.

Our experience in the real world of health care shows us that nurse managers are now expected to understand a great deal about the financial management of organizations for which they work. What they do know is often learned on the job—often without any conceptual basis. Many nurse managers do not know a great deal about financial management, but it is our experience that most of them want to know more. They have found that an understanding of financial management would be a great asset to them in their management function.

This book is for the nurses who want to know what questions to ask the finance department and what answers to give the finance department in response to its questions. Even more importantly, it is for nurses who want to manage better. All levels of nursing management benefit from an improved understanding of financial management concepts.

What about *Budgeting Concepts for Nurse Managers*,[1] written by one of this book's authors? Why write another financial management book? The budgeting book is one of great depth but limited scope. It considers only issues related to budgeting. Financial management extends beyond the realm of budgeting. When the second edition of *Budgeting Concepts for Nurse Managers* was being prepared, the idea for this book was conceived. Some reviewers argued that the first edition of the budget book was inadequate in scope. It did not discuss financial statements, economics, or business plans. It avoided numerous other financial management issues. Other reviewers argued that its narrow focus was its strength. Ultimately a decision was made to maintain *Budgeting Concepts for Nurse Managers* as a budgeting book but also to write a broader, more inclusive text that could serve to cover the many aspects of financial management that are of growing interest to nurses.

Why are the existing financial management texts written for business schools inadequate for this purpose? Our experience as teachers suggests to us that people learn concepts best when the examples are relevant to them. This book is not only about financial management but also about nursing and the problems and opportunities that confront nurses in providing nursing care. Business school courses often use "widget" production as the basis for their examples.

---

[1]Steven A. Finkler, *Budgeting Concepts for Nurse Managers*, Second Edition, W.B. Saunders, Philadelphia, 1992.

Although the financial concepts of producing widgets are similar to those for the delivery of health care services, widgets are not people. Producing widgets and treating patients are inherently, fundamentally, different.

Making financial management concepts come alive to the reader requires some connection between the concept and its ultimate application. We have tried to make that connection in the nursing examples used throughout this book.

This book has been designed for use both as a textbook for graduate students and as a reference for practicing nurse managers who are seeking a better understanding of financial management. Topic coverage includes all the financial management areas with which we think nurse managers should be familiar.

In preparing the book, we chose to err on the side of inclusiveness rather than on the side of omission. In our attempt to achieve completeness, more topics are included in the book than may be covered in some one-semester graduate courses on financial management for nurses. The book is particularly broad in its inclusion of topics such as economics, strategic planning, quantitative decision-making tools, and marketing. To the extent that any course skips over chapters, the students will still find those chapters to be valuable reference material for reading and study at a later date.

Some areas are discussed in greater depth than others. The level of detail for each topic reflects our belief about the depth required by a nurse manager. Each chapter has an extensive list of suggested readings if the reader wants more depth in a particular subject area. In an attempt to provide a coherent whole, chapters refer to pertinent material in other chapters. However, each chapter is virtually self-contained, so the reader can choose to read a single chapter on a particular topic or read chapters in a different order than presented.

This book is not meant to prepare the nurse manager to replace financial managers in health care organizations but rather to prepare the nurse manager for a collegial relationship with financial managers. For example, the book covers business planning. That does not mean that each nurse manager will single-handedly have to prepare a full 100-page business plan. While that may be the case in a limited number of instances, many nurse managers are more likely to need to be able to *participate* in the development of business plans. As a nurse manager you may be aided by consultants, by your own staff, or by the organization's finance department. Nurse managers need to know what a business plan is, what is in a business plan, what is important about it, how to read it, and how to make a decision based on it.

We envision this book's being used in a graduate course in financial management for nurses. It is our expectation that a faculty member can use this book in the order it is written. However, we have attempted to allow flexibility in recognition of the fact that graduate programs prepare different levels of nurse managers and have different core course requirements. Some programs have prerequisites; others may provide an entire required course on some of the topics to which we devoted a chapter such as the health care environment or economics. If students are already familiar with the content, it is not necessary to assign these chapters. We have attempted to prepare a book that can meet the needs of a variety of nursing programs, as well as those of practitioners. On the other hand, the chapters on topics such as management (Chapter

3) or marketing (Chapter 18) do not provide the depth that one would find in an entire textbook written on those topics. Given the financial management focus of this book, we are only attempting to provide an overview of those areas for students who have not yet taken a course in those areas and a refresher for those who have.

The topics covered are appropriate for programs that prepare chief nurse executives (CNEs) and for programs that prepare midlevel nurse managers as well. For programs preparing midlevel managers the instructor may not wish to assign all chapters. Individual instructors may choose to modify their coverage of chapters based on their students' specific needs.

An instructor's manual is available to go with this book. The manual includes questions for discussion as well as problems and their solutions. Course instructors can order a copy of the manual through the W.B. Saunders textbook department. The questions and problems can be used for homework assignments, in class, or for examinations.

Part I of the book includes chapters on the environment faced by health care organizations, how financial management fits in the health care organization, and key issues in applied economics. We believe an understanding of the material in these chapters is fundamental to the study of financial management in health care. An instructor may choose to skip some or all of the chapters in this part if the material the chapter(s) contains is a prerequisite to entry in the program or is covered elsewhere in the curriculum.

Part II discusses financial accounting, including accounting principles and analysis of financial statements. To understand costing and budgeting, we believe the midlevel nurse manager needs to be familiar with the basic accounting concepts in the first chapter in this part (Chapter 5). A thorough understanding of financial statements and financial statement analysis (Chapter 6), however, is more appropriate to the chief nursing executive (CNE) level.

Part III discusses cost analysis. We believe that Chapters 7 and 8 contain content necessary for all levels of nurse managers. Chapter 9, measuring the costs of recruiting and retaining staff, may not be necessary for all midlevel nurse managers.

Part IV focuses on planning and control. The management role of making plans and then attempting to carry out those plans to the extent possible is central to the role of all managers. The chapters in this part of the book therefore contain material with which all levels of nurse managers should be familiar.

Part V deals with management of the organization's financial resources. It includes concepts such as management of cash, loans, and accounts receivable. This content will be of greater interest to managers approaching the CNE level.

Part VI discusses a variety of additional management tools. Although all levels of nurse managers should be at least generally familiar with these concepts, the CNE should have a more thorough understanding of them.

Part VII addresses the future of financial management with respect to nurse managers, and we believe it should be read by all levels of nurse managers.

We would like to express our thanks to the many people who helped with the preparation of this book. First we thank the many nurses whom we have taught and with whom we have worked. They have shared their knowledge and insights about the real world of financial management encountered by nurses in health organizations. A special group of nurses are those who participated in the New Jersey Nursing Incentive Reimbursement Awards program. We learned a great deal from that project and its participating nurses. Our colleagues at New York University, as always, tolerated our obsessiveness with this book and our occasional lack of attention to programs and research that they felt had a higher priority.

We very much appreciate the comments and suggestions made by the following individuals who reviewed the entire manuscript:

> **Helen M. Castillo**, PhD, RN, CNA
> Associate Professor of Nursing
> University of Texas at El Paso
> El Paso, Texas
> Adjunct Associate Professor of Nursing
> Vanderbilt University
> Nashville, Tennessee

> **Elizabeth A. Mottet**, MS, RN
> Doctoral Student, Philip Y. Hahn School of Nursing
> University of San Diego
> Formerly Director of Nursing Research, Education, and Quality Assurance
> UCSD Medical Center
> San Diego, California

> **June A. Schmele**, PhD, RN
> Associate Professor
> University of Oklahoma College of Nursing
> Oklahoma City, Oklahoma

To our spouses we are particularly grateful. Lilli Finkler has suffered through this process several times before. She has learned that a book is like a black hole into which every moment of time is sucked, leaving very little for the rest of the family. Tony Kovner is a valued colleague. His critiques of both content and style made this a better book. He is the health care manager we all hope to be. However, he is most appreciated as a loving husband, who encouraged the writing of this book, even though it meant his wife would not always be there when he needed her.

Finally, we would like to thank our readers. We thank you not only for reading this book but also for helping to improve it. We encourage you to contact us with comments, suggestions, examples, or corrections.[2] All material we receive that is used in a subsequent edition will be acknowledged in that future edition. ❖

Steven A. Finkler

Christine T. Kovner

---

[2]Send all communications to Prof. Steven A. Finkler, Ph.D., C.P.A., Robert F. Wagner Graduate School of Public Service, New York University, Tisch Hall—Room 600, 40 West Fourth Street, New York, NY 10012-1118.

About the Authors

STEVEN A. FINKLER, Ph.D., C.P.A.

Steven A. Finkler is Professor of Public and Health Administration, Accounting, and Financial Management in the Program in Health Management and Policy at New York University's Robert F. Wagner Graduate School of Public Service. He is also editor of the monthly publication, *Hospital Cost Management and Accounting.*

An award-winning teacher and author, **Prof. Finkler** is currently engaged in a variety of research projects in the areas of health care economics and accounting. Among his current research activities are an evaluation of the New Jersey Nursing Incentives Reimbursement Awards program, and a study sponsored by the National Institute of Health examining the impact of home care by nurses on high-risk pregnant women.

In addition to this book, **Prof. Finkler** has authored more than one hundred publications including *Budgeting Concepts for Nurse Managers* (Second Edition, 1992), *Finance and Accounting for Nonfinancial Managers* (Revised Edition, 1992); articles in *The Journal of Nursing Administration, The New England Journal of Medicine, Nursing Economics, Journal of Neonatal Nursing, Western Journal of Nursing Research, O.R. Nurse Managers' Network, Health Services Research, Medical Care, Healthcare Financial Management, Health Care Management Review,* and other journals; and a chapter in *Managing Hospitals: Lessons from the Johnson & Johnson—Wharton Fellows Program in Management for Nurses.*

Prof. Finkler received a B.S. in Economics and M.S. in Accounting from the Wharton School. His Master's Degree in Economics and Ph.D. in Business Administration were awarded by Stanford University. **Prof. Finkler,** who is also a certified public accountant, worked for several years as an auditor with Ernst and Young and was on the faculty of the Wharton School for six years before joining New York University in 1984.

CHRISTINE T. KOVNER, Ph.D., RN, FAAN

Christine Tassone Kovner, PhD, RN, is an Associate Professor in the Division of Nursing, School of Education, Health, Nursing and Arts Professions, New York University, and a Research Associate at New York University Medical Center. She has over twenty years' experience in nursing in a variety of settings. **Prof. Kovner** received her B.S.N. from Columbia University, her M.S.N. from the University of Pennsylvania, and her Ph.D. from New York University. At New York University she teaches courses on public health nursing.

Most recently **Prof. Kovner** was the Co-principal Investigator of the evaluation of the New Jersey Nursing Incentives Reimbursement Awards. This New Jersey initiative provided $18 million in funding to 37 hospitals to implement innovations in the delivery of nursing care.

She is a reviewer for *Nursing Research* and *Applied Nursing Research* as well as the author of numerous journal articles and chapters on nursing resource use. Her publications include "Nursing," in *Health Care Delivery in the United*

States, "Public health nursing costs in home care," "Co-morbidity, age, and hospital utilization among elderly Medicare patients," "Measuring indirect nursing costs," and "Effects of computers on nursing resource use. Do computers save nurses time?"

Prof. Kovner recently served on two committees for the New York State Department of Health. They were the Health Personnel Utilization and Productivity Committee and the Hospital Information Systems Workgroup. **Prof. Kovner** is a fellow of the American Academy of Nursing.

Contents

Chapter 3 ❖ **The Role of Financial Management Within the Health Care Organization**   42

Chapter 4 ❖ Key Issues in Applied Economics   67

Chapter 9 ❖ Costs and Other Issues Related to Recruiting and Retaining Staff 236

PART IV
PLANNING AND CONTROL 257

Chapter 10 ❖ Strategic Management 259

Chapter 13 ❖ Controlling Operating Results 348

PART V
MANAGING FINANCIAL RESOURCES 387

Chapter 14 ❖ Short-Term Financial Resources 389

**PART VI
ADDITIONAL MANAGEMENT TOOLS 429**

**Chapter 16 ❖ The Role of Management Information Systems
and Computers in Financial
Management 431**

Chapter 17 ❖ Forecasting and Other Methods for Decision Making   458

Chapter 18   ❖ Marketing   506

PART VII
THE FUTURE 539

Chapter 19 ❖ **Nursing and Financial Management: Current Issues and Future Directions 541**

A FINANCIAL MANAGEMENT FRAMEWORK

CHAPTER

1

Introduction and Overview

CHAPTER GOALS

The goals of this chapter are to:

- ◆ Provide the reader with an introduction to financial management
- ◆ Clarify the various components of financial management
- ◆ Give the reader a road map for the study of financial management

INTRODUCTION

Few professions have seen as dramatic a change in role over the last several decades as that of the nurse manager. The nurse manager of the 1960s was predominantly a clinical manager. The role focused on ensuring the adequacy of the clinical care provided to patients. The manager was expected to accomplish those clinical activities with the resources provided.

Today, the nurse manager still must accomplish that primary clinical function; it remains the essence of nursing. The responsibilities of the job, however, are much greater. Managers must be able to determine the resources they will need and then argue convincingly to get their share of resources from a limited total amount available to the organization.

The accuracy with which resource needs are projected and the efficiency with which care is provided must be much greater in the current environment. Health care services cost more than ever, and the pressures to control costs are greater than ever as well. As a result, the financial aspects of the job of every nurse manager are growing and becoming more sophisticated each year. Nurses are expected to develop and justify budgets, to use appropriate computer technology, and to minimize the cost of staff and supplies.

Many of the nonclinical managerial aspects of nursing relate to the financial management of the nursing unit, department, and the health care organization itself. This book covers a wide range of financial management topics. It is designed to meet the needs of nurse managers of all levels throughout the health care organization. As was discussed in the preface, some readers may wish to selectively choose chapters that are most relevant to their needs. This overview chapter provides a more in-depth guide to the book and should aid the reader in making an informed choice for approaching this subject matter.

A FINANCIAL MANAGEMENT FRAMEWORK

Part I of this book is designed to set the stage for the study of financial management. It contains three chapters in addition to this one. Chapter 2 focuses on the environment in which health care organizations exist. The next chapter establishes the relationships between financial management and nurse managers. The last chapter in this section provides a fundamental discussion of the principles and tools of microeconomics.

The Health Care Environment

Every organization must act within the confines of an existing environment. Some health care organizations are the sole providers of health care services in their geographic region. Other providers have significant amounts of competition. In some areas it is easier to hire new staff than in other areas. Chapter 2 of this book discusses some of the essential elements of the environment of health care organizations.

Who are the key players in the health care industry? Who buys services? Who sells them? Who pays for them? What legal bodies make regulations that impact on what health care organizations can do?

The health care industry is highly regulated. This has created an especially difficult environment in which to operate an organization. Before one can begin to address the financial management of health care organizations, it is first important to tackle the issue of government, regulation, and competition.

Recently many new types of organizations have emerged and grown with a focus on helping society control burgeoning health care costs. These include not only health maintenance organizations but also preferred provider organizations and managed care companies. These organizations are discussed in Chapter 2, which provides the foundations that the nurse needs as background before addressing the more specific financial management techniques.

Financial Management and the Health Care Organization

In addition to understanding the environment within which health care organizations operate, it is useful for managers and prospective managers to understand the structure of organizations and how financial management is related to that structure. That is the focus of Chapter 3.

Health care organizations are generally structured as hierarchies. Too many people work in most organizations for them all to report to one individual. Therefore a pyramid structure is often established, with the care givers reporting to a manager, who in turn reports to another manager higher in the pyramid, or hierarchial structure.

Increasingly, health care organizations are also using matrix management. Matrix management is a system in which a manager has responsibility cutting across department lines. For example, product-line management has been receiving growing attention since the 1980s. A health care product line is a specific type or group of patients. In product-line management a manager is responsible for a product line, including all services needed to provide care to patients in that product line. This requires a cooperative relationship among the product-line manager and both the managers and staff of all of the organization's departments. Bear in mind that the staff will need to respond to both the product-line managers and also the unit or department manager.

Although matrix management is used in some health care organizations, Chapter 3 will focus on the traditional hierarchical management structure that is used in the majority of health care organizations. Much of the chapter discussion focuses on issues related to the degree of centralization created by such structure. It also considers the official and actual authority of specific individuals within the organization. Equally critical is the discussion of the distinction between the line and staff roles in an organization. Within that context, the role of finance is discussed. The role of the chief financial officer and the finance department staff is explained and contrasted with the roles of nurse managers at various levels in the organization.

Economics

Accounting and finance are applied areas of microeconomics. The theory of economics forms the foundations upon which all financial management is ultimately built. The essence of economics is that society has a limited amount of resources with competing demands for them. The economic system attempts to allocate those resources in an optimal fashion.

Chapter 4 introduces the building blocks used in economics. The critical building blocks—economic goods, marginal utility, marginal cost, supply and demand, and economies of scale—are discussed. This leads into an examination of the workings of a free enterprise system.

In the free enterprise system one cannot separate human motivation from the actions of human beings. The economic system will always be the result of the interplay of resource allocation with the actions of people. As a result, it is necessary to consider the issue of incentives and their role in achieving market efficiency.

The economic system, even a free enterprise system, cannot always be relied upon to generate a perfect outcome. In fact, there may be times when the system simply fails to achieve a socially optimal result. The existence of monopolies, the absence of full information, the impact of insurance systems, and other factors may lead to less than desirable outcomes. Chapter 4 addresses these issues of market failure and of society's attempts to intervene to generate a more equitable outcome.

Economics has a bearing on nursing. It forms the framework from which resources are allocated. Chapter 4 also specifically addresses issues related to the market for nursing labor: Why do nursing shortages occur from time to time and then diminish? Is there some logic or rationale that can explain how the economic system leads to such shortages and then resolves them?

FINANCIAL ACCOUNTING

Accounting has often been referred to as "the language of business." One needs to be conversant with the basic principles of accounting to conduct any of the various aspects of financial management. Therefore, once the reader has the general background of the chapters in Part I, the next step in Part II is to focus on basic accounting issues.

The two principal areas of accounting are managerial accounting and financial accounting. Managerial accounting refers to the generation of any financial information that would be useful to managers in their role managing part of an organization. Most of this book will focus on managerial accounting issues.

The nurse manager also needs to understand financial accounting. Part II contains two chapters on financial accounting issues. Financial accounting provides the foundations of accounting. It focuses on generating financial information about the results of operations and the financial condition of the organization.

Financial accounting originated largely to provide information to outsiders who were lending money to an organization or investing in it, but the information generated is extremely useful for the organization's internal managers as well. Nurse managers who can assess and use this information will be at an advantage. Chapter 5 looks at the basic principles of accounting, and Chapter 6 provides a more advanced look at the analysis of financial statements.

Accounting Principles

Accounting does not represent a science. Surprisingly, accounting professors teach that accounting is closer to an art than a science. No fundamental laws of nature govern accounting. One generally agreed upon principle forms the keystone upon which all accounting is built, however: The books must balance.

This concept has become so pervasively accepted and known that the reader of this book likely takes it for granted. Everyone knows you must balance the books. But what does that really mean? Does it mean that you must break even, that you must balance the revenues against the expenses of each organization or individual? No. Clearly, some organizations make money, while others lose money. What does it mean when one says that the books must balance?

Balancing the books refers to the basic equation of accounting that describes the relationship between the valuable resources possessed by the organization and the claims on those resources by creditors and owners of the organization. That equation becomes the basis for ledgers and journals and the other technical elements of an accounting system. Chapter 5 will introduce the reader to the equation of accounting and to the concepts of assets, equities, revenues, expenses, journal entries, ledgers, and generally accepted accounting principles. These concepts impact on every manager in most health care organizations. A fundamental understanding of these concepts is essential to understand financial management.

Financial Statement Analysis

At higher levels of management, the focus of a manager's interest in financial management must broaden. The tools of financial management become not only an integral element for being able to efficiently manage a unit or department but also the messengers of the general financial well-being of the organization.

Can the organization afford to provide nurses with a substantial raise? Can the organization reasonably be expected to replace old ICU monitors with new ones? Is the organization acting in a prudent manner that will allow for its continued existence? These are just a few examples of the types of issues that become relevant as one moves up through the ranks of nursing management. The answers to those questions require information about the general financial condition of the organization.

Chapter 6 focuses on issues of analysis of financial statement information. What do the income statements and balance sheets of organizations really tell the reader? Are other elements of information also important? Are there ways to use raw financial statement information to make it more informative?

COST ANALYSIS

One of the most critical areas of financial management is the analysis and control of costs. The surplus (profit) or deficit (loss) of an organization each year depends on both its revenues and its costs. Both elements—revenues and costs—require managerial thought and attention. Cost management has been an essential role of nurse managers at all levels for a number of years. Part III examines issues related to costs.

Cost Management

The first chapter in Part III, Chapter 7, deals with basic issues of cost management. All levels of management encounter these issues in their normal activities.

The chapter introduces definitions of critical terms. The concepts of fixed, variable, marginal, and relevant costs are discussed at some length. The nature and behavior of costs are covered in this chapter, with emphasis on the relationship between patient volume and costs. As volume changes over time, managers must be able to understand and predict the impact that such changes will have on costs. Techniques are provided for such prediction or estimation of future costs.

In the last decade the health care industry has become more entrepreneurial. In an effort to find the resources to subsidize services offered at a loss, many health care organizations, even not-for-profit ones, are constantly searching for profitable ventures. The last section of Chapter 7 provides a methodology to determine when a program or project or service will have sufficient volume to break even, i.e., to be financially self-sufficient. Such an approach is frequently used by organizations to determine whether to undertake a proposed new venture.

Determining the Cost of Health Care Services

Chapter 8 moves from basic cost concepts to the broader issue of cost measurement with two primary focuses. One is on how health care organizations collect cost information by unit or department and assign those costs to patients. The second is on how to cost out nursing services.

The Medicare step-down cost-finding and rate-setting methodology is presented in Chapter 8 and contrasted with more recently developed costing methods. Attention is also paid to understanding product-line costing. Issues of patient classification systems and staffing are considered. Standard costing techniques are also discussed.

Costing out nursing has become a topic of much interest to nurse managers. As hospitals are forced to operate in a constrained financial atmosphere, chief executive officers look to nurse managers at all levels to take a greater role in controlling costs. To do this, nurse managers need a better understanding of the costs of providing nursing care. Such an understanding can also be useful in addressing the issue of financial reimbursement for nursing services.

Recruiting and Retaining Staff

The last chapter in this part of the book addresses a concern that peaks during nursing shortages but requires managerial attention regardless of whether there is a current shortage of nurses. That is the issue of measuring and managing the costs of recruiting and retaining staff.

There is little question that personnel is the single greatest cost in health care. Attracting and retaining qualified staff are essential to maintaining a desired quality-of-care level. Because of the high cost of recruiting nurses, the recruitment and retention of nurses has now become a financial management issue.

What can management do to keep key levels of satisfaction high? What are the tools and approaches an organization can utilize in attracting new nurses? What alternative sources of personnel are there? How much does nurse recruitment cost, and how does one measure that cost? These are the issues that Chapter 9 focuses on.

PLANNING AND CONTROL

Planning and control are elements central to the success of any organization. Planning helps the organization to know where it wants to go and to develop a plan to get there. Control helps to ensure that the plan that has been adopted is carried out.

Part IV devotes four chapters to this important topic. These chapters specifically address strategic planning, budgeting concepts, operating budget preparation, and the control of operating results.

Strategic Planning

Strategic planning is an emerging field that is an outgrowth of the long-range planning of the 1950s. *Strategic management* is the process of integrating strategic thought throughout the management process. Organizational success largely depends on the care with which the organization acts strategically. Knowing an organization's strengths and weaknesses and being aware of its opportunities and threats are the critical elements upon which the field of strategic management has been built.

Strategic planning is discussed in Chapter 10. How are strategic plans defined? Why are they prepared? What benefits can the organization hope to achieve from strategic management? The chapter also discusses some specific elements of strategic management: long-range plans, program budgets, and business plans.

Budgeting Concepts and Budget Preparation

The budgeting aspect of planning is explored in the middle two chapters of Part IV. Chapter 11 provides an overview of the various types of organizational budgets and of the budget process. Chapter 12 provides greater depth on the preparation of the operating budget.

The types of budgets examined include operating, long-range, capital, product-line, program, zero-base, cash, and special purpose. Each type of budget has an integral role in planning for health care organizations.

The budget process is much broader than the actual preparation of each unit's budget. The process includes preparing a timetable; doing an environmental review; and developing goals, objectives, assumptions, and priorities. It also includes budget negotiation and revision.

Capital budgeting is becoming more complicated in the health care industry. Recent changes in the way Medicare reimburses hospitals for their capital items have placed a greater burden on hospitals to examine the financial implications of their capital acquisitions more closely. The technical appendix to Chapter 11 discusses sophisticated analytical approaches to capital budget evaluation. The methods discussed include the present cost approach, net present value, and internal rate of return.

Chapter 12 looks at specific issues related to preparation of operating budgets. The starting point for preparing the operating budget is the estimated workload. One must first consider how many patients, and in what mix, are likely before a determination can be made of the resources needed to care for those patients.

The largest and most complicated element of the budgeting process relates to personnel costs. The major part of this chapter is devoted to examining the issues related to staffing and to calculating labor costs. Costs of other-than-personnel services (OTPS) and budgeting for revenues are also covered in the chapter.

The last section of the chapter deals with budget implementation. A budget loses much of its value if it is largely ignored after being approved. It is vital that managers think specifically of the actions that must be taken to implement their budgets.

Controlling Operating Results

Implementation of the budget, however, does not mean that everything will come out according to the plan. Chapter 13 discusses the issue of control. That discussion includes the provision of specific tools of variance analysis, which are used to help managers to discover variations from the original plan and to keep outcomes as close to the plan as possible.

Traditional variance analysis compares the actual results to the budgeted plan. Information is provided for each line item of each budget for the most recent month and cumulatively for the year-to-date. Chapter 13 also introduces the concept of flexible budgeting. That is a variance analysis technique that provides better insight into the likely causes of observed variances. By subdividing variances into their underlying components, the manager is able to identify the major influences that generated the variation from the budget.

MANAGING FINANCIAL RESOURCES

All managers of health care organizations manage resources. Determining what personnel and other resources to use and how to use them is a managerial function. Organizations have many types of resources. The people working for any health care organization are valuable resources, as is the reputation for quality. The financial resources of the organization—specifically, its money—are another. To the same extent that clinical resources must be carefully used, financial resources must be managed in an efficient manner.

Decisions concerning where and how to get money are one element of managing financial resources. Some resources in proprietary organizations come from investments owners make in the organization. In not-for-profit organizations a common source of financial resources is charitable donations. Profits are a potential source of financial resources for all types of health care organizations. In the last half of this century it has also become common for health care organizations to borrow much of the money they need.

Organizations have financial resources, which they must manage efficiently. Decisions must be made concerning how much cash to have on hand. Management techniques must be employed to ensure that cash is received as promptly as possible. In addition, managers must ensure that cash is available when needed for payrolls or interest payments. This need to have control over the inflow and outflow of cash necessitates careful management of receivables, inventories, marketable securities, payables, and leases.

While some readers may assume that the management of financial resources is the strict domain of financial managers, that is not the case. For example, a financial manager can do little to control inventory levels. The nurse manager is in a much better position to make determinations regarding necessary inventory levels and to enforce policies established to avoid unnecessary stockpiling of inventory. Inventory usage directly affects the amount of money available to the organization. Nurse managers and financial managers must work together in the management of financial resources to arrive at an optimal outcome for the organization.

Part V of this book is divided into two chapters. The first chapter focuses directly on the management of the short-term financial resources of the organization. The second chapter is concerned with the long-term financing of health care organizations.

Short-term Financial Resources

Short-term relates to resources that appear in the current asset and current liability sections of the balance sheet. (NOTE: The balance sheet is discussed in Chapter 5.) Such resources generally provide or require cash within a relatively short time, usually less than a year. These short-term resources and short-term sources of resources are referred to as the organization's *working capital*. Working capital is discussed in Chapter 14.

Long-term Financing

Long-term financing relates to the alternatives the organization has for acquiring financial resources that will not have to be repaid for more than a year. To be able to acquire capital assets—buildings and equipment—the organization must know that it can acquire money that does not have to be repaid in a short time. The choices it makes regarding such long-term financing can have dramatic effects on the ability of the organization to provide health care services and to compete in the health care marketplace. The aspects of financial management related to long-term financing are discussed in Chapter 15.

ADDITIONAL MANAGEMENT TOOLS

The health care sector has rapidly become complex. To keep up, managers must constantly expand and improve their capabilities. Part VI of this book examines some additional management tools that can help a nurse manager to cope with the complicated environment of health care.

The chapters in this part focus on computerization and information systems, forecasting and other methods for decision making, and marketing. Each of these may be thought of as peripheral to traditional financial management, yet each represents a topic of direct current interest to nursing managers.

Management Information Systems and Computers

Computers and the information they can generate represent the subject matter of Chapter 16. In the 1990s the question is no longer whether nursing will use computers. Just the first few years of the decade have shown an explosion of computer applications not only to clinical nursing but also to financial management.

The number of uses for computers in nursing management continues to grow. Computers are used to prepare budgets, to examine variances, to write letters and papers, to forecast patient volume and acuity, and so on.

Chapter 16 provides some basic information about computers and information systems. It discusses the definition and nature of computer hardware (equipment) and software (programs). It also looks into some of the common uses of computers to generate information to aid nurse managers in their jobs.

Forecasting and Other Decision-making Methods

One essential role of managers is to make decisions. Forecasting methods can be used to provide managers with information about the future. That information can be used to make a variety of decisions. Chapter 17 discusses a number of quantitative and qualitative approaches to forecasting. These include computerized techniques as well as the less high-tech but often equally effective Delphi and Nominal Group approaches.

Chapter 17 also provides an explanation of expected value, linear programming, inventory control, Gantt, Critical Path Method (CPM), and the Program Evaluation and Review Technique (PERT). Each of these items represents a technique for generating information for managerial decision making that has proven effective over a period of years and range of applications.

Marketing

Health care services sell themselves. When patients are sick, they seek out care. Is it appropriate to try to "sell" health care services? Does marketing have a role in health care? The concept of marketing brings with it the ethical question of whether marketing can be justified in the health care industry. The authors believe that much of the ethical question stems from misunderstanding the objectives of modern marketing.

The role of marketing is to assess customer needs and then to respond to them. Many people perceive marketing as simply developing advertising to sell a specific product regardless of whether consumers need it. In that perception, the seller has something and wants to convince the potential customer to buy it. In a broader view of the marketing function, the role is quite different. The customers include not only potential patients but also those individuals with whom nurses come into contact within the organization. Marketing determines what the potential customer needs. This allows the organization to produce services that fill that need. Advertising is a way to communicate that the organization is prepared to offer what the customer wants or needs.

Advertising is a very small element of marketing. Managers must understand who their customer is. They must understand what needs exist and how those needs can best be satisfied.

Certainly, the organization wants the customer to buy from it rather than from another organization. To that extent the reality of competition must be considered. The main focus of the chapter, however, is on the elements of marketing that allow the organization to use market research to be dynamic and to adaptatively respond to the changing needs of its patients. Failure to use marketing is more likely to result in selling patients services that they do not need than wise marketing management is.

How does this relate to nurses? Nurses are often the ones who most shape the product produced by health care organizations. If the patients are not getting what they need, the care provided should change. If that is to happen, it is critical for nursing to be as involved as possible in determining what the patients do need and how best to fulfill that need. Marketing is discussed in Chapter 18.

NURSING AND FINANCIAL MANAGEMENT—CURRENT ISSUES AND FUTURE DIRECTIONS

The role of nurses in health care organizations has been rapidly evolving over the last several decades. Few nurse managers who left the profession in the 1970s would recognize it today. The level of responsibility for issues with financial management content has increased dramatically for nurses at all levels of health care organizations.

We doubt that the rate of change is going to decrease in the near future. The share of the total economy consumed by health care services has been dramatically escalating over the last three decades. Each year that this trend continues, the pressures to control health care spending grow stronger. Those pressures translate into more and more pressure on nurse managers to provide high-quality care in a cost-effective manner.

Nurses will respond to that need for greater efficiency by becoming more knowledgeable and by taking on an ever-increasing financial management role. To be able to control costs, nurse managers will need to know what those costs are. They will need timely, accurate cost information.

The last chapter of this book relates to the issue of futures. What will be the evolving role of financial management in nursing management in the future? How will financial management impact on the chief nurse executive in the future? The mid-level nurse manager? The nurse entrepreneur? The nurse policy maker? We believe that today we are only seeing the beginning of the role of nurse managers with respect to financial management.

2

The Health Care Environment

CHAPTER GOALS

The goals of this chapter are to:

- Describe the health care system
- Explain the role of each major participant group in the health care system
- Explain the financing system for health care services
- Explain how different health care providers are paid for the services they provide
- Discuss approaches developed in the last several decades to stem the growth in health care costs
- Analyze the implications of the health care environment for nurse managers

❖

INTRODUCTION

Before discussing the specific tools of financial management, it is important for this book to provide the reader with an overview of the health care system. That will allow the reader to better relate the techniques of financial management to the organizations that use them. Providing such an overview is the role of this chapter.

The health care system is based on an intricate set of relationships among a number of different participants. The participants are extremely varied, including not only those who give care and those who receive health care services but also those who regulate the care that is provided and those who provide payments that supplement those made by the consumers. The actions of the participants in the health care system are affected by the economic and regulatory environment of the local, regional, and national society. The economic and regulatory environment changes continuously and is influenced by political as well as economic factors. These factors interplay with technological and other scientific advances in the capabilities of health care organizations to provide the highest level quality of care.

The traditional interplay among the nurse, physician, and patient is just a small part of the larger health care system. There are many different types of providers of care. Some are individually based, such as nurses and physicians; some are institutionally based, such as hospitals and nursing homes; some are organizationally based, such as health maintenance organizations (HMOs) and home care agencies; and some are societally based, such as government-sponsored care for veterans and the military.

The health care system takes into account the needs of a broad base of consumers. These include the typical acute care hospital patients, but they also include those in need of drug rehabilitation, extended convalescent care, permanent nursing home care, mental health care, dental care, rehabilitative therapy, home care, and a myriad of other health care services.

The care that providers supply to consumers is subject to a complex web of regulations. For the most part such regulations stem from an intention to protect consumers. Professional nurses believe that they are skilled and know what care is needed and how to provide it. The regulatory environment often seems to be an unneeded intrusion of politicians into an area in which they have little knowledge and even less expertise. The reason for the regulations is not generally to control the activities of the competent trained individual but to protect consumers from the untrained or incompetent. The well-educated nurse pays a high price for compliance with regulations. In providing care in accordance with regulations, however, one must consider what untrained, unqualified providers of care might do in an unregulated environment.

Care is paid for in a complex manner, under a set of changing rules, by a diverse group of payers. We have already reached a stage where individuals directly pay for only about a quarter of the health care services they receive. The cost of care has become too great for individuals to bear. One hospitalization can easily wipe out the life savings of a family. Therefore we have developed a system that uses pooled resources, many individuals each contributing some money so that the tremendous costs of a serious illness can be paid for by those pooled resources.

The nurse manager can benefit by being aware of constraints and opportunities that the environment offers. Financial decisions must take into account not only the current environment but also anticipated changes that may affect that environment in the future. Today there may be limitations on changes that nurse managers can make to run their units and departments in a more efficient manner. Over time, however, regulations change, and those constraints may fade away. Other regulations arise to pose new challenges.

This chapter begins with a description of the major participants in the health care system. Next it addresses the principal issues related to paying for health care services. Finally, several current approaches to controlling the costs of health services are addressed. Included in this last topic is a discussion of the development and growth of HMOs, preferred provider organizations (PPOs), and other managed care approaches.

THE KEY PARTICIPANTS IN THE HEALTH CARE SYSTEM

Essentially, there are five key groups of participants in the health care system:

1. Providers,
2. Suppliers,
3. Consumers,
4. Regulators,
5. Payers

The providers are those individuals and organizations that actually deliver health care services to patients. The suppliers are the manufacturers and distributors of the equipment and supplies consumed in the process of providing care. The consumers are those individuals who receive health care services (or would, if they had adequate access to care). The regulators are those bodies that create rules with which health care suppliers and providers must comply. Finally, the payers are those individuals and organizations that pay for the care provided.

The remainder of this section will discuss the providers, suppliers, consumers, regulators, and payers in somewhat more depth.

Providers

The providers of health care services include all people and organizations that produce and distribute health care services. Included among providers are health professionals such as nurses and physicians, as well as health care organizations such as hospitals, nursing homes, and home health agencies. The government is also a major provider of health care services.

When discussing the health care environment providers are often grouped together as if they were one entity. However, there are a variety of providers who often have different and competing interests. The traditional providers and those about whom the most is written are nurses, physicians, hospitals, and the government.

Nurses

Most nurses work for hospitals, but many work in other settings, such as nursing homes, home care agencies, surgicenters, clinics, HMOs, physician office practices, hospices, and schools.

Nurses who are affiliated with hospitals are almost always salaried or hourly wage employees. They work in nursing units that are part of the nursing department. The nursing department reports to the chief operating officer or chief executive officer. The organizational structure of nursing within health care organizations is addressed in Chapter 3.

The primary role of the staff nurse is to provide direct hands-on care to patients. That role has been modified over the years. In addition to hands-on care, nurses plan and coordinate the care that patients receive. They also act in a supervisory capacity, managing other individuals—aides, technicians, and LPNs—who are directly providing care to patients. The many professional activities that fall within the domain of nursing are well known to most of the readers of this book.

Nurses are generally interested in providing the best quality of care for patients. They often believe that only educated health professionals can assess the type and quality of care that should be or is being provided to patients. And they generally believe that nursing should have autonomy over its own professional practice.

The fact that nurses are generally employees and their income is usually related to the amount of time they work, rather than to the number of care episodes they provide, must be considered in understanding nurses' incentives. The commonly touted need to control costs in health care organizations may have a lower priority for nurses than providing excellent patient care. Many nurses see their role as providing the best possible care. They consider it the role of other managers of the organization to find the resources necessary for nurses to provide that care. On the other hand, nurse managers see the financial management of resources as a key component in their role.

Although, as noted above, the majority of nurses work in acute care hospitals, nurses do have a variety of options when it comes to selecting a work setting. Each opportunity has its own specific characteristics and advantages and disadvantages. For example, the salaries paid to nurses working as employees in physicians' offices are often lower than those paid in other settings. The working hours tend to be better, however, and often the stress related to the job is lower. Some nurses work as consultants. They tend to work long hours and to earn higher salaries, but they may lose most, if not all, patient contact. Some nurses work for insurance companies, evaluating claims. They may also lose patient contact, but they work very stable, normal, nine-to-five hours with less overtime and stress. Other nurses work as independent nurse practitioners or entrepreneurs, setting their own time schedules.

Physicians

Physicians provide health care both in and out of the hospital. They are generally paid for each episode of care that they provide. The two predominant locales for the provision of care by physicians are their offices and hospitals.

In their offices, physicians are generally owners or co-owners, although sometimes they are employees working for another physician. Often the structure of the physicians' office is corporate. By forming a corporation, the physician limits personal liability. The corporation owning the practice is liable for paying for equipment, rent, supplies, and salaries.

Some essential health care procedures and supplies are used by physicians in their offices regardless of cost. For example, they always use sterile needles. On the other hand, physicians often add facilities to their office practice only if they feel they are financially justified. The addition of an x-ray machine for taking chest x-rays in an internist's office will usually occur only if it is seen as being a profit enhancement. Otherwise patients will be referred to a radiologist.

In most cases, physicians are "guests" at the hospital, rather than employees. This creates an unusual set of incentives. Most technological improvements in the quality of care offered by the hospital are paid for by the hospital. Therefore, the same physician who might not replace an existing office x-ray machine with the latest model available each year is still likely to demand that the hospital purchase the latest equipment. The hospital's acquisition of such equipment will not cost the physician anything. In some cases, the equipment can reduce physicians' time treating each patient or allow physicians to provide additional types of treatments, enhancing their income.

To be sure, physicians also have the motivation of desiring that their patients receive the best care possible. The fact that physicians do not personally pay for the technological and other quality-of-care enhancements at hospitals inherently must alter their incentives, however. Being a "guest" rather than an owner has implications for their view of financial structure of the hospital. It is in the physicians' interest for the hospital to stay in business, but there is often little perceived reason not to try to convince the hospital to acquire the latest technology to ensure that patients have the best quality of care.

Physicians can be extremely persuasive because of their role in advising patients where to go for treatment. The physician represents the primary source of patients for most hospitals. A physician affiliated with two or three hospitals, as many are, then has the ability to steer patients toward any of those hospitals. In most cases, one would hope, the physician chooses some hospital characteristics that makes it most suitable for each specific patient's needs. Physicians, however, sometimes use their control over patient admissions to gain specific concessions from hospitals.

This power of admissions that physicians have is one of the most important forces in the hospital industry. This control over admissions also affects nursing home admissions, home agencies' patient referrals, and referrals to other physician specialists. In trying to understand the actions of participants in the health care system, it is essential to understand this key role that physicians play in directing patients where to go for their care.

Hospitals

Hospitals serve two primary functions. They house sophisticated technological equipment, and they are locations where patients can receive 24-hour-per-day nursing care for acute episodes. Society centralizes services, locating essential pieces of equipment and skilled personnel resources in specific locations—acute care hospitals. Patients with acute health problems go to hospitals for diagnostic and therapeutic treatment. A wide range of health care professionals can make use of sophisticated clinical supplies and technologies to provide patient care.

The hospital is an organizational entity with an existence apart from the individual professionals who provide care within its walls. Some hospitals are organized as for-profit companies. Some hospitals are owned by governments. The majority of hospitals in this country are established as voluntaries. That means that they are not-for-profit organizations, not run by governments or government agencies. Any profits that they earn are reinvested for the benefit of the local community. Some hospitals are established as subsidiaries of larger not-for-profit organizations, such as religious organizations or universities.

The hospital's leadership consists of health care professionals and a board of directors or trustees. That board is generally made up of respected members of the community. Those board members are often not health care professionals.

The hospital's professional leadership, together with the board, establishes overriding goals and directions for the organization. It also provides oversight to ensure that the organization acts to achieve those goals. Most hospitals have as part of their primary mission the provision of the highest quality of care possible. Hospitals, however, also have limited resources. In recognition of that fact, the achievement of all goals is tempered by the need to stay in business. If the hospital financially fails and stops providing service, that result will be less desirable than providing only acceptable rather than the highest-quality care.

Government

The three levels of government—local, state, and national—are large providers of health care services. The federal government runs a significant hospital system for the military and the federal prison system. It also operates the national Veterans Administration system. State governments often operate a variety of health care facilities including hospitals for mental health and clinics and hospitals for prisoners. Many cities and counties operate public hospitals.

Public hospitals have existed for many decades in this country. Local governments often become actively involved as providers of health care services. For example, the New York City Health and Hospitals Corporation owns and operates eleven acute care hospitals, five long-term care facilities, and over thirty outpatient facilities. The New York City Emergency Services Agency operates an ambulance service that provides emergency response services to a population of over 7 million individuals.

The government generally provides only those services that it believes will not otherwise be provided. As we will discuss later, the government also has a role as a payer for care. That role is partly intended to ensure adequate access. Nonetheless, there are clearly situations where access is still not adequate without the direct intervention of the government as a provider of care. In some of those cases the government directly provides the care.

Other Providers

Many other types of providers of health care services have not been discussed here. These include those in which nurses have a significant role, such as nursing homes and home care agencies, and those where nurses have little or no role, such as the dental offices. Each type of provider has its own unique perspectives and problems.

Many providers share commonalities and have differences from those described above. For example, physical therapists may work for a salary at a hospital as nurses do or be paid on a per treatment basis as physicians are. Some home health agencies have a goal of making profits, while others are not-for-profit voluntary organizations.

Nurses who work for home health agencies may be paid a salary or be paid for each visit they provide, similar to the way physicians are paid. It is important to note the variety of providers with competing goals and interests. Even some providers working for other providers may have conflicting interests. These goals may conflict in the area of finance; physicians may make money if the hospital expends resources and loses money. For example, the addition of a lithotripter machine will probably increase the income of urologists at the hospital. The machine itself may be so expensive, however, that the hospital will lose money on the lithotripsy patients.

Other conflicts arise in the area of quality of care; hospitals may want to cut professional hours per patient day, while the nursing staff has a primary goal increasing the quality of patient care. The differences in the underlying goals of each provider may carry over to the strategies that each provider uses to achieve its goals.

Suppliers

The second key participant in the health care system is the supplier. This group includes the manufacturers and distributors of all supplies and equipment used in health care organizations.

Often suppliers are not even considered when one discusses the key participants in the health care system. They are virtually always for-profit corporations that are part of the general industrialized complex. Are they related to health care? Suppliers have billions of dollars of sales each year. One cannot ignore their role.

Suppliers do not just provide the health care industry with the items that providers need to care for their patients. Suppliers also invent new technologies. That innovative role is a significant issue in understanding the environment in which the health care system operates.

On the one hand, there is tremendous pressure to contain the growth in health care costs. Health care before the introduction of Medicare, just a quarter-century ago, consumed just 4% of every dollar earned in this country. By 1992, at least 12% of all society's earnings was being spent on health care. This is not merely the result of inflation. Not only is much more money spent on health care services but also a much larger share of all money earned is spent on health care. For example, in 1965 an individual earning $15,000 spent $600 on average for health care services. In 1992, if the same individual were earning $45,000 (because of the increase in wage rates), the money spent on health care would not increase proportionately to $1,800, but would have risen to $5,400! This amount includes direct payments by the individual, payments for insurance, and taxes paid to the government to support programs such as Medicare and Medicaid. Much of the growth in costs is related to new innovations that allow the health care system to do more things to provide care.

Often new technologies are extremely expensive. The suppliers therefore have taken an active role that at the same time improves the quality of care that can be provided but also increases the costs of providing it.

Consumers

Consumers are the individuals who use health care services. Consumers use a variety of types of services, ranging from preventive and advisory through diagnostic, therapeutic, and rehabilitative. In some cases they include monitoring or custodial care.

Consumers are becoming increasingly knowledgeable about the services they want from health care providers. Nevertheless, there is a huge gap in knowledge between the health care professional and the consumer of health care services. As a result, individual consumers often rely heavily on health care professionals to advise them.

Most nurses view consumers as individual clients. Nurses are educated to encourage clients to participate actively in their care. Therefore nurses work with patients to select treatment options and to choose where care will be provided.

This may not always be the case with other providers. Physicians in particular have tremendous power over consumers because of the physicians' specialized knowledge. As discussed earlier, physicians can use this to their advantage, and perhaps their patients', by convincing hospitals to provide resources in exchange for patient admissions.

Although one usually thinks of patients as individuals, in recent years consumers have increasingly tried collective action. In the 1980s consumer groups such as the American Association of Retired Persons (AARP) actively lobbied for health care options that are in the interest of the represented group. Because many of these groups represent constituencies of voters, governments often respond to them.

Regulators

The regulatory environment in which the health care system exists is dominated by rules and regulations that affect the actions and activities of health care providers, payers, and consumers. Some regulations even regulate the activities of regulators in a technical tangle of rules that often seems to distract the health care system from the activity of providing health care services.

Regulations are generally thought of in terms of a governmental order that has the force of law. The government (at local, state, and federal levels), as part of its role to protect the public, has an interest in maintaining the public's health. To achieve that end a number of regulations are issued. Although regulations are generally not specifically laws, they are often promulgated by governmental agencies to carry out laws. Health care providers must obey the regulations or else be subject to specific legal sanctions. In some instances the sanctions have strong implications for reimbursement. This would be the case, for instance, if a hospital were not eligible to receive Medicaid payments if it failed to comply with a certain state regulation.

The United States Constitution identifies the federal government's responsibility to protect the health and welfare of the people. In recent years this has been broadly interpreted by the federal government to develop increasing safeguards for the public's health. For the federal government this includes things such as regulating pharmacologic agents and monitoring communicable diseases.

In its role as a payer for health services (discussed later in this chapter) the federal government has developed regulations for providers of health care services that are paid for with federal dollars. For example, the federal government has created a number of regulations that specify who can participate in Medicare. These regulations affect providers, consumers, and even those organizations that the federal government contracts with to process Medicare claims for payment.

The state regulatory function varies widely from state to state. In part this regulatory influence is derived from the state's function to regulate those services for which it pays, such as those provided under Medicaid. In part the regulations derive from the state's interest in protecting the public through the licensure of those professionals and organizations that provide health care. Regulations vary from rules that decree the square footage of patient rooms in hospitals, to the ratio of nurses to patients in an intensive care unit, to the information that must be provided to patients before they are discharged from hospitals.

Licensure is one of the widely applied regulations. It is not without controversy, however. Every state has laws concerning the licensing of health professionals and health care organizations that provide care. Some economists have argued that such licensing is unnecessary. Instead, they suggest disclosure. Health care organizations would have to provide consumers with information about their training or accreditation, their experience, and their outcome rates. Then consumers could decide what providers to use and how high a price they are willing to pay. Society, however, continues to insist upon licensure. The arguments in favor are that many consumers are not well informed and that licensure ensures minimum practice levels. Further, the damage that could be done by an untrained, unexamined provider is too great to warrant the risk.

Local government regulations often cover areas related to construction, fire safety, and how to handle a death. For example, in most states, regulations prevent nurses from being able to declare a patient dead. Often such regulations result from lobbying efforts by special interest groups such as the American Medical Association (AMA) rather than from an underlying need to protect the consumer.

Since the government, as discussed earlier, is a large provider of health care services, it is interesting to realize that the government in some instances is regulating itself. Often, the federal government is exempt from local law. Therefore, the building codes and licensing regulations that affect a voluntary hospital may not affect a military hospital. On the other hand, the Medicare payment regulations developed at the federal level affect payments made to county-owned and operated hospitals and other health care facilities.

Only the government has the legal authority to issue regulations and to mandate adherence to them. Health providers are also subject to the regulations of voluntary accreditation and certification bodies, such as the Joint Commission on Accreditation of Healthcare Organizations (JCAHO). While adherence to the standards of these organizations is voluntary, societal and fiscal pressure are such that few hospitals elect not to be accredited by JCAHO, and few surgeons choose not to be certified by their specialty board.

Nurse managers and nursing associations can do a number of things to influence the adoption of regulations at all levels of government and by associations such as JCAHO. That topic is discussed in Chapter 19. Change is slow, however, and not always possible.

Nurse managers must make the effort to become familiar with the various regulations that impact on their organization, department, and unit. They must reflect on how those regulations affect not only day-to-day operations but also the management decisions that they can make. Since regulations vary so much from state to state, it is important for nurse managers to know the regulations in the state in which they practice. In general there is a belief that government regulation is increasing and will likely continue to increase. There is little consensus on whether this regulation is positive or negative for the health care system.

Payers

The last major group of participants in the health care system consists of the individuals and organizations that pay for the health care services consumed. In our health care system, often the consumer of health care services does not pay for them directly. The most common types of payers are individuals, insurance companies, employers, and governments.

In 1989 national health expenditures were $604.1 billion.[1] The rate of increase in spending on health care services continues to be well in excess of the general inflation rate. Unlike other goods and services, health care costs are usually not paid for by the person using the service. The single largest payer group for health care services is the government. Among Medicare, Medicaid, and other direct government payments for health care services, the government pays for 40% of the care.[2] Insurers and employers are the next largest payer for care, followed by individuals paying for their own care. About 36% of health care costs are paid for by private insurance and charitable funds. Only about 24% of all personal health expenditures are paid for by self-pay patients *"out of pocket."*[3] These services and goods include over-the-counter medications, prescriptions, physician services, private duty nursing service, and institutional care.

Individual Consumers

In most aspects of our society, individuals are obligated to pay for the resources they consume. In health care, however, that is only the case for the minority of payments. Most of the money paid to health care providers does not come directly from individuals.

Given the very high cost of health care services, this should not be surprising. If a $200,000 house burns down, it is unlikely that it will be rebuilt with money directly from the owner. It is much more likely that the owner was paying an annual insurance premium of $500 to protect the house in case of a fire. Many people each pay $500, but only a few houses burn down. The insurance then pays the $200,000 to rebuild the house.

Similarly, those individuals who have health insurance call upon that insurance to pay for the major health care services they consume. Health insurance is discussed below. What about the individual who has not been paying premiums and does not have insurance? If a person's house burns down and it is uninsured, there are two main choices. Rebuild it with your own money if you have it, or do without a new house if you do not.

Those individuals who pay providers directly for health care services are referred to as *self-pay* patients. They often are charged the highest rates. They are also the most likely to default on their payment obligations because the high cost of care is beyond their personal means.

Approximately 37 million Americans have no health insurance and are forced to pay for all their care (or seek care from public facilities that do not require payment).[4] Other Americans, even though they have insurance for some health care costs, pay for certain kinds of care because their insurance does not cover it. This often includes preventive care, such as annual gynecologic examinations or mammograms. It also often includes eyeglasses, medications (both prescription and nonprescription), and many home health services.

Any payers other than the individual consumers who receive the care are often called *third-party payers*. This is because the care provided to an individual

---

[1]Robert Wood Johnson Foundation, *Challenges in Health Care: A Chartbook Perspective 1991*, Princeton, NJ, 1991, p. 89.
[2]Ibid. p. 100.
[3]Ibid. p. 100.
[4]Ibid. p. 102.

is paid for not by the consumer or the provider but by a "third" party. The most common third-party payers are insurers, employers, and the government.

Insurers

Insurance companies take money from individuals and employers, pool the money, and then pay providers when the insured individuals consume health care services. Some insurance companies operate as for-profit corporations. Other insurers are not-for-profit, existing to provide service rather than to profit from the provision of that service. Still other insurers are formed as mutual companies, returning any profits earned to their insured population in the form of dividends or reduced premiums.

The most dominant private insurer is Blue Cross/Blue Shield. Historically the Blues have accounted for approximately 30% of all health care payments in the country. Blue Cross generally pays for hospital care, while Blue Shield makes payments for physician services. Blue Cross was founded in 1932 during the depression. Its principal mission was to collect insurance premiums to ensure that hospitals would be paid for the care they provided. Consumer protection was only a secondary goal. Today insuring consumers for their health care needs has become the primary focus.

There are really many separate regional Blue Cross and Blue Shield companies, which are relatively independent. Most serve only one state or a part of one state. They are linked together in a coverage network. If a Blue Cross–insured resident of New Jersey were to get sick while visiting Chicago, the Blue Cross company in Chicago would pay the local hospital and then pass on the charges to the Blue Cross company in New Jersey.

There are some very substantial benefits of this arrangement to the payer and ultimately to the insured individuals. Because Blue Cross is so large, it is able to demand discounted rates from many health care providers. If hospitals refuse to negotiate a discount, then Blue Cross can tell its insured members that they will not be paid for care received from that provider. In fact, this has happened on occasion. Losing payments for all patients who are covered by the Blues can present a substantial financial blow to a health care provider.

The negotiated discount from normal charges becomes formalized through a contract drawn up between the Blues and the health care provider. The discount is referred to as a *contractual allowance* because it is a discount from standard rates, as allowed for in the contract between the payer and the provider.

When the resident of New Jersey gets sick in Chicago, the rate paid is that negotiated by the Blue Cross company that covers the Chicago area. That discount is then passed along to the New Jersey Blue Cross company. This provides market power (see the discussion of monopoly buying power in Chapter 4) on a national level.

Today there are also many private, for-profit insurance companies such as Prudential, Aetna, and Equicor that provide insurance coverage for health care services. Such insurers each cover a much smaller number of people than the Blues. In most cases they do not have the market power to negotiate discounts in the way that Blue Cross does. Therefore, they generally pay the charges set by the providers. Often, however, they limit their payments to customary or reasonable charges.

Employers

Employers, especially larger ones, have included health care benefits as a fringe benefit for many years. To a great extent that benefit used to consist of buying health insurance for the employee. For large companies, however, there are enough employees to reasonably anticipate likely claims. In such cases, employers are starting to provide health care insurance benefits to the employees, without contracting with an insurance company to take the risk.

Consider if the employer had decided to offer its employees fire insurance. If the employer has 20,000 employees, it might reasonably determine from historical patterns that in any given year between five and ten houses will burn down among its 20,000 employees. Rather than buying insurance for each employee, the company may find it cheaper to simply reimburse the employees whose houses burn down. Suppose, hypothetically, that there is an average $200,000 loss when a house burns down. Ten fires would cost the company $2 million. Paying $500 for a policy for each of the 20,000 employees, however, would cost the company $10 million. It is cheaper to bear the risk directly.

The same thing has now taken place with health insurance. The employer still provides the benefit to the employee. As long as the health care services are paid for, the employee probably does not even know if an insurance company or the employer takes the risk.

Many aspects of health care insurance claims are very complicated. Was the treatment appropriate? Was it provided by a qualified individual? Is the charge appropriate? Because of these complexities, there has been a growing trend for insurance companies to work for employers as a conduit of payments from employers to health care providers.

The insurance company uses its expertise to process health insurance claims, but the employer does not buy insurance. It pays the insurance company an administrative fee for processing the claims. The employer pays all the actual costs for the claims. This gives the employer a strong incentive to limit covered benefits and to try to get employees to restrain their use of health care services.

Governments

The last major payer group for health care is governments. Governments not only regulate care and provide care but they are also the largest payer for care. The most notable area that the government is involved in is Medicare and Medicaid. Medicare services are paid for by the federal government, while Medicaid services are paid for by a combination of federal and state and sometimes local payments. (These two programs are discussed further in the next section.) There are also many other federal, state, and local programs that pay health care providers for services.

The federal government pays for about 30% of health care, while state and local government combined pay for about 10% of all health care.[5] The federal government pays for and provides all health care, including dental care for members of the military. The federal government pays for and provides a more limited range of benefits for veterans. The veterans' coverage is substantial, if obtained at the Veterans Administration facilities. The federal government also provides health care for Native Americans and for federal prisoners. On a more

---

[5]Erik Echholm, "Rescuing Health Care," *New York Times*, May 12, 1991, pp. 1, 12.

limited basis the federal government provides health care in a variety of special situations, such as hospital care at the Hospital Center of the National Institutes of Health.

Most state governments provide and pay for health care in institutions for the developmentally disabled and mentally ill. Many city and county governments provide and pay for health care in locally owned hospitals and clinics that have historically provided care to the medically indigent. In addition, most local governments provide minimal services of immunizations and treatment of sexually transmitted disease. Some jurisdictions provide care for children and for communicable diseases.

Other programs are usually directed at vulnerable or at-risk populations such as substance abusers, pregnant women, HIV-positive people, and children at high risk. These programs are subject to whims of local political forces and do not have the breadth of coverage and permanence of programs such as Medicare and Medicaid.

As a payer for health care services, the government takes money, usually raised from taxes, and uses it to pay for health services. In a sense this is a pooling of money, similar to an insurance system, except that often there is a redistributive element. The taxes come from individuals who are not as likely to receive the health care services paid for by the government. Government payments to providers are only for covered groups of individuals that the government has specifically identified.

FINANCING THE HEALTH CARE SYSTEM

Many individuals and organizations provide health care services because they want to help people stay healthy or get well. However, the economic reality is that most providers would not be able to provide care unless they were compensated. As is the case for other consumer goods and services, health care services represent a product that must be paid for. It is important for nurse managers to understand the major sources of revenues for health care providers.

The Medicare and Medicaid Programs

By far the most pervasive role of government in the payment for health care is as a third-party payer. This role is primarily a result of Titles 18 and 19 of the Social Security Act of 1965. These laws created Medicare and Medicaid, which commenced in 1966.

Under Title 18 the federal government administers an insurance program for the elderly and permanently disabled called Medicare. It is divided into two separate elements referred to as Parts A and B. Part A of the program provides payment for hospital care. It is financed by taxes on earnings. Part B, the medical care portion of the program, is optional and is financed by premiums from potential patients. The amount of payments to hospitals and physicians is decided at the federal level.

The Medicare program is administered by the Health Care Financing Administration (HCFA). The actual payment system is carried out through the assignment of a number of *fiscal intermediaries*. These organizations receive an administrative fee from the government for processing bills received from providers. The intermediary receives money from HCFA and pays it to the providers based on approved claims. Often insurance companies such as Blue Cross act as intermediaries, benefiting from their own expertise in processing health care claims.

Under Title 19 the federal government runs the Medicaid program for the medically indigent. The program is financed by federal general tax revenues and state contributions. The percentage share paid by the federal government varies from state to state. The program is optional for states. Those states which choose to participate must pay for a minimal level of services for eligible participants. All states are currently participating. States may also cover other services in addition to the federally mandated minimum. Services paid for under this title vary widely from state to state. Reimbursement rates are decided by each state and also vary widely.

In the quarter-century that these programs have existed, their presence has had a dramatic effect on shaping the way health care is delivered. The original intent was to improve access to care for the indigent and aged, two underserved populations. Through these programs the government, as a major payer, has gained increasing control of what care is provided to whom and how it is provided. Many believe that these programs are the most important factor in the dramatically rising health care costs over the last twenty-five years.

The Insurance System

Insurance has become a major source of financing for the health care system. It is second only to the government in terms of the amount of money it pays to health care providers. Most Americans have private health insurance, usually provided by employers. Some individuals buy their own health insurance.

As noted earlier, in some cases insurance companies are taking the risk of high claims. In other cases the insurance companies just process the claims, and the employers retain the risk. In either event, the ultimate consumer has the protection of insurance.

Insurance is an organized way to share the risk of the costs associated with undesirable events. An insurance *premium* is paid to buy protection against the negative event. If it occurs, the insurer provides a payment to cover the loss. In this way the risk of a major financial loss is spread among all the people paying into the system, and only those "unfortunate" enough to require health care services use this pooled money.

Health insurance most often covers services (benefits) rather than being an *indemnity* plan, which provides a dollar amount for a specific medical condition. The policy states that the insurer will provide payment for specified procedures and activities of certain specified health care providers. Historically, insurers provided a standard set of benefits. Currently employers negotiate with insurers to provide an array of benefits for a set price. This price is usually based on the previous experience of the group being insured (*group rated*).

In contrast, some plans are *community rated*. In such a plan the premium is based on the general experience of the community rather than a specific group. Some argue that community rating is the only fair way to share risks. Otherwise there will be an attempt to load very high insurance costs on a very small group with a high expense experience. This to some extent defeats the purpose of insurance. Others argue that community rating is inherently discriminatory, making low-risk individuals pay for the high losses experienced by distinctly different groups. Sometimes insurers handle this problem by using community rating but adding surcharges for high-risk individuals, such as smokers.

Beneficiaries often complain that "my insurance doesn't cover that" or nurses complain "the insurance company won't pay for a nurse to do that procedure." While it is accurate that the insurance company will not pay, it is important to remember that the decision about benefits is made based on the costs of coverage. If more items are included, the costs to the insurer will be higher and the premium will have to be raised. In the case of insurance benefits received through an individual's employer, it is the employer who ultimately decides what benefits will be included in the coverage.

Moral Hazard

In theory, insurance is an ideal way to deal with the random risk of large losses. Even though some people pay a premium year after year and never collect, they have benefited from the peace of mind of knowing that they are protected from a devastating loss.

In practice, however, there are a number of problems with health insurance. Most of these problems relate to a phenomenon known as *moral hazard*. A moral hazard reflects the fact that once insured, an individual's behavior may change.

Consider an extreme example: Why buy a fire extinguisher for your house once it is insured against fire? This example is extreme because it is unlikely that fire insurance can ever adequately reimburse someone for the loss of a home. Personal, sentimental items may have little dollar value but are very meaningful to their owner. Therefore it is unlikely that an individual would fail to own a fire extinguisher just because the house is insured. Yet fire insurance companies often offer a discount on the premium for working fire alarms or extinguishers. Apparently, even in this extreme situation, the insurers have found that moral hazard exists.

In health care the problems are significantly greater. We might argue that no one is likely to smoke, simply because they know they have the safety of insurance to cover treatment for lung cancer. Yet there are other ways that health insurance policyholders can influence to some extent the number and cost of undesirable events that befall them.

Many health care services may be optional. These cover a wide range including some types of mental health services, some elective procedures, or even whether to go to a doctor for a cold. Health insurance creates a problem related to buying in an economical fashion. If a person has to pay for services, that person is likely not to consume services unless they are worth the price. If a physician charges $60 or $70 for an office visit and the patient must pay that out-of-pocket, the patient will think twice as to whether it is really necessary to see the physician. Once the patient has insurance, the price for the visit could drop to $0. At that price, all the individual is giving up is time. There is a moral hazard effect because the individual changes behavior from what it would be without insurance.

Sometimes insurers turn this to the advantage of all concerned. Many dental plans pay 100% benefits for routine preventive care but lesser percentages for other types of treatments. It is unusual for insurance to cover small losses that have a high likelihood of occurrence. The administrative costs are too high to try to pool money to cover semiannual dental checkups. However, the theory is that by providing full coverage for dental cleanings and examinations, more people will follow a plan of routine oral examinations, reducing the likelihood of larger dental claims for more extreme treatment later.

In contrast, routine physical exams are not covered by most health insurance policies. Apparently there is not as strong a belief that encouraging routine physicals will reduce high treatment costs for medical problems later.

Coinsurance, Deductibles, and Co-payments

In an effort to overcome the problems of moral hazard, insurance companies often require that beneficiaries pay *coinsurance*, a *co-payment*, and/or *deductibles*. These are a variety of attempts to make consumers bear enough of a portion of the cost of health care services to keep them from using the services as if they had a price of $0.

A deductible is an amount of money someone must pay before the insurer will pay anything for care. Generally the way this works is that the insurer requires the consumer to pay the first $100 or $200 for care each year before becoming eligible for any benefits. This can prevent an individual from making unneeded trips to the physician for minor complaints. However, if something really serious is wrong, the individual is likely to seek care, even if he or she must pay for the first several hundred dollars of cost. In the current financial environment, it would not be surprising to see the deductible rise to as high as $500.

A co-payment is a dollar amount that must be paid each time a service is used. This approach is very common among HMOs (discussed later in this chapter). Co-payments are usually several dollars. They are so minor that one is unlikely to fail to seek care when really needed. However, their presence is a reminder to the consumer that care is not free. Some believe that even a small co-payment discourages unnecessary patient use of health care services.

Coinsurance is a portion of each health care payment that is the responsibility of the consumer. It is similar to co-payments but tends to be much more substantive. Generally, coinsurance is stated in terms of a percentage that the consumer must pay. The percentages generally range from 10 to 30.

Insurers and the businesses that pay for insurance use these mechanisms to decrease the use of "unnecessary care." They believe that if the beneficiary must pay some of the cost, he or she will not seek care for conditions that are self-limiting or do not require medical or nursing care. Others argue that these mechanisms prevent people from seeking care early when treatment could be effective and could prevent more expensive care later.

When there are no deductibles, co-payments, or coinsurance, the insurer must pay all health care claims that are valid. This is referred to as *first-dollar coverage*.

Customary and Reasonable Coverage

Whether first-dollar coverage is in effect or not, insurers often place some limitations on how much they will pay for services. This is most commonly accomplished through use of limitations at the level of *customary and reasonable charges*.

Customary charges are based on surveys of what providers in an area are charging. Insurance companies can carry out these surveys simply by reviewing all bills that they receive over a period of time from a particular geographic region. The insurance company decides that any bills that exceed the average charge by a certain amount are excessive. The company then only reimburses up to a level that it determines is reasonable.

In some cases insurance policies contain specific limitations on payment amounts. For example, it is not uncommon for insurance to have a 50% coinsurance rate on mental health care benefits **and** a limit of $40 per visit. In a high-priced area such as New York, psychiatrists commonly charge $150 per session. With a $40 cap and 50% coinsurance, the benefit paid would only be $20, and the patient would be responsible for the remaining $130. It is not clear to what extent this is because insurers believe there is great moral hazard in the utilization of mental health care service, versus the extent to which mental health services are not seen as being as valuable or necessary as acute care hospital treatment, or even a physician office visit for a runny nose.

Other Sources of Financing

Between the government and insurance payments, we have covered nearly three-quarters of the money that goes into the health care system. Of the remaining monies going into the health care system, the bulk are paid for by individuals. Even though only about a quarter of all money is paid directly by consumers, this still represents well over $100 billion each year. Some health care is paid for from philanthropic gifts.

Many payments are small amounts for over-the-counter drugs or prescriptions or an occasional physician visit. Also included here are items such as uninsured dental or routine eye care and eyeglasses. Such items are paid for out-of-pocket by the large majority of citizens.

Self-pay dollars for hospital and other more expensive care generally come from the lower and upper classes of society. The rich tend to pay for many items that health insurance finds beyond the customary and reasonable limits. The working poor tend to have inadequate health insurance. They are too well off to benefit from many programs designed for the indigent but not well off enough to have a comprehensive health insurance plan. Many workers have no health insurance at all.

The last major source of funding for health care services is philanthropy. Historically, the charitable sector of society considered health care services one of its most important concerns. A lot of dollars still flow into health care organizations from philanthropic sources, although this represents a much smaller share of the total than it once did.

The reason for the decline is largely the growing role of the government and insurance. Nearly half of all health care payments come from the government. This is a much larger share than was paid by the government only thirty years ago. Further, despite the high number of uninsured Americans, there is also a growing number who do have insurance.

An additional factor has been the rapid growth of the for-profit sector in health care. Nearly one-third of all hospital beds in the country are now in hospitals that are for-profit. Most of those beds are owned by large multihospital for-profit corporations.

As the industry has become more for-profit oriented and as other sources of funding have increased, the role of philanthropy as a major financer of health care services has gradually declined.

PAYING HEALTH CARE PROVIDERS

The preceding section addressed the issue of where the resources come from for paying health care providers. Different providers are paid in different ways. We now turn our attention to the payment systems for providers. We will focus in particular on hospitals, the largest providers of health care services.

In most industries goods and services are produced at a certain cost to the provider. Providers then add a "profit" for the cost of doing business and to cover their investment. The cost plus the profit is used to establish a charge. Consumers then choose to buy or not buy the product. If a company is making a large profit, other potential providers may decide to enter the industry. Competition increases, and prices are lowered (see a discussion of this process in Chapter 4). If prices become too low, some providers will no longer be able to make a profit. They will leave the industry. Eventually an equilibrium is reached at a stable set of prices, with additional competitors neither entering nor leaving the industry.

Hospital Payment

Hospital prices are not set by the process of market economics just described. The above description suggests that people are free to enter and leave the market at will. Obviously one cannot easily set up a hospital. Even if one had the money to buy or build a hospital building and equip it, a number of state permissions would be required. The need for such permissions tends to restrict entry into the industry.

These restrictions were developed at least in part because society and elected government officials believed that health care services have special characteristics. People who buy health care services do not have the knowledge to choose among providers the way consumers can choose among hotels. Once in a hospital consumers do not have the knowledge to choose which tests they should have as they might choose which services to have in a hotel. Furthermore, the need for health care services is often sudden and unexpected and does not involve a choice. Therefore there must be a certainty that providers are competent and will provide an acceptable level of care.

Not only do we not reach a price equilibrium because of a lack of free entry into the hospital industry but prices are also controlled to a great extent by the government. Both Medicare and Medicaid impose their own pricing on hospitals.

In the last decade there has been a dramatic shift in focus on the part of Medicare payments nationwide and Medicaid payments in a few states. This movement is from a cost-based system of hospital payment to a prospective payment system. We will discuss both the old cost-based system, which is still used for paying many types of providers, and the new prospective payment system, which is used to pay for most Medicare inpatients, as well as some other hospital patients. This section will also address the issue of charity care.

Cost-based Reimbursement

Until 1983 most government payers and Blue Cross paid hospitals based on a reimbursement of their costs. Hospital accountants calculated total costs to provide care and divided that amount by the quantity of care provided. Costs were calculated for most hospital services, such as the cost per chest x-ray, per diagnostic test, and for room and board.

Even for-profit insurers and self-pay patients often paid a price based on costs. The finance department would take costs for units of service and add a factor to develop a charge. Self-pay patients and insurers paid based on those charges.

Medicare, Medicaid, and Blue Cross each established their own definitions of allowable costs. They then paid hospitals based on the amount of those costs incurred on behalf of Medicare, Medicaid, and Blue Cross patients. The Medicare guidelines were nationwide, while the allowable costs and reimbursement levels for Medicaid varied from state to state. Blue Cross definitions varied from one Blue Cross company to another around the country. The system of payment became known as *cost reimbursement*. The difference between the full charge for a service and the cost reimbursed is referred to as a *contractual allowance*.

For the nurse there was little incentive to reduce the cost of care in this system. If supplies were used, they were billed to patients or included in the daily room and board charge. If the unit needed more nurses to care for sicker patients, they could be hired. Obviously, the system was not this simplistic. At times there were not enough nurses to be hired. An even more significant issue was that some hospitals had large numbers of uninsured patients, from whom reimbursement of costs could not be ensured.

Charity Care

Hospitals in our society are not permitted to turn away patients in need of acute care. There have been unfortunate examples of hospitals that used extremely narrow definitions of what represents an acute episode requiring hospital care. Many hospitals have been more open in admitting all patients who truly are in need of care. Patients who either could not pay (indigent) or did not pay (bad debts) have created financial problems that were addressed in a number of ways. These included government subsidies, philanthropy, and cross-subsidizations.

For hospitals with very high rates of poor patients, many governments developed "disproportionate share arrangements." These approaches provided extra payments to hospitals that had very large numbers of poor patients. Often these arrangements were financed by taxing hospitals with fewer poor patients to provide a subsidy to those hospitals with more poor patients.

Philanthropy also covered some of the cost. However, as noted earlier, as the government role has increased, the role of philanthropy in paying for care has declined.

Finally, charges in excess of cost on some insured and self-pay patients resulted in enough revenues to offset the losses on bad debts and charity care patients. This is often referred to as *cross-subsidization*. Payments from one group of patients cover costs for another group of patients. Many would argue that the costs of poor patients should be borne by society through a general tax. The cross-subsidization approach is one where only those individuals who have to be hospitalized are taxed for the care of the poor.

The role of charity care by hospitals is unclear. In some states, such as New Jersey, all inpatients who pay for their care either directly or through a third party (except for Medicare) bear the cost of all indigent patients through a surcharge on their hospital charges.[6] One could therefore argue that not-for-profit hospitals in New Jersey do not provide charity care. In that case, why would hospitals have not-for-profit status and be exempt from taxes? That is a question that has become a nationwide controversy in the last decade.

In recent years changes in financial reporting requirements have been passed that focus on charity care. As of the writing of this book, each year hospitals will have to indicate on their audited financial statements the amount of charity care that they have provided. This should reveal the extent to which hospitals are providing care to the needy and also some information on how that care is financed.

While there are skeptics who do not believe that hospitals provide much charity care, in some cases the burden of charity care has overwhelmed hospitals. A number of hospitals have had to merge or go out of business over time. Such mergers accelerated after the introduction of prospective payment systems.

Prospective Payment Systems

Following the implementation of Medicare and Medicaid in 1966 the cost of hospital care began to escalate dramatically. Since government was paying a large share of these costs, it was in the goverment's (and taxpayers') interest to slow this escalation of costs. In 1983, Congress authorized HCFA to pay hospitals for Medicare inpatients on the basis of a prospective payment system (PPS) called *Diagnosis Related Groups (DRGs)*. A similar system is being developed for hospital outpatients and other ambulatory care. *Prospective payment* means that a hospital has predetermined prices for services rather than simply being reimbursed for whatever costs are incurred.

Developed at Yale University, DRGs are a classification system that groups similar patients into categories that reflect the amount of care required. These groups were constructed to reflect patients with similar medical diagnoses who spent about the same amount of time in the hospital. As of the writing of this book there are 468 different Medicare DRGs based on factors including medical diagnosis, whether the patient had an operating room procedure, the patient's age, complications, and co-morbidity.

It should be noted that a DRG is not assigned to a patient until the patient is discharged. The DRG assigned is based on the illness that required the admission. In most cases a good estimation of what the DRG will be can be made at admission.

Some states have adopted DRGs for Medicaid payments. In some cases, such as the system in New York, refinements were made that enlarged the number of DRGs to be more reflective of diagnoses that are of less import to Medicare. In particular, New York added a number of DRGs in the areas of maternity and AIDS.

Under the DRG payment system hospitals are no longer paid on the basis of the cost of care but are paid a predetermined amount based on the patient's DRG. If the patient's hospital stay costs the hospital more than the DRG rate, the hospital loses the difference. If the stay costs less than the rate, the hospital

---

[6]As this book goes to press, the New Jersey system of surcharges has been challenged in the federal courts. This may lead to a drastic change in the way hospitals are paid in that state.

keeps the surplus. The rates paid are based on the national costs of each DRG, adjusted for annual inflation and expected productivity gains.

The federal DRG payment system applies only to Medicare patients. However, some states, such as New York and New Jersey, have a similar system that applies to all payers (*all-payer system*). Other states have adopted DRGs for their Medicaid payments. In rare instances, such as in Maryland, DRGs are not used for any patients. Instead, a state-designated alternative system is in effect. And for certain specialty hospitals (such as pediatric, pyschiatric, and oncology) DRGs are not used. But, for the most part, DRGS are becoming a dominant force in hospital payment.

For nurses the rules have now changed. The total revenue to the hospital for a given patient is fixed regardless of the costs incurred in treating that patient. It *does* matter how many catheter kits are used. It *does* matter if the patient has one less x-ray, because those items cost the hospital money. Most important, it matters how long the patient stays in the hospital. The most important predictor of hospital cost is the patient's length of stay. If on average it costs $600 per day to stay in a hospital, the patient who stays two extra days will cost the hospital as much as $1,200 more than the patient who stays fewer days. Consequently, there is increasing pressure on nurse managers to decrease patient length of stay. In those organizations where the nurse manager is fiscally accountable for the unit, it is vital for the manager to understand the importance of the reimbursement system.

Nurse Payment

Almost 70% of nurses work in hospitals, and most nurses in hospitals are paid an hourly wage by their employer. Overtime is paid for hours worked in addition to base. Nurse managers are likely to be paid a salary. In general they are not paid overtime but are given compensatory time off. In fact, most nurse managers work more than their scheduled hours without additional compensation.

Several hospitals are now experimenting with alternate payment systems for staff nurses. These include paying nurses a salary with no additional compensation for overtime; paying nurses a salary plus bonus, based on the productivity of the nursing unit; and paying a group of nurses a set amount of money to provide care for a specified period of time. As hospital management attempts to increase productivity, it is anticipated that alternate methods of payment will expand.

Many nurses work in organizations other than hospitals. In most cases they are employees working for an annual salary or on an hourly basis. In some cases there are profit-sharing arrangements or bonuses. Nurses in some home health settings are paid on a per visit basis. Nurses are rarely paid directly by insurers or consumers of care. Most often, these payments are made to an organization, which then pays the nurse.

Some nurses are self-employed and receive payment directly from patients or insurers. Private duty nurses often are paid directly, as are nurse psychotherapists. Nurse practitioners, nurse psychotherapists, and nurse midwives are sometimes paid directly by insurers. For the last ten years professional nurses have been lobbying for "third-party reimbursement for nurses." Nurses argue that they should be reimbursed in the same way physicians are. They provide the nursing care. They argue that they should be able to authorize care and should be directly reimbursed for it.

There is substantial evidence that when nurses provide care that would otherwise be provided by physicians, money is saved. Examples are prenatal care or well-child care. (No empirical studies could be located that discussed the impact of reimbursing nursing care that was not substitutive). However, the concept of direct payment to nurses has met with resistance from payers. Payers apparently believe this care will be additive and will increase total health care costs rather than lowering them.

However, it should be noted that the benefit structure of employees' health insurance is determined by the employer, not the government. Therefore if employers wanted this benefit and were willing to pay for it, their insurers would provide it. It would appear that the nursing profession could make substantial progress in the area of payments for nurses, if it lobbied effectively.

Physician Payment

Physicians have traditionally been paid by patients, either directly or through the patient's insurance company. Their income is usually directly related to the number of care episodes they provide. In recent years, however, a number of changes in physician payment have been occurring.

First, the percentage of physicians who are salaried employees has been growing dramatically. Physicians have long been salaried employees in some hospitals, e.g., some academic medical centers. However, as the costs of opening a practice continue to increase, fewer physicians have been opening their own practices. Within ten years it is possible that the majority of physicians may be salaried employees.

Another major change in physician payment was introduced by Medicare early in the 1990s. This change reoriented the payment scale for different types of physicians. The intent was to reemphasize the importance of cognitive skills and to deemphasize the importance of procedures. Medicare hoped to provide higher payments to physicians for making diagnoses and lower payments to physicians for performing surgery and other high-tech procedures. At this point it is too early to make any assessments about the impact of the change in the payment scales.

Home Health Agency Payment

Home health agencies are paid by government, insurers, and directly by patients. Most agencies bill on a per visit basis for professional nursing services and on an hourly basis for unskilled aide care. Certified home care agencies provide skilled nursing care and other services. They are authorized to receive direct payment from Medicare for the services they provide. In addition, they receive payment from Medicaid, insurers, and directly from patients.

Home care agencies that are not certified to receive payment from Medicare may receive payments from Medicaid, other third-party payers, and directly from patients. Both certified and noncertified agencies are reimbursed by third-party payers on a cost basis. In essence, the agency calculates its allowable costs, divides by the number of visits, and then calculates a per visit charge. Assuming that this reimbursement per visit covers their costs, it is in the agencies' interest to provide more rather than fewer visits. Agencies may not be able to cover their costs. Some costs are not "allowable" by the third-party payers. Some agencies provide care to people who have no insurance and cannot pay.

Home health care costs have been escalating, and it is anticipated that before the next edition of this book is published, some form of episode-of-care reimbursement may be instituted.

Nursing Home Payment

Although nursing homes provide short-term care for patients recovering from injuries such as a hip fracture, most nursing home residents are institutionalized for approximately two years. Paying for long-term care is a major national policy issue for the 1990s. Most nursing home care is paid for by Medicaid. However, in most cases people are not eligible for Medicaid until they have used up all their life savings and become impoverished.

METHODS USED TO CONTROL PAYMENTS FOR CARE

With the rapid rise of health care costs over the quarter-century since the introduction of Medicare and Medicaid, there has been a growing push to control spending. This has given rise to a number of approaches. Most prominent among them is the development of HMOs, PPOs, and managed care efforts.

Health Maintenance Organizations (HMOs)

HMOs provide health care services to individuals or groups in exchange for a monthly payment. The payment is the same whether the individual uses services or not. This contrasts with the fee-for-service approach in which an individual pays specifically for those health care services consumed. HMOs were first popularized in the 1960s as a way to contain health care costs and to improve the health of people. However, the basic type of organization had existed for many decades prior to the 1960s. Two noteworthy examples are the Kaiser-Permanente Health Plan, which is a dominant force in the west, and the large Health Insurance Plan (HIP) in New York. HMOs currently cover 13% of the population.[7] The developers believed that the insurance system was designed to pay for "sickness care." Most insurance pays only for care for people who are sick. Why not develop an insurance system that would pay to keep people well?

In HMOs, preventive care is paid for and there is an emphasis on keeping people well and out of the hospital. Not only should HMOs improve care but they also have the potential to lower costs by eliminating unnecessary care and by detecting health problems early.

For this system to work there needs to be an incentive for physicians (the *gatekeepers*) to use less expensive outpatient care and to hospitalize patients only when necessary. The incentive used is money. In most HMOs physician groups are paid on a *capitation basis*. This means they are paid a flat fee per patient, regardless of the amount of care that the patient consumes.

Patients pay a flat premium, or capitation charge, called the PMPM (per member per month charge). If the population stays well and does not use a

---

[7]Patrice Duggan, "Power Shift," *Forbes*, February 18, 1991, p. 80.

lot of health services, the physician group shares in the money that is not spent. However, the physicians are at risk. If the patient population consumes a lot of health care resources, physician payments are lowered.

From the patients' point of view, there is usually little or no charge for most health care visits. Preventive care is encouraged. The patient does not have to pay the doctor and then get reimbursed.

There are two principal types of HMOs. These are the group model and individual practitioner association (IPA) approaches. In the group model, all the HMO's physicians are employees of the HMO. They provide care only to patients of the HMO in HMO-owned facilities and affiliated hospitals. All HMO members get their care from a physician who is part of the group. This substantially limits choice in selecting a physician.

In the IPA model, physicians have their own private practice and treat many of their patients on a traditional *fee-for-service* basis. That means that they charge those patients for each episode of care and each service provided. However, for members of the IPA HMO that chose the physician as their primary provider, the physician provides the care in exchange for a portion of the HMO's PMPM charge. The IPA model keeps the physicians at risk. They earn less if the covered HMO members consume a lot of health care services. They earn a higher amount if HMO members consume relatively few services.

IPAs tend to have far more affiliated physicians than group model plans. In the group approach, the HMO must have enough members to keep its physicians busy. The IPA model allows the physicians to have their own non-HMO patients. Therefore, an HMO with the same number of members can offer a much larger number of physicians. This provides more choice to members of the HMO. Further, it uses the physicians' offices. Therefore the HMO doesn't have to make nearly as large an investment in clinical offices and equipment.

However, some observers feel that IPA doctors are not as committed to the ideals of the HMO approach as are members of a group model HMO. There is a large rift in the industry between those dedicated HMO physicians who believe that HMOs can not only be less expensive but can also provide more appropriate care and those physicians who view HMO IPA affiliation as just another way to get more patients into their offices.

For HMOs to work, patients must get all their care from physicians affiliated with the HMO. If patients could go to other providers, those providers might order expensive tests or hospitalization when outpatient care and less expensive tests would do. Therefore, most HMOs view the primary care physician as a gatekeeper. This primary physician prevents patients from consuming unnecessary treatments by specialists and from gaining unneeded admissions to the hospital.

In addition, most HMOs have arrangements with specific hospitals to provide care. Often the HMO negotiates a discounted rate for hospital care. In such cases patients' choice of hospitals becomes limited.

Many consumers do not like HMO restrictions on choice of physician and hospital. In addition, because of their comprehensive coverage, HMOs have tended to be more expensive than other insurance plans. As a result, HMOs, while gradually expanding, have never experienced the dramatic growth that had been predicted for them.

Preferred Provider Organizations (PPOs)

PPOs are arrangements between providers (physicians, hospitals, etc.) and third-party payers. The providers agree to provide care for set prices, usually less than the current prevailing rate. The payers agree to steer large numbers of patients to that provider. Incentives are given to insured individuals that encourage them to receive their health care services from these preferred providers.

Arrangements to get discounts from preferred providers are most often made by insurers or employers. In some cases state governments negotiate PPO arrangements for Medicaid care.

If clients choose to receive care from a preferred provider, they often have lower out-of-pocket expenses. For example, the coinsurance for each episode of care may be 0% or 10% if the preferred provider is used, but 20% or 30% if the preferred provider is not used. Sometimes deductibles are waived if care is from the preferred provider. Although the systems restrict the provider options for patients, many employers prefer this method because it lowers expenses. Insurers (and the employers who pay their premiums) believe that PPOs decrease costs.

There is a saying in the PPO industry that "if you've seen one PPO, you've seen one PPO." Each arrangement tends to be unique. It is very difficult to make generalizations about the different PPOs that exist.

Managed Care

Managed care is a system in which someone acts as an intermediary between the patient and the provider of services. The role of physician as "gatekeeper" was discussed above. In a managed care system, a designated person (often called the case manager) rather than the physician authorizes the provision of the services. While a major goal of managed care is to decrease costs by decreasing unnecessary services, case management can also ensure that patients get appropriate and timely care.

Many insurance companies now have managed care. They may require prior approval for all but emergency care and refuse to pay for care that was not authorized. Managed care programs often require second opinions for surgical procedures, and may require that only certain facilities and providers be used.

IMPLICATIONS FOR NURSE MANAGERS

Managers cannot effectively operate in a vacuum. The purpose of this chapter was to discuss the various elements of the health care system to provide an explanation of the environment in which nurse managers work.

There are a number of key players or participants in the health care system. These include not only the providers of care and the patients but also the health care suppliers, regulators, and payers. In health care much of what an organization and professional can or cannot do is influenced by forces external to the organization. These forces may be government regulatory bodies, insurance companies, or consumer groups. Changes in payment systems to health care organizations have implications for how care is provided. Changes in the regulation of health professionals have implications for what ancillary workers can and cannot do. Without considering the role of each participant and the relationships among all the participants, one risks making decisions that do not take all relevant factors into account.

Many things are done by health care providers that may not make obvious sense. Some of these things can be understood if the manager considers the system of financing the health care system. Health care providers have become very dependent on revenues from Medicare, Medicaid, insurance, and self-pay patients. However, the payments being made have placed a great stress on the economy.

In reaction to that financial stress, the government has focused on prospective payment. Insurers have placed hurdles such as coinsurance, deductibles, co-payments, and limits on customary and reasonable charges. With decreasing funding from philanthropic sources, providers must be ever more diligent to carefully remain financially solvent. The main payers are attempting to restrict payments, while at the same time a growing number of patients are not covered, even by government indigent programs, and cannot afford to pay for their care.

In further response to the need to control health care costs, there has been a rise in approaches to manage these costs. The most prominent among these are HMOs, PPOs, and managed care. Each of these has the potential to come into direct contact with the role of the nurse manager in most health care provider organizations. Dealing with such cost containment alternatives is going to require nurse managers to become more conscious than ever of the costs of running units and departments. There is likely to be a growing need for information that can be used in the negotiations and decisions that relate to HMOs, PPOs, and other managed care efforts.

KEY CONCEPTS ❖

Key participants Major groups involved in the organization and delivery of health care are the providers, suppliers, consumers, regulators, and payers.

> **Providers** Health workers such as nurses or physicians and health care organizations such as nursing homes or hospitals that dispense health care services to people. The most important providers of care are hospitals, nurses, physicians, and the government. However, there are many other types of providers that are essential to providing the total range of health care services. Different providers have different goals and incentives and behave in different fashions.

> **Suppliers** Manufacturers and distributors of supplies and equipment used by health care providers. Suppliers have a dramatic impact on the health care industry as a result of their development on new technologies.

> **Consumers** Individuals who receive health care services. Generally consumers of health care are less knowledgeable about health care purchases than they are about the purchase of other goods and services.

> **Regulators** Federal, state, and local governments have the legal authority to regulate the health care industry as part of their function of protecting

the public. Health providers are also subject to the regulations of voluntary accreditation and certification bodies, such as the Joint Commission on Accreditation of Healthcare Organizations (JCAHO).

Payers   Individuals or organizations that pay for health care services provided to consumers. The most common groups of payers are individuals, insurers, employers, and the government.

Third-party payer   Organization or government ("third parties") that pays for health care services consumed by individuals.

Contractual allowances   Discounts from normal charges that are given to large payers of health care services.

Health care financing   Government is the largest payer for health care services, providing about 40% of the funding. Insurers and employers are the next largest group, followed by individuals.

Medicare and Medicaid   Government programs that pay for health care services for the aged, permanently disabled, and some indigent individuals. The Medicare program is administered by HCFA, and payments to providers are made through fiscal intermediaries.

Insurance system   Most Americans have private health insurance. In exchange for a premium, often paid for by an employer, individuals receive health insurance coverage. The premium rates are set based either on the experience of a specific group (group rated) or the community as a whole (community rated). To discourage unnecessary use of health care services, insurance usually has deductibles, co-payments, and coinsurance.

>   **Deductible**   Amount the individual must pay each year before insurance begins to pay for care. This payment is usually several hundred dollars.

>   **Co-payment**   Dollar amount that must be paid by the individual each time a health service is used. For example, some pharmaceutical plans require that a $3 fee be paid for each prescription.

>   **Coinsurance**   Percentage of the charges that must be paid by the beneficiary, usually 20%.

Out of pocket   Money that people expend directly for health care services not covered by insurance or other third-party sources.

Customary and reasonable charges   Limits set by insurers on the amount that they will consider for payment, based on surveys of typical charges in the community.

Cost-based reimbursement   Payments made to providers based on a reimbursement to the provider for the cost incurred in providing care.

Prospective payment   Payments made to providers based on a fixed price for each specific type of patient. Payments are not actually made in advance of treatment.

Diagnosis Related Groups (DRGs)   Medicare prospective payment system. Patients are placed into specific groups (DRGs) based on their principal diagnosis, surgical procedures, age, and other factors. Payment for each patient within a specific group is the same. The payment is a predetermined fixed amount and is not dependent on the amount of costs incurred in treating the patient.

All-payer system   System where all payers use the same payment method. In states such as New York and New Jersey, a DRG-based prospective payment system is applied for all hospital inpatients, regardless of payer.

Health maintenance organization   Health care organization that agrees to provide health care on a capitation basis. The HMO is paid a set fee per member per month to provide all specified health care services to enrolled patients.

Preferred provider organization   Organization that agrees to provide care for a group of individuals, such as an employee group, based on a negotiated set of fees. These fees are often lower than the prevailing fees in the community. In contrast to HMOs, the providers are paid on a fee-for-service basis.

Managed care   System for organizing the delivery of care in which someone other than the provider of care controls the services the patient uses. These systems are usually used to control and limit the use of services. However, they are also used so that people do not get unnecessary care, which subjects the patient to unnecessary risk.

SUGGESTED READINGS ————————————————————

Berk, Marc Lewis, Alan Monheit, and Michael M. Hagen, "How the U.S. Spent Its Health Care Dollar: 1929–1980," *Health Affairs*, Vol. 7, No. 4, Fall 1988, pp. 46–59.

Bishop, C. E., and S. L. Karon, *Composition of Home Health Care Expenditure Growth*, Bigel Institute for Health Policy, Waltham, MA, 1987.

Ermann, D., and J. Gabel, "Multi-Hospital Systems: Issues and Empirical Findings," *Health Affairs*, Vol. 3, No. 1, Spring 1984, p. 50.

Feder, James, Jack Hadley, and Stephan Zuckerman, "How Did Medicare's Prospective Payment System Affect Hospitals?" *New England Journal of Medicine*, Vol. 317, No. 14, pp. 867–873, October 1, 1987.

Fuchs, Victor, *Who Shall Live?* Basic Books, New York, 1974.

General Accounting Office, *Long Term Care for the Elderly* (HRD-89-4), Author, Washington, DC, 1988.

Ginzberg, Eli, and Matthew P. Drennan, *The Health Sector: Its Significance for the Economy of New York City*, Commonwealth Fund, New York, 1985.

Gray, Branford H. (ed.), *For-Profit Enterprise in Health Care*, Institute of Medicine, National Academy Press, Washington, DC, 1986.

Hawes, Charles A., and Charles D. Phillips, "The Changing Structure of the Nursing Home Industry and the Impact of Ownership on Quality, Cost, and Access," B. H. Gray (ed.), *For-Profit Enterprise in Health Care*, National Academy Press, Washington, DC, 1986.

Himmelstein, Daniel U., and Steffie Woolhandler, "Cost without Benefit: Administrative Waste in U.S. Health Care," *New England Journal of Medicine*, Vol. 314, No. 7, pp. 441–445, February 13, 1986.

Institute of Medicine, *Improving the Quality of Care in Nursing Homes*, National Academy Press, Washington, DC, 1986.

Levit, Katherine R., and Mark S. Freeland, "National Medical Care Spending," *Health Affairs*, Vol. 7, Winter, 1988, pp. 124–136.

Levit, Katherine R., Mark S. Freeland, and Daniel R. Waldo, "Health Spending and Ability to Pay: Business, Individuals, and Government," *Health Care Financing Review*, Vol. 10, No. 3, Spring, 1989, pp. 1–11.

Robinson, James, and Harold Luft, "Competition, Regulation and Hospital Costs, 1982–1986," *Journal of the American Medical Association*, Vol. 260, No. 18, November 11, 1988, p. 2676.

Rosenberg, Charles E., *The Care of Strangers*, Basic Books, New York, 1987.

Starr, Paul, *The Social Transformation of American Medicine*, Basic Books, New York, 1982.

3

The Role of Financial Management Within the Health Care Organization

CHAPTER GOALS

The goals of this chapter are to:

- Explain the role of management in organizations
- Explain the structural hierarchy of organizations in theory and practice
- Distinguish between formal and informal lines of authority and between the line and staff roles of managers
- Assess the advantages and disadvantages of centralized versus decentralized management approaches
- Describe the role of financial managers in health care organizations
- Describe the financial responsibilities of the chief nurse executive and other nurse managers
- Discuss the interactions between nurse managers and financial managers in health care organizations
- Introduce and explain the concept of responsibility accounting, including cost and revenue centers
- Discuss issues of politics in budget determinations
- Describe the role of networking

❖

INTRODUCTION

The primary role of nurses is the delivery of patient care. Nurses are educated for that set of activities, and for most nurses it is the reason they chose nursing.

Historically, anything to do with money or financial resources was seen by most nurses as the purview of administration. Most nurses did not know about budgets or organizational resources and did not want to know about them. They wanted to keep people healthy and provide nursing care to those who were not healthy. Some nurses had to be involved with money; they became "nursing administrators." According to some nursing leaders, a number of these nurses even abandoned nursing and became hospital administrators.

Over the last quarter-century, however, there has been increasing pressure for health care organizations to control costs and to provide care efficiently. Health care organizations tried to accomplish this with as little nursing intervention in the area of management of resources as possible. In most cases, financial managers tried to simply provide nursing departments with a budget and to tell nurse managers to hold to the budgeted level of spending. That approach proved unworkable.

Managers who spend the money know the most about the resources that are needed. They must be involved in the planning process if the budget is to be a realistic document. To control costs, nursing departments and units must be directly involved in a wide array of financial activities. In some organizations this means that nurses are taking on an increasing burden of financial calculations. In other organizations nurses are hiring nonclinical individuals with MBA degrees to work for them as staff members. Those individuals do the actual financial calculations. In either case, ultimately nurses are responsible for the content of those calculations. Nurse managers must have sufficient financial skills either to develop or else to supervise the development of financial information needed to run their departments. This is necessary not only to provide acceptable quality of care but also to provide that care on a cost-effective basis.

In today's health care environment, it is acceptable for nurses to know and to be concerned about the organization's money. A growing number of programs in schools of nursing, both on an undergraduate and graduate level, are including financial management in their programs.

This chapter is intended to explain the role of financial management in the structure of organizations and how nursing and nurse managers fit into that organizational structure from a financial management perspective. To accomplish that we will include issues such as lines of authority, formal and informal linkages, interrelationships among managers, and the role of politics and power in health care organizations.

THE ROLE OF MANAGEMENT

Health care organizations include a wide variety of providers of health care services, such as hospitals, nursing homes, home health agencies, and others such as nursing centers. Regardless of the type of organization, certain management functions must be carried out. Three of the most important of these are planning, control, and decision making.

Planning is essential for the efficient management of the organization. Through planning managers consider possible options available to the organization and steer its path. Without planning the organization drifts like a rudderless ship. With planning the organization is able to set a direction and make progress in moving toward it. Strategic planning and budgeting, two topics covered in this book, are essential elements of the planning process.

Control is a critical management task. Once the plan has been established, it must be implemented. Control refers to the managerial tasks related to ensuring that the plans of the organization are carried out as closely as possible. Control is necessary for carrying out the plans, assessing progress, and determining what can be done when progress is not satisfactory.

Decision making is perhaps the most overriding role of management. Plans will not carry any weight unless someone makes decisions that are necessary to carry them out. Control will lack authority if no one makes decisions to correct problems that arise when the plan is not met. Organizations do not progress without change. Change cannot occur without someone's having the authority to make decisions and exercising that authority.

These basic elements of the role of management apply to all managers within the organization. Only when managers apply these principles can organizations most efficiently achieve their goals.

THE HIERARCHY OF HEALTH CARE ORGANIZATIONS

To make plans, control the organization, and make and carry out decisions, each organization has a managerial *hierarchy*. The hierarchy establishes the authority and responsibility that different individuals have within the organization.

Each organization has a governing board, generally referred to as the board of trustees or board of directors. The board has the ultimate responsibility for the decisions made by the organization. The board is generally made up of respected individuals from the community and business world. Most of the board members are *not* full-time employees of the organization.

Ultimately the financial condition of the organization is the responsibility of the board. Therefore it has the final approval over the adoption of the annual budget. It also provides the direction for setting that budget. The board adopts a mission statement that sets the overall direction of the organization. It also adopts goals and objectives that tell the organization's managers what they should be trying to do to accomplish the mission. An administrator, often called the chief executive officer (CEO) or president, reports to the board and is responsible for managing the organization. As is typical in bureaucratic organizations, a variety of managers report to the CEO.

The Top Management Team

It is unusual to find any moderate to large organization that can be run by one manager; too many different functions must be carried out. As a result, there are many managers, each with a specialized set of activities and scope of authority. For the single top manager to know what each manager is doing, there is a hierarchy of managers. Instructions may be passed down through the hierarchy, along with the authority to carry out the instructions. To facilitate this process, many organizations form a top management team, which acts together on making major organizational decisions. In addition, information is passed up through the hierarchy. For example, various nurse managers often directly observe events about which the higher levels of management should be informed.

Many large organizations have an associate administrator as part of this team, often called the chief operating officer (COO) or executive vice-president for operations, who is responsible for the day-to-day operations of the organization. The team also includes a chief financial officer (CFO), who is responsible for the financial aspects of running the organization. The CEO, COO, and CFO attend board meetings. The CEO is often a member of the board.

Until the recent past the chief nurse executive was called the director of nursing. In recent years, the titles vice-president for nursing and vice-president for patient services have gained widespread use. The titles chief nurse executive (CNE) and chief nursing officer (CNO) are also used. There is still a wide gap, however, between some organizations that treat the CNE as a key member of the top management team consisting of the CEO, COO, CFO, and CNE, and those which treat the CNE on a par with a number of other department heads who report to a member of the top management team. The trend is recognition of the special role played by the CNE, who controls approximately half of most health care organizations' budgets and an even greater share of the organizations' salaries. In more and more health care organizations the CNE is included in the top management team and is taking on functions such as attending board meetings and participating in the organization's most important decisions.

There is some controversy in nursing over the appropriateness of this trend. As the CNE becomes part of the top management team, the responsibility of that position shifts from responsibility for and management of the nursing department to responsibility for and management of the organization. Instead of looking downward at the nursing department, CNEs are starting to look outward at the overall actions of the organization and how they affect the organization as a whole. The result is that nursing is gaining in prestige as a member of the inner circle of management. The CNE is privy to more information and is a key player in the most important decisions of the organization. However, some would argue that the role that CNEs serve in such situations lessens their ability to be an advocate for the needs of nursing in the organization. The role removes the CNE even further from the patient and from an awareness of the needs of staff nurses.

The authors of this book believe that the trend is appropriate. Nursing controls too great a part of the resources of health care organization to be excluded from the key decisions that affect the organization. However, we also believe that CNEs must be cognizant of the difficult position in which this trend places them and must make a special effort to ensure that the needs of the organization are balanced with the needs of the nursing department and its managers and staff.

Line vs. Staff Authority

To carry out its mission and its specific goals and objectives, the organization has a hierarchy of managers who are supervised by the CEO or by the top management team. The types of managers that exist in an organization can be divided into two major classes based on their *line* or *staff function*. The line function is the element of running an organization that is related directly to the production of its goods and services. In the case of health care organizations, the line function is carried out by the managers and departments that provide patient care. Most nurse managers are considered *line managers*. Their managerial efforts go to the direct care of patients.

In contrast, the staff function concerns providing auxiliary assistance or service to the line managers and their departments. Finance officers are *staff managers*. The role of finance as a staff department is to carry out necessary functions for running the organization that are indirect to the provision of care. Finance makes sure that there is money to buy the things that the organization needs and to pay for them. It also provides necessary information about the finances of the organization.

Line managers do not report to staff managers. Therefore the finance department does not have authority over any line operations of the organization. Nevertheless, the information provided by finance is often used by line managers to help them make more effective managerial decisions. Nursing managers must understand the staff role played by finance and make use of them as a resource.

To better understand the distinction between staff and line authority, one must understand the framework of both formal and informal lines of authority and responsibility within an organization.

Formal Lines of Authority

Organizations have formal chains of command that define lines of authority and responsibility. Of primary interest in this book is how the nursing department fits within the overall organizational structure and its relationship to the organization's financial management.

The formal lines of authority for most organizations are specified in the form of an organization chart. An organization chart provides a diagrammatic perspective of the interrelationships. Each position identified on the chart has supervision over the individuals below it in the chart connected by solid lines. Each position reports to those above. Other individuals on the same level in the chart are in a similar level of the organizational hierarchy. There is often communication between individuals on the same level, but there is not a direct reporting relationship.

It is also common to have formal relationships that exist but do not represent the same degree of authority or control. For instance, a manager at one level in the organization may report to a line manager directly above. The director of the dietary department may report to the chief operating officer. The director of dietary may also report information on a regular basis to the chief of the medical board, who is concerned about the impact of nutrition on the quality of care. However, the chief of the medical board is not the supervisor of the dietary manager and has only limited ability to make decisions in that area and to give instructions to dietary. Such formal but limited relationships are indicated on organization charts by the use of dashed rather than solid lines.

Informal lines of authority may also exist. However, they are completely outside the official policy of the organization. They would not appear on the organization chart at all.

The most complex health care organizational structures are found within hospitals. Figure 3–1 shows an organizational chart for a hospital of moderate size. Solid lines indicate direct paths of formal authority and responsibility. As can be seen in the figure, the vice-president for nursing reports to the executive vice-president, who reports to the president, who reports to the board of

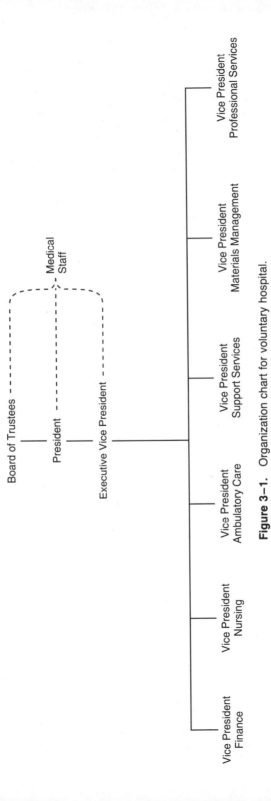

Figure 3–1. Organization chart for voluntary hospital.

trustees. The vice-president for nursing is on the same level as the five other senior management staff.

It is worthy of note that while the CFO is a highly placed individual in the organization, only financial departments report to that individual. None of the direct providers of care report to the CFO.

Figure 3–2 shows the organizational chart of the nursing department within a major medical center (not shown on the chart). In this organization, the CNE reports to the CEO of the medical center. Within the nursing department are associate directors of the various clinical services. Both these organizations follow traditional organizational models with nursing as a separate department and most nurses who work in the organization reporting through nursing. Note, however, that the operating room (O.R.) director reports to the executive director of nursing in the medical center (Fig. 3–2).

Figure 3–2. New York University Medical Center nursing and related departments organizational chart.

As noted in Chapter 2, the medical staff at most hospitals are not employees of the hospital. Most hospitals have voluntary medical staffs. Therefore they also are not part of the direct-line hierarchy in the hospital. Nevertheless, a hospital cannot function without a medical staff any more than it can function without a nursing staff. Therefore, there are established relationships between the medical staff and the employees of the organization.

The dotted line in Figure 3–1 indicates the relationship of the medical staff to the hospital. Most hospitals have a medical board, which has responsibility for the quality of medical care in the organization. While JCAHO and state regulations require that this be a formal relationship, the relationship is not the same as that of employee/employer.

Figure 3–3 shows the organizational chart of a large government-owned hospital. In this organizational chart it should be noted that physicians are employees of the hospital and therefore directly accountable to the chief executive officer.

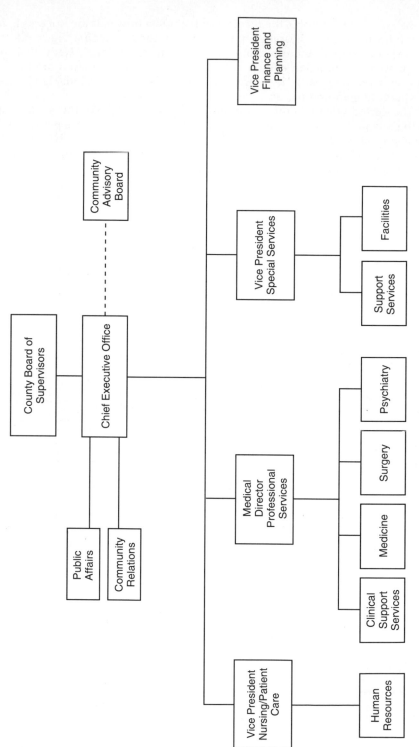

Figure 3–3. Organization chart for government hospital.

Informal Lines of Authority

The organization charts shown above include only the formal relationships. Informal relationships are not part of the official authority structure of the organization. As such, they come and go, often with the individual in a specific position. Informal relationships develop gradually over time. Although they have no official standing, often they become an accepted part of the way an organization operates.

Most texts of organizational theory point out that informal lines of authority are often as important, if not more so, as the formal lines of authority. Informal lines of authority are based on the history of the organization, the key players in the organization, and resources controlled by the various players. Depending on the specific history in any particular health care organization, in some organizations the CNE may have more or less authority and responsibility than the organizational chart indicates. This could develop over time from the presence of a CNE with a particularly strong personality. The gains of one occupant of a position may even carry over to the successor. So may the losses.

Not long ago in many health care organizations, the director of nursing was an individual who believed that nursing was a strictly clinical function. As such, this director relied heavily on the finance department to handle all issues related to money and resources. Even if the formal structure of the organization gave the director of nursing certain authority, it was often not taken. Informal structures then took over, filling the void. As such directors are replaced over time with CNEs who believe that they should have greater control over nursing resources, it often requires a battle to regain the authority that officially resides in the nursing department. Informal structures can be as hard to overcome as formal ones.

In some organizations, individual key players may have special relationships. The CNE may be married to the chief of surgery. This personal relationship allows each access to information that he or she might not normally have. These two players may then form a coalition for certain decisions.

In other cases key employees have a special relationship with people important to the hospital. The director of volunteers may be the brother of the major employer in town. The employer pays for care of employees who use the hospital. In some organizations, key players share a common history: they went to school together; they both worked together at another hospital prior to coming to this hospital; they may socialize at a place of worship. Each of these special relationships has implications for the sharing of information and support that occurs in the process of running a hospital.

A third source of informal authority is control of resources. A common maxim is, "He who controls information, controls the organization." Financial information is an example of information frequently not shared in organizations. Another resource includes employees. The nursing department usually is the largest hospital department in terms of employees.

But number of employees may not be as influential as bottom-line results. Nursing is generally seen as a cost center rather than a profit center. Nursing must work to keep its expenses within budgeted expectations. Certain other departments are profit centers. The results of activities in those departments may be reflected in a departmental profit. Historically the profit generated is used as a bargaining chip when resource allocation decisions are made. This means that some managers may be able to exercise greater influence than others. In some cases, managers may bypass the formal lines of authority and jump over one or more levels in the organization, using their power to gain resources to achieve their goals.

Other elements also serve to reinforce informal lines of authority. Physicians admit patients to the hospital. Patients represent revenue. Therefore, physicians have power. The implicit (and sometimes explicit) threat to refer their patients elsewhere allows the medical board to have significant impact in decisions.

Often informal relationships are worked out in hospitals to exchange services. For example, the head nurse on 3 North makes sure that when the mother of the supervisor of housekeeping is a patient in the hospital, she receives special attention. When 3 North needs extra housekeeping help, the housekeeping department may be more responsive.

Centralized vs. Decentralized Organizations

Health care organizations tend to be centralized and bureaucratic. As they became more complex and employed more specialized workers, authority for decision making became centralized. There is, however, a growing trend toward decentralization in many of these organizations. The unit-based council developed in many shared-governance models in nursing is an example of decentralization. As Finkler states, "To a great extent the degree of decentralization rests upon the confidence top management has in the management team throughout the hospital, and on the quality of the performance measurement system in place."[1]

One author suggests that management should be limited to no more than five layers and prefers no more than three.[2] He argues for increased authority and responsibility for unit managers, including higher spending authority.

Decentralization enhances the development of unit-based managers, puts authority for making decisions with the people who have the current information, allows management by exception rather than by rule, and allows a quick response to both client need and environmental change.

For an organization to grow and thrive it must continually develop its management staff. Decentralization permits the organization to foster management skills and identify those successful managers who can be promoted within the organization. A second advantage of decentralization is that the best information on which to make decisions is often at the unit level. Unit managers are in constant contact with clients and staff. They know and understand the needs of these groups better than a nurse manager sitting in a central office.

A third advantage of decentralization is the ability to decentralize exceptions to rules. Although large bureaucratic organizations need policies and rules, exceptions are inevitably necessary. Decentralization allows exceptions to be made at the unit level when appropriate.

Finally, timeliness is enhanced in a decentralized organization. Centralized organizations take a great amount of time to make decisions as information

---

[1]Steven A. Finkler, "Responsibility Centers," *Hospital Cost Management and Accounting*, Vol. 3, No. 9, December, 1991, p. 1.

[2]Tom Peters, *Thriving on Chaos*, New York, Alfred A. Knopf. 1987, p. 359.

moves up and then back down through the organizational hierarchy. In a decentralized organization, decisions can be made in a more timely and efficient manner.

Although there is a trend toward decentralization, it does have disadvantages. Health care organizations function in a highly regulated environment. This environment requires accountability to a myriad of details. External regulators have requirements on everything from how supplies should be stored to what to tell a patient before discharge. In decentralized hospitals a system for ensuring regulatory compliance may be the greatest challenge.

Other problems exist as well. Decentralization requires that top managment provide the necessary education to train managers. Inevitably, managers will make errors. Communication is a critical factor in decentralization.

Because more decentralized decisions are made, there must be a working communication system so that top management is informed of decisions in a timely fashion. It is likely that unit-based managers and top managers will have conflicting goals. The unit-based nurse manager will have as a goal providing high-quality care at the least stress to the staff. Although those goals are consistent with top management, the cost of providing this care will be of less concern to the nurse manager than to top administration. Systems have to be put in place to motivate the unit manager to achieve the organization's goals and/or a framework for unit managers to participate in setting organizational goals.

Nurse managers at the unit level will likely make some mistakes, if they are human. The organization must tolerate some mistakes and have in place a system to assist managers to learn from, rather than be punished for, exercising judgments.

To successfully achieve decentralization requires a commitment from the organization for education. Most unit managers in health care organizations have a baccalaureate degree at most and few years of experience. Yet the expectations for management skills are those of someone with graduate education. This is particularly apparent with regard to financial decision making. To the authors' knowledge budgeting concepts are not taught in undergraduate nursing programs, yet it is often these undergraduates who in three to five years become the nurse manager of a unit.

For decentralization to work there must be a commitment from the organization to have unit-based managers who have the appropriate management skills, including financial management.

THE ROLE OF THE CFO AND OTHER FINANCIAL MANAGERS

The CFO is in charge of all the financial functions of the organization. As discussed in Chapter 1, the financial resources of cash and investments and their sources—loans, contributions, and retained profits—are the domain of the finance function. This includes those related to the sources and investment of the organization's financial resources. The generation of accounting information for external reports is the function of financial accounting. The generation of accounting information for use by the organization's own managers is the function of managerial accounting. Financial managers also must consider the organization's internal control system. The CFO is responsible for all these functions.

The Finance Function

All organizations, whether in the health care industry or not, must manage their financial resources. These resources include *cash, marketable investments,* and *accounts receivable.* Finance is also responsible for managing the sources of these resources, such as notes and accounts payable, loans, and payroll. The finance function includes making and maintaining relationships with banks and other sources of funds for the organization.

Cash must be managed. This includes safeguarding it against misappropriation, ensuring that cash resources are handled efficiently, and ensuring that the organization has sufficient cash for its needs. In the finance function, financial managers consider the timing of cash inflows and outflows from the organization. If it becomes apparent that there will be insufficient cash at times to meet the organization's needs, then arrangements must be made to get additional cash. This may require arranging for loans or pushing harder on fund-raising efforts.

Finance also actively works to maximize the benefit of accounts receivable. Accounts receivable are amounts owed to the organization for the care it has provided. Those amounts might be owed by individuals, insurance companies, or the government. Careful management is required to ensure that the organization collects all possible receivables in a timely manner. Eventually some receivables will prove to be uncollectible. All large organizations have some bad debts. Active management, however, can minimize bad debts. Active management can also result in receivables' being collected as quickly as possible. The sooner receivables are collected, the sooner the money is in the organization's bank accounts earning interest for it.

When money is collected for the patient care provided, it is either immediately spent or invested. Part of the finance function is to make decisions regarding appropriate investments. It requires care to determine how to invest the money so as to earn a high return for the organization, while safeguarding the money so that the risk of any investment is minimal. Health care organizations do not want to miss the chance to earn high returns on available cash, nor can they afford to lose their investment by taking excessive risks.

Finance officers also manage cash indirectly by managing the payment of the organization's obligations. In some cases, to keep cash invested (earning a return for the organization) the finance managers will defer payment of obligations for a period of time. A choice may be made to pay the telephone bill a month late. This choice must be balanced against the possible negative consequences of the action. The phone bill must not be paid so late that telephone service is discontinued; supplies bills must not be paid so late that suppliers stop providing needed clinical supplies to the organization.

If it becomes apparent that there will be insufficient cash to meet obligations, even with borrowing, fund-raising, and management of receivables and payables, then finance officers will raise the possibility of cost cutting throughout the organization. Such cost cutting cannot be authorized without the approval of the CEO. The CFO is not directly above the department managers in the chart of organization.

Therefore, decisions such as requiring cost cutting must be made by the CEO and COO. Ultimately, the CEO is responsible to the board. If the organization becomes bankrupt because of insufficient cash to pay obligations as due, that is the CEO's responsibility. On the other hand, if quality of patient care declines because of cost cutting aimed at saving cash, that is also the CEO's responsibility. As a result, the CEO will at times approve requests by the CFO to take actions that affect the departments providing care.

More often, the CEO will push to find other financing alternatives that do not impact on care. While most nurse managers become aware of efforts to cut costs to reduce cash expenses, they are not aware of the other efforts. Negotiations with banks to expand the amount they will lend, or with suppliers requesting that they allow deferred payments, are kept within the finance area. In most organizations, a wide variety of approaches will be assessed and attempted before cost cutting that might affect patient care is implemented.

In the final analysis, however, the finance department can only ensure the long-run existence of the organization if total spending is kept to a level that can be met by total receipts. Since even borrowing money requires cash payments (at least interest), the finance department's efforts to control the organization's sources and uses of money will ultimately impact on the operations of the clinical and administrative departments.

The Financial Accounting Function

The financial accounting function of the organization's finance department is very different from the finance function. Financial accounting has nothing to do with the decisions of whether to borrow money and, if so, how much and from where. Nor does it concern the efficient management of cash resources, accounts receivable, investments, or obligations of the organization. It is concerned with collecting information about the finances of the organization and translating that information into a form that can be reported to interested individuals outside the organization.

A wide range of individuals is interested in the finances of health care organizations. These include government regulators and payers, possible donors, suppliers, and lenders. A great deal of effort by the finance department is consumed by the various reporting requirements of different outside users.

The Managerial Accounting Function

Of particular interest to nurse managers is the managerial accounting function of the financial managers of the organization. This function relates to providing financial information that can be used to better manage the organization. This is a give-and-take process. Financial managers are often requesting financial information from nurse managers. However, managerial accounting should be a two-way street. Nurse managers need to learn how to get useful managerial accounting information from financial managers. Understanding the role of managerial accounting should help in that regard.

The first key element of managerial accounting is to aid in the general management role of planning. Planning is an essential role of management. The organization carries out much of its planning via the budgeting process. The financial managers are responsible for putting together an overall financial plan for the organization that achieves certain goals. Those goals may include growth, expansion of services, or just financial stability. From the perspective of the financial manager, the plans of all the departments must be aggregated to generate a plan for the organization that is workable.

Managerial accounting is also concerned with the role of management in the area of control. To implement a plan there must be a variety of control reports that managers use. These reports can ensure that suppliers only get paid for items actually delivered and that employees only get paid for an appropriate number of hours or days. The reports may focus on the spending of each department and each area of each department. From the perspective of the finance department, enough information is generated for control to allow the top management team to have the information it desires.

Other managers in the organization, however, have the right to request information in a form that is useful for their control needs. Nurse managers should place demands on accounting to provide information that is both timely and useful. Realize that information does not make decisions; managers do. But managers cannot take actions to control spending if they do not have information about what is happening. Therefore there should be a demand for all the information that is needed and for that information to be in a usable format.

Note that there is a stress on the usability of data. It is not simply an issue of there being too little information. Certainly, receiving too little information leaves managers without the ability to make informed decisions. However, too much information may obscure the relevant data needed to make an appropriate decision. Line managers must work with the finance department to specify what information is needed and what presentation would be most useful.

One of the most critical problems of management in health care organizations is that too often finance tells line managers what information they need and the format it will be provided in. There is a terrible lack of communication in most organizations. Line managers do not get the information they need, and staff feels abused because the information that they provide is not used. There should be a major effort to have periodic meetings between staff and line managers to discuss whether the information generated by staff meets the needs of the line managers and, if not, why not.

The Internal Control Function

The last major element of the financial management function relates to internal control. *Internal control* refers to the process and systems that ensure that decisions made in the organization are appropriate and receive appropriate authorization. This requires a system of accounting and administrative controls. According to noted accounting authorities,

> *Accounting control* comprises the methods and procedures that are mainly concerned with the authorization of transactions, the safeguarding of assets, and the accuracy of accounting records. Good accounting controls help *increase* efficiency; they help *decrease* waste, unintentional errors, and fraud.
>
> *Administrative control* comprises the plan of organization (for example, the formal organization chart concerning who reports to whom) and all methods and procedures that help management planning and control of operations. Examples are departmental budgeting procedures and performance reports.[3]

---

[3]Charles T. Horngren and George Foster, *Cost Accounting—A Managerial Emphasis*, 6th edition, Prentice-Hall, Englewood Cliffs, NJ, 1987, p. 910.

It is extremely important that health care organizations not waste any of their resources. Accounting controls must be able to minimize the chances that thefts will occur or that other errors will take place that will detract from the organization's resources. Fraud and embezzlement must of course be prevented to the extent possible. Therefore there must be a system of checks and balances that prevents the possibility of one person's withdrawing significant sums of money and misappropriating them. Generally, two signatures are needed for the disbursement of cash, so that there is less chance of theft.

Organizations can help minimize risks by following a few general rules:
♦ hiring qualified, reliable people
♦ creating a separation of functions that prevents the disbursement of cash based on authorization by one individual
♦ requiring authorization before disbursement of resources
♦ requiring documentation of all financial transactions
♦ establishing formal procedures
♦ creating physical protection, such as safes and locks
♦ enforcing vacation and rotation-of-duties policies that ensure that more than one person carries out each task related to money each year
♦ bonding employees (i.e., purchasing insurance policies to protect the organization against theft by the employee)
♦ providing for an independent check of financial transactions.

No organization can ever be guaranteed that it will not lose financial resources. However, it is the role of the financial managers of the organization to establish controls that minimize the possibility of such losses' occurring.

THE ROLE OF THE CNE IN FINANCIAL MANAGEMENT

In identifying the knowledge and skills required for nurse managers Mark, Turner, and Englebardt differentiate two levels.[4] They describe the nurse *executive* as the senior nurse responsible for managing nursing in the entire organization and the nurse *manager* as responsible for an area or program within the organization. We prefer the generic term nurse manager to refer to both and use the term CNE when referring to the nurse executive, while using mid-level or first-line manager when referring to those nurses who manage parts of the organization.

This section discusses the role of the CNE in the financial management of the organization and of the nursing division. As discussed earlier in this chapter, financial management includes the management of the financial resources of the organization. This includes not only cash and obligations but ultimately the expenses incurred by the organization and the revenue it generates. In almost all health care organizations the CNE has the authority and responsibility for the expenses incurred by the nursing department. In some health care organizations the CNE also has responsibility for the generation of revenues.

Responsibility for expenses means that the CNE is the person who is ultimately answerable for all expenses incurred by the department. The CNE is

[4]Barbara A. Mark, Jean T. Turner, and Sheila Englebardt, "Knowledge and Skills for Nurse Administrators," *Nursing and Health Care*, Vol. 11, No. 1, April, 1990, pp. 185–189.

directly involved in the negotiation process that establishes the level of re-sources that will be available for the department and is accountable for any spending above or below the planned level.

Responsibility is starting to extend to revenues as well. Few hospitals hold the CNE accountable for revenues. However, many other types of organizations, such as home health agencies, assign the CNE the authority and responsibility for both expenses incurred and revenues generated. For example, home health agencies are reimbursed on a per visit basis. The manager sets appropriate standards for visits per nurse and charges per visit and authorizes other expenses. In such cases he or she becomes accountable not only for the amount spent but also for the revenues.

In addition to their responsibility for nursing, many hospital CNEs, often those with the title vice-president for patient services, are responsible for non-nursing departments. These often include the emergency room and the operating room and sometimes departments such as social work or other professional services. In many home health agencies the CNE is responsible for all services provided by the agency. In many organizations the CNE is responsible for new product development, such as an outreach program to the elderly or development of ambulatory surgery.

As a member of the senior management team the CNE must have the financial skills of equivalent senior managers. The CNE should have a thorough grounding in applied economics, be familiar with basic accounting principles, and have the skills to analyze financial statements. In addition to these basic skills, the CNE must be highly competent in cost management. To do this the manager must understand how to determine the cost of nursing services. To effectively manage costs it is necessary for the CNE to be effective at strategic planning and controlling operating results.

As a member of the senior management team the CNE must understand the management of the financial resources of the organization. This includes working-capital management and sources of financial resources. All but the smallest health care organizations have financial officers. CNEs need not be financial officers; however, they must understand financial management enough to ask the right questions, comprehend the answers, and participate in senior management decisions about financial management.

THE ROLE OF MID-LEVEL NURSE MANAGERS IN FINANCIAL MANAGEMENT

The authority and responsibility of mid-level nurse managers (e.g., clinical assistant director of nursing, supervisor) varies widely from one health care organization to another. In small nursing agencies, the mid-level nurse manager is responsible for costs and revenue. The manager of eight public health nurses in a home health agency may be responsible not only for personnel and related expenses but also for the amount of revenue generated by the staff. In most hospitals, however, the mid-level nurse managers are responsible only for direct expenses in their area. A recent study indicates that 56% of hospitals have decentralized budgeting to the head nurse at the unit level.[5]

---

[5]Gayle N. Poteet, Linda C. Hodges, and Nanette Goddard, "Financial Responsibilities and Preparation of Chief Nurse Executives," *Nursing Economics*, Vol. 9, No. 5, Sept./Oct., 1991, pp. 305–309.

The level of decentralization will determine the knowledge and skills needed by mid-level and first-line nurse managers. It is clear that first-line nurse managers require budgeting skills. While these managers do not require all the knowledge and skills of the CNE, they should be familiar with most of the concepts.

In preparation for writing this book, the authors interviewed a number of CNEs, mid-level, and first-line managers. Those we spoke with differentiated the depth of knowledge required among levels of nurse managers more than they differentiated among content areas. Most of those we spoke with agreed that in addition to budgeting, the mid-level managers must have basic knowledge about applied economics and the financing of health care. In addition, they should understand cost management, including the basic principles of determining the cost of nursing care. Mid-level managers should have skills in both strategic planning and forecasting. Most of those we interviewed believed that mid-level and first-line managers needed skills in inventory control at the level for which they were responsible but did not need skills in managing other short- or long-term financial resources. They did not think this group needed to be able to read a financial statement. All agreed that the level of skills required depends on the type of organization and level of decentralization of the organization.

For example, many mid-level managers should have skills in securing grants for demonstration projects, research, or ongoing financial needs, while most mid-level managers would not need to understand corporate stock issuance or bond ratings.

To competently manage the unit or program, nurse managers need financial skills for planning, control, and decision making. Using forecasting skills they can estimate services to be delivered in the future and likely labor and supplies needed to provide the services (or evaluate the forecasts provided by other parts of the organization). With this information and solid budgeting skills they can prepare a budget and, more important, interpret the variance reports either created by themselves or supplied centrally.

INTERACTIONS BETWEEN FISCAL AND NURSE MANAGERS

As discussed above, nurse managers have lateral relationships with fiscal managers. As the CNEs in many organizations assume a role as part of the top management team, they become peers of the fiscal officers. At all levels of the organization, however, nurse managers have no formal authority to require information or services. Although the CEO may require that fiscal managers provide information to nurse managers, often the format is not presented in a way that is useful to nurse managers. Therefore a collegial relationship between nursing and finance is essential.

Relationships between fiscal departments and nursing are strained in some organizations. Many fiscal officers continue to believe that nurse managers do not need a substantial amount of financial management information. People in the fiscal department may feel threatened when nurse managers ask questions. One CNE told us that when she pointed out systematic inaccuracies in the data she was receiving from the fiscal department, the CFO became hostile. She eventually was fired, in part because she was raising questions that were uncomfortable.

A substantial amount of team building, informal communication, and networking is necessary for nurse managers and fiscal departments to generate and use financial information that is useful for the organization. It is up to both nursing and finance to work in a cooperative manner. In some cases nursing may have to invest in the nursing/finance relationship for a while before dividends start to be received. Nevertheless, establishing a good working relationship with the people who work in finance can be worth the investment.

RESPONSIBILITY ACCOUNTING

The previous sections have focused on the role of financial managers, the role of nurse managers, and their interactions. There has been a presumption that all managers attempt to the best of their abilities to carry out their activities in the best interests of the organization. The organization, however, needs a way to assess the performance of its managers. That is the role of responsibility accounting. *Responsibility accounting* is an attempt to measure financial outcomes and to assign those outcomes to the individual or department responsible for them. In that way, performance can be assessed.

It is important to note that the performance of a manager is not necessarily the same as the performance of a unit or department. The distinction is primarily concerned with the issue of ability to control outcomes. The philosophy of responsibility accounting is that managers should be held accountable for things that they can control and should not be held accountable for things that are beyond their control. Therefore, there should always be an attempt to evaluate a unit or department's performance separately from its manager.

For instance, top management may be concerned that the cost of providing care exceeded expectations because an unexpected shortage of nurses resulted in the use of additional overtime and high-cost per diem agency nurses. In that case, the performance of the nursing units will likely be below expectations. On the other hand, the unit managers should be evaluated on how well they managed the situation. In light of the shortage of nurses, did they make economical choices about when to use overtime, when to hire per diem agency nurses, and when to leave a position unfilled for a shift?

Nurses should always bear this principle in mind, both in their interactions within the nursing department and between the nursing department and the remainder of the organization. Managers should only be held accountable for the things that they can control. Without implementation of such a philosophy managers develop a pervasive negative attitude. When they are considered to have failed because of causes beyond their control, they lose all incentive to attempt to be efficient in the use of resources that are within their control. Why work hard when you will fail no matter what you do?

Managers must also believe that they will be evaluated in a fair manner. In essence, they must trust that the system will generate a fair evaluation of their performance. The performance evaluation of managers in most health care organizations centers on the use of responsibility centers.

Responsibility Centers

A *responsibility center* is a part of the organization, such as a department or a unit, for which a manager is assigned responsibility. There are three general categories of responsibility centers: cost, revenue, and profit.

A cost center has responsibility only for the control of expenses. Most nursing units are cost centers. This makes sense given the basic concept of responsibility equal to control. The typical first-line nurse manager cannot exercise any control over revenues. This manager does not generate patients, nor is that position responsible for the prices charged to patients. Therefore it is logical to hold that individual accountable only for expenses.

Units that are solely revenue centers are rare. That would imply that they can control revenues but have no control over expenses. Usually marketing departments are considered revenue centers because the organization wants to see specifically how much revenue the marketing effort is generating.

The most common alternative to a unit that is a cost center is a profit center. A profit center is responsible for both revenues and costs. Therefore it is both a cost center and a revenue center. It is responsible for the expenses it incurs as well as the revenues it generates. Most hospital operating rooms are profit centers. However, hospital terminology differs from that used in most industries. The hospital industry, traditionally not-for-profit, prefers to avoid use of the term profit and therefore to avoid use of the term profit center. It has become the practice in health care organizations to use the term *revenue center* to refer to all responsibility units that are both revenue centers and cost centers.

One weakness of hospital management has been its perception of the results of cost centers and revenue centers. Resources have often been more tightly constrained for cost centers than for revenue centers. The reason for this is that cost centers at the end of a year showed a large balance of expense without any counterbalancing revenue. Revenue centers, on the other hand, showed revenue and expense. Many revenue centers show profits. Those profits have been used as a justification for more liberal allocation of resources to those departments. Similarly, managers of revenue centers have at times been perceived as being better managers. This has worked unfairly against nursing departments, which are cost centers.

That approach tends to be somewhat irrational. Expenses are not inherently bad and do not indicate poor management. Patient care cannot be provided without incurring expenses, and there would be no revenue at all without incurring the expenses of departments such as nursing. On the other hand, the existence of profits does not necessarily indicate good management. Evaluations of managers should be based on a standard of comparison. That standard is generally the budget. Both cost and revenue centers should be evaluated against the budgeted amount to assess the performance of the manager.

Even this approach is somewhat simplistic. The budget is based on an expectation of what will happen. If patient volume increases, then expectations need to be adjusted. More patients result in more revenues but more expenses as well. Managers must be evaluated in comparison to the budget after it has been adjusted for patient volume and, if possible, patient acuity. The ultimate goal is to evaluate the contribution of the manager, apart from the factors that are outside the manager's control. That is the only way that managers will perceive that the organizational structure is fair. Fairness is a necessary perception to get the maximum effort from managers.

INCENTIVES AND MOTIVATION

The issue of fairness in the evaluation of managers raises the entire question of goals and attitudes. Organizations are made up of people, as much as they are made up of buildings and equipment, if not more so. Individuals, however, have their own interests as persons as well as employees. It is possible that their own interests will conflict with those of the organization that employs them. In that case it is vital to attempt to achieve goal congruence. *Goal congruence* simply means that the wants and desires of the organization and its employees are consistent. Organizations develop a set of incentives for their employees. The goal of those incentives is to encourage employees to work toward achieving the organization's goals.

Large organizations tend to have many layers of management. Each manager in each layer must work constantly to achieve the goals of the organization to have the most effective results. However, there is reason to believe that in most organizations, managers may have reason not to work in the best interests of the organization. This is because what is in the best interests of the organization may not be in the best interests of the individual manager.

Most nurses entered the profession out of a desire to help people and to serve. They did not expect to get rich from being a nurse. Nevertheless, an individual manager may want a big salary, a large office with fancy furniture, and a large staff. The organization would prefer for the manager to work on a low salary in a small office with old furniture and a minimally sized staff. Individuals are not bad because they would prefer more money and more perquisites. The organization is not bad because it wants to conserve its resources so it can use them to provide more patient care. Yet there must be some meeting of the minds or there will be a constant tension between the wishes of the individuals and the wishes of the organization.

Goal congruence is the meeting of the minds. It is achieved in most cases through a system of incentives. The organization must put forth a system of incentives that makes it worthwhile for the individual to do what is in the interests of the organization. First-line nurse managers must find a way to provide incentives to the nursing staff. Mid-level nurse managers must find incentives for first-line nurse managers. Associate directors of nursing must find incentives for mid-level managers. CNEs must find incentives for the associate and assistant directors of nursing.

Incentives can be provided in a variety of ways. Some organizations use bonuses. Others use merit pay increases. Another approach is to provide managers with a letter from their supervisor discussing budget performance. Often simple, explicit recognition of a manager's hard work to achieve the organization's goals is a sufficient motivating tool to gain the benefits of goal congruence. The question of incentives and motivation is discussed further in Chapter 13.

POWER AND POLITICS

Power, authority, and influence have no standard definitions. Several authors have noted that "influence is the process by which one person follows another's advice, suggestion, or order; power is a personal or positional attribute that enables one to influence; and authority is only one of several bases of power—one granted to an influencer-manager by higher organizational officials."[6] These authors suggest that power can take many forms and suggest six:

♦ Coercive power is based on fear of punishment.
♦ Reward power is based on hope for reward.
♦ Legitimate power is based on the belief that the influencer has formal authority.
♦ Referent power is based on the charismatic leader traits.
♦ Expert power is based on the leader's special expertise.
♦ Finally, representative power is based on the democratic delegation of power to a leader.

It is postulated that referent and expert power are most important for managers of professionals. That is, the managers of professionals will be most effective in influencing if they are charismatic leaders and are seen as experts by others.[7]

Access to information and resources in health care organizations can serve as a base for power development. Because health care organizations are often large and complex, it is difficult to have all the information required to make many decisions. Thus, those who control the information are in a position to be powerful and to influence decision making.

Control of financial information by "administration" and the power associated with it has been seen by many as a reason for the level of nurses' influence in the organization. While the cynic might argue this control has been intentional, other would argue that many nurses have not sought this information. As nurses understand financial management and gain access to and develop financial information, their ability to influence decision making may improve.

NETWORKING

Because managers are often dependent on others over whom they have no authority, the use of power is critical to the effective manager. Effective managers develop relationships with people in the organization whom they depend on for information and with whom they build coalitions to influence the goals and resource allocation of the organization.

Networking was the buzz word of the 1980s. "I'm going to a networking event," "I'm networking at lunch today" was heard in health organizations. Networks have been described as horizontal as well as vertical. For most managers lateral relationships are often more important than vertical relationships in achieving goals. For example, for the unit manager in a hospital, resources

---

[6]David R. Hampton, Charles E. Summer, and Ross A. Webber, *Organizational Behavior and the Practice of Management*. Glenview, IL, Scott, Foresman, & Company, 1987, p. 150.
[7]Ibid.

required from dietary and housekeeping are critical to running the unit. Typically the nurse manager has no direct authority over the housekeepers and dietary aides who perform activities on the unit. Nurse managers must therefore rely on their lateral supervisors, peers, and subordinates to effectively achieve the unit's goals.

Numerous articles have appeared in the nursing literature about networking, what it is, how to do it, and blessing it as a strategy. It is also argued that trade is the basis of networking. Managers trade information and services. They trade the ability to get things done. Effective managers work on building relationships with others, so that when they need something (information, services) they can get it. This occurs both within and outside the organization.

IMPLICATIONS FOR NURSE MANAGERS

As discussed above, the control of information about both revenues and expenses is the key to financial control. In organizations where this information is not shared, control is not possible. A second factor is responsibility and authority for revenues in addition to the responsibility for expenses. Efforts on the part of both fiscal managers and nurse managers to share information and cooperate are necessary for successfully managing an organization.

KEY CONCEPTS

Management's role   Most essential elements are planning, control, and decision making.

Board of trustees or board of directors   Governing body that has the ultimate responsibility for the decisions made by the organization. The board sets the overall direction and adopts goals and objectives for the organization. The chief executive officer reports to the board and is responsible for managing the organization.

Managerial hierarchy   Structure that establishes the authority and responsibility of different individuals within the organization. The board is at the top, with the CEO reporting to the board. The COO reports to the CEO. The CFO and CNE may report to either the CEO or COO, depending on the specific organization. The COO, CFO, and CNE each have a number of managers who report directly to them.

Line and staff functions   Line function is the element of running a health care organization that is related directly to the provision of patient care. Nurse managers are considered line managers. In contrast, the staff function concerns providing auxiliary assistance or service to the line managers and their departments. Finance officers are staff managers.

Lines of authority   Formal lines of authority may be either direct (full authority) such as the associate director of nursing reporting to the CNE, or indirect (limited authority) such as the director of dietary reporting to the chief of the medical staff. Informal lines of authority carry no official authority but may have a substantial de facto impact.

Chief financial officer (CFO)   In charge of all the financial functions of the organization. These include those related to the sources and investment of the organization's financial resources, the generation of accounting information for making external reports, and the generation of accounting information for use by line managers. It also includes the function of internal control.

Chief nurse executive (CNE)   In charge of all nursing functions in the organization. This primarily includes all nursing care provided to clients. Other responsibilities include managing the human and financial resources of the nursing department to achieve the health care mission of the department.

Mid-level nurse manager   Responsible for nursing functions on more than one nursing unit or area. This includes all nursing care provided to clients. Other responsibilities include managing the human resources for the manager's area of responsibility. Responsibilities usually include financial management.

First-line manager   Responsible for one patient care unit, area, or group of nursing staff. This includes all nursing care provided to clients. Other responsibilities may include some financial management.

Responsibility accounting   Attempt to measure financial outcomes and assign those outcomes to the individual or department responsible for them. The performance of a manager is not necessarily the same as the performance of a unit or department. Managers should be held accountable only for things that they can control.

Responsibility center   Part of the organization, such as a department or a unit, for which a manager is assigned responsibility. Health care organization responsibility centers are generally divided into cost centers and revenue centers.

Power   "A personal or positional attribute that enables one to influence."[8] Access to information and resources in health care organizations can serve as a base for power development. Thus those who control the information are in a position to be powerful and influence decision making. Control of financial information is sometimes used to influence decisions.

Networking   Effective managers develop relationships with people in the organization on whom they depend for information and with whom they build coalitions to influence the goals and resource allocation of the organization. The relationships are often made informally through a shared history (e.g., attending school together) or through a shared professional experience (e.g., participation in professional association activities). Trade is often the basis of networking. A person with information or services such as financial information may trade that information for something such as a prompt reply when a request is made.

---

[8]David R. Hampton, Charles E. Summer, and Ross A. Webber, *Organizational Behavior and the Practice of Management*, Glenview, IL, Scott, Foresman, and Company, 1987, p. 150.

SUGGESTED READINGS ❖

Anthony, Robert N., and David Young, *Management Control in Nonprofit Organizations*, 4th edition, Richard D. Irwin, Inc., Homewood, IL, 1988.

Berman, Howard J., Lewis E. Weeks, and Steven F. Kukla, *The Financial Management of Hospitals*, 7th edition, Health Administration Press, Ann Arbor, MI, 1990.

Blaney, Doris R., and Charles J. Hobson, "Developing Financial Management Skills: An Educational Approach," *Journal of Nursing Administration*, June 1988, Vol. 18, No. 6, pp. 13–17.

Botsford, J., "The Successful Managers: Using Knowledge and Savvy in Financial Management," *AORN Journal*, August 1988, Vol. 48, No. 2, pp. 290–294.

Brooten, Dorothy A., *Managerial Leadership in Nursing*, J.B. Lippincott Company, Philadelphia, 1984.

Dominiak, Geraldine F., and Joseph G. Louderback, *Managerial Accounting*, 5th edition, PWS-Kent Publishing Co., Boston, 1988.

Fields, Willa L., "Mentoring in Nursing: A Historical Approach," *Nursing Outlook*, Vol. 39, No. 6, November/December 1991, pp. 257–261.

Flarey, Dominick, "The Nurse Executive and the Governing Board: Synergy for a New Era," *Journal of Nursing Administration*, Vol. 21, No. 12, pp. 11–17.

Gitman, Lawrence, *Principles of Managerial Finance*, Harper Collins Publishers, New York, 1990.

Hampton, David R., Charles E. Summer, and Ross A. Webber, *Organizational Behavior and the Practice of Management*, Scott, Foresman and Company, Glenview, IL, 1987.

Hansen, Donald B., *Management Accounting*, PWS-Kent Publishing Co., Boston, 1990.

Johnson, M.S., "Preparing Nurse Executives for Financial Management," *Nursing Administration Quarterly*, Fall 1987, Vol. 12, No. 1, pp. 67–73.

Kersey, James H., Jr., "Responsibility Accounting: Making Decisions Efficiently," *Nursing Management*, May 1985, Vol. 16, No. 5, pp. 14–17.

Kersey, James H., Jr., "Increasing the Nursing Manager's Fiscal Responsibility," *Nursing Management*, Vol. 19, No. 10, October 1988, pp. 30–32.

Peters, Tom, *Thriving on Chaos*, Alfred A. Knopf, New York, 1987.

Stevens, Barbara J., "What Is the Executive's Role In Budgeting for Her Department?" *Journal of Nursing Administration*, Vol. 11, No. 7, July 1981, pp. 22–24.

Vergara, Gail, H., and Joan Bourke, "Reward Employees, Achieve Goals with Incentive Compensation," *Healthcare Financial Management*, Vol. 39, No. 8, August 1985, pp. 50–52.

Williams, Frank, "Employee Incentive Systems," in *Handbook of Health Care Accounting and Finance*, Vol. I, William O. Cleverley (ed.), Aspen Systems, Rockville, MD, 1982, pp. 395–412.

4

Key Issues in Applied Economics

CHAPTER GOALS

The goals of this chapter are to:

♦ Introduce applied economics and discuss the notion of scarce resources

♦ Define economic goods and services and the role of utility in determining the demand for goods and services

♦ Explain the law of supply and demand and the functioning of free markets

♦ Define the concept of elasticity of demand

♦ Define and explain economies of scale

♦ Consider the role of incentives in economic behavior

♦ Discuss market efficiency and market failure

♦ Distinguish between redistribution of resources to improve economic efficiency versus redistribution for improved equity

♦ Explain the economic view of the market for nurses and periodic nursing shortages

♦ Discuss the implications of economics for nurse managers

INTRODUCTION

Economics is the study of how scarce resources are allocated among their possible uses. The resources available to health care have been growing. Each year a substantially greater amount of money is spent on health care services. However, the competing uses for those resources have been growing even faster.

67

Costly new drugs and technologies strain the capacity of society to pay the costs of health care. The nursing shortage, which began in the mid to late 1980s, led to substantial increases in nursing salaries, further increasing the cost of health care services. Americans have been consuming both more care and more expensive care. Maintaining and improving the quality of health services costs an ever-increasing amount, even if the care is provided in a totally efficient manner.

At the same time, the growing federal government deficits of the 1980s and 1990s and the recession that began in 1990 placed ever-increasing pressures on federal and state governments to restrict the amount of money they spent on health care services. Since Medicare and Medicaid constitute a substantial portion of all health care payments, such efforts to restrict costs have a dramatic role in shaping health care in our society. A knowledge of economics will help the nurse manager understand the rationale behind government programs and regulations.

How are the pressures to increase spending reconciled with the constraints to control spending? Fundamentally that is a question of applied economics, the topic of this chapter. As a management or policy tool, economics is used to help individuals, organizations, and society make optimal use of their limited resources.

The tools of economics are developed from a structure built upon the analysis of the behavior of individuals and organizations. Building upon that analysis this chapter discusses how the law of supply and demand governs how a free market operates. The specific prices charged for products are based on the cost of producing the product. Another important pricing factor is how strongly consumers react to changes in prices. These concepts are discussed in this chapter. Next the chapter focuses on the role of incentives. Individual behavior is often reactive. Therefore, it is possible for an organization or the government to generate desired behavior by creating appropriate incentives.

After the discussion of incentives, the chapter concentrates on issues of market efficiency in the provision of health care services. The basic notions of market efficiency and of redistribution of society's scarce resources are first discussed, then a variety of issues related to the failure of the free market are explored.

The chapter concludes with a discussion of how economists might view the reasons for periodic nursing shortages and of the implications of applied economics for nurse managers.

FUNDAMENTAL CONCEPTS OF ECONOMICS

Economics is the study of the allocation of scarce resources among alternative possible uses. Included in such study are the actions and behaviors of patients, insurance companies, providers of health care services, and the government. Given the limited nature of resources, efficient use of resources is desired. By studying behavior, economists are able to attempt to ensure that resources are used in an optimal manner.

Economic Goods

Consumers purchase *goods or services* provided by suppliers. These goods or services are referred to as economic goods. Goods and services are any items that consumers wish to acquire or to use. Such goods and services provide a benefit to the consumer. Consumers generally acquire goods and services through an exchange. While it is possible to *barter* or exchange some goods or services for other goods or services, most exchanges are facilitated by the use of money. Each good or service has a price in money.

Consumers have a combination of wealth and income available to make purchases. *Wealth* is the value of all of the resources the consumer currently owns. *Income* is the increase in wealth, or the amount of additional resources the consumer gains over a period of time. Additional dollars of income may come either from working or from profits on investments. The wealth and income of all consumers is limited. No one can afford to buy everything. Therefore consumers make choices among the things they purchase.

Utility

When consumers purchase goods and services, they gain a benefit from them. The benefit may be physical. For example, without food and water one would die. There is a clear physical benefit from acquiring enough food and water to survive. Other benefits are psychic. Chocolate may be perceived by some to be a pleasurable food. It is not required for subsistence, but it may well be desired. Economists refer to the physical and psychic benefit one receives from goods or services as the *utility* of those items. The more benefit received, the greater the utility.

Utility helps determine how much an individual would be willing to pay to acquire a good or service. Suppose that the price of water is 10¢ a glass. Water is needed for survival, so its utility to the consumer may well exceed 10¢ by a substantial amount. If the utility exceeds the price, then the consumer will buy the water at the ten cent price.

Suppose that the price of chocolate were $1 per bar. One person may not be wild about chocolate. Given the limitation of that person's total wealth and income, a chocolate bar may have utility that makes the chocolate's value only 50¢. That person would not buy the bar for $1. Other people may get such high psychic benefit from chocolate that they would be willing to pay up to $5 a bar. Some people would buy chocolate for $1. Not everyone receives the same utility from a specific good or service. In other words, the value of different goods and services is different to different people.

The more income an individual has, the more he or she can buy. However, income can also take a nondollar form. Each year individuals receive a dollar salary from their job, and they also gain some leisure time. That leisure time is itself a form of income. Leisure represents an economic good. It can be consumed. Or, like other economic goods, leisure time can be exchanged. A nurse may choose (in some cases) to work more overtime to make more money. In that case the nurse has decided that there is something that can be purchased with the extra money earned that is worth more than the extra eight hours is worth as leisure time. The additional utility of the extra dollars exceeds the utility of the leisure time.

It is assumed that rational individuals will act so as to maximize their total utility. To maximize total utility, a mix of goods must be consumed so that the last unit of each type of item consumed yields the same marginal utility per dollar spent. This accomplishes the purchase of a set of goods and services that, in aggregate, provides the most benefit.

Marginal Utility

As an individual makes purchases, actions are taken as if the *marginal utility* (or *marginal benefit*) of each additional purchase is evaluated. The marginal benefit represents the additional benefit or utility gained from a purchase of one more unit of a particular item. A person may have a very high marginal utility for one glass of water. However, a second glass of water is not worth quite so much. The twentieth glass of water on a given day may not have much additional utility at all.

How much water is the individual likely to consume? The consumer will select a set of goods and services so that the last unit of each yields the same marginal benefit per dollar spent. By doing this, total utility will be maximized. Any other combination of goods and services would mean that some money was spent on items that provided less utility per dollar than could have been obtained from another item.

Not all individuals have the same marginal utility values. If we were evaluating chocolate, some individuals would value the first piece more highly than others would. The same is true for the second, tenth, and hundredth piece. This is true for any good. However, by aggregating information about the marginal benefit or utility for all individuals, we can develop information about the overall demand for the good or service.

Marginal Cost

Economists call the price paid for the good or service the *marginal cost*. It tells what it costs the consumer to purchase one more unit of that item. As a result of the argument just presented about utility, economists conclude that any consumer can maximize utility by setting the marginal benefit of purchases equal to the marginal cost. That is, one purchases units of each good or service until the marginal benefit of another unit is just equal to the marginal cost.

This is also a useful concept for suppliers. They will make a profit when the price they charge exceeds the cost of making the good or providing the service. Therefore we would not expect to see a service sold at less than the marginal cost of the resources needed to produce it. Pricing based on marginal costs is discussed further in Chapter 7.

Savings

What if the consumer has made a series of purchases but feels that the benefit from an additional purchase of any item is not worth the price charged, even though there is still some money left over? In that case, the individual receives more benefit from saving money than from spending it. Many individuals reach a point where the utility of saving money exceeds the utility of additional expenditures. What benefits can be realized from saving money? Several examples of the benefits individuals have from saving as opposed to direct consumption are protection against future unemployment, creation of a pool of money for a future vacation or retirement, and accumulaton of money for a child's college education.

SUPPLY AND DEMAND
Free Enterprise

Economics is governed by the law of supply and demand. *Supply* is the amount of good or service that all suppliers in aggregate would like to provide for any given price. *Demand* is the amount of the good or service that consumers would be willing to acquire at any given price. The United States economy is based on a system of free enterprise or capitalism. In such a system any individual can choose whether to invest wealth or capital in a business venture. That venture provides goods and services to the public. Workers can choose whether to work for that venture at the wages offered. Consumers can choose whether to buy the products of the venture at the seller's price. The central theme of the system is freedom of choice.

In theory such a system would also result in an optimal use of society's scarce resources. Supply and demand are automatically equated by a process known as the *market mechanism.* Suppose that there are consumers who would like to purchase a product and suppliers who would like to sell that product. That represents the basis for there to be a *market* for that product. A *free market* (the basis for the capitalistic system) is simply a situation where sellers are free to charge whatever price they would like for their product, and buyers are free to purchase or not purchase at the price sellers are charging. Exchange may take place if the buyers and the sellers reach a mutually agreeable price.

In a free market system, suppliers compete with each other for the inputs—labor, materials, and capital—and to sell their outputs. Competition may take a number of forms. One hospital might compete for nurses by offering them better working conditions. Another might offer more holidays and vacations. One hospital might compete for patients by emphasizing quality of care. Another might stress the convenience of using their facilities. Throughout the economy, the most widely used basis of competition is price. Higher wages are paid to attract employees, and lower prices are charged to attract customers.

In practice, free markets do not always exist, and unregulated competition does not always result in an optimal use of society's scarce resources. If prices are not set by the results of active competition, but instead by an individual seller or buyer or by a regulator such as the government, then the market is not a free market. Buyers may still have the option of buying at the stated price. But sellers are not free to set whatever price they choose. This chapter will discuss market failure and regulatory intervention at greater length later.

An Example of Supply and Demand

For simplicity, consider a health care product for which there is clearly a free market: toothpaste. This preventive health care item fits all the various requirements for a free market. It is widely available, there are a number of competitors, and consumers have a fair degree of choice in whether to make a purchase. Suppose that the suppliers of toothpaste were to charge $5 per tube. At a price that high, many companies would be willing to supply toothpaste because there would be substantial profits. However, very few people would want toothpaste so badly that they would be willing to pay the price. Some people might, but not many. Suppliers would be trying to sell more toothpaste than people are willing to buy.

Suppose that there is a total demand of 100 tubes of toothpaste at the $5 price, but there are ten suppliers who would each like to sell 100 tubes. Obviously, they cannot each sell 100 tubes. They could each sell ten tubes, but at that low volume the costs of setting up for production would be so high that it would not be worthwhile. An *equilibrium* is a situation in which the quantity of a good or service offered at the stated price is the same as the quantity that buyers want to purchase at that price. An equilibrium is a stable situation. Buyers and sellers are in agreement, and prices fluctuate little, if at all. If supply and demand are not equal at a given price, then the market is in a *disequilibrium* condition. When there is a disequilibrium, as there is in this toothpaste example, there is pressure to either raise or lower the price until an equilibrium is achieved.

One supplier will undoubtedly cut its price in an effort to corner the market. Other suppliers will follow suit or else choose not to produce that product.[1] Eventually a point is reached where the quantity buyers demand at a given price is the same as the supply at that price, in a fully functioning free market.

The amount of any item that a given consumer wants does depend on the price of that item. However, it depends on other factors as well. The utility of water is much higher if that is the only liquid available than it would be if the consumer also had a choice of milk, wine, and soft drinks. Such other items are referred to as *substitutes*. The demand of an individual for a specific good or service is also determined in light of the amount of wealth and income a consumer has, and the specific preferences of the individual. The aggregate demand for a good or service depends on how these factors impact on all consumers.

Suppose that the price offered by toothpaste suppliers dropped to $3. At that lower price, more people are willing to buy toothpaste. Assume the quantity demanded at that price is 420 tubes. The suppliers lowered the price in an effort to compete for the original demand for 100 tubes. At the lower price the number of tubes demanded has increased. On the other hand, at a price of $3, the profits per tube are not as great. Some suppliers will leave the industry. At that lower price suppliers only want to sell 600 tubes rather than 1,000. But 600 tubes offered at that price is still greater than the 420 tubes demanded at that price. The market is not yet in equilibrium.

Price will fall further. At a price of $2.50 buyers want to buy 500 tubes, and sellers want to offer 500 tubes. The demand and supply are now the same, and they are in equilibrium. It is possible to draw a graph that estimates how many tubes of toothpaste would be demanded by consumers for any given price. The *demand curve*, D, indicates the quantity of toothpaste (horizontal axis) that would be desired by consumers for any given price (vertical axis). Similarly, the *supply curve*, S, indicates the quantity that would be offered by suppliers at any given price. Figure 4–1 presents both the demand and supply curves on one graph. Equilibrium is achieved when the demand and supply curves intersect. Only at that point is there a price that generates exactly the same

---

[1]Note that if a supplier does not match the lower price other suppliers offer, then no one will buy from that supplier in a fully functioning free market. Why pay more for exactly the same item? Examples of multiple prices do exist, however. For instance, convenience stores charge higher prices but do not go out of business. This is because the products offered are not identical. In addition to toothpaste, the convenience store is also offering convenience.

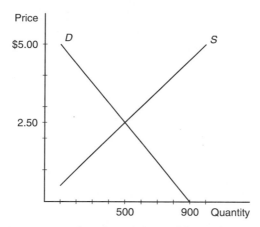

Figure 4–1. Supply and demand for toothpaste.

amount of demand and supply. What is the total dollar size of the toothpaste industry? In equilibrium, there are a total of 500 tubes sold at $2.50 per tube. Therefore, multiplying the quantity times the price, we find that the industry generates $1,250 of charges or revenue.

Note that there is some unfilled demand, even at the equilibrium. The demand curve continues to a volume of 900 tubes. That means that the consumers could use 900 tubes. But what is the price at 900 tubes? It is zero. The demand would only be that high if the product were offered for free.

ELASTICITY OF DEMAND

In the above toothpaste example, the quantity demanded rose steadily as the price fell. It is a general assumption of economics that demand and price are *inversely* related. That is, as price goes down, the quantity demanded rises, or as price rises, the quantity demanded declines. However, an open question is how much more will be demanded as the price declines. Suppliers find this to be a very interesting question. Are profits likely to rise more if prices are raised, or lowered? How responsive is a change in demand to a change in price?

The obvious solution is to look at the supply and demand curves and determine how much would be demanded at any given price. However, the specific demand curve for each product, such as that seen in Figure 4–1, is not generally known. Economists draw the diagrams such as those as an analytical tool, to study what would happen if a certain pattern of demand existed. Measurement of demand is much more difficult to accomplish. Generally demand curves are estimated based on a combination of available evidence and suppositions or assumptions.

On the basis of such estimates, economists attempt to determine whether demand is elastic or inelastic. *Elastic* demand is a situation in which an increase or decrease in price results in a proportionately greater change in demand. *Inelastic* demand is a situation in which a decrease in price results in a proportionately smaller decrease in demand.

Suppose that a product's price were cut by 10%. If the increase in demand is more than 10%, the demand is said to be elastic. The more the quantity demanded increases, the more elastic the demand is. Similarly, if the price of the product were increased by 10% and the quantity demanded fell by more than 10%, the demand would be considered elastic.

If the quantity demanded were to rise by very little in response to a decline in price, it would hardly be worthwhile for the supplier to cut the price. All customers would get the lower price, but the supplier would get very few new customers. On the other hand, if demand were very elastic, a small price cut would result in a large number of additional customers. In that case the price cut might be worthwhile.

Certain types of health care services have generally been considered to be very inelastic. When consumers are sick, they want medical care. They tend to be not very sensitive to the price. For example, if a consumer needs a visiting nurse to come to the house, the difference in charge between $40 and $44 may not affect demand substantially.

Suppose that a for-profit home health agency wished to increase its profits. Currently the average cost to the agency to provide each visit is $38, and the average price charged per visit is $40. The agency provides 1,000 visits per month and makes a profit of $2,000 per month ($40 price less $38 cost equals a profit of $2 per visit, times 1,000 visits equals a profit of $2,000).

What would happen if the price were raised by 10%, to $44? If the demand is inelastic, the number of visits might fall by only 5%. In the case the agency would only have 950 visits (a 5% decrease in volume), but the price for each one would be $44 (a 10% rise in price). The profit of $6 per visit ($44 price less $38 cost) for 950 visits would be far greater than the profit of $2 per visit for 1,000 visits.

On the other hand, suppose that there is a competing visiting nurse association that charges only $40 for a similar service. In that case, the demand for the for-profit agency's services might be highly elastic. The 10% price increase could result in a 90% decrease in the quantity demanded. The profit of $6 per visit on 100 visits would not be as good as the profit of $2 per visit on 1,000 visits. Elasticity of demand depends not only on how essential the good or service is but also on the existence of competition in the marketplace.

ECONOMIES OF SCALE

A critical concept in health economics is *economies of scale*. Many decisions nurse managers make require a knowledge of the cost per patient. However, that cost is not constant. The cost per patient varies due to economies of scale. Economies of scale refer to changes in the cost per patient as the number of patients changes. Having more patients is referred to as a larger scale of operations.

All organizations tend to have some costs that are *fixed* and some that are *variable*. The fixed costs stay the same as the volume of patients increases. For example, rent on a nursing home building remains the same regardless of whether the nursing home is half, three-quarters, or 100% full. Variable costs increase as the quantity of patients increases. When one considers all the costs of providing care, the cost per patient decreases as the number of patients goes up. This is because there are more patients to share the fixed costs.

Increasing Returns to Scale

Suppose that the fixed costs for a nursing home include rent, heat, and the salary of the administrator, for a total of $100,000 per month. Variable costs include nursing staff, medications, and dietary, for a total of $70 per patient day (PD). If there are 2,000 patient days a month, the cost per patient day is $120, as follows:

Total Fixed Cost:	$100,000
Total Variable Cost: $70/day × 2,000 PD's	140,000
Total Cost:	$240,000
Divided by Total Patient Days	÷ 2,000
Total Cost per Patient Day	$120

However, what if there were 4,000 patients days a month? The fixed cost would still be $100,000. The total variable cost would be $280,000 ($70 per patient day × 4,000 patient days). The total cost would be $380,000. The cost per patient day would now be only $95 ($380,000 divided by 4,000 patient days). The cost per patient day has declined as a result of economies of scale, sometimes referred to as *increasing returns to scale*. Large volumes make it less costly to treat each patient because of the sharing of fixed costs by the larger number of patients.

Decreasing Returns to Scale

At extremely large volumes, however, *decreasing returns to scale* are encountered. Decreasing returns refers to the fact that at very large volumes the cost per patient tends to increase. There are several reasons for this. For one thing, when full capacity is reached (e.g., all beds are full), it becomes very costly to add a new facility. Another problem is that at very large size, it becomes more expensive to acquire resources. There may not be any nurses available to staff the extra volume, and this may drive up the costs of labor.

The implications of this is that there is a least cost volume for any organization. At that volume all economies of scale have been realized, but decreasing returns to scale have not yet set in (see Fig. 4–2). Cost C represents the least cost per patient. That cost occurs at a volume of Q patients.

ECONOMICS AND INCENTIVES

In the earlier hypothetical toothpaste example, each individual consumer or supplier acted in his or her own best interest. Suppliers decided whether they wanted to provide a product at different prices. The consumers decided whether they wanted to buy the product at various prices. The decision of each consumer or supplier individually was aggregated to derive a total demand curve and a total supply curve. The lesson that individuals act in their own best interests is central to economics. And in turn it leads to an important lesson about incentives.

Whenever an action is taken, whether by the government, an organization, or an individual, that action may impact on other individuals or organizations. Much as in physics, for every action there is a corresponding reaction. Managers and policymakers must be aware that the actions that they take may give individuals and organizations incentives to behave in a certain way.

Figure 4–2. Economies of scale.

For instance, many health care insurance companies use deductibles and coinsurance. A deductible is a portion of an individual's health care cost that the individual must pay before the insurance covers any of that individual's costs. Coinsurance is a percentage of each health care bill that the individual must pay out-of-pocket. Why are these used? The rationale is that if individuals have full insurance for all costs, they will use health care services for many little problems that don't need medical attention. By making the individuals bear some of the cost, they have a personal financial incentive to be more judicious in the use of health services. The lower the cost to the individual consumer, the greater the demand, as evidenced by demand curves.

The issue of incentives is a concept of economics that has wide applications. Should your employer offer bonuses? One reason to do so is to give the individual an incentive to work harder in the interests of the organization. The bonus provides the individual with more resources. Those resources can be used for more consumption or saving to result in greater total utility.

Consider another example. Should hospitals be paid on a cost reimbursement basis? For many years that is how Medicare paid hospitals. It was determined, however, that this gave hospitals an incentive to have high costs. Therefore the cost reimbursement system was replaced with DRGs. The DRG system does not reimburse the hospital for its costs. It pays a fixed amount, based on the type of patient, regardless of length of stay or cost.[2] The hope was that DRGs would give hospitals an incentive to shorten lengths of stay and decrease costs.

MARKET EFFICIENCY

One can view the health services field as having three key economic questions:

---

[2]For patients who have unusually long lengths of stay there is a supplemental payment. However, that payment is kept very low so that hospitals do not have an incentive to extend patient stays.

1. How much?
2. How?
3. For whom?

How much health services are to be provided? How are they to be produced? And who will receive them? The first two questions relate to efficiency of production. The third question relates to distribution of society's scarce resources. The efficiency of the market is judged by how well it responds to these three questions.

In the case of a fully functioning free market, the three questions would solve themselves. How much production would depend on the supply and demand curves. Finding the equilibrium price and quantity would determine how much.

The how would also be solved at the equilibrium point. The supplier who is most efficient at the task would be able to offer the service at the lowest cost. As price declines until supply and demand intersect, the less efficient producers will drop out of the competition. When equilibrium is achieved it means that the existing suppliers must be using efficient techniques, or they would have been forced out of business. This means that *technical efficiency* would be achieved. Technical efficiency means that the services are produced using the minimum possible amount of resources for the level of quantity and quality of output achieved.

For whom is also solved by the equilibrium. Any potential buyers who are able and willing to pay the equilibrium price or higher will receive the goods or services. Anyone who can or would only pay less than that price would not. This represents *distributional efficiency*. The market efficiently distributes goods based on the utility of the various consumers.

However, market efficiency does not address the issue of equity or fairness. Is the free market outcome fair for those who are poor? The question of fairness raises the issue of redistribution of resources.

REDISTRIBUTION OF RESOURCES

Government and management tend to have very different objectives. The management of an organization may desire to determine how to best provide patient treatment. It uses economics to find the least cost ways to provide a particular level or type of care. This is technical efficiency. The government is interested in distributional efficiency and equity. Could society be made better off by redistribution of resources?

Collective Action

Resource redistribution is more than simply taking resources from the rich to help the poor. It is based on a much wider notion of welfare than the use of welfare payments to the poor. The government taxes everyone so that it can have public sewer systems, police, and fire protection. For any one individual it would be too expensive to buy his or her own individual police department or fire department. The government acts as a central collection organization, taking contributions (taxes) from each individual and putting them all together to be able to do what any one person cannot, such as having fire and police protection. There is little disagreement that such protection is needed and worthwhile.

This is an example of distributional efficiency through government collective action. The government optimizes the result through its redistribution of resources, making everyone better off than they would be without the intervention.

Equity Improvement

A more controversial aspect of resource redistribution concerns taxing one group of individuals to provide a benefit to another group. For example, the taxes on the working class tend to support the Medicare payments made for the elderly. This makes some individuals better off, but some worse off.

Should such redistribution from current workers to the aged take place? That is a value judgment, not an economic calculation. In the fire or police example, collective action makes everyone better off. Attempts to improve societal equity often improve the utility of some people at the expense of others. How much such redistribution should take place? Again, that is a value judgment. Society must make those value decisions. Then economics can focus on whether the money is being used efficiently to achieve society's goals.

MARKET FAILURE

Except for issues of collective action or equity improvement requiring resource redistribution, the free market is generally assumed to be an efficient mechanism. Left to its own devices, it should always find the equilibrium between supply and demand. However, it is often contended that the marketplace for health care services is not perfectly efficient. There is a condition referred to as a *market failure*. Market failure means that the market does not function fully and freely. This results in an inability to reach the supply and demand equilibrium without intervention. The government often steps in to try to correct market failure.

Market failure can result from a number of different factors. Sometimes government intervention itself is responsible for the failure. Another factor is lack of full information on the part of the consumer. Yet another is failure of consumer actions to fully account for the market price because consumers are not directly responsible for full payment for their health care service consumption. Market failure can be caused by lack of full competition. This occurs if either sellers or buyers have monopoly power. Finally, failure can occur when the actions of individuals do not result in an optimal level of output because their actions do not consider externalities that they generate. All these factors are discussed here.

Government Intervention

Free market economics does not generally result in satisfying all demand. It only results in providing products to consumers who are able and willing to pay a high enough price to make it worth the while of producers to supply the product. In the health care marketplace, society has generally agreed that at least some elements of health care should be provided to individuals who cannot afford to pay for their care. This represents an equity redistribution of resources based on a value judgment by society.

In redistributing the resources, an attempt should be made to avoid creating market distortions as much as possible. The consequences of redistribution should be carefully analyzed. Consider, for example, the fact that society does ensure that an individual in terrible pain with an abscessed tooth who appears at an emergency room receives care for that tooth, for free if necessary. This is accomplished either through government payment for the services or through legislation mandating that the care be offered whether the patient can afford to pay the charge or not.

Suppose that a member of Congress argued that the nation was spending $2,000 for emergency care of poor individuals with tooth abscesses that could be saved had those individuals had toothpaste. In our earlier example we noted that at equilibrium, 500 tubes of toothpaste are purchased at $2.50 a tube. However, if toothpaste were free, 900 tubes would have been consumed. There is an unmet demand of 400 tubes because of the $2.50 price. The member of Congress might note that this unmet need is the result of people being too poor to spend their meager resources on toothpaste. At $2.50 a tube, it would cost the government only $1,000 to buy 400 tubes of toothpaste. This is half as much as is being spent on avoidable emergency care. Therefore, it would be both cheaper and more socially responsible and morally correct to distribute toothpaste and avoid all those abscesses. Is that a correct economic analysis?

What happens if the government acts as a buyer for the health care service, be it toothpaste or emergency abscess care? Will the supply curve change? No. The suppliers have calculated their costs, and the curve indicates how much supply they will offer at any given price. What about the demand curve? If the government says that it will buy the care for poor people, then the amount of care demanded at any specific price has changed. To ensure that everyone has toothpaste, 900 tubes must be purchased. The supply curve in Figure 4–3 indicates that the price at which that volume will be available is $4.50 per tube.

What are the implications of this government decision? First of all, society must raise taxes by enough to cover the cost of toothpaste provided to those who did not buy it at the market price of $2.50. Since the free market equilibrium was 500 tubes, this means that the government must buy 400 tubes. At what price? Assuming that the government pays the market price, it would have to pay $4.50 per tube.

However, the government has also introduced another change. At the higher price of $4.50 per tube, the original demand is less than 500 tubes. It is only 180 tubes (see Fig. 4–3). There are a number of people who were able to buy the toothpaste at a price of $2.50, but who are unwilling or unable to pay $4.50 for it. The government policy, however, will ensure that they get the toothpaste by buying it for them. Thus, in the new equilibrium there are 180 tubes of toothpaste bought by consumers at a price of $4.50 per tube, and 720 tubes bought by the government at a price of $4.50 per tube.

Prices have nearly doubled as a result of the government intervention. The number of people providing their own care has fallen from 500 to 180. The 180 are each paying nearly twice as much. Additionally, there will be a tax of $3,240 to pay for the 720 tubes at $4.50 per tube. This compares with the $2,000 tax that was paid to take care of abscesses. It turns out that the new policy of

Figure 4–3. Supply and demand for toothpaste with government intervention.

toothpaste instead of abscesses will be substantially more expensive, not less expensive as had been proposed.

What is the total size of the toothpaste industry? There are 900 tubes sold at $4.50 per tube, for a total charge of $4,050. Earlier there had been 500 tubes sold for $2.50 each for a total of $1,250. The good intentions of the government to provide direct care to avoid tooth abscesses has caused the number of tubes sold to nearly double and the revenues of the industry to increase nearly fourfold. Is it any surprise that health care costs rose dramatically in the decades following the introduction of Medicare and Medicaid?

Therefore, is it obvious that Medicare and Medicaid were mistakes? No, it is not. Perhaps society should be willing to spend substantial additional amounts of money to avoid tooth abscesses, diseases, morbidity, and mortality. Economics is a science, not a political party. Economics is essential because it allows us to analyze the impact of a policy.

Economists would argue that it is inappropriate to adopt a new policy, such as government payment for toothpaste, without considering the likely economic implications of that policy action. Once the costs of the action are known, economics does *not* make recommendations for or against the policy.

Lack of Full Information

A critical factor causing widespread market failure in health care is the fact that the consumer typically has far less information than the seller. This lack of information makes it difficult for the buyer to make a rational, informed decision.

Consider an extreme hypothetical example. A consumer has a cough, and the doctor examines him. The doctor concludes that there is a 99.9% chance that the patient simply has a cold. If the patient has a cold, the cough will probably go away in a week or two. After two weeks perhaps 5% of the patients will still have a cough.

If the cough does not go away, the doctor could then prescribe an x-ray to determine if the patient has some more serious condition, such as tuberculosis or lung cancer. Assume that in one in a thousand cases, there is a more serious condition.

What if the doctor, who happens to own an x-ray machine in his office, prescribes a chest x-ray for each person with a cough. The doctor has a personal incentive to do this, since a profit can be earned on each of 1,000 x-rays. Waiting two weeks, and then prescribing an x-ray for the 5% who are still coughing, will result in only fifty x-rays. In either case the doctor diagnoses the serious condition. However, in one way he can earn far more money.

Assume that no patient will have a significant detriment by waiting the two weeks for the x-ray. When the physician recommends an x-ray, the patient is usually not an informed buyer. The physician recommends that the x-ray be taken to rule out any serious problem. The unknowing patients agree to the x-ray.

Had the patients been fully informed that they could save their money, wait two weeks, and then come back with no risk, many might opt to do so. The lack of complete information takes away an important element of choice from the patient.

This type of market failure can be corrected by a system of regulations. For example, the government could dictate when it is appropriate to prescribe a chest x-ray. The government has provided such restrictive regulations only very reluctantly. The health services community has argued, successfully to a great extent, that the potential risk to the health of patients from extremely high regulation outweighs the economic benefits of reductions in inappropriate utilization.

Lack of Direct Patient Payment

The failure of the market to be efficient due to a lack of information is further exacerbated by the fact that many patients have Medicare, Medicaid, Blue Cross, or some other insurance plan that will pay part or all of the cost of the x-ray. The high cost of health care services has induced many individuals to acquire health insurance. Health insurance represents a pooling of resources, much as in the case of the fire and police protection example.

On the surface, insurance is clearly a good thing. Rather than some people being lucky and healthy and having little if any cost, while some are unlucky and ill and have costs that wipe out their life savings, everyone pays a set insurance premium, such as $2,000 per year. However, there are problems with insurance. Once the individuals have purchased the insurance, there is little incentive for them not to consume great amounts of health care services. The issue of incentives and insurance co-payments and deductibles was discussed earlier.

The impact of insurance is similar to the example in which the government purchased toothpaste. Once individuals are fully insured (with neither deductible nor co-payment), the price to them for healthcare services drops to zero. In that case, their demand is based on a price of zero. Market failure results in a suboptimal use of resources. Health resources are consumed until their marginal utility is nearly zero, because of the zero cost.

Monopoly Power

Market failure is often associated with a lack of full competition. The basic foundations of free markets assume that there are a large number of buyers and a large number of suppliers for any good or service. If there is only one seller, that seller is referred to as a monopoly. Sometimes there are natural monopolies, where it only makes sense to have one supplier. Many public utilities fall into that category. Duplication of power plants and power lines would be technically wasteful. In such cases, government regulates prices to prevent the supplier from charging an excessive amount.

In small communities, hospitals may effectively be natural monopolies. It is too costly to build more than one hospital for the community. In that case the hospital has the potential to charge substantially more than a hospital in a city with 100 hospitals. In the latter case an individual wanting elective surgery could shop around for a hospital offering a reasonable price.

Another element of market failure in health care is the fact that consumers often use the health care facilities and organizations used by their physician. Rather than having to compete directly for patients, hospitals, nursing homes, and home care agencies need only compete for physician referrals. Once the physician makes a recommendation, the patient is often locked in, even if there are other suppliers available. When it comes to the patient's health, especially if there is any chance of death or permanent disability, each health care provider is viewed as being unique. For example, if the patient hears that a surgeon is good, the patient will be reluctant to shop around for another surgeon who is cheaper or who operates at a less expensive hospital. Thus, monopoly power sometimes exists for health care providers even in the absence of single supplier monopolies.

If there is monopoly power, the price may not be driven down to a normal equilibrium level. The monopoly might find that more profits can be made at a higher price. Figure 4–4 considers this situation. The equilibrium is at the intersection of the supply and demand curves, with price P1 and quantity Q1. However, what if the monopoly charges price P2? Consumers will only purchase quantity Q2 at that higher price. However, the price is so high that the monopoly may make more profit selling less volume at a high price than by selling a higher volume at the equilibrium price. This is a result of the relatively inelastic demand for health care services. High rises in price may not lower the quantity demanded substantially. If there were competition, prices would fall to the equilibrium level. Without competition it pays for the provider to keep the price above that level.

Figure 4–4. Example of monopoly power.

The government has traditionally tried to regulate public utility monopoly prices by fixing them at level P1. At that level consumers purchase Q1 quantity of services, and a free market outcome is achieved through intervention.

To the extent that the government pays health care providers directly for Medicare and Medicaid, the government is involved directly in setting the prices it is willing to pay. However, full regulation of health care pricing has not yet taken place, as it has in the case of public utilities. That means that many health care providers may have the ability to set artificially high prices to generate excessive profits.

Monopsony Power

At the same time, however, insurance companies and employers are starting to exercise the power of large buyers. Blue Cross has exercised such power for many years. Just as it is possible to have a monopoly where there is only one seller, it is possible for there to be just one buyer. If there is only one buyer, it is called a *monopsony* situation.

In recent years, there has been a great proliferation of *preferred provider organizations*, as discussed in Chapter 2. Insurance companies or employers direct their members or employees to use these providers of health care in exchange for lower prices. In effect, the insurance companies are behaving as monopsonists. They control the buying of health care services for their populations. That provides them with market power to help them gain a better purchase price for the services.

Just as a supplier with monopoly power can dictate the price at which it sells a good or service, a monopsonist can dictate the price it pays to buy a good or service. For instance, suppose that the only employer for nurses in a geographic area was the local hospital. That hospital would be a monopsony.

The monposony buyer pays low wages, which reduces the amount of supply. Fewer nurses are willing to work at such low wages. However, the savings from the lower wage offsets the financial losses from the inability to hire more staff. This may result in less care being provided. It is conceivable that part of the reason nursing shortages are frequently observed is that health care providers maintain an artificially low wage level for nurses because of their exercise of monopsony power.

Government-induced Inefficiency

Another problem creating market failure is the potential lack of incentive on the part of health care organizations to minimize costs of production. The government is often the cause of this technical inefficiency. This is because many government programs pay health care organizations their costs for providing care to specific groups of patients. For example, home care agencies are paid whatever their costs are, up to a maximum amount.

Without economic analysis, it might seem quite prudent for the government to reimburse an organization for its costs. It should save money, since the government won't have to pay for any profit. However, it provides a perverse incentive. It encourages organizations to have a high cost. Why work hard to control costs if you will be paid whatever you spend. There is no reward for low cost. History has shown that schemes that reimburse costs are not good tools for restraining the growth of health care costs.

Externalities

A last principal cause of market failure is the existence of *externalities*. Externalities exist when an action by an individual or organization has secondary impacts on others that are not taken into account. For example, if a factory pollutes the skies, it may have found the cheapest way to produce its product, but as a side effect its pollution hurts other people. Externalities may present additional costs or benefits to those affected. If a person goes to a hospital and is cured of a contagious disease, it benefits all those who might have caught the disease from that person.

If external costs and benefits are not taken into account, then a nonoptimal amount of output may be produced. There could be too much pollution, or too little health care. This represents a market failure. There needs to be a mechanism to correct the output level. In the case of pollution, the factory can be fined for polluting to make it realize the full costs of the pollution, including its negative external impacts on others. This can cause it to reduce its output of pollution. In the case of health care, the government can tax all individuals for the positive external benefits they receive and use the money collected to pay subsidies for health care.

In fact, the government does take that approach frequently. The government role is essential because of its ability to take collective action. As in the cases of police and fire protection, the government can use collective action to benefit society.

THE MARKET FOR NURSES

A problem that has plagued the health care industry periodically for decades is a shortage of nurses. These shortages have come and gone, with at least some shortages being noted in every decade since World War II. A critical issue is determination of whether nursing shortages occur because of market failure or whether the market is in fact functioning normally. The answer has serious ramifications for what the government should do to alleviate nursing shortages when they occur.

It is often argued that the primary cause of most nursing shortages is not a decreasing supply, but rather an increasing demand. The number of nurses needed increases more rapidly than the supply. The result of an increase in demand with supply unchanged would be a shift of the demand curve from D to D' in Figure 4–5A. The new equilibrium, B, has a substantially higher wage than the original equilibrium, A. This higher wage entices more individuals to become educated as nurses. With higher wages, the profession is relatively more attractive than it was at the lower wage. This results, after a number of years, in an increased supply of nurses. Figure 4–5B shows the eventual shift in the supply curve as newly trained nurses enter the work force. The new supply, S', removes the pressure for salaries to rise (faster than the general level of wages in society). And a new equilibrium exists at point C.

Note that the equilibrium at C has a lower wage than that at point B. Wages, however, often do not adjust downward. Instead, a period of time may occur during which wages rise extremely slowly, if at all. The higher supply removes the pressure on employers to raise wages.

Figure 4–5A. Increase in demand for nurses.

Figure 4–5B. Increase in supply of nurses.

In fact, more nursing, Q3 as compared to Q2, is available. And, if the price stays at P2, then an even greater quantity of nursing would be available. Consider where the P2 price would intersect with the S′ curve. It is at a quantity substantially higher than Q2 or Q3. Therefore, whenever nursing shortages end, there tends to be a period of time during which nursing salaries rise slowly.

This analysis assumes that everyone has reasonably complete information. It is not likely, however, that employers know how much salaries must rise to reach an equilibrium. Therefore, they raise salaries, but not enough, and then wait for the long-run education of more nurses. After several years, if the number of nurses being educated has not risen sufficiently, wages will again rise, gradually seeking the level at which enough nurses will be educated to meet the demand. If demand is continuing to rise during this period, it is difficult for supply to catch up.

The problem is made more complicated by the fact that other industries are also trying to attract qualified labor. The economic analysis of one industry is incomplete because it fails to consider possible increases in demand and wages in other industries.

Therefore, the observed shortages of nurses could be the result of lack of information about the price at which sufficient individuals will be enticed into the industry. Or it could be the result of a moving target. Increasing demand, plus wage increases in other industries, could create a situation where prices are rising to attract more nurses, but simply not fast enough to eliminate the shortage. Both of these arguments revolve around the lag in perceptions until people realize that higher wages are available for nurses, followed by the lag in educating new nurses.

On the other hand, if this were the case, there should be increases in the numbers of students in nursing schools. It would be easy enough for the health care industry to consider if wages are high enough by examining whether more students are applying to nursing schools and continuing to raise wages until applications start to rise.

If that is not the case, then one might argue that the larger employers of nurses were acting in a monopsonist fashion, artificially keeping wages low, and enduring a shortage of nurses in exchange for avoiding a higher total payroll cost.

IMPLICATIONS FOR NURSE MANAGERS

Accounting and finance are often viewed as elements of applied economics. We live in a society that has its entire financial structure built around a system of economics. That economic system permeates all institutions and organizations. It dictates the allocation of society's scarce resources.

The health care system, however, is largely an example of the failure of the economic system. Lack of information, monopoly power, and a variety of other factors cause the laws of supply and demand to fail to achieve a normal free market equilibrium level. These failures lead to a need for a government role to help achieve efficient economic resource allocation.

Externalities and the power of collective behavior hold a special role in health care because of the value to everyone of living in a society that is basically healthy. This means that there is a further need for government intervention.

Compounding the need for a government role even further is the fact that most members of society believe that some degree of resource redistribution is essential for equity as well as for efficiency. This can allow the poorest members of society to be guaranteed at least a minimal level of health care services.

Within this complicated economic environment are nurses—nurses who want to know why hospitals do not provide more resources to their departments; nurses who want to know why salaries cannot be raised to levels that compensate more adequately for their skills and the sacrifices they make; nurses who want to know why everyone isn't guaranteed the highest level of care.

The answers to these questions are complex. However, an understanding of the basic law of supply and demand and the inherent limited nature of all resources is a starting point in obtaining answers to these questions. The complications of market failure further explain why health care is one of the most highly regulated industries and why health care is sometimes viewed as best provided by a not-for-profit organization with a mission of providing care, rather than a mission of maximizing profits.

As the reader goes through the remaining chapters of this book, the laws of supply and demand and the scarcity of resources should be kept in mind. The importance of incentives in understanding the likely behavior of individuals should be considered. The efficiency generated by economies of scale should be thought of. The elements of economics are fundamental to the realm of financial management issues faced by nurse managers.

KEY CONCEPTS ⸻⸻⸻⸻⸻⸻⸻⸻⸻⸻⸻⸻⸻⸻

Economics Study of how scarce resources are allocated among their possible uses. As a management or policy tool, economics is used to ensure that individuals, organizations, and society make optimal use of their limited resources.

Economic goods   Goods or services acquired by consumers that provide physical or psychic benefit. Goods or services are generally acquired through an exchange process.

Utility   Benefit gained by consumers from either consuming or saving resources. Marginal utility is the additional utility gained from consuming one more unit of a particular good or service. Total utility is maximized by purchasing a set of goods and services such that the marginal utility or marginal benefit is the same for each item.

Supply and demand   Supply is the amount of a good or service that all suppliers in aggregate would like to provide at any given price. Demand is the amount of the good or service that consumers would be willing to acquire at any given price. At an equilibrium price, the quantity offered and the quantity demanded are identical.

Free enterprise, capitalism, or market economy   System where each individual can choose whether to invest wealth or capital in a business venture; workers can choose whether to work for that venture at the wages offered; and consumers can choose whether to buy the products of the venture at the requested price.

Elasticity of demand   Degree to which demand increases in response to a price decrease, or decreases in response to a price increase. In general, the demand for health services is considered highly inelastic.

Economies of scale   Cost of providing a good or service falls as quantity increases because fixed costs are shared by the larger volume. However, eventually large volume may lead to decreasing returns to scale, due to capacity constraints or shortages of labor or supplies.

Incentives   Economics assumes that individuals and organizations act in their own best interests. Incentives such as health insurance deductibles are used to make it be in the individual's interest to act in a desired manner. They are often used by management to result in an improved use of an organization's scarce resources, or by government to improve the use of society's scarce resources.

Market efficiency   In a fully functioning free market economy, resources are optimally allocated and used as a result of the supply-and-demand mechanism.

Redistribution of resources   Even in a relatively efficient market, some government redistribution of resources can provide collective action that makes everyone better off, such as the provision of police and fire protection. Economic analysis can determine which redistributions can make everyone better off and no one worse off. Other redistributions of resources are done to improve equity. They may make some individuals better off and some worse off. Such redistribution requires an equity value judgment. Economics cannot determine a "correct" level of redistribution.

Market failure   Situations in which the free market does not operate efficiently. Market failure may be the result of:

> **Government intervention**   The role of the government in guaranteeing basic medical care to all individuals creates a distortion in the normal

equilibrium, the effects of which should be minimized to the extent possible.

Lack of full information There is a tremendous gap between the knowledge of the patient and the health care provider concerning what services are needed and how important they are. This lack of information prevents the consumer from making a rational, informed decision.

Lack of direct patient payment The existence of health insurance allows individuals to consume more services than they would if they had to directly pay the full cost of the services.

Monopoly or monopsony power Organizations with monopoly or monopsony power can sometimes make excess profits by maintaining prices of final products at a level higher than an equilibrium level and the prices of inputs below the equilibrium level.

Government-induced inefficiency Decreases in technical efficiency may occur as a result of government reimbursement to health providers based on the cost of care provided.

Externalities An action by an individual or organization may have secondary impacts on others that are not taken into account. These side effects may present additional costs or benefits to those affected.

SUGGESTED READINGS ❖

Aiken, L.H., and C.F. Mullinix, "The Nurse Shortage: Myth or Reality?" *The New England Journal of Medicine*, Vol. 317, No. 10, September 3, 1987, pp. 641–645.

Cleverley, William O., *Essentials of Health Care Finance*, Aspen Publishers, Rockville, MD, 1986.

Feldstein, Paul J., *Health Care Economics*, 3rd edition, John Wiley & Sons, New York, 1988.

Hicks, Lanis L., Kenneth Bopp, and Richard Speck, "Forecasting Demand for Hospital Services in an Unstable Environment," *Nursing Economics*, Vol. 5, No. 6, November/December 1987, pp. 304–310.

Nyberg, Jan, "The Effects of Care and Economics on Nursing Practice," *Journal of Nursing Administration*, Vol. 20, No. 5, May 1990, pp. 13–18.

Strasen, Leann, *Key Business Skills for Nurse Managers*, J.B. Lippincott, New York, 1987.

II

FINANCIAL ACCOUNTING

Financial accounting is the area of financial management that focuses on collecting and reporting information about the financial position of an organization and the results of its activities. Chapter 5 discusses the basic principles and terms of accounting and addresses the compilation of accounting information into financial reports that can be used by the organization's managers and other interested individuals. Chapter 6 explains the techniques commonly used to analyze and interpret the financial position of an organization and the financial results of its activities. ❖

5

Accounting Principles

CHAPTER GOALS

The goals of this chapter are to:

♦ Explain why accounting is important to health care organizations

♦ Describe the basic framework of accounting, including the fundamental equation of accounting

♦ Introduce the balance sheet and income statement

♦ Define a wide range of common accounting terminology

♦ Explain the process of recording accounting information and then summarizing and reporting that information

♦ Introduce and define the most common and important generally accepted accounting principles

♦ Describe the use of fund accounting in not-for-profit health care organizations

♦ Discuss the implications of financial accounting for nurse managers

❖

INTRODUCTION

Accounting is a system that lets us keep "account" of things. Health care organizations have formalized accounting systems to track the financial well-being and financial success of the organization. The financial well-being and profitability of an organization may not be the most important elements of the organization's *mission*. (See Chapter 10 for a discussion of organizational mission.) The primary goals of the organization may relate to the types of care provided and the population served. The provider of health care services may not be hoping to financially profit from the provision of care. The financial well-being and financial success of the organization are critical, however, because they relate to the viability of the organization and its ability to meet the central elements of its mission.

Unless satisfactory financial results are achieved, at best the organization will be unable to acquire the latest technologies or expand services; at worst, to pay its bills. The organization will then have to cease providing any care at all.

Therefore, a critical job of financial managers is to compile a set of financial reports, called *financial statements,* that convey to the reader information about the organization's financial position and the results of its activities. This information can be used by banks to decide whether to lend money to the organization, by philanthropists to determine whether to give it money, and by suppliers to decide whether to extend it credit. They can also be used by the organization's managers to decide whether the organization's financial results are satisfactory and how they could be improved.

The information contained in these reports can help nurse managers to know whether the organization has sufficient resources to provide larger raises, more staff, or capital expenditure requests or whether the organization will need to substantially cut expenses just to avoid going out of business. Power is often said to reside with those who possess information. Certainly, an ability to understand and interpret the financial results of the organization is critical to ensuring that nursing receives an appropriate share of available organizational resources. Thus, the study of financial accounting and the financial statements generated is not just an "academic" exercise but rather provides nurse managers with tools necessary for critical analysis of the financial status of the organization.

All organizations have a great number of financial transactions. A small home health care agency has thousands of events during the year that have a financial impact. A large medical center may have tens of millions of such events. The job of accounting is to develop a system that can record each of the many events that have financial implications, summarize them, and report them in a manner that is useful to managers and other interested individuals.

This task is accomplished via the techniques of *financial accounting.* Financial accounting is a system that records historical financial information, summarizes it, and provides reports of what financial events have occurred and of what the financial impact of those events has been. Accounting is not a science. It is based upon a generally accepted set of conventions, rules, and terminology.

This chapter will start with an explanation of the basic framework upon which modern accounting rests. Next it will introduce the central financial statements, which are called:

- Statement of financial position (or balance sheet)
- Statement of revenues and expenses (or income statement)
- Statement of changes in fund balances
- Statement of cash flows.

Understanding these financial statements is difficult, if for no other reason than that the accounting terminology they use is new to some readers. A section on terminology is provided in this chapter.

The chapter then moves on to discuss how financial information is recorded and reported by health care organizations. Such reporting often follows a set of rules referred to as generally accepted accounting principles (GAAP). Several of the most important of these principles are discussed. Not-for-profit health care organizations use a unique approach to recording and reporting information. That approach is a technique called fund accounting. The essential principles of fund accounting are discussed in the chapter. The chapter then concludes with a brief discussion of accounting's implications for nurse managers.

THE BASIC FRAMEWORK OF ACCOUNTING

Accounting systems are established based upon one widely accepted *axiom*. This axiom is the basic equation of accounting:

$$\text{Assets} = \text{Liabilities} + \text{Owner's equity}$$

Assets are valuable resources that are owned by the organization. They may be either physical, having substance and form, such as a table or building, or intangible, such as the reputation the organization has gained for providing high-quality health care services. *Liabilities* are legal financial obligations the organization has to outsiders. Essentially they represent money that the organization owes to someone. These liabilities represent claims against the organization's assets. *Owner's equity* represents the amount of an organization's assets that the organization itself or its owners own.

The left-hand side of the equation represents all the valuable resources of the organization and is simply referred to as the asset side of the equation. The right-hand side of the equation represents all the claims against those valuable resources. These claims, both from outsiders and from owners, are referred to as equities. Therefore the right-hand side of the equation is referred to as the equity side. The equation is often referred to as the organization's assets and equities.

The owner's equity is a *residual* amount. When one subtracts the claims of outsiders from the total value of the organization's assets, whatever is left belongs to the organization or its owners. Imagine if you were to buy a house for $200,000 by placing $40,000 as a down payment and borrowing $160,000 from a bank. The $200,000 would represent the value of the house, which is an asset. The $160,000 would represent the mortgage obligation, which is a liability, and the $40,000 would be considered your *equity* in the house, which is an owner's equity. Note that if the house value were to rise or fall, the liability would remain unchanged. If the house suddenly became worth $250,000, the liability would still be $160,000, and your equity in the house would have risen to $90,000.

Since the owner's equity is a residual value, which rises and falls in response to changes in the assets and liabilities, the equation will always remain in balance. The owner's equity balance will be whatever it must be for the equation to be in balance. That forms the basis for all bookkeeping or accounting.

For proprietary or for-profit organizations, the owners may be sole proprietors, partners, or stockholders, depending on whether the organization is legally established as a *proprietorship, partnership,* or *corporation.* The owner's equity belongs to the owners of the organization. In the case of a not-for-profit organization, there is no owner per se. The organization exists for the good of the community at large. No individuals are entitled to benefit from any profits that might be generated by the organization. For not-for-profit organizations, the owner's equity is referred to as the *fund balance.* This represents the balance of the funds after liabilities have been subtracted from assets.

THE CENTRAL FINANCIAL STATEMENTS

Financial information is conveyed to its ultimate users in the form of reports referred to as financial statements. The four key statements are the statement of financial position (the balance sheet), the statement of revenues and expenses (the income statement), the statement of changes in fund balances, and the statement of cash flows. We will discuss the first two now; the remaining two will be introduced in Chapter 6.

The Balance Sheet

The most essential of the organization's financial reports is a document officially called the statement of financial position. This document is frequently referred to as the balance sheet. The role of the balance sheet is to indicate the financial position of the organization at a specific point.

The balance sheet summarizes the fundamental equation of accounting. The assets are shown on the left side (or top) of the statement. The equities (liabilities plus owner's equity or fund balance) are shown on the right side (or bottom) of the statement. A balance sheet for the hypothetical ABC Health Care organization appears in Table 5–1. The basic structure of financial statements is similar for different types of organizations.[1] Note that the total of the assets and the equities must always be equal. This is a result of the fundamental equation of accounting, which is required to always be in balance.

The Income Statement

When services are provided to patients, a charge is generally made. The monies that are received or are expected to be received in exchange for the services are called *revenues*. The costs of providing those services are *expenses*. The revenues less the expenses represent the profit or loss of the organization.

Most organizations in industries other than health care refer to a statement that compares revenues to expenses as an income statement. This is logical because revenue less expense is defined as being *net income* or *profit*. However, the not-for-profit firms in the health care industry have historically preferred not to use the words profit or income because they imply that the organization is profiting from the provision of health care. Instead, the income statement is often referred to as the statement of revenues and expenses. It is sometimes called the activity statement. The net income is often referred to as the excess of revenues over expenses.

In practice, most not-for-profit organizations do earn a profit. This book uses the term not-for-profit rather than the common term nonprofit. The term nonprofit implies that the organization does not make a profit. That is not a correct inference. A key goal of for-profit companies is to earn a profit. In not-

---

[1] There are some differences in the specific detail of financial statements, depending on the type of organization. These differences reflect the diverse nature of health care organizations. The accounting industry official guide for accounting for health care organizations (*Audits of Providers of Health Care Services*, AICPA, NY, 1990) includes illustrative financial statements for hospitals, nursing homes, continuing care retirement communities, home health agencies, health maintenance organizations, and ambulatory care organizations.

❖ **TABLE 5–1**

ABC Health Care
Statement of Financial Position
as of June 30, 1993
(000s omitted)

Assets		Equities	
Current Assets		**Current Liabilities**	
Cash	$ 150	Wages payable	$ 1,123
Marketable securities	220	Accounts payable	2,430
Accounts receivable, *net* of		Notes payable	500
$436 allowance for bad		Deferred revenue	300
debts	2,319	Taxes payable	145
Inventory	832	Total current liabilities	$ 4,498
Prepaid assets	46		
Total current assets	$ 3,567	**Long-Term Liabilities**	
		Mortgage payable	$ 3,560
Fixed Assets		Bonds payable	20,000
Property, plant,		Total long-term liabilities	$23,560
and equipment $43,470			
Less accumulated		**Fund Balance**	
depreciation 17,356		Board-designated sinking	
Net property, plant, and		fund	$ 1,737
equipment	$26,114	Unrestricted fund balance	5,195
Sinking fund	1,737	Total fund balance	$ 6,932
Investments	341		
Goodwill	3,231		
Total fixed assets	$31,423		
Total Assets	$34,990	**Total Equities**	$34,990

for-profit organizations, a profit may be earned, but that profit is not the primary goal.

However, profits *are* a necessary element for all health care organizations for several reasons. First, to fulfill their mission many health care organizations must adopt new, expensive technologies as they become available. Profits earned on current patients help to pay for the adoption of new technology tomorrow. Second, many health care organizations want to expand both the range of services they offer and the number of people served. Such expansion requires the reinvestment of profits. Finally, the impact of inflation is to constantly increase the cost of replacing buildings and equipment as they wear out. Some profits must be earned to allow for replacements at higher prices.

Therefore, not-for-profit health care organizations do not exist for the purpose of making a profit, but making a profit does not represent improper behavior. Rather, it is indicative of an organization that will remain healthy enough to continue to provide services to its community.

An example of an income statement, or statement of revenues and expenses for the hypothetical ABC Health Care appears in Table 5–2.

❖ **TABLE 5–2**

ABC Health Care
Statement of Revenues and Expenses
for the Fiscal Year Ending June 30, 1993
(000s omitted)

Revenues	
Patient revenues	$18,230
Other operating revenues	1,919
Total	$20,149
Expenses	
Wages for clinical services	$10,325
Patient care supplies and food	934
Housekeeping services	654
Operation and maintenance of plant	1,221
Administrative services	2,343
Depreciation and amortization	1,433
Bad debt expense	436
Interest	2,333
Total	$19,679
Excess of Revenues over Expenses	$ 470

ACCOUNTING TERMINOLOGY

Accounting is often referred to as the language of business. Numerous accounting terms become part of the everyday vocabulary of running an organization. Given the background you now have in the basic framework of accounting and the balance sheet and statement of revenues and expenses, we can turn our attention to introducing a large number of the most common terms.

Accounting Terms for Assets

Some of the most common terms related to assets include:
- Liquid or liquidity
- Current assets
- Cash equivalents
- Marketable securities
- Fixed or long-term assets
- Liquidate
- Accounts receivable
- Allowance for uncollectible accounts or allowance for bad debts
- Prepaid assets
- Depreciate
- Depreciation
- Accumulated depreciation
- Sinking fund
- Goodwill
- Intangible
- Amortization

All these terms will be discussed in this section. Consider Table 5–1. One of the first things to note about the balance sheet is the remark "000s omitted" (in the heading of the statement). This means that all numbers have been rounded off to the nearest thousand dollars. For example, cash of $150 is really cash of $150,000. There are several reasons for this optional rounding. One reason is that the financial statement is less cumbersome to read if some rounding is done. More important is the fact that financial statements are not as accurate as most people assume. Most accounting systems have many clerical errors. To eliminate all the errors would be extremely costly. Therefore, financial statements should be thought of as being reasonably, not precisely, accurate. Rounding off the numbers for presentation purposes helps to convey the fact that the numbers are not exact measures.

The balance sheet presents the organization's assets in order of liquidity, from the most liquid to the least liquid. *Liquid assets* are cash or other assets that can quickly be converted to cash to pay the liabilities of the organization. Buildings and equipment, rent paid in advance, and investments set aside for future building expansions are examples of illiquid assets (having little liquidity). Organizations that have a great amount of cash and other liquid assets are relatively safer than those which are "illiquid." The most liquid assets are placed near the top of the balance sheet to give them prominence. This is done because one primary purpose of financial statements is to convey the financial stability of the organization—its ability to continue in business.

The first section on the asset side of the balance sheet is *current assets*. These are the resources that are cash, can be converted to cash within one year, or will be used up within one year. Current assets are often referred to as short-term or near-term assets. Current assets are more liquid than those assets which are not current. *Current liabilities* are those obligations which must be paid within one year.

Within the current assets category, assets are grouped by liquidity. The first asset listed is cash. Cash includes not only money on hand but also *cash equivalents*, such as savings and checking accounts and short-term certificates of deposit. The next item is *marketable securities*. This includes investments in stocks and bonds. Similar investments are also included on the balance sheet under the heading of fixed asset or long-term asset investments. *Fixed or long-term assets* are those assets which will not be used up or converted to cash within one year. The primary difference between marketable securities and fixed asset investments is intent. If management intends to sell or *liquidate* the stocks or bonds within one year of the balance sheet date, they are marketable securities. If the intent is to hold onto those securities for more than a year, they are fixed asset investments.

The next current asset listed after marketable securities is *accounts receivable*. These are amounts owed to the organization by purchasers of the organization's goods or services. Often a transaction occurs "on account." This means that payment is not made immediately. Instead, an account is opened that keeps track of the transaction until the payment is made. For the provider of the service there is an account receivable. For the consumer of the service there is a mirror image, referred to as an account payable.

Accounts receivable are shown on the balance sheet "net." This refers to the fact that health care organizations often have bad debts. That is, there are some patients for whom payment is never received, even though the patient was expected to be able to pay for the care. Although the health care provider may not know who will not pay, an estimate must be made, and the amount of receivables shown on the balance sheet should only be the net amount that the organization estimates it will receive. If the gross amount of receivables outstanding were shown on the balance sheet, there would be an overestimate of the value of that asset. Therefore, there is established an *allowance for uncollectible accounts*, sometimes called an *allowance for bad debts*. In Table 5–1, the total accounts receivable are $2,755,000, but when we subtract an estimated uncollectible portion of receivables equal to $436,000, the net accounts receivable are shown as $2,319,000.

Inventory is the next item listed in current assets. This represents the various supplies that will be used to provide goods or services. If a home health agency sells walkers and wheelchairs to its clients, it may keep a stock of them on hand. Also a wide variety of medical supplies such as sutures is needed for the patients to be treated. Those items which are purchased and then used in providing services are not considered expenses as soon as they are purchased. Rather, they become a valuable resource, inventory, which becomes an expense only as it is used up.

The last item shown in current assets in Table 5–1 is *prepaid assets*. This represents assets that have been paid for and have not yet been used but will be used within one year. This includes items such as fire insurance premiums or rent paid in advance. These items are not expected to be converted back into cash, but they will be used up within one year, so they are considered current assets.

Fixed assets are listed on the balance sheet after current assets. Fixed assets consist primarily of property, plant, and equipment. This refers to the land, buildings, and pieces of equipment owned by the organization. Land is expected to last forever. However, buildings and equipment physically wear out with the passage of time. From an accounting perspective, they are said to *depreciate*, or decline in value or productive capability.

Suppose that a building costs $40 million when it is new, and it is expected to last for forty years. Rather than show the entire cost of the building as an expense in the year it is purchased, accountants require that the cost be spread out over the expected useful lifetime of the building. The allocation of the $40 million cost over forty years is referred to as *depreciation*. The amount of the original cost allocated as an expense each year is the depreciation expense for that year. The total amount of depreciation that has been taken over the years the organization has owned the asset is referred to as the *accumulated depreciation*.

For instance, if the organization is taking depreciation expense of $1 million per year on the $40 million building, and they have owned the building for ten years, then the accumulated depreciation would be $10 million and the net value would be $30 million. The financial statement would show the original cost, the accumulated depreciation, and the net value. Note, however, that financial statements do not list each building and each piece of equipment. Instead, all similar items are combined and shown as one summary amount. On Table 5–1, the property, plant, and equipment might represent the buildings owned by the organization, the land, and all pieces of equipment.

During the years that buildings and equipment get old, the organization tries to charge enough for its services to be able to collect an adequate amount of money to replace these assets when they have exhausted their useful life. However, sometimes the organization spends that money for current activities rather than saving it to replace long-term assets. To ensure adequate accumulation of resources for future major investments in buildings and equipment, the organization will sometimes establish a *sinking fund*. This is simply a segregated group of investments that can only be used for a specified purpose, generally replacement of plant and equipment or repayment of a loan taken to purchase that building and equipment.

The only asset on the example balance sheet that has not yet been discussed is *goodwill*. This is an *intangible* asset. It represents a measure of the value of the organization that goes beyond its specific physical assets. This includes good relationships with suppliers, a favorable reputation for high-quality care, and other similar values that are not easily quantified. Although most organizations have goodwill, they do not show it or any other intangible assets on their financial statements. This is because accountants have trouble measuring the true value of an organization's goodwill.

The only time that intangible assets appear on a financial statement is if the organization has purchased the intangible asset from someone else. Generally this occurs when one organization acquires another organization and has paid more than the value of that organization's specific tangible assets. In that case, accountants assume that the excess paid must have been a payment for the general goodwill of the organization. Otherwise, rather than buy the organization, one would have simply purchased similar tangible assets. Therefore, the excess paid is shown as goodwill, and the cost of the goodwill is depreciated over a period of time.

The term depreciation, however, is only used for identifiable physical assets. Depreciation of intangible items is referred to as *amortization*. Amortize means to "spread out or allocate." The cost of the intangible asset is spread out or allocated over the expected useful lifetime of the asset.

Accounting Terms for Equities

Equities consist of liabilities and owner's equity. The terms to be discussed in this section include:

- Current liabilities
- Long-term liabilities
- Wages payable
- Accounts payable
- Notes payable
- Taxes payable
- FICA
- Deferred revenues
- Mortgage payable
- Bonds payable
- Unrestricted fund balance
- Restricted fund balance, or board-designated

Liabilities are divided on the balance sheet into current liabilities and long-term liabilities. As noted earlier, current liabilities are obligations that are expected to be paid within one year. Long-term liabilities are obligations that are not expected to be paid within the coming year.

Current liabilities in Table 5–1 include wages payable, accounts payable, notes payable, deferred revenue, and taxes payable. Wages payable simply represent amounts that are owed to employees. Accounts payable generally represent amounts owed to suppliers (such as pharmaceutical or medical supply companies). Notes payable represent obligations to repay a loan. Depending on when the loan must be repaid, some notes payable are long-term liabilities. Taxes payable represent taxes owed to a local or federal government. Even if an organization is not-for-profit, it will likely have tax obligations. These usually relate to payroll deductions for employee income taxes and Social Security taxes (FICA) as well as unemployment and workmen's compensation taxes.

Deferred revenues are somewhat more complex. These represent payments that the organization has received in advance of providing its services. For example, suppose that under an arrangement with an employer in the area, your organization will provide primary care to that employer's employees. The employer makes quarterly payments in advance. The payment at the end of this year covers care provided in the first three months of next year. The money has been received, but the organization has not yet delivered any care. This money received will represent revenue in the future, but that recognition is deferred until the quarter of a year has passed and the services have been provided. Until then this "deferred revenue" is treated as a liability. This is because the organization is liable to repay the money it received if it does not keep its part of the bargain and provide the agreed-upon care.

Table 5–1 indicates two types of long-term liability: *mortgage payable* and *bonds payable*. A mortgage payable represents a loan secured by a specific asset. Mortgage payments, including interest and a portion of the liability balance, are generally made monthly. If the organization defaults on its required payments, the lender can take the asset and sell it to recover the balance of the loan.

A bond payable represents a formal borrowing arrangement where a certificate represents the debt. The certificate is legally transferable. For instance, one person lends money to a hospital and receives the bond certificate. The individual can sell that certificate to another person. The hospital is then obligated to repay the money borrowed to the new owner of the bond. Often, interest on bonds is paid only twice a year (semiannually), and the principal amount borrowed is not repaid at all until the maturity or termination date of the bond. Bondholders often are general creditors. Their loan to the organization is secured in general by all the assets of the organization rather than by a specific asset. When insufficient cash is available to make bondholder payments, the organization is often forced into bankruptcy. Therefore bonds may be a riskier way for organizations to borrow money than mortgages. However, the interest rate paid on bonds is often lower than would be obtainable with a mortgage.

The last equity section on the balance sheet is fund balance. In for-profit corporations, this would be called the stockholders' equity section of the statement. The fund balance represents the residual. After recording all assets and subtracting all liabilities, any remaining balance is the fund balance. Note that the fund balance does not represent an available source of cash. This balance represents a claim of ownership of assets. All the valuable resources of the firm are on the asset side of the balance sheet.

The board of trustees or directors of the organization can direct specific uses for some of the residual value of the organization. In Table 5–1 the fund balance has been divided into a general, unrestricted portion and a board-designated or board-restricted portion. The restriction the board has established in this case is to ensure that assets are put aside for reinvestment in buildings and equipment. Therefore there is a board-designated sinking fund. On the asset side of the balance sheet, a portion of the assets has in fact been segregated to be invested in this sinking fund. It should be noted that restrictions made by the board can also be removed by the board.

Accounting Terms for Revenues and Expenses

Table 5–2 presents a statement of revenues and expenses for discussion. The terms to be discussed based on this statement include:
♦ Revenues
♦ Gross revenues vs. net revenues
♦ Operating revenues
♦ Contractual allowances
♦ Gifts, donations, and contributions
♦ Wage, patient care supply, depreciation, administrative, and other operating expenses
♦ Bad debts
♦ Charity care

The decade of the 1990s has seen a number of important changes in health care financial statements.[2] Before 1990, health care organizations started their statement of revenues and expenses with gross patient revenues. Gross revenues are the charges for all service care provided. However, in many cases, health care organizations received less than 100% of their charges from some payers. Some were too poor to pay anything (charity care); some patients just never paid their bill (bad debts); and some payers received discounted prices (contractual allowances). Therefore, statements of revenues and expenses would subtract from patient revenues an amount for contractual allowances, bad debts, and charity care. This approach is no longer permitted.

Consider a car dealership that negotiates on the price at which each car is sold. Would the auto dealer report revenue as the total of the actual amounts that all the cars were sold for, or the total of the sticker (list) prices? Clearly, the sales are the sum of the negotiated prices, not the artificially high list prices shown on the car stickers. The old health care approach was comparable to showing the total of the sticker prices of the cars rather than the total of the agreed-upon prices.

Under the current generally accepted accounting principles (GAAP), the statement of revenues and expenses starts with net patient service revenues and other operating revenues (such as gift shop or cafeteria sales). Patients who pay for their own care—as opposed to having Medicare, Medicaid, or Blue Cross insurance—may well pay a different price than these large "third-party payers" do. In many cases governments and large customers (such as Blue Cross) pay a rate lower than the hospital charges. These discounts are referred to as *contractual allowances*. Sometimes they are mandated by law rather than resulting from a contractual agreement. The current accounting rules

---

[2]*Audits of Providers of Health Care Services*, American Institute of Certified Public Accountants, New York, 1990.

require that patient revenues be shown after discounts have been deducted. The amount of contractual allowances does not have to be shown on financial statements.

One major controversy in health care accounting is whether gifts and donations should be considered part of normal operating activities or should be segregated and shown elsewhere on the statement of revenues and expenses. The general rule is that all revenues are included in operating revenues, unless they are incidental and peripheral to the organization, in which case they are shown after operating expenses have been subtracted from operating revenues to determine profits from operations.

Some health care managers would contend that fund-raising is incidental. It is not related to *why* the organization exists. The operating expenses should show the cost for the organization to provide care. The operating revenues should show the money earned by providing that care. The subtraction of operating expenses from operating revenues should show the extent to which the organization is able to stand on its own two feet. That is, it should show whether the organization is financially independent of gifts because it earns enough to cover its expenses.

Others contend that not-for-profit organizations routinely rely on contributions for part of their revenues. Such gifts are not peripheral or incidental but are essential to the continued normal functioning of the organization.

As a result of these contrasting views, financial statements prepared in accordance with GAAP may result in substantially different presentations of financial information by different organizations. Not only gifts and donations but also items such as rental income, cafeteria income, and gift shop income may or may not be included in operating revenues. This makes it difficult to compare the financial statements of different health care organizations. Over the last twenty years there have been many attempts to arrive at uniform reporting by health care organizations to improve comparability of financial statements from organization to organization. Because of the individual unique characteristics of each organization, these efforts have never succeeded.

Expenses are subtracted from revenues on the statement of revenues and expenses. Expenses are the costs related to generating the revenues of the organization. These include wages, patient care supplies, depreciation, administrative costs, and a wide variety of other types of costs.

Bad debts are shown on the financial statement as an operating expense. Thus the care provided to patients who ultimately do not pay the hospital, although they were expected to pay, are included as revenues. They are then subtracted as a bad debt expense. This contrasts with the accounting treatment for charity care. Most health care organizations provide at least some care to individuals who they do not expect will be able to pay for that care. Under the rules of accounting that went into effect in 1990 charity care is excluded from revenues.

A major controversy started in the late 1980s regarding the appropriateness of tax-free not-for-profit status of health care organizations.[3] The amount of

---

[3]For example, the cover page of the *New York Times* on December 18, 1990, carried a headline, "Tax Exemption of Nonprofit Hospitals Scrutinized." The article discussed congressional and IRS investigations of whether not-for-profit hospitals provided enough charity care to justify their tax-exempt status.

charity care provided is one piece of information that is critical for those interested in this controversy. Under the new accounting rules the amount of charity care provided must be disclosed, either on the financial statement in parentheses or in the notes that accompany the financial statements (see Chapter 6 for a discussion of such notes). It is incumbent on each health care organization to carefully define the difference between bad debts and charity care.

THE RECORDING AND REPORTING PROCESS

How does one develop financial statements? The statements are based on recording each individual event that has a financial impact on the organization, then aggregating that information, and finally developing a summarized form to convey it.

Journal Entries

When a financial event occurs, it is recorded in a *general journal*. The general journal is called the book of original entry because it is the first place that the accounting system makes recognition of the event. When the event is recorded, it is called a *journal entry*. The general journal provides a complete chronological financial history of the organization.

The entries are recorded in the journal using *double-entry accounting*. This term would seem to imply that the entry is recorded twice. That is not the case. Journal entries are made based on the fundamental equation of accounting. That equation begins the year in balance. Every financial event must leave the equation in balance. For instance, suppose that a patient pays the organization $100 in cash. How does that affect the financial records of the organization? Clearly, the organization's cash has risen by $100. But if we simply record a cash increase of $100, can the equation remain in balance?

Consider the impact on the equation:

$$\frac{\text{Assets}}{\text{Cash} \quad +\$100} = \frac{\text{Liabilities}}{} + \frac{\text{Fund balance}}{}$$

Cash has increased the left side of the equation by $100, but the right side is unchanged. The equation does not balance. The term double-entry accounting refers to the fact that whenever one change is made to the accounting equation, at least one other change must be made as well. In this case, suppose that the patient had just received the care. The $100 is revenue for the organization. Revenues represent an increase in fund balance. Therefore the change to the equation should have been the following double entry:

$$\frac{\text{Assets}}{\text{Cash} \quad +\$100} = \frac{\text{Liabilities}}{} + \frac{\text{Fund balance}}{\text{Revenues} \quad +\$100}$$

Suppose that the patient had received care two months ago and was just now paying for that care. At the time the care was provided the organization would have recorded the revenue because it was legally entitled to be paid for the care provided. At that time it would also have recorded an account receivable, an asset representing the legal right to receive payment. What would be recorded when the payment was received?

$$\underline{\text{Assets}} = \underline{\text{Liabilities}} + \underline{\text{Fund balance}}$$

Assets	
Cash	+$100
Accounts receivable	−$100

The left side of the equation has increased due to the receipt of cash and decreased due to the reduction in the account receivable from the patient. The equation remains in balance. Double-entry bookkeeping does not require both sides of the equation to change; it only requires the equation to still balance after the transaction. In this manner, any financial event can be recorded, leaving the fundamental equation in balance.

As a technical way to minimize arithmetic errors, accountants use *debits* and *credits* (abbreviated *Dr.* and *Cr.* based on the Latin roots of the words). A debit is simply an increase in an item on the left side of the equation. A credit is simply an increase in an item on the right side of the equation. Decreases are the opposite—for example, a decrease in an asset is a credit. The bookkeeping rule, debits must equal credits, is a way to help ensure that the equation is in balance.

For example, an increase on the left side of the equation and an increase on the right side will cause both debits and credits to increase by a like amount. An increase on the left side and a matching decrease on the left side will also cause debits and credits to increase by a like amount, since assets increase with a debit and decrease with a credit.

The use of debits and credits is a technical device and does not have any real substance. Nevertheless, because assets can either be debited or credited, depending on whether they rise or fall, as can equities, the technique is complicated. It is further complicated by the fact that the organization looks at the world from its viewpoint, while we generally look at the world from our own viewpoint. For instance, when we receive a debit memo from the bank, it reduces our cash balance. Therefore cash would seem to decrease with a debit.

However, cash is an asset, and assets increase with a debit. A decrease should be a credit! The seeming paradox is caused by the fact that we view the world from our perspective, not the bank's. When you have money in a bank, you have essentially loaned that money to the bank. The bank has a liability (right side of the equation) to pay you back. The bank issues a debit memo, meaning that it owes you less money. Its liability to you has decreased. When a liability decreases, the result is a debit. This views the world from the perspective of the bank. From *your* perspective, however, your asset has decreased. That results in a credit on your records.

The bookkeeping use of debits and credits is further complicated by the fact that the same term can mean something good or bad. If your organization provided care and received payment, that is financially good. Revenue (an equity) goes up with a credit. Therefore a credit is a good event. Cash (an asset) goes up with a debit. Therefore a debit is a good event. However, when you pay cash, the asset amount decreases. That is a credit, and is not necessarily good. The lay usage that a credit is good ("He's a credit to the organization") is ambiguous. (Is he a credit like revenue or a credit like money leaving our account?)

When journal entries are made, they are sometimes specified in detail in a *subsidiary journal,* with only a summary being entered in the general journal. For example, if the organization treats 100 patients on a given day, the many entries related to the revenue and accounts receivable from each patient may be recorded in the subsidiary revenue journal, with only a total summary amount being shown in the general journal.

Ledgers

Although the journal provides a complete permanent financial chronological history, it is somewhat cumbersome to use. If one wanted to know how much cash the organization had, one would have to go back to each journal entry, see whether it changed the cash balance, and sum all the journal entries that had an impact on cash. To simplify this process, accounting uses a set of *ledgers.*

A ledger is referred to as a book of accounts. Each page in the book represents a different item that we would like to keep track of or keep "account" of. When the journal entry is recorded, each item in the journal entry is *posted* to a ledger account. Posting means to copy over or transfer the item. Thus, when a patient pays $100 that had been owed for two months, in addition to the journal entry shown above, the accountant would also add $100 to the cash ledger account and deduct $100 from the accounts receivable ledger account. At some point if we would like to know how much cash we have, we do not have to go through all the individual journal entries. Instead we can simply go to the ledger and look at the balance in the cash account.

As with the journal, there are also *subsidiary ledgers.* Thus, the general ledger would not have a page for each patient who owes the organization money but rather one master account for accounts receivable. However, a subsidiary accounts receivable ledger would keep track of the balance owed to the organization by each and every patient.

In today's computerized environment, only smaller organizations (small home care agencies, for example) keep manual journals and ledgers. Instead, these records are generally maintained in computer files. Whether the accounting system is manual or computerized, journals and ledgers are essential tools for recording financial events.

Reporting Information

When journals and ledgers are maintained, it is a straightforward process to report the financial results of the organization. At the end of an accounting period, the accumulated balance in each ledger account is reported on the appropriate financial statement. Asset and liability accounts are used to prepare a balance sheet. Revenue and expense accounts are used to prepare a statement of revenues and expenses. The excess of revenues over expenses (i.e., the net income) represents a profit that is retained in the organization. It causes the fund balance at the beginning of the year to increase to its level at the end of the year.

The organization can generally choose a year-end date that is convenient. *Fiscal years* do not have to coincide with the calendar year. In some states there is a regulation that mandates a particular year end. Unless that is the case, most organizations choose to end their year when they are at a relatively slow time, so that the extra bookkeeping needed at year end does not pose an unnecessarily great burden.

The use of ledger account balances to create financial statements allows a tremendous number of financial events to be summarized. The financial statements in turn convey to the user information about the organization's financial condition and the financial results of its activities.

GENERALLY ACCEPTED ACCOUNTING PRINCIPLES

As noted earlier, accounting is a set of rules rather than a clear-cut science. These rules are generally followed by both *internal* and *external accountants*. Each organization has its own accountants who keep track of financial information throughout the year as it occurs. Those accountants are referred to as internal accountants. There are also accountants who work for separate certified public accounting companies. Those accountants are referred to as external accountants or external *auditors*. Many organizations hire certified public accountants (CPAs) to *audit* or examine their financial records once a year.

A CPA is someone who has been licensed by the state. Licensing as a CPA indicates a level of expertise in accounting and auditing. *Auditing* is a function that examines the accuracy and completeness of financial records. In an audit by a CPA the financial records of the organization are examined to discover significant errors, to evaluate the organization's accounting system, and to determine if financial statements have been prepared in accordance with generally accepted accounting principles.

Generally accepted accounting principles (GAAP) are rules established by an organization called the Financial Accounting Standards Board. CPAs are required to indicate whether an audited set of financial statements are in compliance with GAAP. Many health care organizations are required to have financial statements that have been audited by a CPA. Therefore, the majority of health care organizations follow GAAP. Here we want to introduce the reader to a few of the most common and important GAAP. These include:

♦ Entity concept
♦ Going-concern concept
♦ Conservatism
♦ Matching principle and cash vs. accrual accounting
♦ Cost principle
♦ Objective evidence
♦ Materiality
♦ Consistency
♦ Full disclosure

The Entity Concept

The *entity* is the person or organization that is the focus of attention. A large medical center that includes a hospital, nursing school, medical school, and long-term care facility is an entity. Accounting records may be kept for that entity as a whole. However, the hospital, nursing school, medical school, and long-term care facility are also entities. Financial records could be maintained separately for each of these subentities. When financial statements are prepared, it is important to identify the specific identity of the entity to which the statements relate.

All accounting transactions must take the perspective of the entity for whom the financial statements report. For example, suppose that we are interested in learning about the finances of the nursing school. Suppose further that the nursing school purchased some supplies from the hospital but has not paid for them. On the financial records of the entity we are looking at, there would be an account payable to indicate the obligation to pay for the supplies. On the records of the hospital entity there would be an account receivable because it has not yet been paid for the supplies it provided.

Going Concern

The second critical GAAP is that of the *going concern*. There is a presumption when accounting records are generally prepared that the entity is going to continue in business into the future. If in fact there is an expectation that the entity is going to go out of business, a special indication of that fact is required. The reason for this stems from the fact that assets may be valuable to an ongoing organization but have much less value if the organization goes out of business.

Conservatism

The principle of *conservatism* requires that the financial statements give sufficient consideration to the risks faced by the organization. Accountants tend to be optimistic pessimists. They assume that the worst possible events will take place. Then they can be optimistic because things tend to come out as good as expected, if not better.

In practice this means that losses are often anticipated, but gains are never recognized until they have occurred. For instance, suppose a health care organization owns stock in a for-profit company. If the stock falls in value, the organization must show the asset on the balance sheet at the current market value. However, if the stock price rises well above the amount paid for it, the organization can only show the cost of the asset on the balance sheet. This nonparallel treatment of potential gains and losses, which is referred to as *lower of cost or market*, results from the principle of conservatism.

The Matching Principle and Cash vs. Accrual Accounting

The simplest way to record revenues and expenses is on a *cash basis*. When cash is received, revenue is recorded. When cash is paid, expense is recorded. Unfortunately, this easy approach does not necessarily give a fair picture of what has happened to the organization in any given fiscal year. Suppose that we provide care to a patient who immediately pays the organization. However, our staff will not be paid their biweekly salary until the second day of the next year. The profit for the year will be overstated because it does not reflect all the costs of providing the care.

Consider further what happens when a building is purchased on the cash basis of accounting. The entire cost of the building would be an expense in the year we pay for the building. In that year the organization would show a huge loss.

To avoid such results that do not truly reflect how well the organization did in a given year, accountants rely on the matching principle, which gives rise to *accrual accounting*. The matching principle requires that organizations record expenses in the same year as the revenues they help to generate. Thus revenue and related expense are matched. Revenues are recorded in the accounting period that the organization becomes legally entitled to them. Even if the cash is not yet received, the organization accrues (i.e., accumulates or adds) the revenue to other current year revenue to find the total revenue for the year.

Accrual accounting helps to make the organization provide a full picture of current year activities. For example, vacation days that are earned this year, but not yet taken by year end, must be accrued. The vacation expense is recorded as part of the current year expenses because the vacation expense is a part of the cost of the labor that treated patients and generated revenue this year. Accrual accounting also gives rise to depreciation, ensuring that part of the cost of a fixed asset is recorded as an expense in each year that the fixed asset is used to generate revenues rather than all in the year the asset is purchased.

Accrual accounting is more complicated than cash accounting. However, because it provides a fairer picture of what has occurred for each year, it is required for most organizations.

The Cost Principle

The cost of any resource is the amount that the organization pays to acquire that resource. Assets are generally recorded on the balance sheet at a value equal to their cost.

There are some exceptions to this straightforward concept. For example, the principle of conservatism requires the use of lower of cost or market, as noted above. Also, depreciation allocates the original cost of an asset over a period of years. Therefore the net property, plant, and equipment value will appear on the balance sheet at a level lower than the original purchase cost.

The cost principle, seemingly innocuous enough, creates serious problems in the interpretation of balance sheet information. That is because over time the value of many assets may vary from their original cost. For example, land may rise substantially in value. Nevertheless, it remains on the balance sheet at its cost. This is largely the result of the principle of *objective evidence.*

Objective Evidence

The principle of objective evidence holds that information reported on financial statements should be based on objective, verifiable evidence. This is evidence that a wide group of different individuals could all be expected to agree upon.

For example, there could be considerable discussion concerning what a patient monitor is currently worth. Some might argue that it is worth what we paid for it. Others might contend that it is worth what we could sell it for. Another choice is that it is worth the amount we would have to spend if we were to replace it today. Yet another view would be that its value is based on the revenues it allows the organization to generate. Each of these perspectives has some merit. However, most of them are subjective measures.

How much revenue will a hospital generate because it has a particular patient monitor? That is clearly subject to speculation. We cannot know what future revenues will be. How much could we sell the monitor for? Again, a speculative question, unless we actually sell it, which we have no intention of doing. Accountants wish to avoid speculation because it makes it very hard to interpret financial statement information. Was the estimate of value made by an optimist or pessimist? It is much simpler to use objective, verifiable evidence.

As a result, accountants record the value of assets at their cost, since we can generally get agreement on the exact amount that was paid to acquire an asset. On the up side, the user of the financial statement does not have to worry about the introduction of bias in valuing the asset. On the down side, balance sheet information often is not a good measure of what assets are really worth. In many cases the assets that appear on financial statements substantially underestimate the value of the assets owned by the organization.

Materiality

The accounting process requires the recording of thousands, millions, and even billions of individual financial transactions. Practice has shown that it is generally impossible to undertake such a task and expect it to occur error free. In general, errors do occur in any accounting system, and to try to eliminate all errors would be extremely costly. Therefore, accounting systems are designed to try to minimize the number of errors.

How many errors of what size are acceptable? To answer that question, accoutants rely on the concept of *materiality*. Individual error, or all errors in aggregate, if not material in amount can be tolerated. What amount represents a material error? Is it $5, or $500, or $50,000? The answer to that question depends on a number of factors, such as the size of the organization. Accountants do not have a standard dollar cutoff level that can be arbitrarily applied to all organizations. Rather, they focus on the likely users of the financial information. An error in a financial report that would cause a user of the financial statement to change a decision is material.

Suppose that we expect the organization's financial statements to be used by a bank when it decides whether to lend money. Assets overstated by a small amount would probably have no effect on the bank's loan decision. If assets are mistakenly overstated by a substantial amount, the bank might lend money that it would not have loaned if it had known the correct level of assets. That would be a material misstatement of financial position. Therefore, accountants must decide what amount of money, in a given situation, is so large that it would likely affect the decisions of users of the financial statement. Then the accountant must attempt to ensure that if any errors of that magnitude occur, they are discovered and corrected before the financial statements are disseminated.

Note that the final financial statements are therefore not expected to be error free. They are only expected to be free of any material errors.

Consistency

In some instances, organizations have choices among alternative allowable accounting methods. The choice may impact on the balance sheet and statement of revenues and expenses of the organization. In such cases, the organization should be consistent in its choice from year to year. To vacillate would confuse users of the financial statement who might be attempting to compare the organization's financial performance from year to year.

Full Disclosure

Financial statements should be a fair representation of the financial position and results of operations of an organization, in accordance with GAAP. The principle of full disclosure is simply a catchall. This principle requires disclosure of any information that would be needed for the financial statements and accompanying notes, taken as a whole, to present a fair representation of the finances of the organization.

In the case of health care organizations, the principle of full disclosure would require that an audited set of financial statements include a balance sheet and statement of revenues and expenses, both of which have already been discussed. However, such disclosure would also generally require a cash-flow statement, a statement of changes in fund balances, and a set of explanatory notes. These items are discussed in Chapter 6.

FUND ACCOUNTING

Historically, not-for-profit organizations developed specialized accounting methods to deal with the unusual *fiduciary* nature of the organizations. A fiduciary is someone in a position of trust. The fiduciary of a not-for-profit organization controls assets that belong not to him but to the community. For-profit corporations can be expected to be closely monitored by the stockholders of the organization. Not-for-profit organizations have no owners, and therefore there are fewer "watchdogs" making sure that managers work to carry out the mission of the organization. The response to this problem was to divide authority, preventing any one manager of a not-for-profit from having excessive control over the organization and its assets. This divided authority was accomplished by using *fund accounting*.

Fund accounting is a system of separate financial records and controls. Distinct funds are established. Each fund has control over certain portions of the assets of the organization, and each fund has its own separate set of financial records. Typical health care organization funds include the *general operating fund*, which is considered *unrestricted* and can be used for any valid organization purpose. The other funds are typically *restricted*, and their assets can only be used for their stated purpose. These funds include the *endowment fund*, the *building fund*, and a variety of *special purpose funds*, which are generally presented in aggregate. Unlike board-designated restrictions, which are made by the board, and can be removed by the board, donor restrictions can only be removed by the donor.

Historically, a different manager would have control over each fund. This would, for example, prevent the chief operating officer, who was in charge of day-to-day operations, from embezzling the endowment fund. It would also prevent the comingling of funds (i.e., mixing together in one pot). That way donors could be assured that endowment funds would not be used to pay for current activities.

The name fund accounting is logical because the organization divides the resources or funds available to it into separate categories, called funds. The term *fund balance* then results from the idea that when the liabilities of each fund are subtracted from its assets, the remaining amount is the balance owned by the organization, or simply the fund balance. That is the term used in not-for-profit organizations for owner's equity.

Fund accounting is optional for not-for-profit organizations. It is acceptable for all the funds to be combined into one set of records the way for-profit organizations do their accounting. Many believe that fund accounting has become obsolete and perhaps even misleading. Segregation of endowment fund amounts can be achieved without keeping a separate set of records. Over the last half-century the use of separate fiduciaries for each fund has mostly been discontinued. For example, the chief executive officer of most organizations has substantial control over all the organization's funds. Nevertheless, many not-for-profit health care organizations continue to use fund accounting either to avoid change or because they believe that the separation of assets into distinct funds provides benefits to the organization.

The unrestricted balance sheet for the general operating fund would look the same as Table 5–1. Table 5–3 presents an example of the balance sheet presentation for the various restricted funds of a health care organization that uses fund accounting. Statements of revenues and expenses are not presented because only the general operating fund has a statement of revenues and expenses; the restricted funds do not. One criticism of fund accounting is that it is possible for income to go through a restricted fund and never appear on a statement of revenues and expenses. This would be the case if someone made a gift directly to one of the restricted funds. Users of the financial statements could never tell from the statement of revenues and expenses that the gift had been made.

There have been accusations that health care organizations use this loophole to have donations made directly to restricted funds. This makes the organization look poorer than it is to better solicit more donations. The extent to which organizations use this loophole to manipulate their financial statements

❖ **TABLE 5–3**

ABC Health Care
Statement of Financial Position
Restricted Funds
as of June 30, 1993
(000s omitted)

Assets		Equities	
Endowment Fund			
Current			
Cash	$ 523		
Long-term		**Fund balance**	
Investments	12,434	Permanent endowment	$12,957
Total	$12,957	Total	$12,957
Building Replacement and Expansion Fund			
Long-term			
Investments	$ 3,245	**Fund balance**	$ 3,245
Total	$ 3,245	Total	$ 3,245
Special Purpose Funds			
Current			
Cash	$ 523		
Accounts receivable			
(research grants)	124		
Long-term			
Investments	227	**Fund balance**	$ 874
Total	$ 874	Total	$ 874

is not known. In any event, recent accounting rulings have permitted the continued use of fund accounting.

IMPLICATIONS FOR NURSE MANAGERS

Basic accounting concepts are critical tools for nurse managers on two levels. First, nurse managers must be able to communicate with financial managers of the organization. Second, accounting provides information that is of critical value to nurse managers as they partake in helping to steer the overall direction of the organization.

The need to garner resources for nursing and to work with the organization to control the use of resources requires that nurse managers be able to communicate with financial managers. It is necessary for you to be able, at least to some extent, to talk their language. Many aspects of basic accounting become part of the lives of most managers. For example, journal entries are a common bookkeeping element that most managers become familiar with, at least on a mechanical level.

Going beyond that mechanical level and learning about things such as GAAP allows the nurse manager to comprehend why certain things are done, such as depreciating capital equipment. It should also serve to put many of the bookkeeping tasks nurse managers perform into their broader context.

Further, however, nurse managers must look beyond their departments to focus on what the organization as a whole must do to survive and thrive in a difficult economic environment. An understanding of accounting and financial statements is critical to being able to assess the financial position of the organization. That information in turn is needed to be able to participate in an informed manner concerning the critical strategic decisions faced by health care organizations.

Chapter 6 takes the nurse manager a step further in developing a capability to understand the organization's financial situation with a discussion of interpretation and analysis of information contained in financial statements.

KEY CONCEPTS ❖

Accounting   System to track financial events and provide information essential to undertaking the financial well-being and financial success of the organization.

Fundamental equation of accounting   Assets = Liabilities + Fund balance. Assets are the valuable resources owned by the organization; liabilities are amounts the organization owes to outsiders; fund balance, or owner's equity, is the portion of the organization's assets owned by the organization or its owners.

Balance sheet   Financial statement that presents the financial position of the organization at a specific point in time.

Income statement or statement of revenues and expenses   Financial statement that presents the financial results of the organization's activities for a specific period.

Depreciation   Allocation of a portion of the cost of an asset with a multiyear life into each of the years the asset is expected to be used to help generate revenues.

Journal   Book (or computer file) in which the financial events of the organization are recorded in chronological order, following the rules of double-entry accounting, which require every transaction to affect at least two different financial accounts, to keep the fundamental equation of accounting in balance.

Ledgers   Set of individual accounts. Information from the journal is transferred (posted) to the ledger accounts so that the balance in any account can be easily determined and reported on financial statements.

Generally Accepted Accounting Principles (GAAP)   Set of rules adopted by the accounting profession that facilitates interpretation of financial statements by users outside the organization.

Fund accounting   Optional accounting system used by not-for-profit health care organizations that establishes a complete distinct set of accounting records for separate groupings of the organization's assets. These groupings consist of a general unrestricted operating fund and a series of restricted funds set aside for specified purposes such as endowment or new buildings.

SUGGESTED READINGS

Audits of Providers of Health Care Services, American Institute of Certified Public Accountants, New York, 1990.

Beck, Donald F., *Basic Hospital Financial Management*, Aspen Systems Corp., Rockville, MD, 1980.

Berman, Howard J., Lewis E. Weeks, and Steven F. Kukla, *The Financial Management of Hospitals*, 7th edition, Health Administration Press, Ann Arbor, MI, 1990.

Cleverley, William O., *Essentials of Health Care Finance*, 3rd edition, Aspen Publishers, Rockville, MD, 1992.

Davidson, Sydney, C. Stickney, and R. Weil, *Accounting: The Language of Business*, 8th edition, Thomas Horton and Daughters, Inc., Glen Ridge, NJ, 1990.

Defliese, Philip L., Henry R. Jaenicke, Vincent O'Reilly, and Murray B. Hirsch, *Montgomery's Auditing*, John Wiley & Sons, New York, 1990.

Dominiak, Geraldine F., and Joseph G. Louderback, *Managerial Accounting*, 5th edition, PWS-Kent Publishing Co., Boston, 1988.

Ernst & Whinney, *Statements of Cash Flows, Understanding and Implementing FASB Statement No. 95*, January 1988, pp. 1–30.

Eskew, Robert K., and Daniel J. Jensen, *Financial Accounting*, 3rd edition, Random House, New York, 1989.

Finkler, Steven A., "Costs for Reporting vs. Costs for Management and Control: Hospital Implications," *Hospital Cost Accounting Advisor*, Vol. 3, No. 6, November 1987, pp. 1, 7–8.

Finkler, Steven A., *Finance & Accounting for Nonfinancial Managers*, revised edition, Prentice-Hall, Englewood Cliffs, NJ, 1992.

Guy, Dan M., C. Wayne Alderman, and Alan J. Winters, *Auditing*, 2nd edition, Harcourt, Brace, Jovanovich, San Diego, CA, 1990.

Horngren, Charles T., and Gary Sundem, *Introduction to Financial Accounting*, 4th edition, Prentice-Hall, Englewood Cliffs, NJ, 1990.

Levine, Summer N., ed., *Financial Analyst's Handbook*, Volumes I and II, 2nd edition, Dow Jones–Irwin, Homewood, IL, 1987.

Mark, Barbara A., and Howard L. Smith, *Essentials of Finance in Nursing*, Aspen Publishing, Rockville, MD, 1987.

Neumann, Bruce R., James D. Suver, and William N. Zelman, *Financial Management: Concepts and Applications for Health Care Providers*, 2nd edition, National Health Publishing, USA, 1990.

Short, Daniel G., and Glenn A. Welsch, *Fundamentals of Financial Accounting*, 6th edition, Richard D. Irwin, Inc., Homewood, IL, 1990.

Smith, Howard L., and Robert Chatfield, "Managerial Reports, Profits, and Quality of Care: Are They Related?" *Journal of Long-Term Care Administration*, Vol. 13, No. 2, Summer 1985, pp. 65–72.

Sorter, George H., Monroe J. Ingberman, and Hillel M. Maximon, *Financial Accounting*, McGraw-Hill, New York, 1990.

6

Analysis of Financial Statement Information

CHAPTER GOALS

The goals of this chapter are to:

♦ Introduce the techniques for interpretation and analysis of financial statements

♦ Explain the role and nature of an independent audit and the information available in an audited report

♦ Introduce and describe the statement of cash flows

♦ Introduce and describe the statement of changes in fund balance

♦ Discuss the types of information contained in notes that accompany financial statements

♦ Discuss how one assesses the financial performance of an organization, including the use of the statements, notes, and ratio analysis

♦ Provide definitions of common ratios and examples of ratio analysis

♦ Distinguish between financial statements and other management reports

♦ Consider the implications of financial statement analysis for nurse managers

❖

INTRODUCTION

Much of accounting is useful for any manager carrying out the day-in and day-out activities of an organization. Understanding the general financial status of the organization can help managers to better focus their department's efforts to help the overall organization. Additionally, as nurse managers work to gain a more central role in management of the organization as a whole, it becomes

115

important to be able to understand as much as possible about the overall financial well-being of the organization. Nurses want to become part of major decisions, such as whether to add or replace equipment and buildings, and the choice of how to finance such expansions. To get involved in broader issues than the management of a unit or department, it is absolutely necessary to be able to interpret and analyze information about the financial status of the organization.

The previous chapter discussed the fundamental concepts of financial accounting. The framework of accounting, terminology of accounting, balance sheets (statements of financial position), statements of revenues and expenses (income statements), recording and reporting accounting information, GAAP, and fund accounting were all covered. That provides a foundation for understanding the accounting elements of the organization. However, it does not provide the reader with the tools necessary to interpret and analyze the information that the accounting process can make available. Those tools are the subject of this chapter.

One of the most useful financial documents is the annual *audit* report. This report includes key financial statements, notes to the financial statements, and an opinion letter from an independent auditor. The information contained in an audit report provides a solid foundation for gaining an understanding of the historical results and current financial condition of the organization. This chapter will begin with a discussion of the independent audit.

An audit report includes the balance sheet and statement of revenues and expenses, which were discussed in the last chapter. It also generally includes a statement of cash flows and statement of changes in fund balances. Both these statements are essential for gaining a full understanding of the finances of the organization, and a discussion of each is included in the presentation of this chapter.

GAAP require that an audit report contain full disclosure of relevant items. To comply with that principle, audited financial statements include a set of notes that provides vital information in addition to that contained in the financial statements themselves. An explanation of the nature and typical contents of the notes follows the discussion of the statement of cash flows and statement of changes in fund balances.

All managers should first carefully read the auditor's opinion letter, the financial statements themselves, and the notes that accompany them to gain a thorough understanding of the organization's finances. In addition, the technique of ratio analysis is widely used to provide additional insights. This chapter focuses on several critical types of ratios.

Not all information that a manager might desire is in the audit report. Additional financial documents, called management reports, can be generated to provide managers with a wealth of additional data. The chapter concludes with a discussion of management reports and how they differ from traditional financial statements and with a discussion of the implications of this chapter's contents for nurse managers.

THE INDEPENDENT AUDIT

An audit is an examination of the organization's financial statements and supporting documents. Many individuals and businesses need financial information about the organization. This includes the organization's own managers. It also includes philanthropists, banks, bondholders, vendors (i.e., suppliers), and regulatory agencies. Users from outside the organization want to feel certain that they can rely upon the information contained in the financial statements. For this reason many, if not most, health care organizations engage a CPA to perform an independent audit of their financial statements.

There are a number of purposes for an independent audit. The first is to examine the internal controls that the organization has built into its accounting system to minimize arithmetic and other clerical errors and to reduce the chances of embezzlement or fraud. The second is to examine through sampling some accounting records to determine whether it is reasonable to conclude that material errors have not occurred, or to find them and allow them to be corrected if they have occurred. The next purpose is to determine whether the financial statements are a fair representation of the financial results of the organization in accordance with GAAP. The credibility of a health care organization's accounting information is often supported by the results of an independent audit.

When a CPA firm completes an audit, it issues two letters. One is the *management letter* and a second is an *opinion letter*. These letters are essentially the end product of what may represent months of detailed investigation.

The management letter is a letter from the CPA to the board of trustees or directors of the organization. It is generally not disclosed publicly. This letter discusses the strengths and weaknesses of the *internal control* system of the organization. Accountants test records on a very limited basis. It cannot be expected that accountants will uncover all frauds or embezzlements in their limited examination. Therefore it is important for the organization to have a system that limits the opportunity not only for errors but also for theft or fraud. In the management letter the auditor provides advice on how to strengthen the system. Also noted are apparent weaknesses that would cause the organization's activities to be inefficient, although that is not the main focus of a financial audit.[1]

The opinion letter is also addressed to the board of trustees or directors, but this letter is more often presented to interested parties, such as potential creditors. All internal managers have a stake in understanding how well their organization is doing. Therefore all internal managers should make a point of obtaining a copy of the opinion letter and audit report each year. An example of the opinion letter is presented in Exhibit 6–1. The opinion letter in the exhibit notes that financial statements from 1993 and 1992 have been audited. The tables in Chapter 5, for simplicity, showed information for only one year. However, it is general practice to provide at least two years' worth of audited information at a time so that the user can compare the previous year's results with the current year's.

---

[1] It is also possible to engage the CPA or other consultant to conduct an operations audit. Such an audit focuses not on the financial records of the organization but rather on the efficiency with which the organization carries out all the various tasks related to providing its products or services. While such an operations audit is beyond the scope of routine annual financial audits, it may provide the organization with a number of opportunities to improve the way services are provided.

❖ **EXHIBIT 6-1**
Opinion Letter

Report of the Independent Auditors

To the Directors
of ABC Health Care:

We have audited the accompanying balance sheets of ABC Health Care as of June 30, 1993 and 1992, and the related statements of revenue and expense, changes in fund balances, and cash flow for the years then ended. These financial statements are the responsibility of the ABC Health Care's management. Our responsibility is to express an opinion on these financial statements based on our audits.

We conducted our audits in accordance with generally accepted auditing standards. Those standards require that we plan and perform the audit to obtain reasonable assurance about whether the financial statements are free of material misstatement. An audit includes examining, on a test basis, evidence supporting the amounts and disclosures in the financial statements. An audit also includes assessing the accounting principles used and significant estimates made by management, as well as evaluating the overall financial statement presentation. We believe that our audits provide a reasonable basis for our opinion.

In our opinion, the financial statements referred to above present fairly, in all material respects, the financial position of ABC Health Care as of June 30, 1993 and 1992, and the results of its operations and its cash flows for the years then ended in conformity with generally accepted accounting principles.

Steven A. Finkler, CPA
date

The standard opinion letter has three paragraphs: an opening or introductory paragraph, a scope paragraph, and an opinion paragraph. Additional paragraphs are included if unusual circumstances require further explanation. Exhibit 6–1 represents an unqualified or clean opinion. That means that the financial statements are a fair representation in accordance with GAAP.

The opening paragraph describes what the auditor was hired to do. Many CPA firms provide a range of consulting services to health care organizations. This paragraph explains to the user that an audit was undertaken. It also explicitly points out that the health care organization's management bears the ultimate responsibility for the contents of the financial statements. Auditors are merely examining the statements that are management's representation and ultimate responsibility.

The scope paragraph describes in brief what is done as part of an audit of financial statements. This paragraph explains the type of procedures auditors follow in carrying out an audit, including complying with a set of generally accepted auditing standards.

The opinion paragraph describes whether the financial statements provide a fair representation of the financial position, results of operations, and cash flows of the company in the opinion of the auditor. An unqualified opinion, such as this one, indicates that in the opinion of the auditor, exercising due professional care, there is sufficient evidence of conformity to GAAP and there is no condition requiring further clarification. This is referred to as a *clean* opinion.

The auditor may issue an adverse, qualified, or disclaimer opinion if it is not possible to issue a clean opinion. An adverse opinion indicates that the auditor believes that the firm's financial statements are not presented fairly in accordance with GAAP. This is rarely issued; much more frequently management makes changes in the statements to bring them into conformity with GAAP. A disclaimer indicates that the auditor was unable to compile enough evidence to form an opinion on whether the financial statements are a fair representation in accordance with GAAP. A qualified opinion indicates that the financial statements are a fair representation in conformity with GAAP except as relates to a specific particular area.

In some cases the audit opinion letter will also contain additional paragraphs containing explanations. This is generally the case if there is a significant uncertainty or a material change in the application of GAAP. When extra paragraphs are included, the user should be alerted to the need to exhibit caution.

BALANCE SHEETS AND STATEMENTS OF REVENUES AND EXPENSES

Reviewing the auditor's opinion letter is the first step in the analysis of financial statements. Any unusual elements of the letter should be noted for later investigation. The next step is a careful review of the balance sheet and statement of revenues and expenses. These statements were introduced in Chapter 5.

It is important to read through each statement carefully. Are there any numbers that seem out of line, too high or too low? Are there indications of strength or weakness? Do things seem to be improving or getting worse? These two statements alone will be inadequate to gain a full understanding of the organization's finances. However, they provide critical information for starting to gain an overall picture of the organization's financial status.

THE STATEMENT OF CASH FLOWS

An audited report also includes a statement of cash flows. Recall that GAAP have a principle of matching revenues and related expenses in the same accounting period, the one in which the revenues are legally earned. However, the result of that principle is that the statement of revenues and expenses is prepared on an accrual basis. It reports the amount of revenue the organization is entitled to, not how much it has received in cash.

However, the flow of cash in and out of an organization is also critical. It is important to know how much revenue the organization is entitled to. But bills must be paid with cash. Knowing when the revenue is received in cash is critical. One must be able to know if there will be enough cash to undertake desired projects or purchase capital equipment, as well as to know if the organization has sufficient cash to be financially stable. Therefore, a statement of cash flows is generally required.

The balance sheet tells how much cash the organization has at the end of each accounting period. By comparing this balance from year to year one can

❖ TABLE 6–1

ABC Health Care
Statement of Cash Flows
for the Fiscal Years Ending June 30, 1993 and 1992
(000s omitted)

	1993	1992
Cash Flows from Operating Activities		
Collections from patients and third-party payers	$17,825	$16,232
Collections from other operating activities	1,919	1,432
Payments to suppliers	(2,122)	(1,876)
Interest payments	(2,333)	(2,290)
Payments to employees	(14,228)	(12,055)
Net cash from operating activities	$ 1,061	$ 1,443
Cash Flows from Investing Activities		
Transfer of earnings from endowment fund	$ 350	$ 350
Increase in sinking fund	(300)	(280)
Net cash from investing activities	$ 50	$ 70
Cash Flows from Financing Activities		
Payments of mortgage principal	$ (2,000)	$ (1,800)
Borrowing from bank	500	0
Net cash used for financing activities	$ (1,500)	$ (1,800)
Net Increase/(Decrease) in Cash	$ (389)	$ (287)
Cash, Beginning of Year	539	826
Cash, End of Year	$ 150	$ 539

see how much the cash balance has changed. However, that does not explain where the organization gets its cash or how it uses its cash.

It is possible for even a profitable organization to become bankrupt. Financial viability depends not only on whether revenues exceed expenses but also on whether there is enough money in the bank to pay bills as they become due. A major investment in equipment may appear to be financially sensible because over the life of the equipment a profit will be made on the treatment of patients using that equipment. However, in the year the equipment is purchased, cash may be needed to pay for the entire cost of the equipment, even though only one year's worth of depreciation will appear as an expense on the statement of revenues and expenses. The organization may not have the necessary cash.

The statement of cash flows provides information on where the organization's cash comes from and where the cash goes. This provides a substantially improved sense of what things the organization will have sufficient cash to undertake. Table 6–1 presents an example of what a statement of cash flows would look like. (Note that parentheses on a financial statement indicate a subtraction or negative number.)

For the most recent year, which ended on June 30, 1993, what does this statement tell the manager? The organization's receipts came from patient care and, to a lesser extent, from other operating activities. Cash used for operations went primarily into wages, supplies, and interest. However, note from the statement that cash also comes from and is used for investing and financing activities. For example, $350,000 of earnings on endowment fund investments were transferred to the operating fund. Note that the statement of cash flows represents just activities in the general unrestricted operating fund. Most of these transferred funds were set aside in a sinking fund for future replacement of plant and equipment.

It is also interesting to note that for hypothetical ABC Health Care, even though there was a positive cash flow of $1,061,000 from operating activities, the cash for the year declined by $389,000 from a starting balance of $539,000 to an ending balance of $150,000. If cash falls again by $389,000, the organization will run out of cash.

In fact, it would appear that the organization did run out of cash during the current year! Note that there was a $500,000 loan from a bank that was taken out during the year (cash flows from financing activities on Table 6–1). Why did this happen? In trying to interpret financial statements, the first question to ask is whether operating activities are self-sufficient. Is enough cash being generated from those activities to sustain their cost? In this case, the answer

❖ **TABLE 6–2**

ABC Health Care
Statement of Financial Position
as of June 30, 1993 and 1992
(000s omitted)

Assets	1993	1992	Equities	1993	1992
Current Assets			**Current Liabilities**		
Cash	$ 150	$ 539	Wages payable	$ 1,123	$ 1,018
Marketable securities	220	230	Accounts payable	2,430	2,575
Accounts receivable,			Notes payable	500	0
net of $436 and			Deferred revenue	300	0
$328 allowance for			Taxes payable	145	176
bad debts	2,319	1,722	Total current li-		
Inventory	832	342	abilities	$ 4,498	$ 3,769
Prepaid assets	46	52	**Long-term Liabilities**		
Total current					
assets	$ 3,567	$ 2,885	Mortgage paya-		
			ble	$ 3,560	$ 5,560
Fixed Assets			Bonds payable	20,000	20,000
Property, plant, and			Total long-term		
equipment	$43,470	$43,470	liabilities	$23,560	$25,560
Less accumulated			**Fund Balance**		
depreciation	17,356	16,085	Board-designated		
Net property, plant,			sinking fund	$ 1,737	$ 1,437
and equipment	$26,114	$27,385	Unrestricted fund		
Sinking fund	1,737	1,437	balance	5,195	4,675
Investments	341	341	Total fund bal-		
Goodwill	3,231	3,393	ance	$ 6,932	$ 6,112
Total fixed assets	$31,423	$32,556			
Total Assets	$34,990	$35,441	**Total Equities**	$34,990	$35,441

is yes. Even though overall cash is falling, and in fact a loan had to be taken out, there was a positive $1,061,000 cash flow from operations.

The problem appears to be caused by a $2 million payment of mortgage principal. The cash excess from operations was not enough to offset the large mortgage payment. Additional borrowing was necessary. From the point of view of an internal manager, the next important question is whether a similar payment will be required in the coming years and, if so, whether there will be sufficient cash to cover it.

The comparative balance sheets for the ABC Health Care general operating fund appear in Table 6-2. Looking at the long-term liabilities, you will see that at the current rate of payment, it will take nearly two more years to fully pay off the mortgage (i.e., $2 million of principal was paid in 1993, and there is still an outstanding balance of $3,560,000).[2] This is a disturbing fact. It means that if 1994 is about the same as 1993, it will be necessary to borrow another $500,000 from the bank. What if 1994 is worse than 1993?

Trends are extremely important in examining financial information. Is 1994 likely to be better, the same, or worse than 1993? Table 6-3 presents comparative statements of revenue and expense for ABC Health Care. Note from those statements that the excess of revenues over expenses fell dramatically from

---

[2]In actual practice, the mortgage liability would be split into two pieces: (1) the portion to be paid within the next year, which would be shown as a current liability under the title of "current portion of long-term debt," and (2) the portion to be paid more than one year into the future. Therefore the exact amount of mortgage principal to be paid in the coming year would be known by the manager.

❖ TABLE 6-3

ABC Health Care
Statement of Revenues and Expenses
for the Fiscal Years Ending June 30, 1993 and 1992
(000s omitted)

	1993	1992
Revenues		
Patient revenues	$18,230	$17,578
Other operating revenues	1,919	1,432
Total	$20,149	$19,010
Expenses		
Wages for clinical services	$10,325	$ 9,525
Patient care supplies and food	934	802
Housekeeping services	654	589
Operation and maintenance of plant	1,221	1,003
Administrative services	2,343	2,050
Depreciation and amortization	1,433	1,433
Bad debt expense	436	328
Interest	2,333	2,083
Total	$19,679	$17,813
Excess of Revenues over Expenses	$ 470	$ 1,197

1992 to 1993. The cash flow statement (Table 6–1) shows that net cash flow from operating activities fell nearly $400,000 from 1992 to 1993 (i.e., from $1,443,000 to $1,061,000).

Does ABC have a cash crisis now? No. It has cash in the bank. Is it facing a cash flow crisis? That may well be the case. Even though the organization has had only profits in the past and even though it generates a positive cash flow from its activities, it is rapidly draining its cash resources.

What response should be taken? That is a difficult question. ABC has a number of options. It could actively work to cut costs to allow the positive cash flow from activities to better cover its needs to repay the mortgage. Or it could refinance the mortgaged item, spreading smaller payments out farther into the future. The ability to do that would largely depend on the likely remaining useful life of the mortgaged property.

Or it could increase the *unsecured* $500,000 loan that had already been taken out. The organization could use its cash flow statement to show a bank, well in advance of a cash crisis, that there is a current need for additional cash. However, that need will only persist for several years until the mortgage has been completely paid off. At that point, the positive cash flow from operating activities can be used to repay the bank.

If the organization and its managers face the coming cash crunch in advance, a variety of options are open. However, without a document such as the statement of cash flows to examine and analyze, the organization might just think everything is okay. Then, one day, when the cash runs out and the managers have no understanding of why, the consequences may be far more severe, often leading to mass employee layoffs (and reduced patient quality of care) or worse. The process of analysis of financial position allows actions at an early stage when there is time to find the most palatable solution.

THE STATEMENT OF CHANGES IN FUND BALANCE

There is a fourth critical financial statement for health care organizations: the statement of changes in fund balance. It was noted in Chapter 5 that restricted funds do not have statements of revenues and expenses, nor do they have statements of cash flows. However, all funds have an additional statement, which is referred to as the statement of changes in fund balance. This statement reconciles the fund balance from the end of the previous year to the end of the current year.

This statement is extremely valuable because it shows the various items that cause the fund balance to change from year to year in each fund, *including* the restricted funds. For example, gifts made to specific restricted funds would show up here. Table 6–4 presents an example of this statement for the unrestricted and restricted funds of hypothetical ABC Health Care organization. For simplicity, the statement is shown for a period of only one year.

Each fund balance is shown at the start of the year, July 1, 1992, in Table 6–4. This is simply a carryover of the balance from June 30, 1992, the end of the prior year. The first item shown that increases fund balance is the excess of revenues over expenses. This is the profit or loss from the operating fund and affects only the unrestricted operating fund. This one number summarizes

❖ TABLE 6–4

ABC Health Care
Statements of Changes in Fund Balances
for the Fiscal Year Ending June 30, 1993
(000s omitted)

	General Unrestricted Operating Fund	Restricted Funds		
		Endowment Fund	Building Fund	Special Purpose Fund
Fund balance:				
July 1, 1992	$6,112	$12,242	$2,788	$584
Excess of revenues over expenses for 1993	470			
Restricted gifts		131	239	23
Earnings on investments		934	218	41
Restricted grants				226
Transfers between funds	350	(350)		
Fund balance:				
June 30, 1993	$6,932	$12,957	$3,245	$874

all the events from the statement of revenues and expenses. Since the restricted funds do not have a similar statement of revenues and expenses, all activities that affect their fund balance must be shown in detail in this statement of changes in fund balances.

The next item on the statement in Table 6–4 is restricted gifts. Note that unrestricted gifts for the operating fund would be shown on its statement of revenues and expenses and thus would have been included in the excess of revenues over expenses. The amounts shown on this new statement represent only gifts to the restricted funds. These gifts bypass the income statement and will never show up as revenue for the organization.

Earnings on investments appear next. In some cases a portion of the earnings of an endowment fund may be specified to be reinvested, in which case they appear in this statement. To the extent that endowment fund income becomes revenue immediately available for use by the operating fund, it becomes part of the revenues on the operating fund.

Restricted grants appear on this statement. These might include government contracts, research grants, or other grants whose use is restricted to a specific project.

The last item shown is transfers between funds. Transactions between funds are not uncommon. For example, when a building is built using money from the building fund, upon completion the building will be taken off the building fund and added to the operating fund fixed assets. This will have the effect of lowering the fund balance in the building fund and raising it in the operating fund.

NOTES TO THE FINANCIAL STATEMENTS

The purpose of financial statements is to convey information to the users. However, in most instances, the statements themselves are inadequate to provide complete information. Additional information is conveyed by appending notes to the financial statements. The purpose of these notes is to ensure a full disclosure of all relevant information needed for the financial statements to constitute a fair representation of the financial position, results of operations, and cash flows of the organization in accordance with GAAP.

Financial statements without notes may be inadequate for several reasons. In some cases, organizations are allowed a number of different choices of how to record and report financial results, for instance, how to report inventory. Two identical hospitals with exactly the same inventory would report a different asset value on the balance sheet and a different net income, depending on the accounting choice made for reporting inventory. A note must disclose the choice that was made, so that the reader can compare financial statements of different organizations on an informed basis.

Sometimes notes are required to disclose particular types of information that do not otherwise appear on the financial statements. For example, an accounting rule adopted in 1990 requires that financial statements of health care organizations disclose the amount of charity care provided by the organization.[3] This specific information may be of interest to users of the financial statements and in most instances would not be available without the notes that accompany the statements.

On occasion there is some important fact that the statements simply do not capture. For instance, a pending malpractice suit would have no impact on the financial statements. No payment or loss occurs until the case has been decided. However, a large potential loss may be of significant importance to users of the financial statement. Until the case is concluded, the lawsuit represents a *contingent* liability. There may be a liability or there may not; it is contingent on the uncertain outcome of the suit. Disclosure of such a possible loss is made in the notes that accompany the statements.

A typical set of notes begin with a summary of significant accounting policies. This is a general statement covering a wide variety of issues. The entity for whom the statements were prepared is described. Other information might include organizational policy with respect to charity care. Exemption from income taxes might be noted. Accounting treatment of donor pledges that have not yet been received in cash may be explained. Many other items of general background information may be contained as well.

Following the summary of accounting policies will be a number of notes on specific topics. Many organizations will include a note calculating the amount of charity care provided. The relationship between the organization and third-party payers is often intricate, involving the rights of the third parties to conduct their own audits and revise the amounts due. Such relationships often merit a specific note. The property, plant, and equipment information shown on the

---

[3]*Audits of Providers of Health Care Services*, American Institute of Certified Public Accountants, New York, 1990, pp. xiii–xiv.

balance sheet is often presented in a highly summarized form. More detailed information is often provided in a note. Malpractice issues, pension plans, and commitments such as future lease payments represent the most common types of notes. Other notes will also appear to explain unusual circumstances.

While the notes are sometimes quite involved and may seem peripheral to some readers, accountants believe that the information they contain is essential. To help convey that fact, each financial statement has a footnote on the same page as the statement referring the readers to the notes that accompany the financial statements.

RATIO ANALYSIS

In addition to a review of the financial statements themselves and the notes that accompany them, a third major component of interpretation of financial statement information is ratio analysis. A *ratio* is a comparison of the relationship between two numbers. This is accomplished by dividing one number by another. Sometimes the result is multiplied by 100% to convert it into a percentage. A number of examples will be given below. The comparison often yields insights that would otherwise not be gained.

In hospitals and other inpatient facilities, one of the most common ratios is not developed from financial statement information. It is the occupancy factor, which is the number of occupied beds divided by the total number of beds, multiplied by 100%. Suppose that a hospital had 150 occupied beds on average. Is that good or bad? Generally, the more beds occupied, the better from a financial perspective, for reasons related to costs, which will be discussed in Chapter 7. However, that still does not make clear whether 150 is good or bad. If the hospital has only 160 beds, then the occupancy rate is 94% (150 divided by 160 multiplied by 100%), which is very good. If the hospital has 300 beds, then the occupancy rate is only 50% (150 divided by 300 multiplied by 100%), which is not very good. The fact that there are 150 filled beds does not convey very valuable information. However, the ratio of 94% occupancy vs. 50% occupancy is more informative.

The issue of comparisons is at the root of ratio analysis. Not only is one number compared to another, but often ratios are compared to each other. A ratio by itself may not clearly be good or bad. Therefore, in ratio analysis one generally asks the question, "good or bad, relative to what?" The easiest comparison is of a ratio to itself for the same organization over time. Suppose that the current occupancy rate was 70%. Knowing that the occupancy rate for the last three years has fallen from 90% to 80% to 70% tells us something very different about the organization from knowing that the ratio has risen from 50% to 60% to 70%. In both cases the occupancy ratio is 70%, but one would draw very different conclusions about the status of the organization after considering the trends over time.

A second type of comparison is of the ratio for the organization to information for the entire industry. For example, the Health Care Financial Management Association has a financial advisory service that calculates a large number of different financial ratios for hospitals all over the country. A hospital can compare its own ratios to those of other hospitals throughout the country or region. Further, with that service hospitals can compare themselves to others of like size. Other health care industries, such as nursing homes, home care agencies, and nursing schools, have their own associations that sometimes generate ratios on an industry-wide basis.

A third focus for comparison should be to a specific similar competitor. Comparing the ratios for your organization with those of another organization just like yours can provide a number of important insights about differences. Investigation of those areas can yield important information for improving the functioning of your organization.

Before the specific classes of ratios are discussed, several notes of caution are appropriate. First, one cannot rely on the information from just one or a few ratios. Second, keep in mind that ratios draw information from financial statements that often may be misleading.

Any one ratio is much like one mosaic tile. One can tell very little about a mosaic from just one tile. A large number of tiles are needed to develop a pattern. It is quite possible for one ratio to cause a user to draw wrong conclusions. What if a health care organization is in desperate financial condition? As a result of severe financial losses, the organization sells one of its buildings. Immediately after the building is sold, the organization will have a large amount of cash. Ratios that look at liquid assets will imply that the organization is in an extremely strong financial position. With the building gone, however, losses are likely to become even greater. Only a thorough review can provide information on which to base inferences.

Ratios generally use numbers from the financial statements. Financial statements are prepared in accordance with GAAP. GAAP require assets to be valued at their cost. However, often assets are worth far more than their cost. Therefore, ratios that concern assets that have risen in value may be misleading to the user. Another problem is that GAAP allow choices of accounting method in some cases. When one prepares a ratio, the information concerning choice (which is generally specified in the notes) is lost to an extent. When comparisons are made of ratios from different organizations, it is difficult to take into account the differing accounting choices made by those organizations.

Except for the occupancy ratio, the ratios discussed here come from financial statement information. However, as you become familiar with the concept, bear in mind that a ratio is simply a comparison of one number to another. The ratios discussed below are not an exhaustive list. Many additional ratios can be conceived of and calculated. They may be financial, using information from the financial statements; they may be financial, but use information not available on financial statements (perhaps departmental budget information); or they may be nonfinancial, such as the occupancy ratio. Managers should attempt to consider relationships that can generate new informative ratios.

The five major classes of financial statement ratios are common size, liquidity, solvency, efficiency, and profitability. Each of these is discussed below.

Common Size Ratios

The first type of ratio is the common size ratio. Several typical common size ratios are defined in Exhibit 6–2. The goal of common sizing is to make an organization comparable to other organizations of different sizes. For example, the hypothetical ABC Health Care has $150,000 of cash at the end of June 30, 1993 (Table 6–2). Is that the right amount of cash? Organizations want to have neither too little (potential chance of inability to pay bills and bankruptcy) nor

❖ **EXHIBIT 6–2**
Several Key Common Size Ratios

$$\text{Cash to total assets} = \frac{\text{Cash}}{\text{Total assets}}$$

$$\text{Accounts receivable to total assets} = \frac{\text{Accounts receivable}}{\text{Total assets}}$$

$$\text{Current assets to total assets} = \frac{\text{Current assets}}{\text{Total assets}}$$

$$\text{Current liabilities to total equities} = \frac{\text{Current liabilities}}{\text{Total equities}}$$

$$\text{Total expenses to total revenues} = \frac{\text{Total expenses}}{\text{Total revenues}}$$

$$\text{Excess of revenues over expenses to total revenues} = \frac{\text{Excess of revenues over expenses}}{\text{Total revenues}}$$

too much cash (wasted investment opportunities). But how much is appropriate?

Suppose that XYZ Health Care has $300,000 of cash. Does that mean that ABC has too little or that XYZ has too much? Before that question can be answered, the cash balance must be viewed in light of the relative size of both organizations. A larger organization would be expected to need more cash for its activities. We are really interested in which organization has relatively more cash.

The common size ratio helps out by putting everything into perspective based on organizational size. Each asset is divided by total assets to find its ratio as a percentage of total assets. Each liability and fund balance is divided by total equities. Each item on the statement of revenues and expenses is divided by total revenues. Thus, cash for ABC is $150,000, compared to total assets of $34,990,000 (cash and total asset values are from Table 6–2).

$$\text{Cash to total assets} = \frac{\text{Cash}}{\text{Total assets}}$$

$$\text{Cash to total assets } 1993 = \frac{\$150,000}{\$34,990,000} \times 100\%$$

$$= .4\%$$

Dividing the cash by total assets and multiplying by 100% to convert to a percentage, we find that ABC's cash is four-tenths of 1% of its assets. Assume that XYZ has total assets of $15 million. Its $300,000 of cash would then be 2% of total assets. Assume that XYZ's 2% cash to total assets ratio has been fairly stable over the last few years. That is, it was about 2% in the prior several years as well as the most recent year.

We still do not know if XYZ has too much cash or ABC too little. However, now the relative portions of assets held in cash are known. This one ratio alerts management to the possibility that cash levels may be too low. This would tend to confirm some of the conclusions drawn from an examination of the cash flows statement. At the end of 1992, ABC's cash of $539,000 was 1.5% of total assets. From 1992 to 1993 the cash to total assets ratio fell from 1.5% to .4%. This downward trend over time further confirms the possibility that ABC is dangerously low on cash.

In a similar fashion, a common size ratio can be developed for each class of asset, liability, fund balance, revenue, and expense. For example, interest of $2,333,000 is 12% of total revenues (see Table 6–3, $2,333,000 divided by $20,149,000 multiplied by 100%) for 1993. For the previous year, interest was 11%. This rise is slight but might reflect the increasing dependence ABC has on borrowed resources. Again, a comparison with XYZ or with the industry, also showing trend information over time, would be useful.

Liquidity Ratios

One key focal point of any ratio analysis is an attempt to determine whether the organization has sufficient assets that are cash or will become cash soon to pay current liabilities as they come due. The common size cash ratio is one attempt to look at liquidity. In addition, a class of ratios focuses specifically on the question of liquidity. Several common liquidity ratios are defined in Exhibit 6–3.

The most widely used liquidity ratio is the current ratio. This compares current assets to current liabilities. Rules of thumb are often dangerous, since each industry and each organization within an industry have special circumstances. Nevertheless, a rule of thumb of a current ratio of 2.0 has become widely accepted. This would imply $2 of current assets for every dollar of current liabilities. The reasoning behind this rule of thumb is that current liabilities generally must be paid within several months. However, current assets may take longer to be converted into cash. For example, inventories must first be consumed in providing patient care to be converted into accounts receivable, and then accounts receivable may take several or more months to be collected.

❖ **EXHIBIT 6–3**
  Several Key Liquidity Ratios

$$\text{Current ratio} = \frac{\text{Current assets}}{\text{Current liabilities}}$$

$$\text{Quick ratio} = \frac{\text{Cash} + \text{Marketable securities} + \text{Accounts receivable}}{\text{Current liabilities}}$$

For ABC Health Care, using information from Table 6–2, the current ratios for 1992 and 1993 were:

$$\text{Current ratio} = \frac{\text{Current assets}}{\text{Current liabilities}}$$

$$\text{Current ratio 1992} = \frac{\$2,885,000}{\$3,769,000}$$

$$= .77$$

$$\text{Current ratio 1993} = \frac{\$3,567,000}{\$4,498,000}$$

$$= .79$$

Over this short period, the ratio was fairly constant. Often it is desirable to view ratios over a longer time frame, perhaps three to five years, to fully observe trends or patterns. Plotting ratios on graphs each year can be particularly helpful. For example, Figure 6–1 shows three possible five-year comparisons for the current ratio for ABC Health Care. Each one tells a story at a glance.

Assume that Figure 6–1B is the actual five-year history of ABC. While there is no clear trend here, the relatively low current ratio (as compared to a rule of thumb of 2.0) is cause for some concern. One would probably have a greater incentive to try to get some comparative industry data to see if this is typical of the industry (e.g., hospital, nursing home, home care agency) in which ABC operates.

Another widely used liquidity ratio is the quick ratio. This ratio, recognizing the time that may be needed before inventory is used up in the normal process of activities, looks at only those current assets which are likely to be quickly available as cash. These are cash itself, marketable securities (which can be sold immediately), and accounts receivable (which can be used as collateral for a loan if necessary). For ABC, the quick ratio over the last two years, using data from Table 6–2, would be:

$$\text{Quick ratio} = \frac{\text{Cash} + \text{Marketable securities} + \text{Accounts receivable}}{\text{Current liabilities}}$$

$$\text{Quick ratio 1992} = \frac{\$539,000 + \$230,000 + \$1,722,000}{\$3,769,000}$$

$$= .66$$

$$\text{Quick ratio 1993} = \frac{\$150,000 + \$220,000 + \$2,319,000}{\$4,498,000}$$

$$= .60$$

A. Improving trend.

B. No discernible trend.

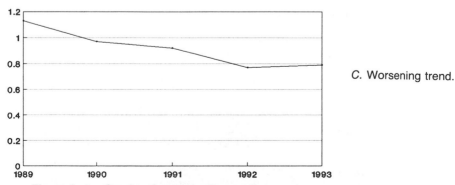

C. Worsening trend.

Figure 6–1.   Graphs of current ratio over five years.

These results are not dramatically different from those of the current ratio. However, there is a falloff in the ratio from 1992 to 1993 that might warrant further attention, especially in light of the other things that have turned up concerning the organization's cash flow. Keep in mind that the major focus of the liquidity ratios is on the ability of the organization to meet its obligations over the coming year.

Solvency Ratios

In contrast, the solvency ratios try to interpret the organization's ability to meet its payment obligations over a longer period of time, such as the next five years. Several common solvency ratios are defined in Exhibit 6–4. These ratios emphasize cash payments that must be made every year to avoid default. Such payments include interest and principal payments on loans.

The total debt to equity ratio is a generic ratio looking at long-term solvency. If this ratio rises to a high level, then creditors are supplying a substantial portion of all resources used by the organization. This in turn makes it more difficult for the organization to borrow further, if it were to become necessary.

For instance, suppose that a for-profit home care agency had $2 million in assets, $1 million of debt, and $1 million of stockholders' equity. The assets might consist of accounts receivable, inventory, buildings, and equipment. Creditors would perceive that there were $2 of assets available to protect every dollar loaned to the organization. Even if the organization fell on hard times, it could sell off assets to pay creditors. In bankruptcy sales, however, buyers know that the seller must sell. Therefore they often pay less than the assets might otherwise be worth.

In this example, even if each asset were sold for only half its balance sheet value, there would be enough money to pay creditors 100% of the amount owed to them. But what if there were $1,500,000 of debt and only $500,000 of stockholders' equity? Then each asset would have to be sold for three-quarters of its balance sheet stated value, not just for half, for creditors to recover their money. This means that creditors are less content if the debt to equity ratio rises.

Discontent on the part of creditors may block the ability to borrow, which in turn may generate a cash crisis. Therefore it is important to monitor and

❖ **EXHIBIT 6–4**
Several Key Solvency Ratios

$$\text{Total debt to equity} = \frac{\text{Current liabilities} + \text{Long-term debt}}{\text{Fund balance}}$$

$$\text{Interest coverage} = \frac{\text{Cash flow from operating activities} + \text{Interest expense}}{\text{Interest expense}}$$

$$\text{Debt service coverage} = \frac{\text{Cash flow from operating activities} + \text{Interest expense}}{\text{Principal payments} + \text{Interest expense}}$$

$$\text{Plant age} = \frac{\text{Accumulated depreciation}}{\text{Annual depreciation expense}}$$

control the debt to equity ratio. Total debt is equivalent to total liabilities. For ABC Health Care:

$$\text{Total debt to equity} = \frac{\text{Current liabilities} + \text{Long-term debt}}{\text{Fund balance}}$$

$$\text{Total debt/Equity 1992} = \frac{\$3,769,000 + \$25,560,000}{\$6,112,000}$$

$$= 4.8$$

$$\text{Total debt/Equity 1993} = \frac{\$4,498,000 + \$23,560,000}{\$6,932,000}$$

$$= 4.0$$

The rule of thumb commonly used for a debt to equity ratio is 1. That implies liabilities of $1 for every $1 of fund balance. In the health care industry, this ratio is often higher, typically going as high as 3. In both 1992 and 1993, the total debt to equity ratio is very high for ABC, as computed above. In 1992 there was almost $5 of debt for each dollar of fund balance. However, the trend is good. Although the ratio remains high, it has fallen dramatically. This is a positive sign. It would tend to indicate that the problems ABC faces are ones related to short-term liquidity but not necessarily to long-term solvency. On the other hand, due to the high level of the debt to equity ratio, it may not be possible for ABC to borrow in the short term to solve its short-term cash liquidity problems.

Examination of the interest coverage ratio provides information on the ability of the organization to meet its current interest payments. Often, failure to meet payments on interest creates the crisis that results in bankruptcy. The top half, or numerator, of this ratio consists of two parts. First, the cash flow from operations is taken from the cash flow statement (Table 6–1). Next, interest paid (also from Table 6–1) is added to this amount. This is because the amount paid for interest obviously was available for that purpose, in addition to the cash that was left over after all expenses, including interest, were paid.

$$\text{Interest coverage} = \frac{\text{Cash flow from operating activities} + \text{Interest expense}}{\text{Interest expense}}$$

$$\text{Interest coverage 1992} = \frac{\$1,443,000 + \$2,290,000}{\$2,290,000}$$

$$= 1.6$$

$$\text{Interest coverage 1993} + \frac{\$1,061,000 + \$2,333,000}{\$2,333,000}$$

$$= 1.5$$

The interest coverage is not particularly encouraging. The cash flow coming into the organization that is available to pay interest is only able to pay the interest due about one and a half times over. This means that if for any reason the cash coming into the organization were to fall by an amount equal to half the amount of interest itself, there might be a default.

This indicates a need to closely examine not only interest but also the required principal payments. The numbers for cash flow from operating activities, cash payments for interest, and principal payments can all be found on the statement of cash flows (Table 6–1). The debt service coverage ratio provides that information:

$$\text{Debt service coverage} = \frac{\text{Cash flow from operating activities} + \text{Interest expense}}{\text{Principal payments} + \text{Interest expense}}$$

$$\text{Debt service coverage 1992} = \frac{\$1,443,000 + \$2,290,000}{\$1,800,000 + \$2,290,000}$$

$$= .91$$

$$\text{Debt service coverage 1993} = \frac{\$1,061,000 + \$2,333,000}{\$2,000,000 + \$2,333,000}$$

$$= .78$$

The debt service coverage ratio paints a bleak picture for ABC. Apparently, to cover both interest and debt principal payments, the organization spends more money than it brings in. In fact, that has been observed to be the case. In 1992, the organization's cash fell by nearly $300,000. In 1993 not only did the cash balance fall by nearly $400,000 but in addition the organization borrowed $500,000 from the bank.

This would *not* appear to be a financially stable position. On the other hand, the large mortgage payments that were made in 1992 and 1993 would appear to continue only for about two more years before the mortgage is fully repaid as noted in the earlier discussion of the cash flow statement. The organization's managers, however, should be specifically taking actions to provide for the cash that will be needed to make those payments. Also, the $20 million bond payable must be examined. When is it due? What plans are being made to repay that principal? Even if the payment is not due for ten years, there should be a plan now on what actions must be taken to ensure that cash will be available to pay the bond liability when it comes due.

Care should be taken in interpreting these ratios, however. As noted before, any one ratio only gives a part of the overall picture. For instance, ABC owns some investments and marketable securities. These are worth over $600,000 and could be used to offset much of the cash shortfall during the coming year, if necessary. Also, the ratio analysis focuses on the financial statements of the general operating fund. However, ABC, as we have seen (Table 5–3, balance sheets for restricted funds), has considerable additional resources with relatively few liabilities. Therefore, there is a tendency for things to look worse for health care organizations that use fund accounting than is in fact the case.

Another focus of solvency ratios is on whether the organization is keeping its plant up to date. A failure to reinvest in physical facilities is often a symptom of an organization that is going to be in financial trouble in the future. Failure to keep facilities up to date often reduces the competitiveness of an organization, worsening the financial problems that caused it to be unable to keep its facilities up to date in the first place.

In the case of ABC Health Care,

$$\text{Plant age} = \frac{\text{Accumulated depreciation}}{\text{Annual depreciation expense}}$$

$$\text{Plant age 1992} = \frac{\$16,085,000}{\$1,433,000}$$

$$= 11.2$$

$$\text{Plant age 1993} = \frac{\$17,356,000}{\$1,433,000}$$

$$= 12.1$$

The accumulated depreciation (from Table 6–2) represents all the depreciation charged over the years on the organization's existing buildings and equipment. By dividing that total by one year's worth of depreciation (from Table 6–3) one can find approximately how many years the assets have been depreciated. It appears that the buildings and equipment for this organization have aged from about eleven years old on average to about twelve years old on average.

In other words, the plant has aged approximately one full year in the last year. That is cause for concern. It means that no significant updating of facilities or addition of equipment has taken place in the last year. If additional buildings or equipment had been purchased, the current depreciation would be higher because there would be depreciation on those new facilities. That in turn would make the ratio lower. The average age of plant would decline or at least rise less rapidly. In light of what is known about the organization's cash situation, this is not surprising. Nor is it a serious problem, unless it is allowed to continue for more than just a few years.

The average age of plant, which uses accumulated depreciation from the balance sheet and depreciation expense from the income statement, is another ratio that would benefit greatly from some comparison with specific competitors and the industry in general. Are ABC's facilities comparatively old or new?

Efficiency Ratios

Ratios can be used as an indicator of whether the organization is running in an efficient manner. This is done on an organization-wide basis. Organizations may have many inefficiencies. The ratio technique will not specifically identify particular inefficiencies. Rather, it can provide some overall measures to assess total relative efficiency of the organization. Several common efficiency ratios are defined in Exhibit 6–5.

The efficiency measure that tends to receive the most attention is days receivables. This is a measure of how long it takes, on average, to collect receivables. Once money has been collected, it can be invested and earn interest or used in some other beneficial way to aid the organization. While money is tied up in uncollected receivables, it provides no direct benefit to the organization. Therefore, generally one wants to keep the average collection period short.

To calculate days receivables, one first measures the patient revenue per day. This simply requires dividing the total patient revenue by the number of days in the year. If the total accounts receivable is then divided by the patient revenue per day, the result is the number of days worth of patient billings that are tied up in accounts receivable. For ABC,

$$\text{Patient revenue per day} = \frac{\text{Patient revenue}}{365}$$

$$\text{Days receivables} = \frac{\text{Accounts receivable}}{\text{Patient revenue per day}}$$

$$\text{Patient revenue per day 1992} = \frac{\$17,578,000}{365} = \$48,159$$

$$\text{Days receivables 1992} = \frac{\$1,722,000}{\$48,159} = 35.8$$

$$\text{Patient revenue per day 1993} = \frac{\$18,230,000}{365} = \$49,945$$

$$\text{Days receivables 1993} = \frac{\$2,319,000}{\$49,945} = 46.4$$

❖ **EXHIBIT 6–5**
Several Key Efficiency Ratios

$$\text{Patient revenue per day} = \frac{\text{Patient revenue}}{365}$$

$$\text{Days receivables} = \frac{\text{Accounts receivable}}{\text{Patient revenue per day}}$$

$$\text{Revenue to assets} = \frac{\text{Total revenue}}{\text{Total assets}}$$

In the health care industry it is not uncommon to take substantial periods of time to be paid for some patients, especially those covered by Medicare and Medicaid. Therefore the 35.8 average days until collection in 1992 would be considered a fairly good result. And without knowing the 1992 ratio, the 46.4 day result for 1993 would not necessarily be considered bad. However, the trend from 1992 to 1993 is not good. It represents a substantial deterioration.

It might be that this was caused by slowing of payments by insurance companies or Medicaid and Medicare. Such slowing may be beyond the control of the organization. Or it might be caused by lack of attention to prompt mailing of bills, accurate documentation of bills, or vigorous collection efforts. Such events should be within the organization's control. Ratios are quite limited. They cannot explain underlying events or causes. However, they are effective at alerting managers to situations that would seem to call for attention.

Another popular efficiency ratio is revenue to assets. This ratio tells how many dollars of revenues have been generated by each dollar invested in assets. It is foolish to waste resources. Therefore, it does not make sense to use far more assets to provide care than are necessary. If your organization generates $1 of revenue for each dollar of assets invested, while other organizations in your field generate $3 of revenue for each dollar of assets, it would seem to imply that your organization is not efficient in the use of its assets. For ABC,

$$\text{Revenue to assets} = \frac{\text{Total revenue}}{\text{Total assets}}$$

$$\text{Revenue to assets 1992} = \frac{\$19,010,000}{\$35,441,000} = \$.54$$

$$\text{Revenue to assets 1993} = \frac{\$20,149,000}{\$34,990,000} = \$.58$$

Without industry comparisons, these numbers tell relatively little. The increase from $.54 to $.58 would seem to be an improvement. However, one must bear in mind the fact that relatively little if any fixed assets were acquired this year. Thus revenues rose without the addition of assets. However, while that makes this ratio look better in the short run, it has other potentially negative long-run consequences. Once again we see that individual ratios cannot be considered by themselves.

Profitability Ratios

The last major class of ratios is profitability ratios. It was noted earlier in this book that it is appropriate for not-for-profit organizations to earn a profit. Even if profits are not part of the organizational mission, they are an essential element to accomplish that mission. Therefore, it is sensible to focus at least some attention on the success the organization has in earning profits. Several common profitability ratios are defined in Exhibit 6–6.

The first two ratios considered in Exhibit 6–6 are simply common size ratios. However, they focus attention directly on profits. The operating margin considers revenues and expenses before unusual gains or losses. That focus keeps attention on the normal day-in and day-out activities of the organization. How-

❖ **EXHIBIT 6–6**
Several Key Profitability Ratios

$$\text{Operating margin} = \frac{\text{Operating income}}{\text{Total revenue}} \times 100\%$$

$$\text{Profit margin} = \frac{\text{Excess of revenues over expenses}}{\text{Total revenue}} \times 100\%$$

$$\text{Return on fund balance} = \frac{\text{Excess of revenues over expenses}}{\text{Fund balance}} \times 100\%$$

ever, it also creates a difficulty with ratios and more generally with the use of financial statements. Financial statements are not uniform across organizations. Is a gift to the organization a normal operating revenue or an unusual gain? Some organizations treat it one way, while others choose to treat it the other way. This weakens the value of ratios for comparison purposes.

The operating margin considers of each dollar of revenues, what percentage is left as a profit before considering unusual items. The profit margin looks at *all* revenues, expenses, gains, and losses and measures what percentage of revenues is left as an excess of revenues over expenses (i.e., net income). Due to the problems with consistent definition of gifts as revenue or gains, it is important to place more weight on the profit margin than on the operating margin when interorganizational comparisons are made. For ABC, there were no unusual gains or losses, so the operating and profit margins are identical. Using data from Table 6–3, they are:

$$\text{Profit margin} = \frac{\text{Excess of revenues over expenses}}{\text{Total revenue}} \times 100\%$$

$$\text{Profit margin 1992} = \frac{\$1,197,000}{\$19,010,000} \times 100\% = 6.3\%$$

$$\text{Profit margin 1993} = \frac{\$470,000}{\$20,149,000} \times 100\% = 2.3\%$$

The profit margin has fallen off considerably. If this is simply a one-year aberration, it may not be important. If it represents a trend of declining profitability, it is important. A ratio such as this represents a warning sign that cannot be ignored.

Another important profit measure is the return on fund balance. Essentially, either the owners (of a for-profit organization) or the community (in the case of a not-for-profit organization) has invested valuable resources in the organization. When one compares the profit to the fund balance, one gets a measure of the financial return the community is earning from its investment. In the case of ABC the ratios are:

$$\text{Return on fund balance} = \frac{\text{Excess of revenues over expenses}}{\text{Fund balance}} \times 100\%$$

$$\text{Return on fund balance 1992} = \frac{\$1,197,000}{\$6,112,000} \times 100\% = 19.6\%$$

$$\text{Return on fund balance 1993} = \frac{\$470,000}{\$6,932,000} \times 100\% = 6.8\%$$

However, this ratio is only a part of the return to the community. The community additionally receives the benefits related to the health care services provided. One should exercise extreme care in using the return on fund balance (also called return on equity) ratio. It does not serve as a full measure of the benefits generated by the use of the assets invested in the organization because it ignores the health benefits to the community.

It is entirely possible to use a wide variety of additional ratios in each of the areas discussed above or to create other ratios. The essence of ratio analysis is to find two numbers that, when compared, yield some beneficial insight.

MANAGEMENT REPORTS

The financial statements generated by the accounting process are potentially of great value to managers of a health care organization. However, it should be noted that they are designed primarily with outside users in mind. They focus on reporting the financial history of the organization. By contrast, management reports focus on the future.

The role of management reports is to provide any information that can aid the manager to improve the organization's future results. Unlike financial accounting reports, which are limited by the specific rules of GAAP, management reports need only be useful. GAAP serve a purpose in providing a sound basis of comparability for outsiders to use. An outsider familiar with GAAP can learn much about the organization from financial statements prepared following GAAP. Internal users of information need not be limited by that desire for comparability or by an ability to understand an organization from the outside.

Another problem with the GAAP financial statements is that they tend to report in a highly summarized fashion. There is no detailed information by department. To operate efficiently, organizations assign responsibility to a large number of unit and department managers. These managers cannot control results without having information specific to their departments. Managers can use department-level information to calculate ratios. Those ratios can then be tracked over time to assess whether there is improvement or deterioration in financial results at the department level.

Therefore it is not only allowable but also desirable for internal managers to request a wide variety of additional financial information. It is possible to structure any set of reports that contain information that management believes would help in managing the organization better. Such reports need not follow GAAP. Throughout the remainder of this book, a number of different financial reports will be discussed that will aid the manager in the process of managing efficiently and effectively.

IMPLICATIONS FOR NURSE MANAGERS

Nurse managers should endeavor to obtain a copy of their organization's financial statements, preferably audited financial statements. There will often be a resistance to providing such statements. Information represents power, and often some individuals do not want to share power. "Why do you need those statements?" they may well ask. "Your concern should be with the management of your department." Yet how can one manage a department in isolation from what is happening to the organization as a whole?

Management of a department takes place within the organization. Often, restrictions are placed on salary increases or capital acquisitions. Are those restrictions justified? If they are, then the financial managers should be pleased to share the financial statements with you to prove how bad things really are. Doing so will be an excellent way to help rally all members of the organization in support of the organization in its financial crisis. On the other hand, if the hard times are really not so hard, then managers have the right to know that, too.

At the highest levels of nursing management, it is critical that the chief nursing executive be a part of the organization's top management team. That job should not be focused on running the nursing department. It should be focused on helping the organization make the correct organization-wide decisions. Understanding the finances of the organization is obviously critical to such decisions.

But even at the lower levels of nursing management, it makes little sense to try to manage in a vacuum. All members of the management team can be more effective the better they understand their organization and its finances.

KEY CONCEPTS ❖

Independent audit   Examination of the organization's financial statements and supporting documents by an outside independent auditor. The audit examines the organization's internal controls, searches for material errors, and determines whether the statements have been prepared in accordance with GAAP.

Opinion letter   Letter from the CPA indicating whether the audited financial statements conform to GAAP.

Analysis of financial statements   Review of the opinion letter, the balance sheet, statement of revenues and expenses, cash flows statement, statement of changes in fund balance, notes to the financial statements, and ratios related to the financial statements.

Statement of cash flows   Financial statement that shows where the organization's cash came from and how it was used over a specific period.

Statement of changes in fund balances   Financial statement that summarizes the items that affect the organization's fund balances for each fund from the beginning to the end of a specific period.

Notes to the financial statements   Supplementary and explanatory information; a critical element of an overall presentation of the organization's financial information. These notes are required to ensure that adequate and full disclosure of all relevant information, in accordance with GAAP, is made.

Ratios   Comparisons of one number to another with the goal of providing some insight or understanding of the finances of the organization that would not be realized from looking at each number individually. Ratios should be compared over time and also to the industry norms and to specific competitors.

Common size ratios   Comparison of financial statement numbers to a key number on the financial statement to take into account the relative size of the organization.

Liquidity ratios   Comparisons aimed at determining the organization's ability to meet its obligations over the coming year.

Solvency ratios   Comparisons aimed at determining the organization's ability to meet its obligations over the long term.

Efficiency ratios   Comparisons aimed at determining the relative efficiency of the organization's use of its resources.

Profitability ratios   Comparisons aimed at determining the relative profitability of the organization.

Management reports   Any report other than the four central financial statements, which are prepared to provide managers with information to aid in their management of the organization.

SUGGESTED READINGS ———————————————————

Audits of Providers of Health Care Services, American Institute of Certified Public Accountants, New York, 1990.

Beck, Donald F., *Basic Hospital Financial Management,* Aspen Systems Corp., Rockville, MD, 1980.

Berman, Howard J., Lewis E. Weeks, and Steven F. Kukla, *The Financial Management of Hospitals,* 7th edition, Health Administration Press, Ann Arbor, MI, 1990.

Cleverley, William O. *Essentials of Health Care Finance,* 3rd edition, Aspen Publishers, Rockville, MD, 1992.

Davidson, Sydney, C. Stickney, and R. Weil. *Accounting: The Language of Business,* 8th edition, Thomas Horton and Daughters, Inc., Glen Ridge, NJ, 1990.

Defliese, Philip L., Henry R. Jaenicke, Vincent O'Reilly, and Murray B. Hirsch, *Montgomery's Auditing,* John Wiley & Sons, New York, NY, 1990.

Ernst & Whinney, *Statement of Cash Flows, Understanding and Implementing FASB Statement No. 95,* January 1988, pp. 1–30.

Finkler, Steven A., "Costs for Reporting vs. Costs for Management and Control: Hospital Implications," *Hospital Cost Accounting Advisor,* Vol. 3, No. 6, November 1987, pp. 1, 7–8.

Finkler, Steven A., *Finance & Accounting for Nonfinancial Managers,* revised edition, Prentice-Hall, Englewood Cliffs, NJ, 1992.

Finkler, Steven A., "Ratio Analysis: Use With Caution," *Health Care Management Review,* Vol. 7, No. 2, Spring 1982, pp. 65–72.

Guy, Dan M., C. Wayne Alderman, and Alan J. Winters, *Auditing,* 2nd edition, Harcourt, Brace, Jovanovich, San Diego, CA, 1990.

Horngren, Charles T., and Gary Sundem, *Introduction to Financial Accounting*, 4th edition, Prentice-Hall, Englewood Cliffs, NJ, 1990.

Levine, Summer N., ed., *Financial Analyst's Handbook*, Volumes I and II, 2nd edition, Dow Jones–Irwin, Homewood, IL, 1987.

Mark, Barbara A., and Howard L. Smith, *Essentials of Finance in Nursing*, Aspen Publishing, Rockville, MD, 1987.

Neumann, Bruce R., James D. Suver, and William N. Zelman, *Financial Management: Concepts and Applications for Health Care Providers*, 2nd edition, National Health Publishing, USA, 1990.

Smith, H.L., and R. Chatfield, "Managerial Reports, Profits, and Quality of Care: Are They Related?" *Journal of Long-Term Care Administration*, Summer 1985, Vol. 13, No. 2, pp. 65–72.

United Hospital Fund, *Hospital Watch*, 55 Fifth Avenue, New York, quarterly.

III

COST ANALYSIS

One of the most critical areas of financial management is analysis and control of costs. Costs represent half the financial equation. The surplus (profit) or deficit (loss) of an organization each year depends on its revenues and its expenses or costs. Both elements—revenues and costs—require managerial thought and attention. Cost management has been an essential role of nurse managers at all levels for a number of years. Revenue management is an area of growing interest for nurse managers.

The first chapter in this part of the book, Chapter 7, deals with basic issues of cost management. The chapter introduces definitions of critical terms. The nature and behavior of costs is discussed. The relationship between patient volume and costs is stressed. Techniques are also provided for the prediction or estimation of future costs. Finally, the chapter provides a methodology to determine when a program or project or service will have sufficient volume to break even, i.e., to be financially self-sufficient.

The next chapter moves from basic cost concepts to the broader issue of cost measurement. There are two primary focuses of Chapter 8. One is how health care organizations collect cost information by cost center and assign that information first to revenue centers and ultimately to patients. The second is how to cost out nursing services.

In that chapter the Medicare step-down cost-finding and rate-setting methodology is presented and contrasted with more recently developed methods. Attention is also placed on understanding product-line costing. Issues of patient classification systems and staffing are considered. Standard costing techniques are also discussed.

Costing out nursing has become a topic of much interest to nurse managers. As hospitals are forced to operate in a constrained financial atmosphere, CEOs look to nurse managers at all levels to take a greater role in controlling costs. Financial reimbursement for nursing services is also discussed.

The last chapter in this part of the book addresses a concern that peaks during periods of nursing shortages but that requires managerial attention regardless of whether there is a current shortage of nurses. That is the issue of measuring the costs of recruiting and retaining staff. Chapter 9 looks at ways to measure those costs and to include them in the budget.

Nurse managers require a solid background in costing out nursing to understand the costs of their units and services. This will aid them in managing staff and other resources effectively. ❖

7

Cost Management

CHAPTER GOALS

The goals of this chapter are to:

- ◆ Define basic cost terms
- ◆ Explain the underlying behavior of costs and the importance of that behavior for decision making
- ◆ Provide tools for cost estimation
- ◆ Explain how costs can be adjusted for the impact of inflation
- ◆ Provide the tool of break-even analysis

❖

INTRODUCTION

Cost control is a major element of the job of all nurse managers. Understanding costs and their behavior provides the manager with the ability to understand the expenses incurred in the cost centers under their authority. The skillful management of costs is an essential element of the financial success of any health care organization. However, cost management is complicated.

Many cost terms commonly used are not well understood. Direct costs, indirect costs, average costs, fixed costs, variable costs, and marginal costs are concepts that managers use and must clearly understand. This chapter stresses the definitions of these and other key terms.

The relationship of fixed and variable costs, discussed in this chapter, is the most fundamental cost concept. The total costs incurred by health care organizations depend directly on the interplay between fixed and variable costs. Building upon those concepts is the issue of volume. Volume ultimately becomes a critical aspect of almost every successful health care organization and of every failing one.

Health care organizations are not static. They are constantly in a state of flux and change. Services are added to the mix offered. Other services are deleted. Some areas of the organization expand, while others contract. To a great extent these changes are dictated by clinical factors. However, with every change there is an impact on organizational cost. In each case managers should determine whether the financial impact of a proposed change will be favorable or unfavorable for the organization. While an unfavorable financial impact may not mean that a service must be deleted, a good manager makes decisions based on as much information as possible. An approach discussed in this chapter, called marginal cost analysis, is critical to generating information for such decisions.

Another important area of cost management is cost estimation. What will costs likely be in the coming year? That question requires careful management attention. This chapter provides several techniques to help in exploring that topic.

The last major topic covered in this chapter is break-even analysis. It addresses the issue of the volume of patients required for a program or service to become financially self-sufficient.

BASIC COST CONCEPTS

The most critical of cost concepts is referred to as *cost behavior*. Cost behavior is the way that costs change in reaction to events within the organization. If patient volume rises by 5%, what do costs do? What if patient volume falls 5%? How can one predict whether total costs will exceed revenues or remain at a level less than revenues? What factors are related to stable costs and what to rising costs?

Cost behavior depends on the specific elements of cost in any cost center or organization. A *cost center* is any unit or department in an organization for which a manager is assigned responsibility for costs. Some types of costs are stable, changing little, if at all, even in response to significant changes in patient work load. Other costs are highly changeable, reacting directly to other changes in the organization.

The goal of this section is to lay out a framework upon which one can develop an understanding of how costs behave in health care organizations.

Definitions

Cost measurement is more complex than one might expect. When someone asks what something costs, accountants have trouble responding with a direct answer. The reason is that the appropriate measure of cost depends substantially on the intended use for the cost information. Finding out what it cost to treat each patient last year is very different from calculating what it might cost to treat one more patient next year. The cost per patient when 100 patients are treated may be very different from the cost per patient when 500 patients are treated.

To make sense in the complicated area, all managers (nurse managers and accountants) must rely heavily upon a consistent set of definitions. These definitions provide the basis of a common language so that when a cost per patient is cited, all managers can interpret that information in the same way and effectively communicate with each other.

> **Service unit** A basic measure of the product or service being produced by the organization, such as discharged patients, patient days, home care visits, emergency room treatments, or hours of operations.

Cost information is often collected on a service unit basis. Managers need to know the cost per service unit. Within one health care organization, a number of different types of service units may exist. For example, the operating room may use hours of operations, while a med/surg unit uses patient days.

Direct costs
a. The costs that are incurred within the organizational unit for which the manager has responsibility are referred to as direct costs of the unit.
b. The costs of resources for direct care of the patient are referred to as the direct costs of patient care.

Indirect costs
a. The costs that are assigned to an organizational unit from elsewhere in the organization are indirect costs for the unit.
b. The costs within a unit that are not incurred for direct patient care are indirect costs of patient care.

Direct costs are a particularly difficult concept because their definition relates to the object of the analysis. If one were interested in the direct cost of patient care in a specific med/surg unit, that cost would not include the cost of the unit manager's time spent on administrative duties or the cost of clerical personnel in the unit. It likewise would not include the cost of a nurse restocking a supply cart. It would, however, include the cost of clinical supplies used as well as the cost of nursing time spent with a patient.

From a different perspective, however, all those costs cited in the previous paragraph are direct costs. That perspective applies when one is contrasting all the costs assigned to a unit or department. For the unit as a whole, all nursing salaries and clerical salaries incurred within the unit are direct costs. Costs assigned to the unit from outside, such as laundry or housekeeping, are indirect costs to the unit. Similarly, a portion of the salary of the chief nurse executive (CNE) and of nursing administration are indirect costs to a specific unit. However, from the perspective of the nursing department as a whole, rather than that of one unit, the salary of the CNE is a direct cost.

Laundry costs would be considered indirect by both the unit manager and the CNE. The labor and other costs of the laundry department are clearly incurred neither directly within individual nursing units nor within the nursing department as a whole, even though nursing may control the amount of laundry it uses. But that does not mean that laundry costs are considered indirect costs by everyone. The manager of the laundry department would consider all costs incurred in that department direct costs. Perspective is critical in the classification of a cost as direct or indirect.

Full cost The total of all costs associated with or in an organizational unit or activity. This includes direct and indirect costs.

For example, all the costs of a hospital would represent its full or total costs. Moving to the department or unit level, it is important to include not only direct costs but also overhead costs. Full costs include an appropriate share of laundry, administration, billing, engineering, medical records, housekeeping, and so forth. The question of what is an appropriate share of costs to assign to each cost center is difficult and will be addressed in the next chapter.

Average cost The full cost divided by the volume of service units.

Many questions faced by managers require information on the cost per patient, per treatment, or per patient day. This represents the average cost. Each cost center may use its own service units and calculate its own average cost.

Fixed costs   Those costs that do not change in total as the volume of service units changes.
Variable costs   Those costs that vary directly with changes in the volume of service units.

The salary of the CNE does not change day by day as the census changes. Therefore the costs of the CNE are fixed costs. Supplies that are used for every patient are variable. The more patients, the more supplies used.

The definition of the service unit measure is crucial in defining fixed and variable costs. For example, while most clinical supplies used in a hospital vary with the number of patient days, surgical supplies are more likely to vary with the number of surgical procedures, and clinic supplies will likely vary with the number of clinic visits.

Relevant range   The normal range of expected activity for the cost center or organization.

Fixed costs are fixed over the relevant range. Suppose that a thirty-bed nursing unit anticipated an average occupancy rate of 75%. It would not be unreasonable to expect the unit to have an 80% occupancy or even an 85% rate. However, a rate of 160% would clearly be beyond the reasonable anticipated rate for that unit. To accommodate that many patients, the hospital would have to add another nursing unit.

Within the normal relevant range, the costs for the salary of the nurse manager would be fixed. However, if the occupancy went to 160%, there might well be an expansion to two units, with a manager for each. The fixed costs would rise. They are only fixed within the relevant range.

Marginal costs   The extra costs incurred as a result of providing one more service unit, such as one extra patient day.

Marginal cost information is critical in the decision-making process. Managers are often interested in how costs change when the number of patients cared for changes. This differs to some extent from variable costs. Suppose that a hospital does not currently provide liver transplantation. What would be the marginal costs of adding liver transplantation to the hospital's range of services?

Since no transplants at all are done currently, it is probable that the hospital would need equipment, supplies, and personnel to provide that service. The supplies represent a variable cost. For each transplant done, the hospital will need additional clinical supplies. However, the equipment represents a fixed cost. Once the equipment is purchased, it will have the capacity to be used for many transplants. Since both the supplies and the equipment are needed to provide the first transplant, both the supplies and equipment costs are marginal costs of adding that service.

If one considers the total costs incurred by an organization before it makes a change and the total costs after it makes the change, the difference in costs represents the marginal costs of that change.

Mixed costs   Costs that contain both fixed and variable cost elements.

An example of a mixed cost would be electricity. The operating room uses some electricity every day to light hallways and for other purposes that are not related at all to the number of patients. That portion of electric usage is a fixed cost. Much of the electricity used by the department is used in the operating suites. The more surgeries, the more electricity used. Therefore it has a variable component as well.

Mixed costs create some problems for managers. If the number of service units for a cost center rose by 10%, one would expect fixed costs to stay unchanged. One would expect variable costs to rise by 10%. Mixed costs would be expected to rise but by some amount greater than zero and less than 10%. Later in this chapter methods will be provided for estimating the change in mixed costs resulting from a change in patient volume.

>   **Step-fixed or step-variable cost**   These are costs that are fixed over small ranges of activity that are less than the relevant range.

Often nursing units require a fixed number of nurses on duty for a range of patients. Within that range of patients, the nursing personnel cost will remain fixed. However, if the number of patients increases by a large enough number, additional personnel will be needed. That personnel level will then be fixed over a new, higher range of activity.

The key to step costs is that they are fixed over volume intervals but do vary *within* the relevant range.

Discussion of Fixed vs. Variable Costs

The total costs of running a department are generally divided into those costs which are fixed and those costs which are variable. The concepts of fixed and variable costs are often conceptualized with the use of graphs. In this example the service unit measure is assumed to be patient days. Figure 7–1 provides an example of fixed costs. Specifically, the graph shows the annual salary for a unit nurse manager for the coming year. The salary is $45,000.[1]

That salary is a fixed cost for the organization. The salary paid to a nurse manager is not dependent on any patient-volume statistic. In Figure 7–1 the vertical axis shows the cost to the institution. As one moves up this axis, costs increase. On the horizontal axis are the number of patient days. The farther to the right one moves, the more patient days the institution has.

Note that the fixed costs appear as a horizontal line. This is because regardless of the volume, the salary for the nurse manager will remain the same. Thus the cost is the same for 8,000 patient days, for 10,000, or for 12,000.

Variable costs, as noted earlier, vary with the volume of service units. Suppose that each patient's temperature is taken twice a day. If the hospital's thermometers use disposable thermometer covers, then one would expect use of disposable covers to vary directly with patient volume. Assuming that each thermometer cover costs $.50 and that two a day are used for each patient, then the cost of those items would be $1 for each patient each day. The more patient days, the more the cost for that disposable item in the total nursing unit budget.

Consider Figure 7–2. This graph plots the cost for disposable thermometer covers as they vary with patient volume. As in Figure 7–1, the vertical axis represents the cost and the horizontal axis represents the patient volume. Unlike Figure 7–1, which showed some positive amount of cost even at a

---

[1]This is a hypothetical number. First-level nurse manager salaries vary with geographic region, institution size, and institution type.

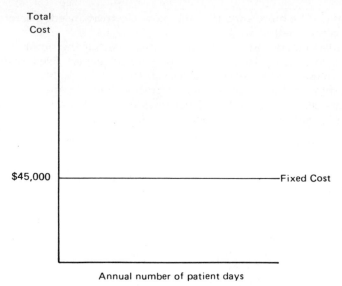

Figure 7–1. Fixed costs: cost for a nurse manager.

volume of zero, this graph shows zero cost at a volume of zero, since zero patient days implies that none of this particular supply will be used. The total variable cost increases by $1 for each extra patient day.

For instance, in Figure 7–3, dotted lines have been inserted to show the cost when there are 10,000 patient days and the cost when there are 50,000 patient

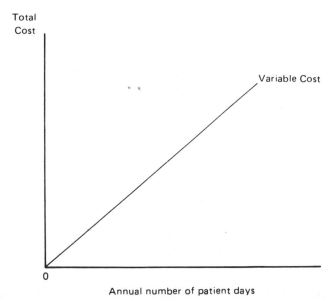

Figure 7–2. Variable costs: costs of a disposable supply item.

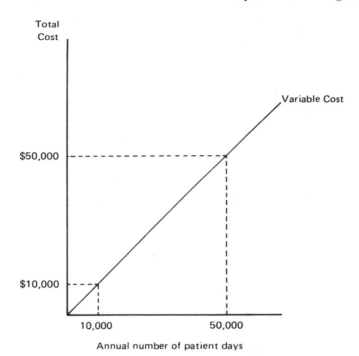

Figure 7–3.   Variable costs: costs of a disposable supply item at volumes of 10,000 and 50,000 patient days.

days. As you can see, $10,000 would be spent on the disposable item if there were 10,000 patient days and $50,000 if there were 50,000 patient days.

The total of the fixed and variable costs is shown in Figure 7–4. This figure combines the fixed costs from Figure 7–1 with the variable costs from Figure 7–2. Note that in the graph the total costs start at $45,000, even if volume is zero because of the fixed costs of the nurse manager.

Cost Graphs and the Relevant Range

One potential problem exists with this type of graphic analysis of fixed and variable costs. That concerns the *relevant range*. As defined earlier, the relevant range represents the likely range of activity covered by a budget.

Variable costs increase proportionately over the relevant range. However, it is unlikely that the hospital will pay $.50 for each disposable thermometer cover at *any* volume level. If purchases increase substantially, the hospital will probably get a price reduction per unit. On the other hand, if purchases decreased substantially, the hospital would possibly have to pay more per unit. However, the variable costs may reasonably be considered to increase proportionately over the relevant range.

It was noted earlier that fixed costs are not fixed over any range of activity. If a nursing unit had zero patient days, the hospital would close the unit and would not have any fixed cost for a nurse manager. If patient volume rose substantially and exceeded the capacity of the unit, the hospital might need

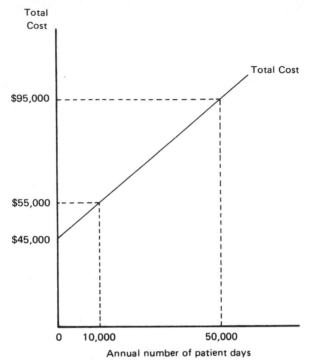

Figure 7–4. Total costs for unit.

to open a second unit and have the additional cost of a second nurse manager. The costs are, however, fixed over the relevant range.

Essentially, variable costs do not increase by exactly the same amount per unit over *any* range of volume, and fixed costs do not remain fixed over *any* range of volume. However, for most budgets, volume expectations for the coming year do not assume drastic changes in volume.

When fixed and variable costs are graphed, the relevant range issue is often ignored, e.g., costs appear fixed over all ranges of activity in the graph. However, the user of the graph should bear in mind that the graph's information is only accurate within the relevant range.

Many costs are *step fixed* and vary within the relevant range but not smoothly. They are fixed over intervals that are shorter than the relevant range. See Figure 7–5 for a graphic representation of step-fixed costs.

For example, staffing patterns may be such that a nursing unit will use five nurses over a range of work load. If that range were exceeded, the unit would have to use six nurses. Clearly, more patient days or greater average acuity requires more nursing care hours. However, if the staffing pattern is about 4.2 hours of nursing time per patient day, the unit would not expect to hire a nurse for an additional 4.2 hours every time the patient-day census increased by one.

As long as there is a staffing chart that tells how many nurses are needed for any volume of patient days, the presence of step costs does not present a major budgeting problem.[2] Generally, because of the use of overtime and agency nurses, a step-fixed pattern of cost is estimated by treating the staffing costs as if they were variable. While this will not give a perfectly precise result, it is usually a reasonable approximation.

The Impact of Volume on Cost per Patient

If a nurse manager were to ask what it costs to treat patients in the unit, accountants would probably answer that it depends. Costs are not unique numbers that are always the same. The cost to treat a patient depends on several critical factors. One of these is the volume of patients for whom care is being provided.

Suppose that a unit has fixed costs of $200,000 and variable costs per patient day of $200. Using this hypothetical data, what is the average cost per patient day? If there are 3,000 patient days for the year, the total costs will be the fixed cost of $200,000 plus $200 per patient day for each of the 3,000 patient days. The variable costs would be $600,000 (i.e., $200 per patient day times 3,000 patient days). The total cost would be $800,000 (i.e., $200,000 fixed cost plus $600,000 variable cost). The cost per patient would be $267 (i.e., $800,000 total cost divided by 3,000 patient days) per patient day.

However, what if there were only 2,500 patient days? Then the variable costs, at $200 per patient day, would be $500,000 and the total cost would be $700,000. In that case the cost per patient day would be $280. The cost is higher because there are fewer patients sharing the fixed costs. Each patient day causes the hospital to spend another $200 of variable costs. The $200,000 fixed cost remains the same regardless of the number of patient days. If there are more patient days, each one shares less of the $200,000 fixed cost. If there are fewer patient days, the fixed cost assigned to each rises.

Table 7–1 calculates the fixed, variable, total, and average cost per patient at a variety of patient volumes.

---

[2]Note that such staffing charts often give the volume of patient days, adjusted for acuity level. See Chapter 12 for a discussion of using acuity for staffing calculations.

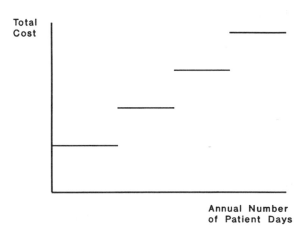

Figure 7–5. Example of step-fixed costs.

❖ **TABLE 7–1**
Fixed, Variable, Total, and Average Costs at Various Patient Volumes

Volume (A)	Fixed Cost (B)	Variable Cost (C = $200 × A)	Total Cost (D = B + C)	Average Cost (E = D/A)
1	$200,000	$ 200	$200,200	$200,200
50	200,000	10,000	210,000	4,200
100	200,000	20,000	220,000	2,200
500	200,000	100,000	300,000	600
1,500	200,000	300,000	500,000	333
2,500	200,000	500,000	700,000	280
3,000	200,000	600,000	800,000	267

Figure 7–6 shows the average cost at different patient volumes. The cost declines as the volume of patient days increases. This is because more patients are sharing the fixed costs. In Chapter 4 this result was referred to as economies of scale.

Suppose there were only 500 patient days. The total variable costs of $200 per patient day would be $100,000, and the total cost would be $300,000. The cost per patient day would be $600—more than double the previous cost per patient results at 2,500 and 3,000 patient days.

In trying to understand costs, it is critical to grasp the concept that because fixed costs do not change in total, the cost per patient or per patient day does

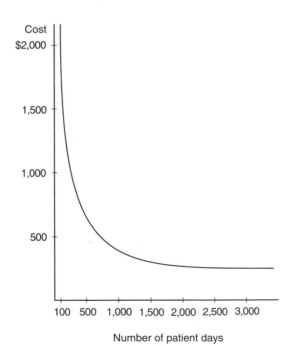

Figure 7–6. Average cost per patient day.

change as volume changes. The greater the volume, the greater the number of patients who are available to share the fixed costs. There is no unique answer to the question, What is the cost per patient day? That question can only be answered by giving the cost per patient day assuming a specific volume of patients. The volume of patients is critical.

One implication of this result is that health care organizations almost always find higher volume preferable to lower volume. As volume increases, the average cost per patient declines. If prices can be maintained at the original level, the declining cost will result in lower losses or higher profits.

Marginal Cost Analysis

Another costing concern is the issue accountants and economists refer to as *marginal cost analysis*. Decisions to change the volume of a service or to change the specific types of services offered should be based on marginal rather than average costs.

If someone were to ask the nurse manager the cost of treating a particular type of patient, the answer should be "it depends." The previous section has pointed out that it depends on the number of patients. It also depends on what the answer will be used for. If the question is just one of historical curiosity, the average cost is an adequate response. However, if the information will be used for decision making, that response may well be incorrect.

Suppose that the hospital was trying to decide whether to negotiate with an HMO to accept additional patients of the same average acuity and mix as the 2,500 patient days the hospital currently has. The HMO has offered $250 per patient day for 500 patient days. From the earlier calculations, the cost per patient for 500 patient days is $600! However, the hospital would not be providing only 500 patient days of care. It already has 2,500 patient days. From the earlier chart, the average cost is $280 per patient day at 2,500 patient days. At 3,000 patient days the average cost would be $267. Given that information, would it pay to accept the additional patients at a price of only $250?

It definitely would. Why should the hospital accept $250, if the additional patient days will cost at least $267? Actually the additional patient days will not cost at least $267. All the patients, on average, will cost that amount. The $267 includes a share of both fixed and variable costs. If the unit is going to treat at least 2,500 patient days regardless of the HMO negotiation outcome, then the fixed costs of $200,000 will be incurred no matter what. The fixed costs will not change if the hospital has the extra 500 patient days.

Decisions such as this one require *marginal analysis*. The "margin" refers to a change from current conditions. A patient on the margin refers to adding one more patient or reducing volume by one patient. Marginal costs are the costs for treating one more patient.

On the *margin* in this case, if the hospital were to take the additional HMO patients, it would have more variable costs but would not have any additional fixed costs (assuming that 3,000 patient days is within the relevant range). Each extra patient causes the hospital to additionally spend only the variable costs of $200 per patient day. That is less than the $250 the HMO has offered to pay. The hospital will be better off by $50 for each additional patient day.

The additional costs incurred for additional patients are often referred to as the *marginal, out-of-pocket,* or *incremental* costs. If fixed costs were to rise because the relevant range was exceeded, those costs would appropriately be included in the incremental costs along with the variable costs. The key element in marginal costing is that the only costs relevant to a decision are those which change as a result of the decision.

The decision may be to add a new service or to close down an existing one. It may be to expand volume (as shown in the above HMO example) or to contract volume. In any case where a decision is being made that contemplates changing patient load, the essential information to be considered is the revenues and costs that change. Effective managerial decisions require that the manager know the amount by which total costs will increase and the amount by which the total revenues will increase or, alternatively, the amount by which both will decrease. Costs that do not change in total for the organization are not relevant to the decision. Fixed costs generally do not increase when additional patients are added (within the relevant range), and therefore they do not impact on the marginal costs.

Marginal cost analysis is sometimes referred to as *relevant costing*. The concept of so-called relevant costing is that all decisions should be made based only on those costs which are relevant to the decision. The simplest way to think about this concept is to consider costs before and after a change. The only relevant costs are those which change as a result of the decision. The approach applies equally to revenues.

In the hospital-HMO example, suppose that prior to the HMO negotiation the hospital was receiving $275 for each of its 2,500 patient days. Total revenue ($275 times 2,500) was $687,500. Total costs were $700,000 (calculated earlier). The hospital was losing $12,500, the amount that the $700,000 total costs exceeded the $687,500 of revenues. If the HMO business is accepted, the additional revenue would be $250 times 500 patient days, or $125,000. The total costs for 3,000 patient days (calculated earlier) are $800,000. The cost increase of going from 2,500 patient days to 3,000 patient days is only $100,000 (i.e., $800,000 total cost for 3,000 patient days vs. $700,000 total cost for 2,500 patient days).

The total costs with the HMO patients are $800,000, and the total revenues are $812,500 (i.e., the original $687,500 plus $125,000 revenue from the HMO). The unit has gone from a loss of $12,500 to a profit of $12,500. The costs have increased by $100,000 while the revenues have increased by $125,000. The amount by which the extra revenues exceed the extra costs for the 500 HMO patients accounts for the turnaround from a loss to a profit. This should not be surprising. The extra revenue per patient day is $250. The additional cost per patient day is $200. The difference between incremental revenue of $250 per patient day and incremental cost of $200 per patient day is a profit of $50 per patient day. This extra profit of $50 for each of the 500 HMO patient days accounts for exactly the $25,000 profit from the HMO patients.

Had the hospital used average cost information for its decision, it would have turned away the extra business and lost the chance to gain a $25,000 profit. The $250 revenue is less than the $267 average cost. However, the average cost is not relevant for such decisions because it incorrectly assumes that each extra patient will cause the hospital to have additional variable and fixed costs. The incremental cost is relevant because it considers only the additional revenues and additional costs that the hospital will have as a result of the proposed change.

Relevant Cost Case Study

Assume that a hospital is trying to decide whether to perform liver transplantations.[3] The finance department has prepared a financial projection of the expenses for the service. It appears in Table 7–2. Which elements of that table are not relevant costs for the decision?

The first questionable item in the financial projection is the cost of the program supervisor. It is quite possible that one individual will in fact be given the responsibility for the liver transplant program. However, one must question whether a new manager will be hired just for that position, or whether the responsibility will be assigned to a manager who would be working on various other things in any case. Does the hospital actually spend more for supervisors if it has this program than it would if it did not? If the answer is that no more money is spent on supervision if the program exists than if it does not, then the cost is not relevant.

The costs of the staff in the operating room during the transplantation are probably relevant. By adding more patients, more nursing staff will be needed. The same is true of the technician. On the other hand, it is not clear that the secretary and orderly are relevant costs. The manager must assess whether the addition of the program will necessitate having an additional full- or part-time secretary and/or orderly. If existing staff carry a heavier burden with no staff additions, the costs are not relevant, unless additional overtime is incurred. In that latter case, it would be the overtime cost that was relevant.

---

[3]This discussion is not intended to be a comprehensive analysis of all the relevant and nonrelevant costs related to liver transplantation. Its purpose is merely to provide the reader with some examples of costs that are not relevant to a particular decision.

❖ **TABLE 7–2**
ABC Hospital Liver Transplant Program Financial Projections

Operating Expenses	
Nurse program supervisor	$ 50,000
OR nurses (RN: circulating, scrub)*	70,000
Technicians*	28,000
Orderlies*	14,000
OR receptionist/secretary*	24,000
Benefits*	40,000
Medical supplies*	120,000
Allocation of building depreciation	10,000
Allocation of OR equipment depreciation	20,000
Telephone allocation*	5,000
Office supplies*	3,000
Allocation of malpractice insurance and overhead not included above*	130,000
Total	$514,000

*Expense items assumed to vary directly with the number of operations.
NOTE: These numbers are hypothetical and do not reflect the true costs related to liver transplantation.

Allocation of building overhead is clearly a nonrelevant cost. The building will depreciate in any case. Unless remodeling was done to accommodate the program or unless the organization must acquire additional space, building depreciation should not be considered in making a decision regarding whether to offer the program. The same is true for equipment depreciation. Assuming that no additional equipment is acquired for the program, the depreciation would not be a relevant cost. On the other hand, some new equipment would likely be required, and the depreciation of any equipment specifically purchased for the program is a relevant cost.

Malpractice insurance is a peculiar item. In some hospitals it is based on past experience. In other hospitals it is based on the sum of the riskiness of the patients and services of the hospital. Liver transplantation has the potential to be a risky operation. However, the patients are aware of that. An assessment must be made concerning whether this program increases the risk of lawsuits and malpractice findings against the hospital. If so, then the malpractice insurance costs will probably increase as a result of the program, and the cost would be considered relevant.

Accountants may still argue that a portion of the nonrelevant cost items must be assigned to the program so that the full costs of the liver transplant program will be known. "All costs must be allocated to all activities to be fair, or else why should any costs be allocated to any activities?" Academics would argue that it is preferable not to allocate any costs rather than to allocate costs in such a way as to result in poor managerial decisions. If it is decided not to do the liver program because of costs allocated to it that are not relevant, then the accounting system is a hindrance to the organization's success. The analysis of the new program must allow the manager to know how much *more* cost the organization will have because it does the program than the costs it will have if it does not do the program.

Whether preexisting costs are allocated to the program or not, the important thing to keep in mind is that when the decision is made whether to have the program, it should be based only on the relevant costs.

COST ESTIMATION TECHNIQUES

One of the most difficult parts of financial management is the prediction of costs. This is an essential component of financial management. Budgets contain cost estimates. Trying to predict how much will be spent on each type of expenditure in the coming year presents great problems for both inexperienced and experienced managers. Yet managers must have ways to estimate such costs.

One approach is to simply look at what happened this year and predict that it will occur again next year, with an increment for inflation. At the other extreme is an approach that says it is desirable to do better next year than this year, so it is appropriate to budget a certain percentage less than was spent this year. In each case, the approach is far too simplistic. A priori, there is no reason to believe that next year will be just like this year, and simply wishing to spend less than this year will not make it so.

Some sort of clear methodology is needed that will allow prediction of what will happen next year based on the past. Some way to formally consider why that prediction may not come true is also needed. Finally, if costs are to be reduced below the predicted outcome, there must be a specific plan that the nurse manager believes can accomplish the cost cutback.

This section will consider several methods of cost estimation. Not all elements of the budget are simply costs. Items such as the number of patient days must be predicted as well. A discussion of general forecasting is presented in Chapter 17. Here the focus will be solely on prediction of costs.

Often, historical information about costs incurred in the past can be a great aid in predicting what costs will be in the future. This is especially true in the case of mixed costs, which have both fixed and variable cost elements. Cost estimation techniques exist that look at historical information and compare the change in cost over time with the change in volume over time to isolate fixed and variable costs.

If costs rise as volume rises, what could account for the increase in costs? Fixed costs, by definition, do not change as volume changes. Therefore, any change in cost as volume changes must be attributable to the variable cost. By seeing how much costs change for a change in volume, it is possible to calculate the variable cost per unit. Once the variable cost per unit is known, the total variable cost for any volume can be determined by multiplying the variable cost per unit by the volume. Then fixed cost can be determined as well. The difference between the total cost for any volume and the total variable cost for that volume is the fixed cost. The fixed and variable cost information can then be used to estimate costs for the coming year, based on a forecast of the volume in the coming year.

There is one critical problem in the flow of logic that allows cost estimation. Changes in cost over time are assumed to be the result only of changes in volume. However, to some extent changes in cost over time are the result of other changes. One possible type of change is evolving clinical practice. For example, lithotripsy may require more IV solutions than a unit needed before its patients had access to that technology. Managers should always adjust any estimates they make for the impact of any changes that they anticipate.

Another problem is inflation. If inflation were a constant percent that was the same each year, one could argue that past inflation could be ignored and inflation would automatically be built into predictions for the future. However, inflation rates tend to fluctuate from year to year. Over a period of years the fluctuations can be substantial. Therefore, to be able to predict fixed and variable costs, the data should be free from the impact of inflation.

Adjusting Costs for Inflation

Suppose that a nurse manager is interested in determining how much the total RN staff costs of the unit will be for the coming fiscal year, 1994.[4] This hypothetical unit is staffed with a minimum of ten full-time equivalents (FTEs) for any volume up to 9,000 patient days at a certain acuity level. The cost of those ten FTEs is fixed because the unit will always have at least that cost. As volume increases above 9,000 patient days, additional nursing time will be needed. In 1992 patient days numbered 9,800 and the cost including fringe benefits was $500,000. In 1993 the patient days totaled 11,000 and the cost was

---

[4]A fiscal year may have a starting point at any convenient date, not necessarily January 1. For example, a fiscal year could begin on July 1 and end on June 30. In that case, fiscal year 1994 would refer to the year from July 1,1993, through June 30, 1994.

$580,000. The cost increase of $80,000 was attributable to both the increased volume and inflation.

Most readers are probably familiar with the consumer price index (CPI). That is the most widely used measure of inflation. The CPI and many other indexes of inflation, such as the hospital market basket index, were developed by or for the federal government. The CPI measures the relative cost of a typical basket of consumer goods. Whatever the basket of goods cost in the base year was considered to be 100% of the cost in that year, or simply 100. The index is revised and a new base year established from time to time. If it costs twice as much to buy the same goods in a year subsequent to the base year, then the index would be 200% of the base year costs, or simply 200.

The U.S. Department of Commerce, Bureau of the Census, annually publishes the Statistical Abstract of the United States. Included in that book are "Indexes of Medical Care Prices." There are several quite useful indexes under that heading, including the index of medical care services and the hospital daily room rate index.

In this example, the nurse manager wants to find the variable cost per patient day of nursing labor for 1994, using current dollars as of the end of fiscal year 1993. If information from 1989 through 1993 is used, the nurse manager would have to find the value of an appropriate index in each of those years. The financial managers in most health care institutions can provide nurse managers with appropriate indexes adjusted for labor costs in the specific geographical area. Failing that, most library reference sections can be of assistance with current index information. Assume that an appropriate index has values as follows:

1989:	258
1990:	287
1991:	318
1992:	357
1993:	395

Suppose also that the following cost and volume information is available:

Year	Patient Days	Cost
1989	8,000	$328,000
1990	8,700	364,000
1991	8,850	404,000
1992	9,800	500,000
1993	11,000	580,000

It appears that costs have risen from 1989 to 1991 even though volume is below 9,000 patient days in each of those years. Because the staffing is fixed at ten FTEs for any volume below 9,000 patient days, the cost is expected to be about the same in each of those three years and to increase only as volume increases above 9,000 patient days, thus requiring more nursing staff. The cost information, however, is not comparable because of the impact of inflation. To make the numbers reasonable for comparison purposes, they must be restated in *constant dollars*, i.e., amounts that have been adjusted for the impact of inflation.

That adjustment can be done by multiplying the cost in any given year by a fraction that represents the current value of the index divided by the value of the index in the year the cost was incurred. This is not a complicated procedure. For example, in 1989 the cost was $328,000. The hypothetical index value is 395 for fiscal year 1993. In 1989 it was 258. Multiply $328,000 by the fraction 395/258. The result is $502,171, which is the 1989 cost adjusted to 1993 dollars. Now the $580,000 spent when there were 11,000 patient days in 1993 can be compared to $502,171, the constant-dollar cost of 8,000 patient days in 1989. In a similar fashion all the data can be restated into 1993 dollars as in Table 7-3.

Inflation accounts for changes in prices. One example of a change in prices is a change in wages. Wage rates are the price an organization pays for labor. From 1989 through 1991 nursing salaries rose substantially, largely as the result of a nationwide shortage of nurses. Note that adjusted for inflation, there was very little change in costs from 1989 to 1991, the period during which the staffing was fixed because patient days were less than 9,000. However, the actual dollars spent in those years, before adjusting for inflation, rose from $328,000 to $404,000. Such an increase might at least partly reflect the impact of rising nursing salaries.

High-Low Cost Estimation

The high-low approach is a relatively simple, quick-and-dirty approach to cost estimation. It is unsophisticated and therefore not terribly accurate, but in many cases it may be good enough. It certainly is better than simply taking a guess.

The key to the high-low method is the fact that fixed costs do not change at all in response to changes in volume. The way the method works is to look at the organization's cost for a specific item over a period of approximately five years. Costs adjusted for inflation should be used, as described above.

The use of five years is arbitrary. It might be more appropriate to use a longer period, but one would not want to use data from much less than five years. Less than five years should be used only if there have been substantial changes in the unit that would make earlier data no longer relevant. For the period chosen, find the highest volume and the lowest volume and compare the costs at these two volumes.

The amount by which the costs changed from the lowest to highest volume should be compared to the amount by which the volume changed. In the example from the previous section, the highest volume in the last five years was 11,000 patient days and the cost for nursing labor that year for the de-

❖ **TABLE 7–3**
Adjusting Costs for Inflation

Year	Patient Days	Original Cost		Index Fraction		Adjusted Cost
1989	8,000	$328,000	×	395/258	=	$502,171
1990	8,700	364,000	×	395/287	=	500,976
1991	8,850	404,000	×	395/318	=	501,824
1992	9,800	500,000	×	395/357	=	553,221
1993	11,000	580,000	×	395/395	=	580,000

These index values are hypothetical. Managers should consult with their organization's financial managers for an appropriate inflation index and its actual values for their specific geographical region.

partment was $580,000. The lowest volume in the last five years was 8,000 patient days and the constant dollar inflation adjusted cost in that year was $502,171. In this case, inflation-adjusted costs increased by $77,829, while volume increased by 3,000 patient days. If $77,829 is divided by 3,000 patient days, the result is $25.94 per patient day. Although it is certainly likely that nursing labor is a step-fixed cost and therefore will not go up by $25.94 for *each* additional patient day, that volume provides a reasonable measure of the amount of additional nursing services needed per patient day when there are significant changes in volume.

If the variable cost per patient day is $25.94, then what is the fixed cost? The yearly total variable is first found by multiplying the variable cost per patient day by the number of patient days ($25.94 × 8,000 = $207,544). The total nursing labor cost for 8,000 patient days was $502,171 in 1989; if $207,544 is the variable cost, then the remainder, $294,627, represents the fixed cost. Similarly, for 11,000 patient days at $25.94 per patient day, the variable cost is $285,373; given a total cost of $580,000 in 1993, the fixed cost would be $294,627. The fixed cost is expected to be the same at either volume level, since by definition it is fixed.

This fixed and variable cost information can be used in preparing next year's budget. If 12,000 patient days are expected, then costs would be expected to rise by $25.94 times 1,000 patient days, or $25,943. The fixed cost portion will not change. Since this information has been calculated using 1993 constant dollars, both the fixed and variable costs would have to be adjusted upward for the expected 1994 salary increases or, more generally, for the expected impact of inflation during the next year.

The high-low method is not terribly accurate because it only considers the experience of two years. One or both of the two years chosen may have had some unusual circumstance that would skew the costs in that year. A superior prediction is possible if some method is used that takes more experience into account. *Regression analysis* is a method that can provide such a prediction.

Regression Analysis

The volume of patient days and the total cost for those days for a number of years can be plotted on a graph. The horizontal axis would represent the volume, and the vertical axis would represent the cost. The result would be a scatter diagram. The series of points on the graph would each represent a volume and the cost at that volume. If a line were drawn through the points, it could be used for future predictions. By selecting any expected volume on the horizontal axis, it would be possible to go vertically up to the line and then from the line move horizontally across to a point on a vertical cost axis. That point would represent the prediction of cost. For example, Figure 7–7 shows a scatter diagram with a line drawn through these points.

The difficulty in drawing the diagonal line connecting those points is properly placing it so that it will give accurate predictions. Regression analysis is a technique that applies mathematical precision to a scatter diagram. Regression technique can select the one line that is effectively closest to all the individual points on the scatter diagram and that will therefore best predict cost for the future. This can fairly accurately break costs down into their fixed and variable components.

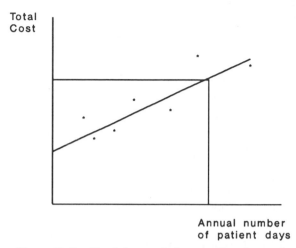

Total
Cost

Annual number
of patient days

Figure 7–7.   Predicting costs from scatter diagram.

Simple linear regression analysis can take all available past information into account in estimating that portion of any cost which is fixed and that portion which is variable. The phrase simple linear regression refers to several issues. First, it is simple in the sense that there is only one *dependent* variable and one *independent* variable. Cost is the dependent variable that is being estimated. Cost depends on the value of the independent variable.

An independent variable is a *causal* factor. For example, the most significant causal factor for nursing costs might be patient days. The more patient days, the greater the costs for nursing. Patient days *cause* costs to be incurred. For the admissions department of the hospital, it would not be patient days but rather the number of patients that is important, since admission time is the same for each patient regardless of the ultimate length of stay.

The second part of the phrase simple linear regression refers to the presumption that cost behavior can be shown in a linear fashion, that is, using a straight line. What if a slightly lower price per disposable supply unit was paid for every increase in volume (e.g., $.75 for one unit, $.7499 per unit for two units, $.74998 per unit for three units, and so on)? In that case, Figure 7–2 would not be an accurate reflection of how variable costs change. It would be necessary to draw a curved line in the graph, but the mathematics involved with curved lines instead of straight lines are far more complicated. Variable costs are generally treated as if they were linear even if that is only an approximation of their true behavior.

Finally, the term regression refers to trying to regress, or bring all the points from the scatter diagram as close as possible to the estimated line.

For example, suppose that the CNE desired to make a rough starting prediction for the total cost of all nursing units in a hospital for the coming year. If last year there were 50,000 patient days and this coming year patient days are expected to be 52,000, then there is a 4% expected increase in the number of patient days. However, it cannot be assumed that all nursing costs will go up by 4% because some costs, like the salary of the CNE, are fixed and will not rise in proportion to the number of patient days.

The high-low method discussed above would be one way to make the prediction, but the high-low method relies on only two data points. Far greater accuracy in breaking out fixed and variable costs would be possible if the past years' costs on a very detailed basis were examined, cost item by cost item, to determine which were fixed and which were variable. That would be a very time-consuming procedure. Gathering information costs money, and even if that information was gathered, there are always some costs that cannot be separated into fixed and variable components without some estimating methodology because they are mixed costs. For example, nonmedical supplies, such as paper, pens, and forms, will be needed to some extent regardless of patient volume. On the other hand, the more patients, the more nonmedical supplies used.

How can costs be divided into their fixed and variable components and less money be spent on gathering information than if each line item from past years was examined? Regression analysis can help to separate these mixed costs.

Mixed Costs and Regression Analysis

Suppose it is known that last year the combined cost of the salary of the nurse manager and the disposable supplies was $95,000 and that the number of patient days was 50,000. This uses the information represented in the graphs presented in Figures 7–1 through 7–3. The volume of patient days is expected to go up to 52,000 next year. Should the $95,000 cost be increased by 4% because volume is increasing by 4%? No, it should not. Some costs are fixed. Only variable costs would increase as volume increases.

One would expect costs to increase by $2,000, or $1 for each extra patient day, because it is known in this simple example that variable costs for the disposable thermometer covers were described as being $1 per patient day. However, in dealing with a more realistic example with many different fixed, variable, and mixed costs, the variable costs per patient day would not necessarily be known. Suppose that the historical information in Table 7-4 were available (already adjusted for inflation using the indexing techniques). If the high-low technique were used to evaluate the fixed and variable costs, there would be a very strange result. The highest cost is $95,000 and the lowest cost is $86,000, so costs have risen by $9,000. At the same time volume has increased

❖ TABLE 7–4
Historical Data for Thermometer Cover Costs

Year	Patient Days	Cost
1984	40,000	$86,000
1985	42,000	87,000
1986	43,000	88,000
1987	44,000	89,000
1988	45,000	90,000
1989	46,000	91,000
1990	47,000	92,000
1991	48,000	93,000
1992	49,000	94,000
1993	50,000	95,000

❖ **TABLE 7-5**
More Likely Historical Cost Pattern

Year	Patient Days	Cost
1984	40,000	$86,000
1985	42,000	86,800
1986	43,000	88,600
1987	44,000	88,800
1988	45,000	90,300
1989	46,000	91,700
1990	47,000	91,900
1991	48,000	93,800
1992	49,000	93,900
1993	50,000	95,000

from 40,000 patient days to 50,000 patient days, or an increase of 10,000. When $9,000 is divided by 10,000 patient days, a variable cost of $.90 per patient day results. Is that an accurate estimate? No, because it is known that the variable cost is $1 per patient day. What might be the cause of the discrepancy?

It is possible that 1984 was the first year that the disposable thermometer cover was used. Perhaps many of them were defective and were thrown away, or perhaps some were wasted because of lack of familiarity with using them. In any case, if more than $1 per patient day was spent on disposables in the low-volume year, then the costs were unduly high in that year. Therefore, the change in cost from 1984 to 1993 looks unrealistically low, and the variable cost measure is unrealistically low.

At the other extreme, had there been unusual waste (perhaps the fault of the nurses, but very possibly due to quality problems with a large batch of the disposable item) in the most recent, high-cost year, the change in cost would look especially high, and the variable cost per unit would have come out to more than $1. As has been stated before, if one relies on just two data points, as the high-low method does, results are subject to the whims of unusual events in either one of those years.

In reality, one would not expect to use exactly $1 per patient day on disposable supplies in any year. For one reason or another, some patients will have their temperature taken only once on a given day. This might be caused by admission to the hospital late in the day, for instance. On the other hand, patients running a fever will undoubtedly have their temperature taken more often. A pattern of costs that is more likely to be observed is shown in Table 7-5.

Simply looking at this list does not provide a lot of insight about fixed and variable costs. Figure 7-8 shows a scatter diagram for these points. By looking at this diagram, one can roughly see how the costs are increasing as volume increases. A straight line cannot go through all the points on this scatter diagram. However, the regression technique uses all the available information to select a line that will provide the best estimate in the absence of any other information.

Regression analysis uses information about the dependent and independent variables in the past to develop an equation for a straight line. As part of that

Figure 7–8. Scatter diagram of total costs for nursing (costs and patient days in thousands).

process it calculates a constant value and a coefficient for the independent variable. If the dependent variable is the cost, then the constant represents the fixed cost and the coefficient of the independent variable represents the variable cost.

Regression analysis is a statistical technique. A detailed discussion of statistics is beyond the scope of this book. However, many mechanical approaches to regression have made it a workable tool in health care institutions. Regression can be performed on many hand-held calculators. A wide variety of statistical programs and spreadsheet programs for personal computers also have regression capability.

Turning back now to the scatter diagram in Figure 7–8, it is possible to use regression analysis to predict what the costs will be for the nursing unit next year if there are 52,000 patient days. Regression analysis will determine a specific line to plot through this scatter diagram that will give the best possible estimate of fixed and variable costs and therefore allow prediction of the cost next year.

Basically the process requires several simple steps. First determine the cost associated with each volume of patient days. For instance, when there were 40,000 patient days, the cost was $86,000. The independent variable, patient days, is often referred to as the X variable because it is plotted on the horizontal axis. The dependent variable, cost, is often referred to as the Y variable because cost is plotted on the vertical axis.

Any computer program used will require that you provide the X values and the Y values for each year. Having provided that information, it is generally only necessary to give a command to compute the regression to complete the process. It is important not to let the extremely quantitative nature of regression theory learned in a statistics course discourage you from attempting to use this tool. In practice very little mathematics are required of the user. Regression is a tool to help you manage better. The major difficulty in using regression is simply a fear of the process.

In the example, regression analysis predicts that the fixed cost is $47,255 and the variable cost is $.96 per unit. Figure 7–9 shows the resulting line. If extended, it would have its intercept at $47,255, increasing with a slope of .96. These figures are not exactly the expected variable cost of $1 per patient day and fixed cost of $45,000 for the salary of the nurse manager. They are, however, better estimates than the ones the high-low method would give us. The high-low approach predicts a fixed cost of $50,000 and variable cost of $.90 per patient day. Regression analysis is an inexpensive, potentially very useful, and relatively simple way of estimating fixed and variable costs and helping to predict the future.

For any number of patient days predicted, it is now possible to multiply by .96 and then add $47,225 to get a forecast of future costs. In many computer regression packages, the process is made even simpler by just requiring that the forecast volume be entered into the computer along with the historical data.

Figure 7–9. Simple linear regression of total costs for nursing (costs and patient days in thousands).

The computer will then generate the estimated cost for the coming year automatically based on the forecast volume. Remember, however, that it is necessary to adjust upward the resulting cost for expected increases due to inflation for the coming year.

While you will soon find this approach quite simple, it is useful only as a tool to aid you in managing. It should not be allowed to take over the role of your judgment. The mathematical model is quite accurate in predicting the future if nothing has changed. It is your role as a manager to know if there are reasons that costs would be likely to change from their past patterns.

For instance, if you knew that 1984 was the first year disposable thermometer covers were used and that there was an awful lot of waste that year, you might want to eliminate that year from the analysis. If you did, your regression results would have shown fixed costs of $44,970 and variable costs of $1.005. Recall that the fixed costs actually were $45,000 and the variable costs were $1. As you can see, the input of judgment into the process can substantially improve the resulting estimates.

When a regression analysis is performed, one statistic that is generally provided by the calculator or the computer is the R-squared (R^2). That value can range from a low of zero to a high of 1.0. If the value is very close to zero, it means that the independent variable does not do a very good job of explaining the changes in the dependent variable. An R-squared of .20, for example, might indicate that patient days are not a very good predictor of nursing cost. On the other hand, an R-squared of .80 would indicate that it is a very good predictor. However, it is possible to become even more exact in estimating costs.

Multiple Regression Analysis

There is a type of regression analysis that is more sophisticated than simple linear regression. It is called *multiple regression* because it allows for use of multiple independent, or causal, variables. The use of simple linear regression can be a substantial aid in estimating future costs because it is so efficient at predicting the fixed cost and the variable cost per unit when there is one major independent variable. Sometimes, however, there will be several key variables. For instance, suppose that the nursing costs vary with the number of patient days but also with the number of patients. That is most probably the case.

Certainly the costs vary with the number of patient days. The more patient days, the more temperatures to be taken, pulses to be checked, medications to be administered, and so on. Yet for each patient there is a health history to be recorded, a chart to be set up, a patient care plan to be established, valuables to be stored, orientation to be given, discharge planning to be done, discharge education, and so on. These costs are not fixed—the more patients, the more time spent on these activities—but they do not vary directly with the number of patient days. Several patients with a long length of stay will cost less than many patients with a short length of stay, even if the total patient days are the same. So it is likely that the cost of a nursing unit varies with both the number of patient days and the number of admissions.

Most hand-held business calculators cannot perform multiple regression. However, most statistical programs for personal computers can handle this easily. Instead of simply entering the X and Y values for each year into the calculator or computer, one enters an X value for the historical information for each of the independent variables as well as the Y value. Then to predict a future cost, provide the computer with, for example, the expected number of patient days and the expected number of patients to predict the expected costs.

Sometimes the multiple regression level of sophistication adds extra work and complexity without substantially changing the results. Recall that when all is said and done, the result is just an estimate; all types of events can happen in the future that will throw off the estimate, no matter how finely tuned it is. It is not necessary to add complexity for its own sake. At times, however, multiple regression can produce information that would not otherwise be available.

For example, there has been more and more attention placed on measures of patient acuity, or the level of intensity of required nursing services. It certainly is clear that the amount of nursing services varies not just with the number of patient days but also with the severity of the patients' illnesses. If data about the number of patient days and the average acuity level are used as independent variables, the accuracy of estimated costs might improve substantially.

Another use for multiple regression is in investigatory work with respect to costs. Suppose that there is a strong feeling by the nursing staff that the way a particular physician practices medicine is extremely costly. This is quite common in the operating room, where particular surgeons often exhibit out-of-the-ordinary behavior. The number of operations by a specific physician each year can be used as an independent variable. Costs increasing as a result of more cases by that physician would show up as a positive coefficient for that independent variable. The nurse manager would then have evidence to support the more general feelings of the staff that the physician is an unusually high resource consumer.

The reader of this book is encouraged to pursue the topic of regression analysis further. This should be done on both a conceptual basis, reviewing the underlying principles and theories of regression analysis, and on a practical basis, using a computer software package to perform some regression analyses. The problems at the end of this chapter contain several exercises that can be completed using a common computer program such as LOTUS 1-2-3.[5]

BREAK-EVEN ANALYSIS

To this point the general behavior of costs (fixed vs. variable) has been discussed, as well as the techniques for cost estimation (high-low and regression). Attention will now be focused on using cost information for understanding whether a particular unit or service will lose money, make money, or just break even. This technique is useful for the evaluation of both new and continuing projects or services.

Nurse managers in many instances find it necessary to be able to determine whether a program or service will be profitable. One key to profitability is volume. Prices are often fixed. Average cost, however, is not fixed. As the number of patients rises, the cost per patient falls because of the sharing of fixed costs. One cannot simply compare price and average cost and determine

---

[5]LOTUS 1-2-3 is a registered trademark of the LOTUS Development Corp.

that a program or unit will make a profit or a loss. To determine whether something will be profitable, it is critical to know the volume of patients.

Break-even analysis is a technique to find the specific volume at which a program or service neither makes nor loses money. Forecast information about the likely volume of the service can be compared to the break-even volume to predict whether there will be profits or losses.

Break-even analysis is based on the following formula:

$$\text{Break-even quantity (Q)} = \frac{\text{Fixed costs (FC)}}{\text{Price (P)} - \text{Variable cost per patient (VC)}}$$

or

$$Q = \frac{FC}{P - VC}$$

where Q is the number of patients needed to just break even, FC is the total fixed cost, P is the price for each patient, and VC is the variable cost per patient. At a quantity lower than Q there would be a loss; at a quantity higher than Q there would be a profit.

The basis for the formula is the underlying relationship between revenues and expenses.[6] If total revenues are greater than expenses, there is a profit. If total revenues are less than expenses, there is a loss. If revenues are just equal to expenses, there is neither profit nor loss and the service is said to just break even.

A Break-even Analysis Example

Suppose that a hospital opens a new home health agency that charges, on average, $50 per visit. The agency has fixed costs of $10,000 and variable costs of $30 per patient visit. If there are no patients at all, there is no revenue, but there are fixed costs of $10,000 and there is a $10,000 loss. If there were 100 patients, there would be $5,000 of revenue ($50 times 100 patients), $10,000 of fixed cost, and $3,000 of variable cost ($30 times 100 patients). Total costs would be $13,000 ($10,000 of fixed cost plus $3,000 of variable cost), while revenues would be $5,000 and the loss $8,000. These data are hypothetical.

Each additional patient brings in $50 of revenue but causes the agency to spend only $30 more. The difference between the $50 price and the $30 variable cost, $20, is called the *contribution margin*. If the contribution margin is positive, it means that each extra unit of activity makes the organization better off by

---

[6]The formula may be derived as follows:
1. Profit = Revenues − Costs, or Profit = Revenues − Fixed costs − Total variable costs.
2. At the break-even quantity, profit is zero, so: 0 = Revenues (R) − Fixed costs (FC) − Total variable costs (TVC)
3. Moving revenue to the left side of the equation and multiplying the equation by −1 yields: R = FC + TVC
4. Revenue is the price per unit (P) multiplied by the quantity of units (Q), and total variable costs are the variable costs per unit (VC) multiplied by the quantity of units (Q): (P × Q) = FC + (VC × Q)
5. Moving the VC to the other side of the equation: (P × Q) − (VC × Q) = FC
6. Factor out the Q from the left side of the equation: Q × (P − VC) = FC
7. Divide both sides of the equation by (P − VC) to yield the formula: Q = FC/(P − VC)

that amount. The contribution margin from each patient can be used to cover fixed costs; if all fixed costs have been covered, it represents a profit.

In this example, when there are 100 patients, there is $20 of contribution margin for each of the 100 patients, or a total contribution margin of $2,000. Note that the loss with zero patients was $10,000, while it was only $8,000 when there were 100 patients. The loss decreased by $2,000, exactly the amount of the total contribution margin for those 100 patients.

How many visits would the agency need to break even? The answer is 500. If each additional patient generates $20 of contribution margin, then 500 patients would generate $10,000 of contribution margin (500 patients times $20 = $10,000), exactly enough to cover the fixed costs of $10,000. If the agency has 500 patients, it will just break even.

This could have been calculated using the formula:

$$Q = \frac{FC}{P - VC}$$

or

$$Q = \frac{\$10,000}{\$50 - \$30} = \frac{\$10,000}{\$20} = 500 \text{ visits}$$

Break-even analysis can also be viewed from a graphic perspective (see Fig. 7–10). The total cost line starts at a level of $10,000 because of the fixed costs. The total revenue line starts at zero because there is no revenue if there are zero patients. Where the revenue line and the cost line intersect, they are equal and the agency just breaks even. Note that at quantities of patients fewer than the break-even point, the cost line is higher than the revenue line. At quantities

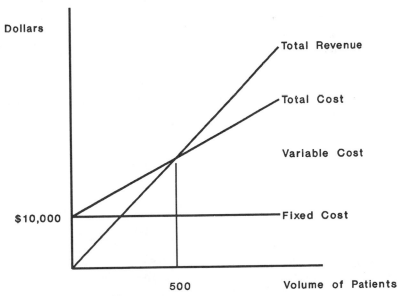

Figure 7–10. Break-even analysis.

TABLE 7–6
Contribution Margin by Type of Patient

	Price (A)	Variable Cost (B)	Contribution Margin (C = A − B)
Complex	$80	$55	$25
Moderate	50	30	20
Simple	30	20	10

of patients greater than the break-even point, the revenue line is higher than the costs and a profit is made.

Prior to the introduction of DRGs, most break-even analyses in hospitals focused on the number of patient days needed to break even. Hospitals do not get paid for extra patient days under the DRG prospective payment system. Therefore there is now greater attention on the total number of patients needed to break even, rather than patient days. Break even can also be performed based on the number of surgeries, clinic visits, or other appropriate service unit volume measure.

When there are different types of patients, break even becomes somewhat more complicated. The formula presented at the beginning of this section assumes that there is only one price and one variable cost and therefore one contribution margin. If there are different types of patients with different prices and different variable costs, it is necessary to find a weighted average contribution margin. That weighted average can be divided into the fixed costs to find the break-even volume for all patients.

For example, suppose that there are three classes of home care visits, which will be referred to here as complex, moderate, and simple. The price for the visits is $80, $50, and $30, and the variable costs for the visits are $55, $30, and $20, respectively. The contribution margin for each type of patient can be calculated by subtracting the variable cost from the price, as shown in Table 7–6.

The crucial piece of information for calculating the break-even point is the relative proportion of each type of visit. Management of the home health agency

TABLE 7–7
Calculation of Weighted Average Contribution Margin

Visit Type	Percentage of Visits		Contribution Margin		Weighted Average Contribution Margin
Complex	20	×	$25	=	$ 5
Moderate	30	×	20	=	6
Simple	50	×	10	=	5
Total weighted average contribution margin					$16

expect that 20% of all visits are complex, 30% are moderate, and 50% are simple. This information can be used to determine a weighted average contribution margin. This requires multiplying each type of visit's individual contribution margin by the percentage of patients that type of visit makes up. The results are added together to get an overall weighted contribution margin, as shown in Table 7–7.

This $16 weighted contribution margin represents the average contribution margin for all types of visits. It can be used to calculate the break-even quantity. Assume that fixed costs are $10,000. The break-even quantity of visits is:

$$Q = \frac{FC}{P - VC} = \frac{FC}{CM}$$

or

$$Q = \frac{\$10,000}{\$16} = 625 \text{ visits}$$

Of the total of 625 visits needed to break even, 20% or 125 would be complex, 30% or 188 would be moderate, and 50% or 312 would be simple.

This method works for three different kinds of patients. What if there were more than three kinds? The same weighted average approach that can be used to find the break-even volume when there are three different types of patients could be used even if there were hundreds of different types of patients, as is the case with the DRG system.

What if there is more than one price for each type of patient? It is possible that Medicaid pays one price, Medicare another, Blue Cross another, and self-pay or commercial insurance yet another. This still can work within the same framework as has been presented. It would be necessary to calculate a weighted average contribution margin treating each payer for each type of patient as a separate group. For example, if Medicaid pays $40 per visit regardless of the type of visit and the other payment rates are the same as indicated earlier, the contribution margin by type of patient by payer would be as shown in Table 7–8.

If it is possible to anticipate the percentage of each type of patient, a weighted average contribution margin can be estimated. Assume that 10% of all patients are Medicaid complex patients and 10% are other complex patients. Assume

❖ **TABLE 7–8**
Contribution Margin by Type of Patient and by Payer

	Price (A)	Variable Cost (B)	Contribution Margin (C = A − B)
Complex Medicaid	$40	$55	($15)
Complex other	80	55	25
Moderate Medicaid	40	30	10
Moderate other	50	30	20
Simple Medicaid	40	20	20
Simple other	30	20	10

that 20% of all patients are Medicaid moderate patients and 10% of all patients are other moderate patients. Assume that 30% of all patients are Medicaid simple patients and that 20% of all patients are other simple patients. The weighted contribution margin would be as shown in Table 7–9.

The break-even volume could then be calculated as follows:

$$Q = \frac{FC}{P - VC} = \frac{FC}{CM}$$

or

$$Q = \frac{\$10,000}{\$13} = 769 \text{ visits}$$

The number of visits of any type could be determined by multiplying the 769 break-even volume times the percentage of patients in any given class. For example, since 30% of the patients are Medicaid simple, 30% of 769, or 231, Medicaid simple patients would be expected at the break-even level.

Using Break-even Analysis for Decision Making

If a particular service is expected to have a volume of activity well in excess of the break-even point, managers have a clear-cut decision to start or continue the service. If the volume is too low to break even, several options exist.

One approach is to lower the volume needed to break even. There are three ways to reduce the required break-even level. One approach is to lower the fixed costs. In some cases it might be possible to do that. Another alternative would be to increase prices. Price increases would increase the contribution margin per patient. That would also have the effect of lowering the break-even point. However, price increases might reduce the expected volume. In that case the price increases would be defeating their purpose. Also, prices are sometimes regulated and beyond the control of the organization. Finally, one could try to reduce the variable cost per unit. This might be accomplished by increased efforts toward improved efficiency.

If it is not feasible to change the fixed costs, price, or variable costs, an organization can try to attract more patients so that the volume will rise above

❖ **TABLE 7–9**
Calculation of Weighted Average Contribution Margin with Multiple Payers

Visit Type	Percentage of Visits		Contribution Margin		Weighted Average Contribution Margin
Complex Medicaid	10	×	($15)	=	($ 1.5)
Complex other	10	×	25	=	2.5
Moderate Medicaid	20	×	10	=	2.0
Moderate other	10	×	20	=	2.0
Simple Medicaid	30	×	20	=	6.0
Simple other	20	×	10	=	2.0
Total weighted average contribution margin					$13.0

the break-even point. In the example presented, what type of patients would be desirable? The most desirable type of visit is for a complex, non-Medicaid patient. That patient yields a contribution margin of $25. The least desirable is a Medicaid complex patient. The contribution margin is negative. For each additional Medicaid complex patient, the agency loses money. In this particular example the most attractive patient has the highest revenue. However, the focus should not be on revenue. If the highest-revenue patient also had extremely high variable costs, that patient might not be so attractive as one with lower revenue and much lower variable costs. The attractiveness of additional patients is determined by how much contribution margin they provide to the organization.

Break-even Analysis Cautions

A few words of caution are advisable when working with break-even analysis. First of all, once a break-even point is calculated, one must decide whether it is likely that actual volume will be sufficient to exceed that point. That will require a volume forecast such as those in Chapter 17. To the extent that the forecast of volume is incorrect, the decision to go ahead with a new service may turn out to be a bad one, even if the break-even analysis is perfect.

Another potential problem is that break-even analysis assumes that prices and costs are constant. If it can be reasonably expected that prices will fall over time, then a higher volume would be needed to keep a service viable, unless variable or fixed costs would be falling as well. On the other hand, if prices are expected to rise faster than costs, then a marginal service today may become profitable over time, even without an increase in volume.

Another consideration is that there is an assumption that the mix of patients will stay constant. Suppose that in the above example, over time there are more and more Medicaid complex patients. The contribution margin for such patients is negative. If the demographics of the population are such that a shift in mix in that direction is likely, then the results of the break-even analysis require very close scrutiny. Will there be enough of those patients to shift a profitable service over to a loss?

As with all budgeting tools, judgment is essential. The nurse manager must through experience, insight, and thought examine the assumptions of any modeling technique and consider the reasonableness of the results. If a result does not seem to make sense, often that is because it does not make sense. However, break-even analysis is a tool that can help give a manager a firm starting point in understanding whether a project or service is likely to be financially viable.

IMPLICATIONS FOR NURSE MANAGERS

Assessing costs is a complex topic. In general, costs do not increase in direct proportion with volume. The implications of this are that if money is lost on a particular program, the solution may be to increase patient volume for that program. More patients do not necessarily mean greater losses. It is possible that volume increases can turn a loss into a profit. Understanding how that can happen requires an understanding of cost behavior. Some costs are fixed, while others are variable. The result of that basic nature of costs is that the cost per patient will decline with increasing volume. The greater the number of patients who share the fixed costs, the lower the average cost per patient. Costing is further complicated by the fact that additional patients do not cause costs to increase by the average cost per patient. Decisions that are in the organization's best interests often require marginal cost analysis.

An important part of the budgeting process is the prediction of costs. Estimated costs for the future can be based upon historical cost information. Some estimation relies upon using the historical information to isolate variable costs from fixed costs. To make such calculations, it is first necessary to convert historical cost information into common or constant dollars. This requires *indexation* of costs for the impact of inflation. Indexation is a process that adjusts a dollar value for the impact of inflation over a period of time by using a *price index*, such as the CPI. A price index is a tool that indicates year-to-year changes in prices. Using indexed historical costs, the results of the cost estimation process will be in constant dollars. In preparing next year's budget, the cost estimate has to be adjusted upward by the anticipated inflation rate over the next year.

Once constant-dollar information is available, cost can be estimated using the high-low method, simple linear regression, or multiple regression analysis. Being able to estimate fixed and variable costs is potentially a valuable tool. To apply the results, however, projections of the estimated number of patients, patient days, acuity level, and so forth are needed. Chapter 17 focuses on the process of forecasting such data.

Break-even analysis is a tool that allows one to focus specifically on the quantity of patients needed for a program, project, or service to be financially viable. Its foundations are in fixed and variable costs. At low volumes of patients, the average cost may surpass the revenue per patient. As the number of patients increases, the cost per patient falls as fixed costs are shared by more patients. Eventually the cost per patient falls below the revenue. Break-even analysis allows the manager to determine what the break-even quantity is so that a reasonable decision can be made about the likely financial viability of a program, project, or service.

From the nurse manager's standpoint, the topics of this chapter have critical implications. At the most basic level, falling volume will mean rising cost per patient. In such cases it is likely that a revenue crisis will exist, and actions to restrain costs should be immediately contemplated. On the other hand, rising volumes represent an opportunity. Not only do they bring in more revenue but they also result in decreasing average cost per patient. Therefore there is the opportunity for profit from more patients and for more profit from each patient. Profits ultimately allow the organization to replace buildings and equipment, add services, add staff, improve quality, and raise salaries.

Additionally, in preparing budgets nurse managers should take into account the behavior of costs. The fact that certain costs vary in proportion while others are fixed may reorient a manager's thinking from the notion that a 10% increase in volume requires 10% more resources. This in turn can allow a manager to prepare budgets in a more sophisticated and exact manner.

Finally, managers should remember that decisions to begin, continue, or stop a program are not made solely on the basis of profit-and-loss projections. Some programs are continued as a community service, and the institution makes a conscious decision to subsidize them from other sources of revenues.

However, such decisions require as much information about anticipated profits or losses as possible.

KEY CONCEPTS ————————————————————————

Service unit   Basic measure of the product or service being produced by the organization, such as discharged patients, patient days, home care visits, emergency room treatments, or hours of operations.

Direct costs   Costs that are incurred within the organizational unit for which the manager has responsibility, or costs that are directly related to patient care.

Indirect costs   Costs that are assigned to an organizational unit from elsewhere in the organization, or unit costs that do not directly relate to patient care.

Full cost   Total of all costs associated with an organizational unit or activity. This includes direct and indirect costs.

Average cost   Full cost divided by the volume of service units.

Fixed costs   Costs that do not change in total as the volume of service units changes.

Variable cost   Costs that vary directly with changes in the volume of service units.

Relevant range   Normal range of expected activity for the cost center or organization.

Marginal costs   Extra costs incurred as a result of providing care to one more service unit, such as for one extra patient day. If one considers the total costs incurred by an organization before it makes a change and the total costs after it makes the change, the difference in costs represents the marginal costs of that change.

Mixed costs   Costs that contain both fixed and variable cost elements.

Impact of volume on cost per patient   Average cost declines as the volume of patients increases because more patients are sharing the fixed costs. Therefore health care organizations almost always find higher volume preferable to lower volume.

Marginal cost analysis   Decisions about changes should be based on the marginal costs of the change. They should not be based on full or average costs.

Cost estimation   Prediction of costs. This process is complicated by the necessity to divide historical mixed costs into their fixed and variable cost components and by the necessity to adjust historical costs for the impact of inflation to use them for predicting future costs.

Adjusting costs for inflation   Part of the change in costs over time is a result of volume changes, but part is due to inflation. To adjust for the impact of inflation, a historical cost must be multiplied by the current value of an appropriate price index divided by the value of that index when the cost was incurred.

Regression analysis   Once historical costs have been adjusted for the impact of inflation, regression analysis can be used to estimate the fixed and variable costs. Costs are the dependent variable, and service units are the independent variable. The constant term of the regression represents fixed costs, and the coefficient of the independent variable represents the variable costs.

Multiple regression analysis and cost estimation   This technique allows superior cost estimates by incorporating information from several independent variables, rather than just one.

Break-even analysis   Technique that allows the user to determine the volume of patients required for a program or service to be financially self-sufficient. At volumes above the break-even point a profit is made, and below that point a loss occurs. Break-even analysis is based on the following formula:

$$\text{The break-even quantity (Q)} = \frac{\text{Fixed costs (FC)}}{\text{Price (P)} - \text{Variable cost per patient (VC)}}$$

Contribution margin   Price minus the variable cost per service unit. This represents the additional financial benefit to the organization from each additional service unit. This benefit can be used to cover fixed costs or provide a profit. A weighted average contribution margin is used for break-even analysis when there is more than one type of service unit or more than one price for each type service unit.

SUGGESTED READINGS ❖

Finkler, Steven A., "Fixed and Variable Costs: The Long and Short of It," *Hospital Cost Accounting Advisor*, Vol. 1, No. 7, December 1985, pp. 1–4.

Finkler, Steven A., "Using Break-Even Analysis Under DRGs," *Hospital Cost Accounting Advisor*, Vol. 1, No. 1, June 1985, pp. 4–6.

Finkler, Steven A., "Using Break-Even Analysis with Step-Fixed Costs," *Hospital Cost Management and Accounting*, Vol. 1, No. 8, November 1989, pp. 1–5.

Finkler, Steven A., "Indexing for Inflation," *Hospital Cost Accounting Advisor*, Vol. 1, No. 2, July 1985, pp. 1, 3, 6–7.

Finkler, Steven A., "Cost Estimation Using Linear Regression," *Hospital Cost Accounting Advisor*, Vol. 1, No. 2, July 1985, pp. 1, 4–6.

Finkler, Steven A., "Breakeven Analysis: Caveats," *Hospital Cost Management and Accounting*, Vol. 1, No. 4, July 1989, pp. 1–5.

Horngren, Charles T., and George Foster, *Cost Accounting: A Managerial Emphasis*, 7th edition, Prentice-Hall, Englewood Cliffs, NJ, 1990.

Kovner, Christine, "Public Health Nursing Costs in Home Care," *Public Health Nursing*, Vol. 6, No. 1, March 1989, pp. 3–7.

CHAPTER

8

Determining Health Care Costs and Rates

CHAPTER GOALS

The goals of this chapter are to:

♦ Clarify the difference between the types of cost information needed for external reporting and the information useful to managers

♦ Explain the traditional cost-finding methodology as required in Medicare cost reports

♦ Survey the literature and approaches to costing out nursing services and provide examples of specific approaches to determining the cost of nursing services

♦ Define productivity and describe measures of nursing productivity

♦ Describe the issues related to determining the costs of different patient product lines

♦ Introduce the concept of standard cost and discuss approaches designed to yield more accurate cost information

♦ Explain the various approaches to rate setting

♦ Discuss variable billing for nursing services

❖

INTRODUCTION

The previous chapter provided the reader with the basic foundations for cost analysis. Fixed, variable, average, and marginal costs were discussed. The chapter explained which costs to use for different types of management decisions. Additionally, Chapter 7 discussed methods for estimating future costs and for calculating whether a program or service would be financially self-sufficient. All these elements represent essential tools in routine management activities. One can think of that material as representing the trees. Now that the reader can identify each different type of tree, it is necessary to step back

179

and look at the forest. This chapter looks at some broader, organization-wide costing issues as well as issues related to setting rates or prices for health care services.

The first section of this chapter considers the difference between cost information generated by the organization to help managers to manage the health care organization and cost information needed for reports provided to persons outside the organization. This is an important distinction, as the needs of internal and external users of information differ significantly.

The requirements for external cost reporting are complex. Traditionally, health care institutions have calculated their costs in what is called a *cost-finding* process, which finds the costs of units of service such as lab tests, x-rays, or routine patient days based on an allocation of *nonrevenue cost center* costs to *revenue centers*. That process generates the information needed to complete Medicare cost reports. Virtually all health care organizations that receive some revenue from Medicare are required to submit such reports. Historically these reports have formed the basis for cost accounting in health care organizations. The information generated by such reports is used to determine department and patient costs.

However, such reports do not provide particularly useful information about the cost of nursing services. To understand the costs of caring for any specific type of patient, one must know the resources consumed by that type of patient and the cost of those resources. One of the most significant elements in that calculation is an understanding of the nursing resources consumed by each different type of patient. Since the early 1980s the nursing profession has placed an ever greater stress on improving the ability to make such calculations. Understanding the costs of nursing services well provides the manager with valuable information for decision making.

The chapter next turns to the issue of productivity. *Productivity* has simply been described as the ratio of *outputs* to *inputs*. To determine this ratio managers must first decide the appropriate outputs and inputs. The largest component of inputs for most health care organizations is nursing personnel. Determining outputs is more complicated. It has been traditionally defined as a unit of service such as a patient day of care or patient encounter such as a visit. However, more recently outputs are being considered episodes of care or even patient outcomes defined as some level of health. Determining productivity ratios will depend on how inputs and outputs are defined.

After addressing productivity, the chapter discusses product-line costing. In the highly competitive health care marketplace managers have found that to remain competitive, they must have information about the costs not only of departments or units but also of treating different types of patients. This has led to a growing emphasis on what is called *product-line costing*. In product-line costing an attempt is made to find the average costs for a given type of patient or group of similar patients. This is done for all costs, not just nursing service costs.

Unfortunately, Medicare cost reports do not necessarily provide an extremely accurate picture of the cost to treat patients. This makes product-line costing difficult to accomplish. As a result, in recent years health care organizations have started to develop various *standard cost* approaches to provide improved cost information for managers, especially with respect to the cost of various types of patients. Product-line and standard costing are both discussed in this chapter.

Rate setting and revenues are also discussed in this chapter. Cost information is the most essential ingredient in the pricing decisions that health care organizations make. When an organization sets prices for its services, it wants to be sure that they are at least as high as the cost of providing those services. If they are not, then losses will be incurred. The amount of revenue received in relation to the costs of providing care is critical to the continued existence of the organization.

Revenues are no longer the sole domain of the financial officer. In the last twenty years there has been a shift in responsibility from finance to nursing for the planning and control of nursing costs. More recently this shifting financial responsibility has been including responsibility for revenues. Nurse managers need to become knowledgeable about the revenue process in health care organizations. In some cases revenues are set outside the organization. For example, the federal government sets Medicare DRG rates. Managers must be able to determine whether the revenue received in such cases will be sufficient to cover all the costs of providing care.

In addition to general rate-setting issues, nursing departments are starting to focus on direct charging for nursing services. Accurate information on the cost of nursing services can be used as a basis for charging for nursing services. Nursing historically has not been a revenue center in most health care organizations. This has been a result of a lack of accurate data about the nursing cost for different patient types. With improved information, nursing can be a revenue department, similar to laboratory or radiology. This issue is also discussed in this chapter.

COSTS FOR REPORTING VS. COSTS FOR MANAGEMENT CONTROL

Managers need to have cost information to manage their responsibility centers. Many decisions that managers must make require information about the costs that their units are incurring. The correctness of the decisions depends to a great extent on the accuracy of the cost information available. Therefore cost-data collection for use by managers should have a high priority.

At the same time, health care organizations are required to comply with a number of external reporting requirements. Earlier in the book the financial statements for external reporting were discussed. In addition to producing financial statements, most health care organizations also are required to complete other reports that focus on the organization's costs. These reports are most commonly prepared for Medicare, Medicaid, and other governmental agencies as well as for some insurance companies. Some HMOs now also require cost reports from hospitals.

External reports are generally required by law or to comply with contractual arrangements. It is important to keep in mind that historically many third-party payments to health care organizations have been based on costs incurred. Prior to the introduction of DRGs, hospitals were reimbursed for their costs by Medicare. As a result, Medicare needed to know the hospital's costs. For outpatients at hospitals and for some other types of health care organizations, Medicare payments are still cost based.

Most health care organizations spend a great deal of energy generating reports that contain the mandated cost information. Unfortunately, in some cases the information contained in the external reports is used for internal management without careful thought to how internal information needs differ from those of the external users.

This problem is not limited to health care organizations. A growing management accounting literature has called for drastic revisions to the process of collecting cost information for internal purposes.[1]

What types of information are inappropriately used for internal management purposes? The answer is many types. Some of the problems are relatively easy to deal with. Others are much more complex and are built into the underlying cost-accounting calculations used throughout the organization.

First, consider an example of an easily solvable problem. Suppose that you are a hospital or nursing home unit manager and that nurses float from their home unit to another, depending on which units are slow and which are busy. In some organizations the nurse continues to be charged to the home unit, even when shifted temporarily to another unit. That results in charges to the home unit for more resources than it consumed, and it undercharges the unit that borrowed the float nurse.

For external reporting purposes it may be adequate to simply show the total cost for the nursing staff. However, the organization needs its managers to control their costs. When it is time to contrast budgeted costs with actual costs, the actual costs should reflect the resources actually consumed on the unit.

How can this problem be solved? A system needs to be put into place that tracks which units nurses are assigned to each day and charges float costs to the unit that actually had the use of the nurses. Such systems are widely, although not universally, used.

A much more difficult problem concerns the use of cost reports for determining the costs of treating different types of patients. Cost reports are complex, difficult documents to complete. There are a number of problems with the information they contain. However, those problems become buried in the calculations, and many managers treat the cost report information as if it were more accurate than it really is. The next section explains the cost-finding process used to develop cost reports. The problems with the process that make its resulting information less than optimal for management use are discussed. Later sections of the chapter discuss alternatives that provide managers with more accurate information.

TRADITIONAL COST-FINDING METHODOLOGY

Health care organizations consume a variety of resources in providing their services. A variety of types of labor, supplies, and equipment are needed to

---

[1]For example, see Thomas Johnson, "The Decline of Cost Management: A Reinterpretation of 20th Century Cost Accounting," *Journal of Cost Management for the Manufacturing Industry,* Spring 1987, Vol. 1, No. 1, pp. 5–12; William L. Ferrara, "The New Cost/Management Accounting: More Questions Than Answers," *Management Accounting,* Vol. 72, No. 4, October 1990, pp. 48–52.

provide care to each patient. The challenge faced by accountants in health care organizations is both to accumulate cost information relating to all the resources used and also to find an efficient, economical way to accurately associate with each patient the costs incurred to treat that patient.

Practically speaking, it is unrealistic to believe that assignment of perfectly accurate costs to each patient is a reasonable expectation. To keep track perfectly would require constant observation of each patient to see how many towels are used, exactly how many minutes of nurse time, technician time, and so on. Cost information costs money to collect. All organizations use accounting shortcuts to save money. However, there is a clear trade-off between how much is spent on cost information and how accurate it is. The more accurate the information, the more it costs. Each organization must decide when the level of information is "good enough." In the future, expanded use of bar coding and computers may make it possible to collect more detailed and accurate information without substantially increasing the cost of data collection.

The simplest cost-finding approach is to simply divide the total dollars spent over a period of time by the number of patients treated over that period. The result is the average cost per patient. That average will be the same for all patients. Clearly, however, such an approach is not good enough. It would be impossible for managers to begin to determine which patients are profitable and which generate losses if such a method were used. If managers worked hard to treat a certain type of patient more efficiently, they would not have any sense of whether that goal were accomplished if the same cost were assigned to all patients regardless of resources consumed. The approach must be more sophisticated.

The Medicare Step-down Approach

The approach most health care organizations use for their cost finding is the one mandated for Medicare cost reports. In that approach all resource consumption is first associated with a cost center. Housekeeping, dietary, pharmacy, intensive care, operating room, and coronary care are examples of cost centers. Each cost center accumulates its direct costs, such as labor and supplies used in the center.

The next step is to allocate all the costs of the nonrevenue cost centers to the revenue centers. Revenue centers are the parts of the organization that specifically charge for their services. For example, patients are generally charged a specific amount for an operation but not for security. Revenue center managers are responsible not only for the costs incurred in their unit or department but also for the revenues. While this creates the burden of additional responsibility, it also adds benefits. If a unit or department is a revenue center, then it can point to an explicit measure of the financial contribution that it earns for the organization. The revenue it generates can be used as an argument for giving additional resources to the center. If given their choice, most managers would want their departments to be classified as revenue centers.

How do health care organizations distinguish between cost centers that are revenue centers and cost centers that are not? The key requirement for a revenue center is that it must be possible to measure different consumption of that center's services by different patients.

For example, each day each patient benefits equally from the presence of a security guard at the front door of the organization. Therefore, there can be one catchall charge per patient per day, called the *per diem*. It will include costs such as the security guard. However, if patients consume different amounts of a resource, we need to have specific charges to reflect those differences. For example, if one patient has surgery and one does not, we need to be able to charge for the operation only the one who had surgery. And we need to be able to charge a greater amount to someone who had a more expensive operation than to someone who had a less expensive operation. Therefore, security is not a revenue center, but the operating room is.

Examples of revenue centers include pharmacy, radiology, the operating room, respiratory therapy, central supply, and the laboratory. Examples of nonrevenue centers include dietary, administration, housekeeping, medical records, and in most cases medical/surgical nursing.

Why is nursing not a revenue center? Clearly, different patients consume different amounts of nursing resources each day. A key ingredient in being a revenue center is that different patients consume different amounts of resources from the center. However, historically there was difficulty in measuring the amount of nursing resources each patient consumed. It would require an observer to follow each patient or each nurse and determine how much nursing resource each patient actually used. With the widespread introduction of patient classification systems in the 1980s this is no longer the case. It is now possible to at least approximate the differing amount of nursing resources consumed by different patients. The issue of making nursing into a revenue center is discussed in the last section of this chapter.

Why must the nonrevenue center costs be allocated to the revenue centers? Health care organizations get their revenues by charging for the services provided. When the prices or rates are set, the organization must consider all its costs. Laundry is not a revenue center. It does not charge the patients a fee for its services. Operating rooms consume large amounts of scrubs and sheets, which must be laundered. If a hospital were to set its operating room prices high enough to recover the cost of operating room nurses but did not consider the cost of the laundry, its prices might not be set high enough to recover all costs incurred by the organization. Therefore, to ensure that the organization sets prices high enough to recover all its costs, the costs of the revenue centers must include all the costs of the nonrevenue cost centers.

Once all the nonrevenue center costs have been assigned to the revenue centers, each revenue center can in turn assign its total direct and indirect costs to the units of service that have been provided to the patients it has treated. One could then aggregate the costs assigned to a specific patient by each of the revenue centers to determine the total cost of treating that patient.

Even though Medicare now pays hospitals on the basis of DRGs rather than a direct cost reimbursement, the Medicare cost report is still completed by hospitals. The cost information from the report is used by the federal government in its process of setting national payment rates for each DRG.

A Detailed Look at the Cost-finding Approach

The steps in traditional cost finding are examined here to provide an understanding of the traditional cost-finding approach and its weaknesses.

Accumulate Direct Costs for Each Cost Center

The first step in the cost-finding process is to accumulate the direct costs of the cost center. For example, consider an operating room (OR), which is a revenue center.

Direct costs in the OR include salaries and wages for regular staff. This includes all supervisory and staff personnel that work in the OR and are included in the OR budget. The OR manager, the scrub and circulating nurses, operating room technicians, orderlies, clerks, and secretaries will all be included. Employee benefits are also included in direct costs.

Other direct costs include the costs for supplies, seminars, agency per diem nurses, and all other items under the direct control of the OR that are normally considered its direct costs.

Determine Bases for Allocation

The laundry department is an example of a nonrevenue cost center. Once its direct costs have been accumulated, they must be assigned to revenue centers. Each center that uses laundry should be charged for a portion of the costs of the laundry. To do this, the manager must first decide upon the basis for the allocation.

The cost of the laundry could be charged in equal shares to each department that uses it. However, that would be quite unfair to departments that use relatively little laundry. Such an allocation would not be good enough.

Other approaches to allocating the cost of laundry would be on the basis of pounds of laundry or pieces of laundry. In fact, most health care organizations that have a laundry department assign laundry costs on the basis of the number of pounds of laundry. All dirty laundry is placed in a laundry cart, which is weighed. Then total laundry costs can be allocated based on the share of total pounds of laundry consumed by each department.

Is that an appropriate basis for the allocation? It is not the best basis. A lab jacket may be more complicated to sort and fold than a sheet. Although four lab jackets may weigh the same total amount as one sheet, they would undoubtedly require more labor than one sheet. Labor is one of the greatest expenses of the laundry department. Therefore, cost accuracy would improve if costing were done on the basis of the number of each type of laundry item. However, it would cost more to keep track of pieces than pounds.

Most health care organizations have decided that pounds of laundry is a good-enough measure. It does effectively assign all the costs of the laundry to the revenue centers. And it does use an allocation basis that takes some, if not perfect, account of relative usage by different cost centers. In any event, the only perfectly accurate measurement would require one staff member to constantly observe each patient to see exactly what laundry that patient used. That would obviously be prohibitively expensive.

It is worth noting that most outside linen services that contract with health care organizations charge a different price for each different type of item. Some charge a price per piece based on the type and number of pieces. Others charge a price per pound, but the price per pound varies by type of item. Laundry companies apparently believe that their costs per pound of laundry are significantly different enough for different types of pieces that they must charge based on the type of piece.

The problem of the specific basis to choose is not limited to the laundry. Other cost centers also have had to make choices. For example, any health care organization that has a building must allocate its annual depreciation to the various cost centers. That is usually done on the basis of square feet. A cost center that physically occupies many square feet would be charged more than one that has fewer square feet.

Actually, it costs more to build certain parts of a facility than other parts. For example, an OR costs about ten times as much per square foot as a patient room. By allocating an equal amount of depreciation per square foot, this means that too little is assigned to the OR and too much to medical/surgical rooms. Ultimately this means that medical patients are overcharged, relative to their resource consumption, and surgical patients are undercharged. However, hospitals have generally decided that an equal depreciation charge per square foot is good enough.

Allocate from Cost Centers to Revenue Centers

All the costs of the nonrevenue cost centers are allocated to the revenue centers using the allocating bases discussed above. Figure 8–1 provides a simplified example of what we are attempting to do with this allocation. In the figure, housekeeping and laundry are nonrevenue centers. Coronary care and pharmacy are revenue centers. Each nonrevenue center must ultimately allocate all its costs to the revenue centers.

Table 8–1 provides a simplified numerical example. As in Figure 8–1, housekeeping and laundry are nonrevenue centers and the coronary care unit (CCU) and pharmacy are revenue centers. The first line in the table shows the direct cost incurred in each of the four centers. The next two lines show the allocation base and how much of the base is related to each department.

Housekeeping cost will be allocated on the basis of square feet; laundry, on the basis of pounds. The table shows the percentage of all square feet that each cost center has and the percentage of all pounds of laundry used by each cost center. The square feet in the housekeeping department and the pounds of laundry done by the laundry for the laundry are excluded because no cost

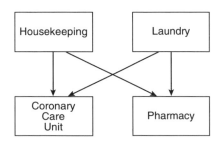

NONREVENUE CENTERS

REVENUE CENTERS

Figure 8–1. Allocating costs.

❖ TABLE 8–1
Cost-base Information for Allocation

| | Nonrevenue Cost Centers | | Revenue Cost Centers | | |
	Housekeeping	Laundry	Coronary Care Unit	Pharmacy	Total Cost
Direct cost	$40,000	$60,000	$500,000	$500,000	$1,100,000
Allocation statistics:					
Housekeeping (square feet)	—	70%	25%	5%	100%
Laundry (pounds)	20%	—	10%	70%	100%

❖ TABLE 8–2
Direct Distribution

| | Nonrevenue Cost Centers | | Revenue Cost Centers | | |
	Housekeeping	Laundry	Coronary Care Unit	Pharmacy	Total Cost
Direct cost	$ 40,000	$ 60,000	$500,000	$500,000	$1,100,000
Allocation:					
Housekeeping (square feet)	−40,000	0	33,333	6,667	0
Laundry (pounds)	0	−60,000	7,500	52,500	0
Totals	$ 0	$ 0	$540,833	$559,167	$1,100,000

center allocates its own costs to itself. Thus, housekeeping services are used 70% by the laundry, 25% by the CCU, and 5% by the pharmacy. Laundry services are used 20% by housekeeping, 10% by the CCU, and 70% by the pharmacy.

Table 8–2 shows an allocation of the direct costs to the revenue centers. The allocation in this table is called a *direct distribution*. In the direct distribution method nonrevenue center costs are allocated only to revenue centers. In making the allocation, a problem arises. Although 25% of the square feet are in the CCU and 5% are in the pharmacy (see Table 8–1), if those percentages are used for the allocation, the full $40,000 of housekeeping cost would not be allocated. This is because 70% of the square feet are in the laundry, and no cost is being allocated to the laundry. This problem is resolved by allocating to the revenue centers based on the remaining square feet after eliminating the nonrevenue centers. Since 30% of the square feet are in all the revenue centers combined and 25% are in the CCU, 25% divided by 30% gives the proportion of the housekeeping cost allocated to the CCU. Similarly, 5% divided by 30% gives the housekeeping cost allocated to the pharmacy; 10% divided by 80% gives the laundry cost allocated to the CCU; and 70% divided by 80% gives the portion of the laundry cost allocated to the pharmacy. For example, 25% divided by 30% multiplied by the $40,000 housekeeping cost results in the $33,333 of cost allocated to the CCU.

There is also an additional complexity because direct distribution fails to take account of the fact that some nonrevenue cost centers provide service to other nonrevenue centers. Housekeeping cleans the laundry. If all housekeeping costs went directly to revenue centers, none would be allocated to the laundry and a distortion in costs would occur. The possible distortion is so great that a direct allocation to revenue centers only is not considered good enough.

Instead an allocation approach is used called the *step-down method*. This is shown in Figure 8–2 and Table 8–3. The step-down method requires the organization to allocate all the cost of a nonrevenue cost center to *all* other cost centers (both revenue and nonrevenue). First one nonrevenue center's costs are allocated to every cost center. Then another nonrevenue center is allocated. As each center is allocated, its cost balance becomes zero and it no longer is

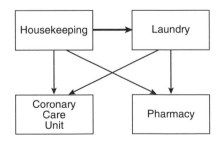

NONREVENUE CENTERS

REVENUE CENTERS

Figure 8–2. Allocating costs by step-down.

❖ **TABLE 8–3**
Step-down Distribution

	Nonrevenue Cost Centers		Revenue Cost Centers		
	Housekeeping	Laundry	Coronary Care Unit	Pharmacy	Total Cost
Direct cost	$ 40,000	$ 60,000	$500,000	$500,000	$1,100,000
Allocation:					
Housekeeping (square feet)	–40,000	28,000	10,000	2,000	0
Subtotal	$ 0	$ 88,000	$510,000	$502,000	$1,100,000
Laundry (pounds)		–88,000	11,000	77,000	0
Totals		$ 0	$521,000	$579,000	$1,100,000

❖ **TABLE 8–4**
Step-down Distribution with Altered Order of Step-down Allocation

	Nonrevenue Cost Centers		Revenue Cost Centers		
	Laundry	Housekeeping	Coronary Care Unit	Pharmacy	Total Cost
Direct cost	$ 60,000	$ 40,000	$500,000	$500,000	$1,100,000
Allocation:					
Laundry (pounds)	–60,000	12,000	6,000	42,000	0
Subtotal	$ 0	$ 52,000	$506,000	$542,000	$1,100,000
Housekeeping (square feet)		–52,000	43,333	8,667	0
Totals		$ 0	$549,333	$550,667	$1,100,000

189

part of the process. In other words, no costs can be allocated to a cost center once it has allocated its costs. Note in Figure 8–2 that housekeeping now would allocate costs to coronary care, pharmacy, *and* laundry. The laundry, however, would only allocate costs to coronary care and pharmacy. Therefore some amount of distortion still remains in the allocation process.

Other more elaborate allocation approaches eliminate most or all of the remaining distortion. These are called the *double distribution* and the *algebraic* or *matrix distribution* approaches. The algebraic or matrix distribution approaches are based on solving a set of simultaneous equations. While the allocation that results from use of such methods is more accurate, it is also more complicated to understand and implement. The hospital industry generally considers step-down allocation good enough.

The use of step-down allocation creates another problem: Should housekeeping be allocated before or after the laundry? The order of the allocation may affect the ultimate outcome. Table 8–4 changes the order of allocation. Laundry is now allocated using step down before housekeeping is allocated. Look at what happened to the ultimate cost in each revenue center. The total CCU cost has risen by $28,333, from $521,000 to $549,333. The pharmacy cost has fallen by $28,333, from $579,000 to $550,667. This is an extreme example, but it demonstrates the distortion possible by changing the order of allocation. In a perfect allocation system the ultimate cost in each revenue center would remain the same regardless of the order in which the nonrevenue center costs are allocated.

Are the actual resources consumed by the organization any different because the order of allocation of nonrevenue centers changed? No. The same total amount of money was spent. The same resources were used. However, the cost of the CCU and the pharmacy can vary because of the accounting methodology used. With the more sophisticated algebraic approach, such variation in costs does not occur. However, the step-down method, as noted, has been considered good enough.

It is possible that the step-down method has allowed health care organizations to manipulate their cost reporting in an attempt to shift costs between revenue centers in an effort to increase reimbursement. For example, many hospitals have both inpatients and outpatients. Medicare inpatients are paid on a fixed DRG payment scale. Although it may change, at the date this book was written outpatient payments for Medicare patients were not based on fixed DRG-type rates. If the order of the step down causes more costs to be allocated to the outpatient areas and fewer costs to be in departments that treat predominately inpatients, total reimbursement will rise.

Part of an institutional cost report is reproduced in the appendix to this chapter. This is from the type of report typically submitted to Medicare and Blue Cross. It shows how the step-down allocation appears for a real organization.

Allocate Costs to Units of Service

Up to this point, the discussion has centered on allocating all costs of the organization into the cost centers that are revenue centers. The next part of the cost-finding process centers on assigning each revenue center's costs to the units of service that it provides. For example, a laboratory assigns its costs to the various lab tests it performs; an operating room assigns its costs to the surgical procedures that take place. There are four approaches to allocating a revenue center's costs to units of service: the per diem, surcharge, hourly rate, and weighted procedure methods.

The per diem method is used if none of the other three methods reasonably applies. The per diem method divides the total costs of the center by the number of patient days, generating a uniform cost per patient day. Although some nursing cost centers do qualify for treatment using the other methods, that tends to be the exception rather than the rule. Most nursing costs are assigned ultimately to per diem categories. There are often different per diems for routine care as opposed to intensive care or coronary care. The major problem with such an approach is that it assumes that each patient consumes exactly the same amount of nursing (or other) resources per patient day. It takes no account of patient severity of illness or nursing requirements. However, the cost-finding process has treated this approach as being good enough.

The surcharge method is commonly used in the pharmacy and medical supplies cost centers. The revenue center compares its costs excluding inventory to the inventory cost and determines a surcharge. For example, if a pharmacy spends $10,000 on all costs except pharmaceuticals and $100,000 on pharmaceuticals, then the surcharge would be 10% (i.e., $10,000 divided by $100,000). As each prescription is filled, the cost would be calculated as the cost of the drug itself, plus 10%. The problem with this approach is that in reality, just because a drug costs ten times as much to buy as another drug does not mean that it requires ten times as much pharmacist time to process. Some organizations overcome this problem partly by using a minimum charge applied to all drugs dispensed. The proverbial hospital $10 aspirin is partly the result of charging a standard minimum amount for processing the aspirin order, storing the aspirin, and dispensing it.

The hourly rate approach measures the amount of service a revenue center provides by time. This method is used by respiratory therapy, physical therapy, ORs and recovery rooms. For example, an OR would divide its total cost (after the step-down allocation) by the total number of hours of procedures to determine a cost per hour. Sometimes the calculations are done in minutes, yielding a cost per surgical minute. The logic of this method is that longer operations consume more resources.

This method is very accurate for a service such as physical therapy, where there is generally only one therapist working with the patient. A problem that arises in using this approach in the OR is that an operation may have just one nurse, two nurses, or two nurses and a technician. Also the supplies and equipment used may not bear a direct relationship to time. It is possible that a two-hour operation might consume far more resources than a three-hour operation. This method, while not very good, had traditionally been considered good enough. In recent years, however, operating rooms are trying alternative approaches. For example, many ORs keep track of person hours, rather than just surgical hours, to account for the number of staff members in the surgical suite.

The last method is the weighted procedure method (sometimes called the relative value unit, or RVU, method). This approach is based upon a special study of the center's costs, which establishes a relative costliness of each type of service the center performs. This method is commonly used in departments such as laboratory or radiology, where there are a specific limited number of services provided, and they are provided in similar fashion each time. A base value is assigned to one type of procedure, and all other procedures are assigned a relative value. Thus if a blood gas is twice as costly as a CBC, the CBC might be assigned a value of 1.0 unit of work and the blood gas a value of 2.0 units of work. In any given month, the values assigned to all the services provided can be summed and divided into the total cost of the revenue center. This yields a cost per unit of work.

For example, suppose that the total costs of the laboratory revenue center after the step-down allocation of nonrevenue centers costs were $5,000. If the laboratory performed 300 blood gasses and 400 CBCs, it performed a total of 1,000 units of work (300 blood gasses $\times$ 2 units of work + 400 CBCs $\times$ 1 unit of work). $5,000 divided by 1,000 units of work is $5 per unit of work. Therefore the $5,000 total laboratory costs would be assigned at a rate of $10 per blood gas (2 units of work $\times$ $5 per unit) and $5 per CBC (1 unit of work $\times$ $5 per unit).

A problem with this approach is that it relies heavily on the assumption that a blood gas is always twice as costly to perform as a CBC. This problem is exacerbated by the fact that many health care organizations use standard relationships based on a survey of institutions rather than measuring the relative costs in their own facility. Since the personnel pay rates and the equipment used will vary from one organization to another, the relative relationships are not likely to be exactly the same at all institutions. However, in comparison to having an accountant observe the resources used each time a lab test is performed, it is considered good enough. While this method is much more accurate than the per diem method, it requires data that would be very difficult and costly to collect for departments such as nursing.

Is Good-enough Cost Finding Good Enough?

For the first two decades under Medicare and Medicaid, the good-enough approximations that resulted from the above cost-finding system were considered acceptable. Most large third-party payers—Medicare, Medicaid, Blue Cross, and private for-profit insurers—have a large mix of patients. If they are overcharged on one patient, they are likely to be undercharged on another. As long as the total costs are not overstated, overcharges and undercharges are likely to average out for large groups of patients. It would not be sensible for them to require health care organizations to spend substantially more money on improved cost accounting. They would then have to bear the cost of the improved cost accounting in addition to the costs of patient care.

With the introduction of DRGs, however, incentives have changed. Hospitals, in particular, are now at risk for the costs they incur. If patients cost more to care for than the DRG payment rate, the hospital suffers a loss. It has become a great interest to hospitals to have accurate methods for finding costs of specific types of patients. With a new type of DRGs on the verge of being introduced for ambulatory care and already introduced in some states for long-term care, improved costing is of interest in most health care organizations.

This means that to the extent possible, still being mindful of the cost of collecting more accurate information, managers of health care organizations would like to improve on the good-enough approximations. They would like to eliminate the inaccuracies of using pounds of laundry instead of pieces or using square feet instead of construction cost for depreciation. They would like to eliminate the distortions created by the order of allocation in the step-down process. They would like to remove the inaccuracies generated by weighted procedure, hourly, surcharge, and per diem assignments of cost.

Can this be done? Probably there will never be a 100% accurate costing system. As computer use in health care organizations increases, the potential exists to make great strides in accurate assignment of patient resource consumption. In the interim, many health care organizations are taking at least intermediate steps to improve their costing. Some of the approaches used are discussed in the remaining sections of this chapter.

COSTING OUT NURSING SERVICES

The essence of the costing problem is that in most hospitals nursing costs are charged to patients as part of a general per diem charge rather than being charged separately on the patient's bill. As a result, all patients in a given unit of the hospital will receive the same daily charge for nursing care services. In terms of providing management with an understanding of the cost implications of different patients, this provides extremely poor information. It implicitly assumes that all patients consume exactly the same amount of nursing care, even though different patients have different nursing care requirements.

Until the 1980s, measurement of differential consumption was, if not impossible, at least too costly to consider. Hospitals are faced with two extreme alternatives. One choice is to take the total annual costs of nursing care and divide that by the number of patients treated for the year to come out with an average cost per patient. At the other extreme, the hospital could hire a data collector to follow each nurse and determine exactly how much of the nurse's time was used by each patient. Figure 8–3 reflects this extreme choice. Alternative A is a very simple and inexpensive approach at one extreme. Alternative Z is an extremely detailed and expensive approach at the other extreme.

What hospital could afford to assign a data collector to each nurse to observe how much time was devoted to each patient? The value of information should always justify its cost. Alternative Z in Figure 8–3 was just too costly to undertake. Figure 8–4 adds a compromise. In most cases a patient with a three-day stay would consume less nursing care than a patient with a fifteen-day stay. If total nursing care costs are divided by total patient days, patients who are in the hospital for more days can be assigned more nursing cost than patients in the hospital for fewer days. This is Alternative B. It is still not nearly so precise and accurate an approach as Alternative Z. However, it is not much more expensive than Alternative A and gives a much better approximation of the nursing care cost for different patients.

However, under Alternative B, which is the approach most hospitals use, the nursing cost is assumed to be the same for all patient days. More days imply more cost, but for the same number of patient days, all patients are assumed to use the same amount of nursing care. While this is much better than Alternative A, it is still a very poor measure of nursing cost. This is the approach currently used by most hospitals.

Solutions to the Costing Problem

How can the cost of each individual patient be better measured without having an accountant follow every nurse? One solution that many hospitals

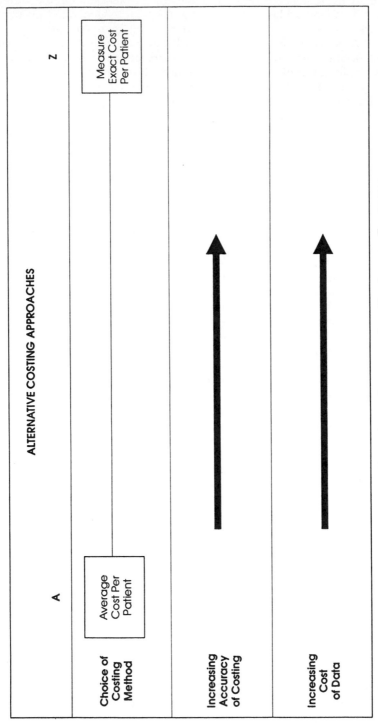

Figure 8–3. Alternative costing approaches: The A versus Z extremes.

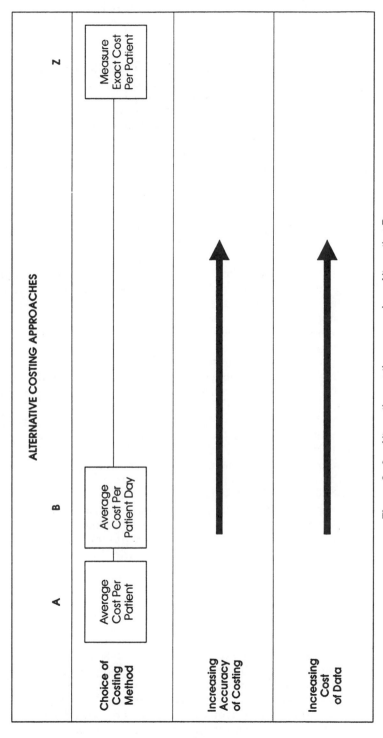

Figure 8–4. Alternative costing approaches: Alternative B.

are beginning to examine is computerization. The addition of computers not only at nursing stations but also by each bedside is seen by many nurses to be the future for all hospitals. Many hospitals are already installing bedside computer terminals.

One use of bedside computer systems will undoubtedly be to better track nursing costs. In Figure 8–5 computers have been added to the continuum from low-accuracy, low-cost information to high-accuracy, high-cost information. This alternative has been labeled Y. With computers, nurses can record not only when they are with each patient but also what they are doing for each patient. The specific cost of the nurse giving care can be associated with the patient by having the computer multiply the time spent by the salary of the particular nurse providing the care. When nurses are doing some indirect activities, such as documenting a patient's record, the computer can also assign that cost to the appropriate patient, since the documentation is being done on the computer.

Substantial progress is currently being made in a variety of areas to ease the input of data into the computer. Uniform price codes (bar coding) are becoming more widely used on a variety of supplies consumed by hospitals. Employee identification cards are being issued in some hospitals with magnetic strips containing the employee number in computer-readable form. This allows nurses to just slide their card into the computer to identify themselves. Light pens are beginning to be replaced with touch-sensitive screens. Such screens allow the user to simply touch a particular item on the screen to select menu choices and enter data.

The result of progress in the computer area is that there will probably soon be bedside terminals widely available that can very accurately capture most of the costs (both direct and many indirect costs) of providing nursing care to specific patients.

Note that Alternative Y is very close to Alternative Z in several respects. The data to be gained is potentially quite accurate and clearly can be very patient specific. For patients who require the presence of a nurse at the bedside for substantial amounts of time, that cost will be captured. It would be able to assign to different patients costs (and ultimately charges) based on their differing consumption of nursing resources. At the same time, however, computerization has the potential to be quite costly. The computers, computer terminals, and other computer hardware must be purchased and installed. Nurses must be trained to use the system. Software has the potential to be the largest cost. A tailored system may be needed to make the computer function well at your specific institution.

Is there a solution to the costing problem that can be used at hospitals that lack bedside computer systems? Many believe that the solution to this problem is patient acuity data. Sophisticated *patient classification systems* have been developed to identify patient acuity levels. These systems assess the differing consumption of nursing care hours by patients with differing acuity levels. Although such systems were a rarity in the early 1980s, today they are a requirement for hospital accreditation. As a result of this requirement most hospitals have in place a working patient classification system. The extent to which they use their classification system is less uniform.

Patient classification systems require rating patients based on the likely nursing resource requirements resulting from their acuity. Sicker patients re-

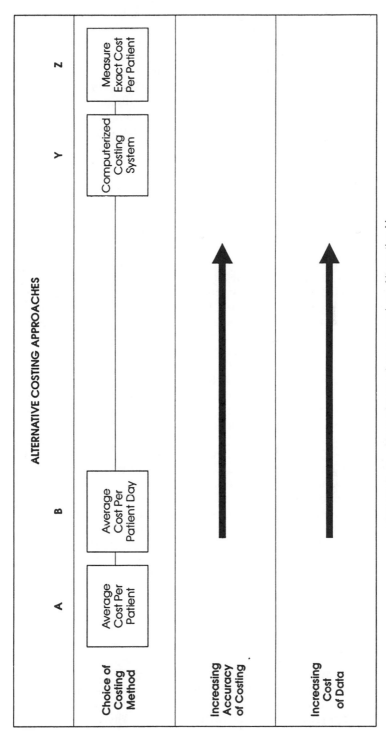

Figure 8–5. Alternative costing approaches: Alternative Y.

quiring more nursing care are assigned higher acuity or higher classification levels. Many hospitals have developed their own systems, while several systems are widely used in hospitals throughout the United States. Patients are rated on scales such as 1 to 5. Scales up to levels of 48 (to represent two hours of nursing care per patient hour in an ICU) exist.

Patient classification will not generally be perfectly accurate measures of the resources needed for each patient. Some patients who are classified as level 2 will require more care than level 2 calls for, and some level 2 patients will require less care than would be expected based on that classification. However, if the system is functioning reasonably well, average patient resource consumption will match what is expected based on the classification system. And certainly it would generally be expected that a level 2 patient will consume resources closer to the level 2 average than to the level 1 average or the level 3 average.

If a mechanism to determine patients' costs based on their patient classification can be established, it will not provide the precise accuracy of Alternative Z. It will not even provide the Alternative Y accuracy that a computer system can generate. However, it can create a new alternative, called X (see Fig. 8–6). Alternative X is inaccurate in that all patients are assigned the same nursing cost for a day at the same classification level. If two patients are both level 2 on a given day, their cost is assumed to be the same, even though it is known that they will probably not consume exactly the same nursing resources. However, Alternative X is much more accurate than Alteratives A and B. Alternative B assumes that the cost is the same per patient day for all patients regardless of acuity.

Alternative X is an improvement because the cost is considered the same per patient day only for patients in the same acuity level. Different costs are assigned to patient days at different acuity levels. Users of Alternative X must recognize that the information has some degree of inaccuracy. However, the system may be accurate enough, given the current high costs of using either Alternative Y or Z. Therefore, patient classification systems can be the basis for a system that allows more accurate estimates of the cost a hospital incurs for nursing care for different types of patients.

Somewhere between X and Y on the scale from A to Z one could place work-load measurement tools. These are variants of patient classification. Work-load measurement tools attempt to determine the nursing care time required for each individual patient each day. The approach of these tools is to identify the time required for each of the types of nursing interventions that take up most of the nurses' time. Each patient is evaluated each day to determine which interventions will be needed. Such tools can track required care hours specific to each patient. This is contrasted with patient classification systems that use an average hour figure for all patients within a broad category or level of care.

Such an approach is not as sophisticated as Alternative Y, where the actual care hours are entered into the computer as the patient receives the care. It is likely that some interventions will take longer than typical for some patients and less time for others. Therefore the cost ultimately assigned to the patient will be based on average times, not actual times. However, the work-load measurement approach is more sophisticated than Alternative X, which uses

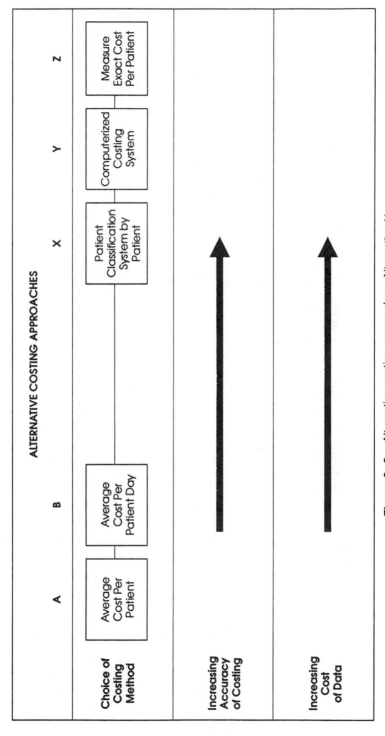

Figure 8–6. Alternative costing approaches: Alternative X.

average nursing care hours for all patients in a given patient classification category.

Although patient classification and work measurement systems can be used to determine the cost of nursing, these systems were initially developed to predict staffing needs, not to determine costs. The nurse managers should be aware that although patients require a designated amount of care, this does not mean that they receive it.

Why Change the Costing Approach?

The mere fact that the ability to improve costing now exists does not in itself explain why a nurse manager would want to more accurately identify costs. What is to be gained from having a more accurate measure of the different costs for nursing care for different types of patients?

A critical benefit from improved costing of nursing services is that the organization can generate information for better management decisions. Is a particular service too costly? What price can be bid for an HMO or PPO contract? Hospital costing has long been based on averages and cross subsidizations. In the current environment, errors in calculations of costs become more serious, as negotiations for discounted prices become more intense. Thus, if the organization's managers are mistaken about the resources a particular class of patient consumes, the ramifications can be quite serious. Less averaging of costs is acceptable today than was acceptable in the past. This means that managers are being pushed along the increasing accuracy of the costing line in Figure 8–6, even though this also moves in the direction of increased cost of data.

In addition, as costing becomes more specific and more accurate, not only can managers deal better with pricing problems but they can also be more efficient in the management of costs. Control of budgets improves as another measure of expected cost becomes available. Flexible budget systems can provide better analysis and control of costs, and productivity can be monitored better if more is known about costs. Not only is it possible to assess how costs should change based on changing numbers of patient days but information about the cost per patient in a given DRG can also be used to assess costs as the number of patients in each DRG changes.

Should Costing Be Linked to DRGs?

If hospitals are going to move in the direction of more accurate costing of nursing services, one of the critical questions is how to categorize the cost. Should there be one nursing cost for medical patients and another for surgical patients? Should the cost for men as opposed to women be determined, or for young people as opposed to old people? Should there be one nursing cost for each type of patient based on ICD code? Should the cost be found by DRG?

The problem managers face is the definition of the product of nursing care. What does nursing produce? If a nurse changes a dressing or gives a patient a medication, are those the products of nursing care? Probably most people would consider those activities to represent only intermediate products. The ultimate product is the health of the patient, not the care provided.

However, health care organizations treat many different kinds of patients. They do not have only one final product: a healthy patient. They have many final products represented by the different patients to whom nurses give care.

Yet currently all patients are costed for nursing care as if they were the same. That needs to be changed. Final products need to be defined so that nurse managers can assess the cost of each. Patients could be divided into categories called *nursing resource groupings* (NRGs), perhaps based on nursing diagnoses. Ideally, the patients should be divided into homogeneous NRGs based on nursing care consumed. Any patient in one NRG would consume a similar set of nursing resources as any other patient in that grouping.

The problem encountered with this approach is how to establish the NRGs. The nursing profession has argued that DRGs are not natural groupings based on the consumption of nursing resources. NRGs and DRGs would not necessarily coincide. Not all DRGs require different nursing resources, so several or many DRGs might fall into one NRG. On the other hand, some DRGs have patients with widely varying nursing needs. Therefore, one DRG might have patients from a number of different NRGs. So the specific NRGs are not the same as the specific DRGs, although there are similarities in the basic concepts. How would NRGs be developed?

Several attempts have been made at developing NRGs. For example, in New Jersey a method called relative intensity measures (RIMs) was studied. However, because of problems in consistency of the measures across hospitals, it never became widely adopted throughout the nursing industry. It will take a great deal of research and testing before any reliable NRG system is developed and becomes widely accepted. It is likely that for at least the next ten years hospitals will be reimbursed on a medical diagnosis–based DRG system. Therefore nursing short-term efforts should be directed at grouping nursing resource use within DRGs or combining DRGs into NRGs.

What should be the basis for costing nursing services in the interim until a NRG type system is in use? One approach is to fall back on Alternative X. A patient classification system can be used to determine how many days a given patient is at each classification level. If the cost of each day at each classification level (discussed later in this chapter) can be determined, the manager can add up the costs to determine the patient's total nursing care cost.

However, this requires determination of the patient classification for every patient for every day. Some hospitals will feel that the advantages of being at Alternative X on the costing accuracy scale are sufficient to warrant this investment in data collection. Doing this will not only improve costing but will also collect information that can be used for calculating acuity variances.[2] Such data are also potentially very beneficial in planning staffing. If the classification for each patient each day is known, the nursing staff can be assigned to the units where they are most needed.

Historically most nursing departments have not made a regular practice of moving nurses from unit to unit in response to information regarding patient classification. There are problems with such an approach in terms of union rules and quality-of-care concerns. However, if resources for the health care industry continue to be extremely tight, hospitals will have to learn to maximize their resources. Nursing staffs will undoubtedly become even more constricted

---

[2]See Chapter 13 and also Steven A. Finkler, *Budgeting Concepts for Nurse Managers*, W.B. Saunders, Philadelphia, 1992, pp. 292–294, and Steven A. Finkler, "Variance Analysis: Part I, Extending Flexible Budget Variance Analysis to Acuity," *Journal of Nursing Administration*, Vol. 21, No. 7/8, July/August 1991, pp. 19–25.

than is already the case, even though the trend toward higher patient acuity will likely increase. It would not be unreasonable to expect that nursing departments are going to have to become more flexible in moving nurses to the units where the need is greatest. That will require knowledge of where the need is. Ongoing daily use of patient classification systems can provide that information. Once collected, the information can be used for specific costing of each patient under Alternative X.

However, many hospitals will not want to spend the resources needed to classify every patient every day. The alternative is to take a sample of patients from each DRG and determine the average nursing cost for patients in each DRG based on a sampling approach. All patients within a specific DRG will not consume the same nursing resources for each day at a specific patient classification level. Nor will all patients in one DRG have the same number of patient days at each classification level or even the same total number of patient days. This approach is based on an average length of stay, an average number of days at each patient classification level, and an average nurse resource consumption within each patient classification level. However, the average amount of nursing resources for each type of DRG can be found.

For example, if a hospital uses a nursing patient classification system with a scale from 1 to 5, a group of patients from each DRG can be sampled to find out, on average, how many days of the patients' stay were at level 1, how many at level 2, and so on. Averaging all patients in a given DRG at a given hospital will not give a measurement alternative accurate enough to be labeled W on the scale from A to Z. Such an estimate of cost would probably be considered R on such a scale. It would not be nearly as accurate as X, but it would be substantially more accurate than Alternatives A and B. This new Alternative R (see Fig. 8–7) would be substantially less expensive than Alternatives X, Y, or Z.

DRGs, although perhaps not ideal for the purpose of costing nursing care, are an adequate categorization for the assignment of average differential nursing costs. Many hospital decisions are based on particular DRGs or clusters of DRGs, so the DRG-based cost information generated will be of considerable management value.

A SPECIFIC APPROACH TO COSTING NURSING SERVICES

Nursing care costs consist of the staff costs of:
♦ Direct patient care
♦ Indirect patient care (supervisors, secretaries, etc.)
♦ Patient care–related costs (e.g., patient and unit supplies)
♦ Overhead (allocated from other departments)
Note that the cost of nursing care is more than just the hourly salary and benefits of the nurse giving care at the bedside. Nursing management, assessment, planning, evaluating, teaching, and discharge planning are also critical elements of nursing care. Additionally, supplies, secretaries, and overhead are elements of overall nursing care cost. A manager could try to determine the costs of each of these elements separately for each category of patient or else do the costing in some more aggregate fashion. Start with the assumption that all nursing department costs are aggregated.

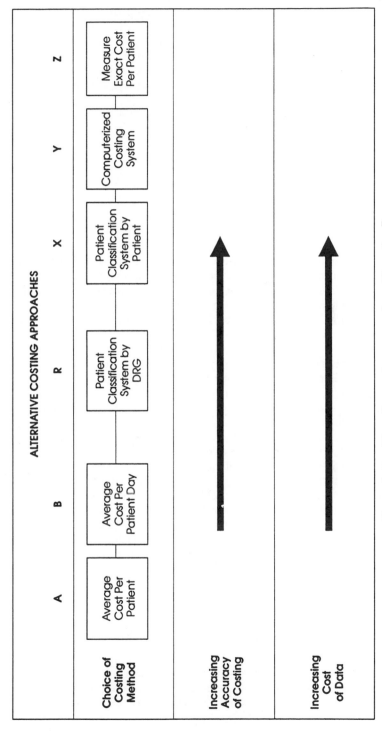

Figure 8–7. Alternative costing approaches: Alternative R.

The key element that allows for improved costing of nursing services is the fact that nursing patient classification systems are currently in place in almost every hospital. Without such systems different patients consume different amounts of resources, but the manager has no way to measure the differential consumption. With a classification system, once a patient has been classified, the manager has some idea about the nursing resources that patient consumes.

For example, suppose that a nursing unit has the following hypothetical patient classification resource guidelines:

Acuity Level	Hours of Care
1	3.0
2	4.0
3	4.8
4	6.6
5	9.0

In developing the patient classification system, various clinical indicators are used to determine if a patient should be classified as a 1, 2, 3, 4, or 5. Once the patient has been classified, the classification system tells how many hours of nursing care should be required to treat that patient. In the above example, a patient classified as a 4 would typically require an average of six and six-tenths hours of care.

Note that the scale is not proportional. A patient classified as a 2 does not require exactly twice as many hours as a 1. While a level 1 needs three hours of care, a level 2 patient needs four hours. Rather than double, this is only 33% more care. A level 3 patient needs four and eight-tenths hours. That is 20% more than a level 2. A level 4 patient requires 38% more care than a level 3. As one moves from level to level, the amount of additional care does not change in proportion. It changes based on the specific classification system and the clinical needs of a patient at each level in that system.

This complicates the cost calculation. If the scale were strictly linear, one could add up all the patient days at each level and divide into total nursing cost to get a cost per unit of patient classification. However, since the scale is not linear, it is necessary to create a relative value unit (RVU) scale. This scale will allow determination of how much care each level requires relative to the care needed for a typical level 1 patient. A patient classified as a 1 will be given a value of 1 on the *relative value scale*. Each other classification level would then be calculated in relative proportion. This can be accomplished by dividing the required hours of care for each level by the number of hours required for level 1. For example:

$$\frac{\text{Level 2}}{\text{Level 1}} = \frac{4.0 \text{ hours}}{3.0 \text{ hours}} = 1.33$$

Therefore the relative value assigned to classification level 2 is 1.33. This value of 1.33 represents the fact that a level 2 patient consumes .33 more nursing care hours than a level 1 patient. Continuing for all classification (acuity) levels:

Acuity Level	Hours of Care	RVU
1	3.0	1.00
2	4.0	1.33
3	4.8	1.60
4	6.6	2.20
5	9.0	3.00

Assuming the following information, the reader will be able to see how the RVU system can be used to develop cost information:

Total nursing costs: $250,000

Number of patient days
at each acuity level: 1   100 days
                              2   220 days
                              3   350 days
                              4   110 days
                              5   40 days

The first step is to determine the total amount of work performed by the nursing department. This is done by multiplying the RVUs for each acuity classification level by the number of days at that level. Using the number of patient days given above and the RVUs calculated above, the total RVUs would be:

Acuity Level	Patient Days	× RVUs =	Total RVUs
1	100	× 1.00	100.00
2	220	× 1.33	292.60
3	350	× 1.60	560.00
4	110	× 2.20	242.00
5	40	× 3.00	120.00
	820		1,314.60

There were 1,314.6 units of nursing work performed. We can divide this into the total nursing cost to find the cost for each RVU of nursing work.

$$\frac{\text{Total nursing costs}}{\text{Total RVUs}} = \text{Cost per RVU}$$

$$\frac{\$250,000}{1,314.60} = \$190.17 \text{ per RVU}$$

Here one can see that the nursing cost for a patient for one day with classification 1 would be $190.17. The cost for a patient with classification 4 would be $190.17 multiplied by 2.20 (the RVU for classification level 4).

How would a manager calculate the nursing cost for a patient from admission to discharge? Suppose that the average DRG 128 patient had a length of stay of seven days, with two days classed as a 1, four days classed as a 2, and one day classed as a 4. The nursing cost for DRG 128 would then be:

Acuity Level	Patient Days	× RVUs	×	Cost per RVU	=	Total Cost
1	2	× 1.00	×	$190.17	=	$ 380.34
2	4	× 1.33	×	190.17	=	1,011.70
3	0	× 1.60	×	190.17	=	0.00
4	1	× 2.20	×	190.17	=	418.37
5	0	× 3.00	×	190.17	=	0.00
	7					$1,810.41

Would all patients in a given DRG be expected to consume the same resources? Not really, but the manager can still be confident that an approach such as this on average for any given DRG will give a much more accurate assignment of cost than simply assigning to every patient in a nursing unit the same daily cost for nursing care.

LIMITATIONS OF THE RVU APPROACH

Patient Classification vs. Other Work-load Measurement

The purpose of the RVU patient classification approach is to provide a workable costing approach accessible to the majority of hospitals in the country. However, it does not generate perfectly accurate measures of cost and is subject to a variety of limitations.

The idea of an alternative to patient classification was discussed earlier. If a work-load measurement tool is in place in a hospital and is being used on an ongoing basis to categorize resource needs of each patient each day, then it can be used to provide cost information that is potentially more accurate. Rather than being limited to perhaps five patient classification levels for a given medical/surgical unit, such an approach collects indicators of hours of resource consumption for each patient. It is more patient specific than the RVU approach. Putting such an approach in place and following through with it on a continuous basis may be a considerable undertaking. However, if it is used, costing is made potentially easier.

Under such an approach the required interventions for each patient are translated into required hours of care. Total nursing care costs for direct and indirect expenses must be calculated as with the RVU system. Dividing total nursing costs by total hours of care generates a cost per hour of care. This cost per hour can be multiplied by the required hours of care for each patient for each day as determined by the system. This will give the cost per patient for each day in the hospital. If aggregate information is desired by DRG, it can be obtained by averaging the costs of each patient in that DRG. However, the majority of hospitals do not have patient-specific work measurement systems in place.

Indirect Nursing Costs

A problem with both the RVU and more detailed work measurement systems as described so far is that this chapter has been implicitly assuming that all nursing costs vary in proportion to the hours of nursing care. Does that make sense for indirect costs? For example, will a sicker patient who requires more direct nursing care also require more indirect nursing care? More charting time? More supplies? More overhead? The answer to these questions depends on the specific situation of your institution.

Is it true that secretarial costs will be greater for more acutely ill patients? It may well be that a simple per diem allocation is a more appropriate way to allocate such costs. Costing could therefore be improved by dividing total nursing costs among those costs which vary with nursing care hours (such as RN staff and LPN staff and perhaps clinical supplies) and those costs which do not vary with nursing care hours (such as office supplies, nurse manager time, and secretarial time). The costs that vary with nursing care hours would be allocated by the RVU or work measurement approaches described above. The other costs could be divided by total patient days and assigned to patients based on their number of patient days.

Staffing Mix

A significant problem is the fact that most nursing classification systems provide required hours of care but do not specify the mix of care. If 30% of all nursing care hours are provided by LPNs, then it is assumed that 30% of the care for each patient is provided by LPNs.

It is possible that one patient at level 2 might require four hours of RN care, while another might require three hours of LPN care and only one hour of RN care. Obviously both of these patients do not consume the same amount of nursing care resources, even if they consume the same number of hours of care. Therefore there will be some distortion of costs unless the hospital uses a system that indicates not only how many hours of care are needed but also how many hours of care by staff type.

This problem is not unique to costing, however. It represents a weakness of patient classification systems. If the hospital does not know the required mix of care providers, the classification system is not going to be useful for staffing decisions. Part of this problem stems from the fact that different hospitals have different views on which functions can be done by different types of staff. However, over time one can expect that classification systems will improve. As they do, this mix problem should become less serious.

In the meantime, managers could attempt to separate the cost of RNs from LPNs and aides and assign those costs separately to patients. Special studies could be undertaken for each DRG to determine whether their care was biased toward more than an average amount of RN care or toward more than an average amount of LPN care. Then the cost of nursing care for that DRG could be adjusted accordingly. Other approaches to handling this problem are discussed below in the section that discusses productivity.

How complex are managers willing to make the costing system? Each health care organization must decide how much it is willing to refine its costing system, realizing that generally the more accurate the costing system, the more expensive. Some managers believe that the historical average nursing cost per patient day is so inaccurate that an RVU-based system is a tremendous improvement, even with the problems cited here.

We have used a hospital as an example. The same principles apply whether the cost determination is for nursing care delivered in the hospital, nursing home, outpatient setting, or patient's home.

MEASURING PRODUCTIVITY

As the pressure to contain costs in health care continues, nurse managers are under increasing pressure to improve productivity. It is not enough to know nursing costs for different patient types. Managers hear the CEO saying "the staff must be more productive," "we've got to use fewer resources," and "do something to improve efficiency." Productivity is defined as the ratio of outputs to inputs and is often notated as an algebraic equation:

$$\text{Productivity} = \frac{\text{Output}}{\text{Input}}$$

Productivity is a ratio and therefore affected by changes in output or input. If output increases and input stays the same, productivity is said to increase. If output stays the same and input decreases, productivity increases. To increase productivity the nurse manager must increase output while decreasing or not changing input, or provide the same output with fewer inputs.

Why must health organizations be more productive? Increasing productivity gives an organization the resources with which to develop and grow. Inflation causes the costs of inputs to increase. Many health care revenue sources, such as Medicare, do not rise as rapidly as inflation. Quality and quantity of care provided can only be maintained if productivity increases.

Although improving productivity is not a simple task in any industry, aspects of nursing care make it particularly complicated. The first step in measuring productivity is to define input and output. Inputs are the resources needed to produce the product. For nursing, inputs usually include nursing staff, equipment, supplies, and the organizational support needed to keep the nursing staff available, such as personnel and recruiting.

Nursing's output or product is more difficult to define. McHugh discusses many of the problems in measuring nursing productivity. She states that a patient day of care, the traditional measure of nursing output, is "really not a nursing output; it is an institutional output and relatively insensitive to nursing productivity."[3]

Although most nurses agree that a healthy patient is the goal of nursing and therefore nursing's output, most nurses recognize that there is wide disagreement on the definition of health. Further, there is wide agreement that the health of a patient is related not only to nursing care but also to the care of other health providers and a myriad of patient characteristics. Thus far, nurse managers (and CEOs) have been satisfied defining nursing output as some measure of what economists call throughput, i.e., what the nurse does for the patient.

For purposes of this chapter, we will discuss productivity as it has been traditionally defined, with output defined as units of service provided. Additionally one must consider how the health care organization is paid. It is critical to consider whether the outcome measure used by payers is the same as that used by the productivity system. If nurses reduce hours of care per patient day but increase the number of patient days and the total number of

---

[3]Mary L. McHugh, "Productivity Measurement in Nursing," *Applied Nursing Research*, Vol. 2, No. 2, 1989, p. 100.

hours of care, is that good or bad? Financially it would likely be good for the organization if it is paid for patient days, but bad if it is paid for the patient on a fixed basis regardless of hours of care or patient days. Under the cost-based reimbursement systems, health care organizations are reimbursed on a per diem or per visit basis. Thus for each day of patient care provided, the organization charges the patient and receives a negotiated reimbursement rate or a regulated rate from a third-party payer or the charge from the patient. If an organization can produce a day of care or a visit with less input, productivity improves. Although this approach to productivity may be appropriate in a reimbursement system that pays based on days of care, the approach is not appropriate for a reimbursement system that reimburses organizations for an episode of care. Thus as reimbursement moves to an episodic basis, nurse managers need to rethink the unit of output.

For example, assume that average hours of nursing care per patient day (HPPD) on a unit were four. A new nurse manager arrives and decreases the HPPD to three and five-tenths HPPD with no change in quality. The manager might be considered efficient. However, using this same case, assume that when HPPD were four the patient stayed in the hospital for six days, thus consuming 24 hours for the entire stay. Under the new efficient manager, the HPPD decreased to three and five-tenths, but the length of stay increased to seven days and the patient therefore used twenty-four and five-tenths hours of nursing care. Is the second nurse manager really more efficient? Clearly, the second manager is less efficient than the first. However, under a per diem–based reimbursement system that pays a fixed amount per patient day, the hospital would receive more income from care provided when the patient received three and five-tenths hours of care per day and stayed for seven days. Thus from the hospital's financial point of view, the less efficient manager would be the better manager. However, as payment systems increasingly are based on an episode of care (e.g., DRGs), a productivity measure based on an episode is necessary.

Since health care organizations in most states continue to be reimbursed (at least for many patients) on a per diem basis, approaches to calculating productivity will be reviewed. Most organizations have or should have a standard for the ratio of output to input. These standards are often developed based on the historical activities of the organization, industry standards developed by provider organizations, and collective bargaining contracts.

For hospitals the usual standard is an identified number of hours per patient day, while in home health agencies the standard is usually nurse visits per day. Standards may be for direct care hours or some combination of direct care and indirect care.

In the simplest case, if the hospital's standard is to provide four hours of direct nursing care per day and 1,000 days of care were provided, it is expected that 4,000 hours (four hours × 1000 days) of care were needed. Assume that 3,000 hours of direct care were actually provided. The unit would be considered 133% productive (4,000 required/3,000 actual = 133%). Assume, however, that 4,500 hours of direct care were actually provided. The unit would then be considered to be 88% productive (4,000 required/4,500 actual = 88%). Note that this measure of productivity ignores quality of care. Being "more productive" could result from understaffing and thus potentially have a negative impact on quality of care.

Nurse managers recognize that not all patients require the same amount of nursing care per day. Thus required care is usually adjusted for a measure of acuity. For example, suppose that a unit has two acuity levels. Based on hospital direct care standards, patients with acuity level 2 require six HPPD and acuity level 1 patients require three HPPD. For one day the unit provides care for fifteen acuity 2 patients and twenty acuity 1 patients; therefore the required hours are calculated as follows:

15 acuity 2 patients × 6 HPPD =   90
20 acuity 1 patients × 3 HPPD =   60

Total hours required for the unit = 150

By determining the actual hours worked, the ratio of hours required to hours worked can be determined. Determining the actual hours worked requires identifying those staff who worked and the hours worked. Some financial managers suggest that all nursing staff are interchangeable. Therefore when calculating productivity they consider all nursing hours equally, whether they are provided by a professional nurse or a nursing assistant. Most nurses would agree that hours of professional nursing care cannot be equated with hours of nursing assistant or even LPN hours; thus some adjustment is made.

One approach is to develop a standard based on the usual staffing mix on the unit and assume the differentiation in level of staff is consistent. Given the variation in staffing both among units and within units on particular days, this approach is usually not meaningful.

Another common approach is to set the standard in terms of RN hours required and consider levels of staff as equivalent to a part of an RN. For example, a CNE might decide that an LPN equals .8 of an RN and a nursing assistant equals .6. Thus, if the patient unit required the equivalent of six professional staff, that staff could be composed of three RNs (3 × 1 = 3), three aides (3 × .6 = 1.8), and one and a half LPNs (1.5 × .8 = 1.2), for a total equivalent staff of six.

The above section described a method for determining productivity if the output is patient day of care. Determining output for an episode of care is far more complicated. In the above example it is assumed that patients can be grouped in categories of care required for each day of care. Although nurse managers agree that these groups are not exact, they are precise enough to be adequate in most cases.

To determine productivity for an episode of care it is necessary to determine standards for episodes. No widely accepted systems have been developed to group patients into categories of nursing care required for their entire stay. The following section outlines some approaches to product-line costing, a variation on episode of care.

PRODUCT-LINE COSTING

One result of the work done on costing nursing services (discussed earlier) is that it is possible to group all patients of one type and find an average cost for that type of patient. In other words, *product-line* costing becomes feasible with this methodology. A product line is a group of patients with some commonality that allows them to be grouped together, such as a common diagnosis.

Many people believe that managers will be given hospital-wide responsibility for both the revenues and expenses related to specific patient product lines. For example, a manager might be responsible for the revenues related to the "obstetrics" product line, as shown in Table 8–5. In that table the manager is accountable for both the variance in the number of discharges and the revenue per discharge. Of course the manager would be responsible for the budgeted and actual costs of the product line as well.

Before one takes the step of costing by product line or budgeting by product line, it is necessary to question what the information will be used for. In terms of running a nursing unit, will knowledge of the cost for all patients in a given DRG be useful? The answer to that question depends a great deal on the types of decisions that a manager or organization faces.

Some authors envision use of cost information by DRG as a way to promote efficiency. For example, consider Table 8–6. In that table the treatment patterns of the two physicians' patients are examined to see if one physician is inefficient.

Alternately, suppose that a hospital is trying to decide whether to accept a group of cardiac patients from an HMO at a discounted price. Knowing the costs for that type of patient would certainly be advantageous in the negotiating process. Often product-line calculations include nursing costs simply as part of the overall per diem cost. The organization can have much better information about different types of patients if it relies on the costing out nursing resource use discussed above in doing product-line calculations.

Direct Care Hours

Product-line information can be used not only for negotiations but also for budgeting. The direct care hours approach to product-line budgeting consists of dividing the patients for a given nursing unit into product lines, determining the number of hours of care required for each product line, and aggregating that information to find the total hours of care needed in the budget. This is a straightforward approach to using product-line information to improve budgeting capability. It represents an alternative to using acuity adjusted patient days for determining nurse staff requirements (as will be discussed in Chapter 12).

In this approach the first step is to separate all patients for a unit into specific groups. These groups, or product lines, could conform to DRGs but do not have to. The next step is to determine how many patients are expected in the coming period in each group. That information can be generated using the forecasting techniques discussed in Chapter 17. Using historical information, forecasting can also be used to predict the average length of stay of the patients in each group.

Once the manager has predictions of the number of patient days in each group and the average length of stay, those two numbers can be multiplied to determine the total number of patient days expected in each product line. The number of patient days can be multiplied by the expected average direct care hours per patient day (HPPD) for patients in the product line to generate the total hours of direct care needed for each specific product line. The total direct care hours for each product line can then be aggregated to determine the total direct care hours needed for the unit for the coming year. Based on that information the unit's budget for staff can be prepared. Table 8–7 presents a simplistic example of this process. In this example sufficient staff must be

Text continued on page 215

❖ TABLE 8–5
Product-line Manager Volume and Revenue Report

Segment	Actual Discharges	Budget Discharges	Variance	Actual Net Revenue per Case	Budget Net Revenue per Case	Net Revenue Variance	Financial Effect
Product Line: Obstetrics/Gynecology							
C-Section	200	100	+100	$3,500	$2,300	+$1,200	$470,000 [F]
Normal deliveries	400	450	(50)	2,000	2,100	(100)	(145,000) [U]
Surgical gynecology	500	500	0	4,500	4,600	(100)	(50,000) [U]
Medical gynecology	100	125	(25)	3,000	3,000	0	(75,000) [U]
General obstetrics	500	400	+100	3,000	3,500	(500)	100,000 [F]
Totals	1,700	1,575	+125				$200,000 [F]

F = Favorable variance   U = Unfavorable variance

Reprinted from Richard Johnson and Daniel McGinty, "Product Line Management Requires Change in Financial Reports," *Healthcare Financial Management*, August 1989, p. 40, with permission of Healthcare Financial Management Association.

❖ TABLE 8–6
Analysis of DRG 152[a]

Description of Services	Dr. Getwell				Dr. Severe	
	Patient 1	Patient 2	Patient 3	Patient 4	Patient 1	Patient 2
Medical surgical bed	$ 460	$ 460	$ 460	$ 460	$ 460	$ 460
Intensive care bed	720	1,440	720	720	720	720
Operating room	420	360	300	300	850	360
Anesthesia	300	300	300	300	425	150
Laboratory:						
Blood work	75	125	50	50	50	50
Tissue test	25	—	75	75	100	100
Urine analysis	35	35	35	—	70	70
Radiology:						
Chest 4 views	45	45	45	—	90	45
Spine, cervical	65	—	65	65	65	65
Nuclear medicine:						
Thyroid washout	95	95	95	210	210	95
Urinary recovery	105	105	105	—	105	105
T-3 uptake	85	85	85	85	85	85
Red-cell survival	40	40	40	40	40	40
Total	$2,470	$3,090	$2,375	$2,305	$3,270	$2,345

[a]Broken out by physician and hospital services ordered for minor small and large bowel procedures.
Reprinted from John Tselepis, "Refined Cost Accounting Produces Better Information," *Healthcare Financial Management*, May 1989, p. 34, with permission of Healthcare Financial Management Association.

❖ TABLE 8–7
Product-line Budgeting for Direct Care Hours

	Forecast Volume of Patients	×	Forecast Average Length of Stay	=	Expected Patient Days	×	Expected Hours per Patient Day	=	Total Hours of Direct Care
Product line 1	200		3		600		5		3,000
Product line 2	50		5		250		6		1,500
Product line 3	100		4		400		3		1,200
Product line 4	300		7		2,100		6		12,600
Product line 5	500		3		1,500		4		6,000
									24,300

budgeted to provide 24,300 direct care hours. The benefit of this process is that it has the potential to accurately provide information on the resources needed by the unit.

The major difficulty with this process is the determination of an accurate measure of average direct care hours per patient day by product line. If that information is inaccurate, the resulting total direct care hours needed will be inaccurate as well. Planning the budget based on a forecast of the number of patients in each product line may be helpful to the manager.

An alternate approach is to determine the total number of days at each patient classification level for all patients in each product line. Using information from the patient classification system, the nursing staff requirements for that product line can be determined. If this is done for all product lines, the total nursing requirements can be determined.

Standard Costs

Most industrial organizations establish standard costs against which performance can be measured. Standard costs represent expectations of what it should cost to produce a good or service, usually on a per unit basis. They are targets, often established based on industrial engineering studies of the resources that should be consumed in the production of the good or service. Standard costing breaks the costs of each product down into its parts. These include direct and indirect costs, divided into their fixed and variable cost components.

It is important to isolate fixed and variable costs in standard costing so that the information can be used for decision making. By dividing costs in that manner the manager can determine the likely *change* in costs resulting from changes in the number of patients treated. Historically, health care organizations have not done very much standard costing. This is because of the fact that each patient is fairly unique, requiring a somewhat customized treatment.

If we could overcome that uniqueness, a number of benefits could be realized from the use of standard costs. They present a basis for comparing actual results to the predetermined standard. They can be used for decisions on HMO contracts, on expanding or contracting services, and on other revisions in the way services are offered. Even though patients are unique, there are standard approaches for most patients with specific problems. Those approaches can form the basis for development of standard costs. Table 8–8 presents an example of what a standard cost would be for a pacemaker implant with AMI. The table accumulates costs per procedure for all types of procedures and for the quantity of each to arrive at a total cost of $11,710 per patient in this product line. Since revenues are estimated at $7,739, there is a projected loss of $3,971.

A central article on product-line standard costing overcomes much of the obstacle to standard costing by focusing on the idea that hospitals treat patients by providing them with a large number of intermediate products.[4] By carefully examining each department, one can make a list of the various intermediate products produced by that department.

For example, a laboratory produces different types of lab tests. Based on this approach, the set of intermediate products consumed by the average pa-

[4]William O. Cleverley, "Product-Costing for Health Care Firms," *Health Care Management Review*, Vol. 12, No. 4, Fall 1987, pp. 39–48.

❖ TABLE 8–8
Product Resource Consumption and Cost Profile Report

| Procedure | | | Standard per Procedure | | | Standard in Total | | | | Margin | |
Number	Name	Usage	Gross Revenue	Cost Variable	Cost Total	Gross Revenue	Cost Variable	Cost Total	Gross	Net
12001110	Acuity class I	1	$ 190	$ 57.89	$ 199.32	$ 190	$ 58	$ 199	$ 132	$ (9)
12001111	Acuity class I (surgical)	1	202	62.30	203.01	202	62	203	140	(1)
12001112	Acuity class II (surgical)	1	258	79.96	260.55	258	80	261	178	(3)
12001113	Acuity class III (surgical)	1	314	97.62	318.11	314	98	318	216	(4)
14001000	Recovery base	1	38	7.58	25.89	38	8	26	30	12
14002000	Recovery less than 60 minutes	1	40	8.53	29.89	40	9	30	31	10
14006000	Recovery 61-90 minutes	1	76	22.76	77.94	76	23	78	53	(2)
31004000	Cardiac output monitor	2	437	222.53	361.27	874	445	723	429	151
31005670	OR time major per hour	1	47	96.82	201.71	47	97	202	(50)	(155)
31005000	Pacemaker	1	4,985	4,353.52	9,013.56	4,985	4,354	9,014	631	(4,029)
31000500	Pacemaker view	3	119	21.32	169.87	357	64	510	293	(153)
33752500	CBC	3	18	3.28	21.93	54	10	66	44	(12)
33754000	Platelet count	1	13	.71	4.74	13	1	5	12	8
35003000	Prothrombin time	1	13	1.16	7.72	13	1	8	12	5
35005000	Cell count differential fluids	1	13	4.22	28.15	13	4	28	9	(15)
35005500	IV service fee	3	3	.35	1.35	9	1	4	8	5
35509000	Demerol 100 MG Ing	8	4	.35	1.35	32	3	11	29	21
35505555	MA CL 0.9 100 MLS	9	11	.24	.91	99	2	8	97	91
35507500	Dex 5 R/L 1000CC	6	11	1.00	1.50	66	6	9	60	57
35508700	Gloves dispense	5	11	.14	1.24	55	1	6	54	49
35509870	Admission kit	1	4	.14	1.24	4	0	1	4	3
	Totals					$7,739	$5,327	$11,710	$2,412	$(3,971)

Source: Ernst & Young.
Reprinted from George Kis and George Bodenger, "Cost Management Information Improves Financial Performance," *Healthcare Financial Management*, May 1989, p. 42, with permission of Healthcare Financial Management Association and with permission of Ernst & Young.

tient in a specific product line can be used to determine the standard costs of that product line. The set of intermediate products consumed by a patient in each product line is referred to as the standard treatment protocol (STP) for that product line.

In this system, each intermediate product line is called a service unit (SU). A chest x-ray would be one type of SU produced by the radiology department. A patient who has three chest x-rays receives three of that SU. A standard cost profile (SCP) must be established for each SU. That profile indicates the cost of producing that SU. That profile would include direct and indirect costs, and it would identify fixed and variable costs.

Conceptually this seems straightforward. The patient care provided by each department is broken down into intermediate products called SUs. The cost of each SU is determined. The average number of each SU from each department is found for each product line. Then the SUs consumed for a product line are multiplied by their cost to determine the total costs for patients in that product line.

A difficulty with the approach is determining SUs for nursing units. One could try to break down nursing care into the various specific activities and then relate those to SUs. Administering a medication could be an SU. Taking a patient's vital signs could be an SU. Charting information about a patient could be an SU. Using hospital computer information systems, it is possible to disaggregate nursing care and assign it to patients in this manner.

Current work in this area focuses on developing critical paths for a patient's hospital stay. Using this approach, the standard care required for patients (usually by DRGs) is determined. During the course of the stay variances from this standard are noted. Some variances are acceptable. For example, the patient's health status is beyond the control of nursing. Other variances are not acceptable, for example, if the patient was not ambulating because nurses did not provide care as outlined in the standard plan. With these data it is possible to determine the ratio of outputs to inputs required (as determined by the standard) and actual (as determined by the actual care provided). Because of the amount of data required to assess productivity in this way, successfully determining productivity for an episode of care usually requires the use of a computer.

For organizations that have sufficiently sophisticated information systems in place, it is possible to determine the average number of vital signs taken for a patient in a specific product line. For most hospitals, such a detailed level of information is not currently cost effective to collect. However, nursing SUs could be based on patient classification. Thus, a patient's day at level 3 could be an SU. A day at level 4 would be a different SU. When the STP is established, it would consider which nursing SUs are typically consumed and how many of each. The costs for those SUs could be determined using the RVU method discussed earlier.

This method is a very ambitious approach to product costing. It is used, but only in a small minority of hospitals. However, it does provide a vision for the future. It suggests an ability to have very detailed information from all parts of the hospital, including nursing, about each product line. The management implications of such information are significant. By examining all the SUs consumed in each department, a team of clinicians might be able to find ways to more efficiently provide care. SUs with a lower SCP might be substituted for more expensive ones. Ways might be found to reduce the number of SUs in various departments. If one considers product-line costing broadly as a tool in the case management of the organization's product lines, the potential benefits of product-line standard costing are significant.

RATE SETTING

In the last decade nurse managers have started to become directly involved in the revenue process of health care organizations. It is no longer sufficient to simply control costs. For health care organizations to prosper, their managers must have an understanding of the processes by which they receive their revenues. Rate setting is the element of financial management that focuses on setting the prices the organization charges for the services it provides.

To some extent, rate setting is outside the control of health care organizations. The federal government sets hospital DRG rates. Additionally, many other rates of health care organizations are mandated by governmental bodies, such as state-controlled Medicaid rates. Nevertheless, the process of developing a *charge master*, i.e., a list of the organization's prices for each of its services, remains a critical element of the management process.

Total Financial Requirements

Health care organizations strive to obtain the financial resources needed to meet their *total financial requirements* (TFR). These requirements are the financial resources needed to provide for the health care needs of the population served by the organization. Clearly, the financial requirements of any organization include sufficient money to cover the current costs of operations. On a broader perspective, however, the financial needs of the organization encompass the need to be able to replace facilities as they become obsolete and to adopt new technologies as they become available.

The total financial requirements of health care organizations have been defined to include five categories[5]:
1. Costs of doing business
2. Costs of staying in business
3. Costs of changing business
4. Returns to capital sources
5. Costs of uncertainty

The costs of doing business are the routine operating costs of the organization, including salaries and expenses. If the organization provides education or research, it must recover enough to pay for those services in addition to patient care. If some payers pay less than the full costs generated on their behalf, other payers must be charged more if the organization is to recover the full costs of doing business.

Costs of staying in business relate to having financial resources needed to operate, to replace assets, and to acquire new technology. Most patients do not pay for their care until after they are discharged. However, the organization must acquire supplies before the patient arrives and must pay salaries concurrent with the patient stay. To stay in business, the organization must there-

---

[5]Bruce R. Neumann, James D. Suver, and William N. Zelman, *Financial Management: Concepts and Applications for Health Care Providers*, National Health Publishing, USA, 1984, p. 313.

fore have a reserve of cash available to tide itself over until revenues are received.

Costs of changing business relate to the modification of existing services and the addition of new services. Health care services do not remain stagnant over time. As the practice of nursing and medicine changes, health care organizations must be flexible enough to delete outmoded services and to add new ones.

Return to capital refers to repaying those who provide the organization with the basic resources to be in business. This includes the money needed to first establish the organization, as well as additional monies provided to allow the organization to acquire buildings and equipment over time. Some of this money is borrowed. In that case return on capital refers to interest on the loan, as well as repaying the principal of the loan. For-profit entities have owners who have invested money. A return to those owners is generally in the form of dividends. In some cases the organization is either community owned or a voluntary, and its original resources came from tax dollars and/or philanthropic sources. In such cases the return on capital may come in the form of subsidized health care services.

Costs of uncertainty refer to the fact that organizations may find themselves with unexpected and unplanned expenses. These include the impact of adverse legal decisions, political decisions, regulatory changes, and similar occurrences.

A stable entity must set rates in such a manner that all these financial requirements are considered. Some payers (such as Medicare) can dictate their prices to the organization. The rates the organization charges the remaining payers must be adequate so that in total the organization has the financial resources it needs. This means that if the organization loses money on Medicare patients, it must attempt to charge a higher price to non-Medicare patients to offset the loss. This is sometimes referred to as a "plug-figure" approach. The organization decides the amount of revenue it needs. It determines how much revenue it will receive from sources over which it has no ability to set prices. Then it plugs in the charges for the remaining patients to achieve the desired revenue.

Unfortunately, this may require the organization to charge a high price for its services. Charging a high price is likely to result in increased bad debts as prices become higher than patients can afford. Increased bad debts mean that charges to the remaining payers must be even higher to offset that loss. This can create a vicious circle, with the organization unable to collect enough to remain financially viable.

Rate-setting Approaches

Neumann, Suver, and Zelman[6] identify three approaches to rate-setting: cost-based, negotiation, and market.

Cost-based reimbursement generally relies upon the cost-finding analysis discussed earlier. Often cost-based payers, such as Medicaid or Blue Cross, dictate that they will pay the lower of cost or charges. If for some reason the organization were to set its charges less than its costs, they would pay the lower amount.

The cost-based approach requires a knowledge of the cost of treating each

---

[6]Ibid. p. 314.

patient. If one is to reimburse the organization for the cost of treating the patient, one must know that cost. However, rather than actually trying to capture the cost of treating any one patient, cost-based payers generally use what is known as the ratio of charges to charges applied to costs, often referred to as the *ratio of cost to charges* (RCC). In this approach it is assumed that a given payer's costs and charges in any revenue center will be approximately the same. Thus, if 30% of all surgical charges are for Medicaid patients, then Medicaid is responsible for 30% of all operating room costs. That 30% can be applied to the total operating room revenue center costs to determine the amount Medicaid must pay.

Looking at this calculation another way, suppose that the operating room had total charges of $1 million and that 30% of those charges, or $300,000, were to Medicaid patients. Since Medicaid pays costs rather than charges, the costs of treating those patients must be determined. Suppose that the total costs of the operating room were $800,000. Costs are 20% lower than charges (i.e., $800,000 is only 80% of $1 million). Therefore Medicaid costs must be only 80% of the $300,000 of charges, or $240,000.

Negotiated rates are becoming fairly commonplace in the health care industry. HMOs, insurance companies, and even large employers are actively negotiating directly with hospitals and other health care providers. Generally, guaranteed patient volume is offered in exchange for discounted prices. Based on the discussions of Chapter 7, negotiated prices should always provide a positive contribution margin to the organization.

The market approach is based on the concepts of supply and demand introduced in Chapter 4. The organization can set any price it wishes. However, if its price is high enough to earn a large profit, that would encourage additional competitors to enter the market and underbid the organization. If the price set is too low, the organization will lose money and eventually go out of business. Health care organizations therefore have to walk a tightrope in setting prices.

Furthermore, there are times when competition may cause the organization to lower some prices and raise others so as not to be perceived as being an expensive provider. For example, suppose that two hospitals in the same area both offer open heart surgery, but that one performs 500 per year while the other performs 50 per year. The charge at the hospital with the higher volume might be significantly less than at the one with low volume because of economies of scale. The low-volume hospital has fewer patients to share the fixed costs of doing open heart surgery (such as the expensive equipment required). It is not unreasonable to expect that the low-volume hospital will lower its charges to match the competition, even if this means that it is charging less than cost.

How will the low-volume hospital survive in that case? It would probably raise charges on a low-cost high-volume item for all patients. For example, it might add a charge of $1 per test for all lab tests done for all patients to offset the reduced charge to open heart surgery patients for their surgery. In this way it would avoid the possibility of being labeled as being very expensive for a high-visibility program such as open heart surgery. If a policymaker were to question the wisdom of allowing a low-volume open heart surgery program to exist, the hospital could counter that it is so efficient that its charges are no higher than those of the high-volume program.

Major payers are aware of such influences on hospital rate setting. That is why cost-based payers often mandate that they pay only the lesser of cost or charges. This allows them to take advantage of competitive situations that result in prices below cost.

Rate setting is a critical area of health care management. Managers must take into account their total financial requirements, the patient mix by type of patient, and the patient mix by type of payer. Balancing these factors is often essential to organizational viability.

FINANCIAL REIMBURSEMENT FOR NURSING SERVICES

Despite the limitations of costing systems, great progress has been made in costing out nursing services. It is now possible to recognize different nursing costs for different patients. That means that it is feasible for nursing to become a revenue center that charges directly for its services. The ability to recognize different consumption of resources by different patients and to charge accordingly is the essential ingredient for a revenue center. Establishment of nursing as a revenue center is feasible as long as different patient classification levels can be assigned different costs.

If an organization's patients are all fixed-fee patients, revenue centers make little sense. For example, a fixed DRG payment to a hospital will not vary if nursing, lab, or radiology varies its charges. If all patients were paid on a DRG basis, eventually there would be no revenue centers. In home health care a fixed payment for an episode of care will not vary if the cost per nursing visit varies.

However, at present most health care organizations still have some patients who pay charges. Even in states with systems that use DRGs for all inpatients, outpatients are often billed on a charge system. Therefore, there are potential benefits if nursing is treated as a revenue center. First, it does charge patients more fairly by charging on a closer approximation of their actual consumption of resources. Second, for hospitals it clearly segregates nursing from room and board. Third, it can help to alleviate the "nursing as a burden" misconception.

As health care organizations find an ever increasing need to manage themselves in a business-like manner, a clearer understanding of both revenues and expenses will be required. The movement toward recasting the nursing function as a revenue center can help in that evolution. Separate costing for different types of patients allows for *variable billing*. Variable billing refers to the fact that the amount billed to each patient per patient day or per visit varies. Instead of simply charging all patients the same amount per day or per visit for their nursing care, different patients will be charged different amounts, based on their differing resource consumption. Once the different costs of caring for different patients are known, they can be charged accordingly.

Variable billing may be a way to better justify hospital bills and in some cases increase overall revenues to the hospital. Variable billing may be beneficial to nursing because it shows in a dramatic way the specific contribution that nursing makes to the overall revenue structure of the hospital.

Home health agencies generally charge on a per visit basis, although nurse managers recognize that different patients require different amounts of care. For example, the patient who requires an insulin injection requires much less care than the HIV patient with opportunistic infections. Most managers assume that the variation will balance. For each visit requiring a substantial amount of time, there will be an "in-and-out" visit to offset it. This approach was adequate in the past when most nurses were paid on a salaried basis. As more and more home health agencies are paying nurses on a per visit basis, this approach may no longer prove workable. Billing may move to a variable basis depending on nursing resources consumed.

IMPLICATIONS FOR NURSE MANAGERS

Nurse managers have a responsibility not only to units and departments but also a broader responsibility to the organization. It is imperative for nurse managers to understand the organization's perspective on cost finding and rate setting.

However, that does not mean that all accounting methods and procedures will always be correct or appropriate. By understanding how the organization conducts its cost accounting, nurse managers can identify situations in which the accounting data are inadequate for their needs. Perhaps all supplies are charged to the nursing department when paid for rather than when consumed. While that would have little impact on external reporting of costs, it makes monthly evaluation of performance difficult. Are the right amounts of supplies being used for the number of patients actually being cared for? That question cannot be answered without cost information related to monthly consumption of resources. Information about how much was paid in a given month for supplies is not useful to the nurse manager.

Once such problems are identified, the accountants of the organization must be informed of the inadequacy of the existing information. Nurse managers and financial managers can then work together to generate and use relevant information to improve the organization's overall management capabilities and results.

Nurse managers cannot lose sight of the fact that a great deal of the organization's revenues depend on following the cost-finding requirements of external payers and providing them with external reports. The reasons for the cost-finding techniques should be understood lest they be condemned for their lack of perfection. At the same time, recognition of their limitations makes clear the need for the nursing profession to step forward in developing its own approaches for costing out nursing services.

This need is made more critical by the introduction of fixed-payment systems such as DRGs. The shift away from cost reimbursement and toward prospective payment makes knowledge about the cost of treating different types of patients essential. Improved costing of nursing services is a vital step toward getting a more accurate cost for each of the organization's product lines.

Whether this will in turn lead to variable billing for nursing services on a universal basis is still unclear. Accurate costing information for nursing does, however, remove the roadblocks to variable billing.

Improving the costing of nursing services has become important to nurse managers for several reasons. One reason is that improved cost information can be used to get an improved understanding of the contribution that nursing makes to the organization as a whole. A second reason is that the information generated by improved costing can be used to help managers make effective decisions and better control the costs of providing nursing services. Third, periodic nursing shortages make it more important to understand the nursing resources needed by patients. Costing information is also useful for examining changes in the way nursing care is provided. For example, the cost impact of primary vs. team nursing or of using different levels of staff can be examined.

The most accurate costing system requires continuous observation of all nurses by data collectors. The cost of such highly accurate costing is prohibitive. However, one can think of a continuum of costing methods. In general, less expensive methods provide less accurate data; more expensive methods provide more accurate data.

Over time fully integrated computer systems may become inexpensive enough to be introduced in most hospitals. Also over time software programs will be developed and perfected to make using the computers easy and efficient. At the time of the writing of this book, however, the software was still not perfected and the cost was still very high. On the other hand, many hospitals are experimenting with such systems.

In the meantime patient classification systems can be used to substantially improve the assignment of nursing costs to patients in an economical way. Combining classification with an RVU system is relatively simple. Once this has been done, all nursing costs can be allocated based on the RVU system, or some costs can be allocated using RVUs while others are assigned to patients based on patient days or some other approach. Each hospital must decide how much refinement to the RVU approach is worthwhile.

It is important to stress that the RVU approach suggested here is not perfect. It has a number of limitations and weaknesses. However, the nurse manager must decide whether these weaknesses are so significant that the method should not be used. The cost information generated, while not perfectly accurate, are likely to be a substantial improvement over costing methods that have historically been used.

Costing out nursing services provides an extremely useful tool for product-line costing and budgeting. Information about product-line costs can show management where profits are being made and where losses are accruing. Product-line information can aid managers substantially in understanding which patients place the greatest burden on the unit and in helping the organization make appropriate decisions regarding changes in its patient mix.

KEY CONCEPTS ❖

Cost information for reporting vs. for management   Managers must be careful to use information appropriate to their needs. Cost information generated for external reports may provide managers with information that will lead to poor managerial decisions.

Traditional cost finding   Allocating the direct costs of nonrevenue centers to other nonrevenue centers and to revenue centers with the goal of ultimately allocating all the organization's costs to its revenue centers. The total direct and indirect costs of the revenue centers are then allocated to units of service. Revenue centers are cost centers that charge for their services. To be a revenue center, the cost center must be able to distinguish the different amount of resources consumed by different patients. The steps in cost finding are:

1. **Accumulation of direct costs for each cost center:**   Costs directly incurred within the cost center.

2. **Determine basis for allocation:** Costs must be allocated on some measurement basis such as pounds or square feet.

3. **Allocate to revenue centers:** The step-down method is widely used to assign nonrevenue center costs to revenue centers.

4. **Allocate revenue center costs to units of service:** Using the weighted procedure, hourly rate, surcharge, and per diem methods.

Costing out nursing services Process of determining the cost of providing nursing care for different patients. This cost has traditionally been included in the room and board charge.

Prospective payment Patients are classified into a variety of categories. The health organization knows in advance what it will be paid for patients in these various categories. The payment is not based on the amount of resources a patient uses.

Patient classification system Scheme for grouping patients into categories. Each category contains patients who require similar amounts of nursing care. Some systems are commercially available, and others are developed by individual health care organizations. Patients are usually classified into one of four or five categories.

Acuity How acutely ill patients are. Usually used in conjunction with the nursing resources required to care for patients. The higher the acuity, generally the more resources needed for care.

Variable billing Amount billed to each patient reflects the amount of resources consumed by that patient. Rather than billing a patient for a patient day of care, patients are billed an amount based on the nursing care hours and supplies actually used.

Productivity Ratio of outputs to inputs.

    Inputs Those resources required to produce outputs. In nursing inputs usually include personnel, supplies, and equipment necessary to care for clients.

    Outputs Products produced by nursing. Traditionally these are identified as patient days of care, visits, and episodes of care. More recently outputs are being defined as patient outcomes such as health and/or wellness.

Product-line costing Determination of the cost of providing care to specific types of patients. This approach is sometimes aided by the use of standard cost techniques such as Cleverley's model of standard treatment protocols.

Rate setting Process of assigning prices to the units of service of the revenue centers. Prices must be set high enough to recover the organization's total financial requirements.

SUGGESTED READINGS

Barhyte, Diana Young, and Gerald L. Glandon, "Issues in Nursing Labor Costs Allocation," *Journal of Nursing Administration*, Vol. 18, No. 12, December 1988, pp. 16–19.

Bennett, James, "Standard Cost Systems Lead to Efficiency and Profitability," *Healthcare Financial Management*, Vol. 39, No. 9, September 1985, pp. 46–54.

Berliner, Callie, and James A. Brimson, *Cost Management for Today's Advanced Manufacturing*, Harvard Business School Press, Boston, 1988.

Berman, Howard J., Lewis E. Weeks, and Steven F. Kukla, *The Financial Management of Hospitals*, 7th edition, Health Administration Press, Ann Arbor, MI, 1990.

Budd, Marjorie C., and Toni Propotnik, "A Computerized System for Staffing, Billing and Productivity Measurement," *Journal of Nursing Administration*, Vol. 19, No. 7, July/August 1989, pp. 17–22.

Cleverley, William O., *Essentials of Health Care Finance*, 3rd edition, Aspen Publishers, Rockville, MD, 1992.

Cleverley, William O., "Product-Costing for Health Care Firms," *Health Care Management Review*, Vol. 12, No. 4, Fall 1987, pp. 39–48.

Cleverley, William O., *Handbook of Health Care Accounting and Finance*, Volumes I and II, 2nd edition, Aspen Systems Corp., Rockville, MD, 1989.

Cooper, Jean, and James Suver, "Product Line Cost Estimation: A Standard Cost Approach," *Healthcare Financial Management*, Vol. 42, No. 4, April 1988, pp. 60–70.

de Mars Martin, Pamela, and Frank J. Boyer, "Developing a Consistent Method for Costing Hospital Services," *Healthcare Financial Management*, Vol. 39, No. 2, February 1985, pp. 30–37.

Dieter, Bryan, "Determining the Cost of Nursing Services," *Hospital Cost Accounting Advisor*, Vol. 2, No. 9, February 1987, pp. 1, 5–7.

Donovan, Marilee Ivers, and Gwendolyn Lewis, "Costs of Nursing Services: Are the Assumptions Valid?" *Nursing Administration Quarterly*, Vol. 12, No. 1, Fall 1987, pp. 1–6.

Edwardson, Sandra R., and Phyllis B. Giovannetti, "A Review of Cost Accounting Methods for Nursing Services," *Nursing Economics*, Vol. 5, No. 3, May/June 1987, pp. 107–117.

Edwardson, Sandra R., and Patricia Nardone, "Resource Use in Home Care Agencies," *Applied Nursing Research*, Vol. 4, No. 1, February 1991, pp. 25–30.

Etheridge, Phyllis, "The Case for Billing by Patient Acuity," *Nursing Management*, Vol. 16, No. 8, August 1985, pp. 38–41.

Ferrara, William L., "The New Cost/Management Accounting: More Questions Than Answers," *Management Accounting*, Vol. 72, No. 4, October 1990, pp. 48–52.

Finkler, Steven A., "Costs for Reporting vs. Costs for Management and Control: Hospital Implications," *Hospital Cost Accounting Advisor*, Vol. 3, No. 6, November 1987, pp. 1, 7–8.

Finkler, Steven A., "Costing Out the Operating Room: A Case Study," *Hospital Cost Accounting Advisor*, Vol. 2, No. 2, July 1986, pp. 1, 6–7.

Finkler, Steven A., "Costing Out Nursing Services," *Hospital Cost Management and Accounting*, Vol. 1, No. 12, March 1990, pp. 1–5.

Finkler, Steven A., "The Distinction Between Cost and Charges," *Annals of Internal Medicine*, Vol. 96, No. 1, January 1982, pp. 102–109.

Finkler, Steven A., *Budgeting Concepts for Nurse Managers*, 2nd edition, W.B. Saunders, Philadelphia, 1992.

Fosbinder, Donna, "Nursing Costs/DRG: A Patient Classification System and Comparative Study," *Journal of Nursing Administration*, Vol. 16, No. 11, November 1986, pp. 18–23.

Grimaldi, Paul L., and Julie A. Micheletti, "RIMs and the Cost of Nursing Care," *Nursing Management*, Vol. 13, No. 12, December 1982, pp. 12–22.

Grimaldi, Paul, "PPS for Operating and Capital Costs," *Nursing Management*, Vol. 22, No. 11, November 1991, pp. 17–19.

Haas, Sheila, "Patient Classification Systems: A Self Fulfillment Prophecy," *Nursing Management*, Vol. 19, No. 5, May 1988, pp. 56–58, 60–62, 81, 84.

Helmer, F. Theodore, and James Suver, "Pictures of Performance: The Key to Improved Nursing Productivity," *Health Care Management Review*, Vol. 13, No. 4, Fall 1988, pp. 65–70.

Hendrickson, Gerry, Terry Doddato, and Christine Kovner, "How Do Nurses Spend Their Time?" *Journal of Nursing Administration,* Vol. 20, No. 3, March 1990, pp. 31–37.

Jacox, A. K., "Determining the Cost and Value of Nursing," *Nursing Administration Quarterly,* Vol. 12, No. 1, Fall 1987, pp. 7–12.

Johnson, Thomas H., "The Decline of Cost Management: A Reinterpretation of 20th Century Cost Accounting," *Journal of Cost Management for the Manufacturing Industry,* Spring 1987, Vol. 1, No. 1, pp. 5–12.

Kaplan, Robert S., "The Four-Stage Model of Cost Systems Design," *Management Accounting,* Vol. 71, No. 8, February 1990, pp. 22–26.

Kerschner, Morley, ed., "Product Costing," *Topics in Health Care Financing,* Vol. 13, No. 4, Summer 1987.

Kovner, Christine T., "Public Health Nursing Costs in Home Care," *Public Health Nursing,* Vol. 6, No. 1, March 1989, pp. 3–7.

Kovner, Christine T., "Measuring Indirect Nursing Costs," *Hospital Cost Accounting Advisor,* Vol. 1, No. 3, June 1989, pp. 6–7.

Knox, J. T., "Direct Reimbursement to Nurse Practitioners: The Importance of the Federal Employees Health Care Freedom of Choice Act," *Nurse Practitioner,* Vol. 13, No. 11, November 1988, pp. 52–54.

McCloskey, Joanne Comi, Diane L. Gardner, and Marion R. Johnson, "Costing Out Nursing Services: An Annotated Bibliography," *Nursing Economics,* Vol. 5, No. 5, September-October 1987, pp. 245–253.

McCloskey, Joanne Comi, "Implications of Costing Out Nursing Services for Reimbursement," *Nursing Management,* Vol. 20, No. 1, January 1989, pp. 44–46, 48–49.

McHugh, Mary L., "Productivity Measurement in Nursing," *Applied Nursing Research,* Vol. 2, No. 2, May 1989, pp. 99–102.

Mowry, M. N., and R. A. Korpman, "Do DRG Reimbursement Rates Reflect Nursing Costs?" *Journal of Nursing Administration,* Vol. 15, Nos. 7 and 8, July/August 1985, pp. 29–35.

Nagaprasann, B., "Patient Classification Systems: Strategies for the 1990's," *Nursing Management,* Vol. 19, No. 3, March 1988, pp. 105–106, 108, 112.

O'Connor, Nancy, "Integrating Patient Classification with Cost Accounting," *Nursing Management,* Vol. 19, No. 10, October 1988, pp. 27–29.

Omachonu, Vincent K., and Ravinder Nanda, "Measuring Productivity: Outcome vs. Output," *Nursing Management,* Vol. 20, No. 4, April 1989, pp. 35–40.

Osterhaus, R. B., and C. M. Justice, "Cost Accounting and Its Role in the Nursing Department," *Healthcare Computing and Communications,* Vol. 3, No. 11, November 1986, pp. 56–60.

Picha, P. K., "The Nursing Link to Cost Accounting—Developing Patient Classification Systems," *Nursing Management,* Vol. 19, No. 5, May 1988, pp. 81, 84i.

Reschak, Gary L., Diana Biordi, Karen Holm, et al., "Accounting for Nursing Costs by DRG," *Journal of Nursing Administration,* Vol. 15, No. 9, September 15, 1985, pp. 15–20.

Rosenbaum, Heidi L., Todd M. Willert, Elizabeth A. Kelly, et al., "Costing Out Nursing Services Based on Acuity," *Journal of Nursing Administration,* Vol. 18, Nos. 7 and 8, July/August 1988, pp. 10–16.

Ruman, James M., and Deanna L. Nelson, "Patient Classification Systems Capture Nursing Costs," *Health Care Financial Management,* Vol. 41, No. 6, July 1987, pp. 84–86.

Schaffer, Paul L., Betsy J. Fraventhal, and Catherine Tower, "Measuring Nursing Costs with Patient Acuity Data," *Topics in Health Care Financing,* Vol. 13, No. 4, Summer 1987, pp. 20–31.

Shaffer, Franklin A., ed., *Costing Out Nursing: Pricing Our Product,* National League for Nursing, New York, 1985.

Shaffer, Franklin A., ed., *Patients & Purse Strings,* National League for Nursing, New York, 1986.

Scherubel, Janet, and Franklin A. Shaffer, eds., *Patients & Purse Strings II,* National League for Nursing, New York, 1988.

Sovie, Margaret D., Michael A. Tarcinale, Alison W. Vanputee, et al., "Amalgam of Nursing Acuity, DRGs and Costs," *Nursing Management*, Vol. 16, No. 3, March 1985, pp. 22–42.

Stanton, Laura J., "Nursing Care and Nursing Products: Revenue or Expenses?" *Journal of Nursing Administration*, Vol. 16, No. 9, September 1986, pp. 29–32.

Strasen, Leann, "Implementing Salary Cost per Unit of Service Productivity Standards," *Journal of Nursing Administration*, Vol. 20, No. 3, March 1990, pp. 6–10.

Stepura, Barbara A., and Kathleen Miller, "Converting Nursing Care Cost to Revenue," *Journal of Nursing Administration*, Vol. 19, No. 5, May 1989, pp. 18–22.

Swansburg, Russell, and Richard Sowell, "A Model for Costing and Pricing Nursing Services," *Nursing Management*, Vol. 23, No. 2, February 1992, pp. 33–39.

Thomas, Surpora, and Robert G. Vaughan, "Costing Nursing Services Using RVU's," *Journal of Nursing Administration*, Vol. 16, No. 2, December 1986, pp. 10–16.

Trofino, Joan, "JCAHO Nursing Standards Nursing Care Hours and LOS per DRG—Part I," *Nursing Management*, Vol. 20, No. 1, January 1989, pp. 29–32.

Trofino, Joan, "JCAHO Nursing Standards Nursing Care Hours and LOS per DRG—Part II," *Nursing Management*, Vol. 20, No. 1, January 1989, pp. 33–35.

Watson, Phyllis M., Mary S. Lower, Susan M. Wells, et al., "Discovering What Nurses Do and What It Costs," *Nursing Management*, Vol. 22, No. 5, May 1991, pp. 38–45.

Wilson, Leslie, Patricia A. Prescott, and Leah Aleksandrowicz, "Nursing: A Major Hospital Cost Component," *Health Services Research*, Vol. 22, No. 6, February 1988, pp. 773–796.

Wood, Charles T., "Relate Hospital Charges to Use of Services," *Harvard Business Review*, Vol. 60, No. 2, March/April 1982, pp. 123–130.

Young, Sue W., Linda M. Daehn, and Christine M. Busch, "Managing Nursing Staff Productivity through Reallocation of Nursing Resources," *Nursing Administration Quarterly*, Vol. 14, No. 3, Spring 1990, pp. 24–30.

Young, Wendy B., Evelyn L. Lehrer, and William D. White, "The Effect of Education on the Practice of Nursing," *IMAGE: Journal of Nursing Scholarship*, Vol. 23, No. 2, Summer 1991, pp. 105–108.

Institutional Cost Report

This appendix presents and discusses several pages from a real institutional cost report. Exhibits 8A–1 through 8A–3 present just a small portion of an institutional cost report form. The actual report was nearly two inches thick. This form was submitted to Empire Blue Cross and Blue Shield, which acts as an agent for HCFA, the federal government agency in charge of Medicare. The institution's cost report is a public document. Exhibit 8A–1 is the cover page of the report.

Exhibit 8A–2 shows a portion of Worksheet B, Part I of the report. This provides the allocation of general services costs. This part of the report, although much more complex and set up somewhat differently, parallels the allocation process made in Table 8–3. In Table 8–3 all cost centers and revenue centers are shown across the top of the table, and the allocation proceeds row by row. In the official cost report, all cost centers and revenue centers are shown as rows. The allocation proceeds column by column.

Notice that in the 0 column on the first page of this exhibit there are $1,322,802 of costs in Row 17D for "nursing administration." These costs must be allocated. However, there are no costs in rows 17E or 17F for "nursing services." Those costs have already been reclassified in an earlier section of the report. That reclassification placed the costs of nursing units directly into departments for which the hospital makes a per diem charge. This includes line 25 "adults and pediatrics," line 26 "intensive care unit," line 27 "coronary care unit," and a number of other departments. The hospital has more than fifty-five departments. The rest of the departments appeared on additional pages not shown here.

Looking across all three pages from Exhibit 8A–2, one can see the pattern created by the process from which it earned the name step-down report. On the third page of Exhibit 8A–2, Worksheet B, Part I, you can see in column 17D that $2,297,296 is being taken out of "nursing administration" and allocated into the departments on lines 25 through 39. Note that the $2,297,296 is greater than the original $1,322,802 of direct costs of nursing administration. That is because nursing administration has received allocations of costs for depreciation, employee benefits, administrative services (other than nursing), plant operations, laundry, housekeeping, and cafeteria on the previous two pages. For example, there is a $21,838 allocation from housekeeping (column 8) into nursing administration.

What is the basis for each cost allocation? Exhibit 8A–3 provides the statistical basis for each allocation. This is Worksheet B-1 of the report. Notice in the headings for each column that the basis is given. For example, in column 1 the basis for allocating the building depreciation is square feet. On the second page of the exhibit, laundry and linen is allocated based on pounds of laundry and dietary is allocated based on meals served. On the last page of the exhibit note that nursing administration is allocated based on time spent on supervision of

❖ EXHIBIT 8A–1

PROVIDER NO.	EICR - EMPIRE BLUE CROSS AND BLUE SHIELD	VERSION: 91.02
PERIOD FROM 01/01/90 TO 12/31/90	IN LIEU OF FORM HCFA-2552-89 (12/89)	05/31/91

WORKSHEET S

	INTERMEDIARY USE ONLY	DATE RECEIVED: _____
HOSPITAL AND HEALTH CARE COST REPORT	__AUDITED ___DESK REVIEWED	INTERMEDIARY NO. ____
CERTIFICATION AND SETTLEMENT SUMMARY		

PART I - CERTIFICATION

INTENTIONAL MISREPRESENTATION OR FALSIFICATION OF ANY INFORMATION CONTAINED IN THIS COST
REPORT MAY BE PUNISHABLE BY FINE AND/OR IMPRISONMENT UNDER FEDERAL LAW

CERTIFICATION BY OFFICER OR ADMINISTRATOR OF PROVIDER(S)

    I HEREBY CERTIFY THAT I HAVE READ THE ABOVE STATEMENT AND THAT I HAVE EXAMINED THE ACCOMPANYING COST REPORT
AND THE BALANCE SHEET AND STATEMENT OF REVENUE AND EXPENSES PREPARED BY MAIMONIDES MEDICAL CENTER (33-0194)
(PROVIDER NAME(S) AND NUMBER(S)) FOR THE COST REPORT PERIOD BEGINNING 01-01-90 AND ENDING 12-31-90, AND THAT TO THE BEST OF
MY KNOWLEDGE AND BELIEF, IT IS A TRUE, CORRECT, AND COMPLETE STATEMENT PREPARED FROM THE BOOKS AND RECORDS OF THE PROVIDER
IN ACCORDANCE WITH APPLICABLE INSTRUCTIONS, EXCEPT AS NOTED.

(SIGNED)
        OFFICER OR ADMINISTRATOR OF PROVIDER(S)

Robert J. Flannery

ROBERT F. FLANNERY
Notary Public, State of New York
No. 24-1247950
Qualified In Kings County
Commission Expires March 30, 1992

President
TITLE

May 31, 1991
DATE

PART II - SETTLEMENT SUMMARY

	TITLE V	TITLE XVIII		TITLE XIX
		A	B	
	1	2	3	4
1 HOSPITAL		11639543	8958664	1
2 SUBPROVIDER I		387055		2
3 SUBPROVIDER II				3
4 SWING BED - SNF				4
5 SWING BED - ICF				5
6 SKILLED NURSING FACILITY				6
7 INTERMEDIATE CARE FACILITY				7
8 HOME HEALTH AGENCY		1091713		8
9 COMPREHENSIVE OUTPATIENT REHABILITATION FACILITY (CORF)				9
10 TOTAL		13118311	8958664	10

THE ABOVE AMOUNTS REPRESENT DUE TO OR DUE FROM THE APPLICABLE PROGRAM FOR THE ELEMENT OF THE COMPLEX INDICATED.

---

nurses. A total of 10,000 hours of supervision has been used, and the amount of hours of supervision required by nurses in each of the departments is shown lower in that column. For example, the nurses in the adults and pediatrics department received 4,934 hours of supervision from the nursing administration department. However, given the exact 10,000 hour total, one must wonder whether all the numbers in that column are approximations.

Worksheet B-1, i.e. Exhibit 8A–3, parallels the information shown in Table 8–1. However, in Table 8–1 percentages were used. In Exhibit 8A–3, the raw numbers are shown. To determine what portion of nursing administration costs to allocate to subsequent departments in the step down, one would have to determine what portion of nursing supervision total hours were consumed by each department. For example, since 4,934 hours of the total of 10,000 (both numbers are from column 17D on the third page of Exhibit 8A–3) were consumed by adults and pediatrics, 49% of the nursing administration costs should be allocated to adults and pediatrics ($4,934/10,000 \times 100\% = 49\%$).

Looking back at the third page of Exhibit 8A–2, we find that of the $2,297,296 in nursing administration when it gets its turn to allocate, $1,113,486 has been allocated to adults and pediatrics (line 25). If we divide $1,113,486 by the total of $2,297,296, we find that it is 49%. The portion of nursing administration that was consumed by adults and pediatrics has in fact been allocated to adults and pediatrics in the step-down process.

❖ EXHIBIT 8A–2

PROVIDER NO.
PERIOD FROM 01/01/90 TO 12/31/90

EICR - EMPIRE BLUE CROSS AND BLUE SHIELD
IN LIEU OF FORM HCFA-2552-89 (12/89)

VERSION: 91.0?
05/31/9?

COST ALLOCATION - GENERAL SERVICE COSTS

WORKSHEET ?
PART I

COST CENTER DESCRIPTION	NET EXP FOR COST ALLOCATION 0	CAP REL COST-BLDGS & FIXTURES 1	CAP REL COST-MOVBL EQUIPMENT 2	EMPLOYEE BENEFITS 3	SUBTOTAL 3A	ADMINIS-TRATIVE & GENERAL 4	OPERATION OF PLANT 6	LAUNDRY & LINEN SERVICE 7	
GENERAL SERVICE COST CENTERS									
1 CAP-REL COSTS-BLDGS & FIXTURES	10057369	10057369							1
2 CAP-REL COSTS-MOVABLE EQUIPMENT	8749151		8749151						2
3 EMPLOYEE BENEFITS	23821018	48726	7411	23877155					3
4 ADMINISTRATIVE AND GENERAL	21995738	2822931	3170817	2803776	30793262	30793262			4
5 MAINTENANCE AND REPAIRS									5
6 OPERATION OF PLANT	7187749	672903	522802	717424	9100878	1478574	10579452		6
7 LAUNDRY AND LINEN SERVICES	1656701	79351	64221	201015	2001288	325139	128899	2455326	7
8 HOUSEKEEPING	4234204	98664	82461	709761	5125090	832648	160270	1601	8
9A DIETARY - RAW FOOD	1975372				1975372	320929			9A
9B DIETARY - OTHER	3555271	280234	46609	686607	4568721	742257	455214	4234	9B
10 CAFETERIA		44201			44201	7181	71800		10
11 MAINTENANCE OF PERSONNEL		209229	23035		232264	37735	339873		11
15 MEDICAL RECORDS AND LIBRARY	2076416	143892	112927	298081	2631316	427497	233739		15
16 SOCIAL SERVICE	970843	30406	3235	178265	1182749	192155	49392		16
17A MEDICAL SUPPLIES AND EXPENSE	6898852		9358	11728	6919938	1124248			17A
17B CENTRAL SERVICES & SUPPLY	756944	63375	103815	103435	1027569	166944	102946		17B
17C PHARMACY	10220289	65672	349540	636502	11272003	1831306	106678		17C
17D NURSING ADMINISTRATION	1322802	124568	164432	103716	1715518	278712	202349	24826	17D
17E INTENSIVE NURSING CARE									17E
17F GENERAL NURSING SERVICE									17F
18 VISUAL AIDS	120322	32484	31911	20973	205690	33417	52767		18
19 NON-PHYSICIAN ANESTHETISTS	307291			59946	367237	59663			19
21 INT-RES-SAL & FRINGES (APPVD)	9139414	83103	34105	1738760	10995382	1786365	134993		21
21A SUPERVISING MDS - TEACHING	4322807			843289	5166096	839310			21A
22 INT-RES-OTHER PGM COSTS (APPVD)									22
22A SUPERVISING PHYSICIANS									22A
INPATIENT ROUTINE SERV COST CENTERS									
25 ADULTS & PEDIATRICS	30439700	2446206	558969	5175185	38620060	6274390	3973635	1333861	25
26 INTENSIVE CARE UNIT	3095455	106906	186535	488044	3876940	629867	173659	229519	26
27 CORONARY CARE UNIT	1358736	31214	238707	248574	1877231	304984	50704	37159	27
28 SURGICAL ICU	1526368	18470	15122	248104	1808064	293747	30003	124329	28
28D NEO-NATAL INTENSIVE CARE UNIT	2137404	32934	76018	353233	2599589	422342	53498	63990	28D
31 SUBPROVIDER I-PSYCHIATRIC	3533373	299154	22919	694223	4549669	739162	485948	40907	31
33 NURSERY	2230959	28450	11804	428740	2699993	438654	46279	136645	33
ANCILLARY SERVICE COST CENTERS									
37 OPERATING ROOM	9535973	241366	619977	1082681	11479997	1865098	392077	342551	37
39 DELIVERY ROOM & LABOR ROOM	2741743	93769	57740	488056	3381308	549344	152319		39
40 ANESTHESIOLOGY	838627	17258	196344	83644	1135873	184540	28034		40
41 RADIOLOGY--DIAGNOSTIC	3137506	255126	785018	316845	4494495	730198	414429	26298	41
43 RADIOISOTOPE	629912	22972	56645	26622	736151	119599	37316		43
43A C.A.T. SCAN	124058	31537	67171	24045	246811	40098	51229		43A
44 LABORATORY	7098960	335020	417404	1029069	8880453	1442763	544209	8387	44
47 BLOOD STORING,PROCESS,TRANSFUS	3127615	108834	68221	198256	3502926	569103	176790		47
49 RESPIRATORY THERAPY	1395321	8404	116276	186508	1706509	277248	13651		49
50 PHYSICAL THERAPY	766384	50596	21374	145677	984031	159871	82188	9311	50
53 ELECTROCARDIOLOGY	3044165	135753	266417	193500	3639835	591346	220519	5239	53
54 ELECTROENCEPHALOGRAPHY	305469	83541	16529	57551	463090	75236	135705		54
55 MED SUPPLIES CHGD TO PATIENTS									55

❖ **EXHIBIT 8A–2** *Continued*

PROVIDER NO.
PERIOD FROM 01/01/90 TO 12/31/90

EICR - EMPIRE BLUE CROSS AND BLUE SHIELD
IN LIEU OF FORM HCFA-2552-89 (12/89)

VERSION: 91.02
05/31/91

COST ALLOCATION - GENERAL SERVICE COSTS

WORKSHEET 8
PART I

COST CENTER DESCRIPTION	HOUSE-KEEPING 8	DIETARY RAW FOOD 9A	DIETARY OTHER 9B	CAFETERIA 10	MAINT OF PERSONNEL 11	MEDICAL RECORDS & LIBRARY 15	SOCIAL SERVICE 16	MEDICAL SUPPLIES & EXPENSE 17A	
GENERAL SERVICE COST CENTERS									
1 CAP-REL COSTS-BLDGS & FIXTURES									1
2 CAP-REL COSTS-MOVABLE EQUIPMENT									2
3 EMPLOYEE BENEFITS									3
4 ADMINISTRATIVE AND GENERAL									4
5 MAINTENANCE AND REPAIRS									5
6 OPERATION OF PLANT									6
7 LAUNDRY AND LINEN SERVICES									7
8 HOUSEKEEPING	6119609								8
9A DIETARY - RAW FOOD		2296301							9A
9B DIETARY - OTHER			5770426						9B
10 CAFETERIA		480708	1207983	1811873					10
11 MAINTENANCE OF PERSONNEL					609872				11
15 MEDICAL RECORDS AND LIBRARY				48458		3341010			15
16 SOCIAL SERVICE				20014			1444310		16
17A MEDICAL SUPPLIES AND EXPENSE								8044186	17A
17B CENTRAL SERVICES & SUPPLY				16547					17B
17C PHARMACY				57914					17C
17D NURSING ADMINISTRATION	21838			54053					17D
17E INTENSIVE NURSING CARE									17E
17F GENERAL NURSING SERVICE									17F
18 VISUAL AIDS									18
19 NON-PHYSICIAN ANESTHETISTS									19
21 INT-RES-SAL & FRINGES (APPVD)	131026			209120	166579				21
21A SUPERVISING MDS - TEACHING									21A
22 INT-RES-OTHER PGM COSTS (APPVD)									22
22A SUPERVISING PHYSICIANS									22A
INPATIENT ROUTINE SERV COST CENTERS									
25 ADULTS & PEDIATRICS	2953137	1410661	3544881	519725	352432	1521162	1049726	4334920	25
26 INTENSIVE CARE UNIT	327566	44227	111138	38688	23404	172730	2166	409319	26
27 CORONARY CARE UNIT		20951	52649	18674		101567	2166	142799	27
28 SURGICAL ICU	65513	19342	48605	21747	5507	125622	2166	327802	28
28D NEO-NATAL INTENSIVE CARE UNIT	131026			30572		75173	53728	143378	28D
31 SUBPROVIDER I-PSYCHIATRIC	494541	173575	436179	68078		153352		219633	31
33 NURSERY	131026			35142		84862		24861	33
ANCILLARY SERVICE COST CENTERS									
37 OPERATING ROOM	196540			101251	4130			1097301	37
39 DELIVERY ROOM & LABOR ROOM	262053			45464				380993	39
40 ANESTHESIOLOGY				11819	16520			170551	40
41 RADIOLOGY--DIAGNOSTIC	163783			48222	8260			23127	41
43 RADIOISOTOPE				2679					43
43A C.A.T. SCAN				2364					43A
44 LABORATORY	98270			122998	8260			64750	44
47 BLOOD STORING,PROCESS,TRANSFUS				24505	8260			18501	47
49 RESPIRATORY THERAPY				22220				42784	49
50 PHYSICAL THERAPY				15286	8260			578	50
53 ELECTROCARDIOLOGY				29784				27754	53
54 ELECTROENCEPHALOGRAPHY				5437					54
55 MED SUPPLIES CHGD TO PATIENTS									55

❖ **EXHIBIT 8A–2** *Continued*

```
PROVIDER NO. 33-0194                              EICR - EMPIRE BLUE CROSS AND BLUE SHIELD    VERSION: 91.02
PERIOD FROM  01/01/90  TO  12/31/90                  IN LIEU OF FORM HCFA-2552-89 (12/89)        05/31/91

        COST ALLOCATION - GENERAL SERVICE COSTS                                             WORKSHEET B
                                                                                              PART I
```

COST CENTER DESCRIPTION	CENTRAL SERVICES & SUPPLY 17B	PHARMACY 17C	NURSING ADMINI-STRATION 17D	VISUAL AIDS 18	NON PHYSI-CIAN ANES-THETISTS 19	I/R-APPRVD SALS & FR BENEFITS 21	SUPERVIS-ING PHY-SICIANS 21A	SUBTOTAL 25	
GENERAL SERVICE COST CENTERS									
1 CAP-REL COSTS-BLDGS & FIXTURES									1
2 CAP-REL COSTS-MOVABLE EQUIPMENT									2
3 EMPLOYEE BENEFITS									3
4 ADMINISTRATIVE AND GENERAL									4
5 MAINTENANCE AND REPAIRS									5
6 OPERATION OF PLANT									6
7 LAUNDRY AND LINEN SERVICES									7
8 HOUSEKEEPING									8
9A DIETARY - RAW FOOD									9A
9B DIETARY - OTHER									9B
10 CAFETERIA									10
11 MAINTENANCE OF PERSONNEL									11
15 MEDICAL RECORDS AND LIBRARY									15
16 SOCIAL SERVICE									16
17A MEDICAL SUPPLIES AND EXPENSE									17A
17B CENTRAL SERVICES & SUPPLY	1314006								17B
17C PHARMACY		13267901							17C
17D NURSING ADMINISTRATION			2297296						17D
17E INTENSIVE NURSING CARE									17E
17F GENERAL NURSING SERVICE									17F
18 VISUAL AIDS				291874					18
19 NON-PHYSICIAN ANESTHETISTS					426900				19
21 INT-RES-SAL & FRINGES (APPVD)		1740				13425205			21
21A SUPERVISING MDS - TEACHING							6005406		21A
22 INT-RES-OTHER PGM COSTS (APPVD)									22
22A SUPERVISING PHYSICIANS									22A
INPATIENT ROUTINE SERV COST CENTERS									
25 ADULTS & PEDIATRICS	859777	10875603	1133486.	291874	356376	6224583	2225394	87855683	25
26 INTENSIVE CARE UNIT	102630	418651	66851			722643		7349998	26
27 CORONARY CARE UNIT	60247	39783	65932			361321		3136167	27
28 SURGICAL ICU	61852	386110	66622			173622		3560653	28
28D NEO-NATAL INTENSIVE CARE UNIT	47221	23973	53297			583041		4280828	28D
31 SUBPROVIDER I-PSYCHIATRIC		148663	586270			430536	159697	8686210	31
33 NURSERY		8428				197084		3802974	33
ANCILLARY SERVICE COST CENTERS									
37 OPERATING ROOM	16547	30758	218243					15744493	37
39 DELIVERY ROOM & LABOR ROOM	5968	14252	106595			509135		5407431	39
40 ANESTHESIOLOGY		113618				750798	107521	2519274	40
41 RADIOLOGY--DIAGNOSTIC	14798	77224				375399		6376233	41
43 RADIOISOTOPE								895745	43
43A C.A.T. SCAN								340502	43A
44 LABORATORY		89				422324	383590	11976093	44
47 BLOOD STORING,PROCESS,TRANSFUS		20					34241	4334346	47
49 RESPIRATORY THERAPY								2062412	49
50 PHYSICAL THERAPY								1259525	50
53 ELECTROCARDIOLOGY	14918	1857						4531252	53
54 ELECTROENCEPHALOGRAPHY						93850	253887	1027205	54
55 MED SUPPLIES CHGD TO PATIENTS									55

❖ **EXHIBIT 8A–3**

PROVIDER NO.
PERIOD FROM 01/01/90 TO 12/31/90

EICR - EMPIRE BLUE CROSS AND BLUE SHIELD
IN LIEU OF FORM HCFA-2552-89 (12/89)

VERSION: 91.02
05/31/91

WORKSHEET B-1

COST ALLOCATION - STATISTICAL BASIS

COST CENTER DESCRIPTION	CAP REL COST-BLDGS & FIXTURES (SQUARE FEET)	CAP REL COST-MOVBL EQUIPMENT (DOLLAR VALUE)	EMPLOYEE BENEFITS (GROSS SALARIES)	RECON-CILIATION	ADMINIS-TRATIVE & GENERAL (ACCUM COST)	MAINT AND REPAIRS (SQUARE FEET)	OPERATION OF PLANT (SQUARE FEET)	
0	1	2	3	3A	4	5	6	
GENERAL SERVICE COST CENTERS								1
1 CAP-REL COSTS-BLDGS & FIXTURES	871246							2
2 CAP-REL COSTS-MOVABLE EQUIPMENT		7143229						3
3 EMPLOYEE BENEFITS	4221	6051	122397259					4
4 ADMINISTRATIVE AND GENERAL	244544	2588807	14372516	-30793262	189537921	244544	244544	5
5 MAINTENANCE AND REPAIRS					622481			6
6 OPERATION OF PLANT	58292	426841	3677607		9100878	58292	564189	7
7 LAUNDRY AND LINEN SERVICES	6874	52433	1030429		2001288	6874	6874	8
8 HOUSEKEEPING	8547	67325	3638327		5125090	8547	8547	9A
9A DIETARY - RAW FOOD					1975372			9B
9B DIETARY - OTHER	24276	38054	3519637		4568721	24276	24276	10
10 CAFETERIA	3829				44201	3829	3829	11
11 MAINTENANCE OF PERSONNEL	18125	18807			232264	18125	18125	15
15 MEDICAL RECORDS AND LIBRARY	12465	92199	1528004		2631316	12465	12465	16
16 SOCIAL SERVICE	2634	2641	913810		1182749	2634	2634	17A
17A MEDICAL SUPPLIES AND EXPENSE		7640	60117		6919938			17B
17B CENTRAL SERVICES & SUPPLY	5490	84760	530222		1027569	5490	5490	17C
17C PHARMACY	5689	285381	3262790		11272003	5689	5689	17D
17D NURSING ADMINISTRATION	10791	134250	531663		1715518	10791	10791	17E
17E INTENSIVE NURSING CARE								17F
17F GENERAL NURSING SERVICE								18
18 VISUAL AIDS	2814	26054	107509		205690	2814	2814	19
19 NON-PHYSICIAN ANESTHETISTS			307291		367237			21
21 INT-RES-SAL & FRINGES (APPVD)	7199	27845	8913107		10995382	7199	7199	21A
21A SUPERVISING MDS - TEACHING			4322807		5166096			22
22 INT-RES-OTHER PGM COSTS (APPVD)								22A
22A SUPERVISING PHYSICIANS								
INPATIENT ROUTINE SERV COST CENTERS								
25 ADULTS & PEDIATRICS	211909	456369	26528559		38620060	211909	211909	25
26 INTENSIVE CARE UNIT	9261	152296	2501774		3876940	9261	9261	26
27 CORONARY CARE UNIT	2704	194892	1274222		1077231	2704	2704	27
28 SURGICAL ICU	1600	12346	1271811		1808064	1600	1600	28
28D NEO-NATAL INTENSIVE CARE UNIT	2853	62065	1810718		2599589	2853	2853	28D
31 SUBPROVIDER I-PSYCHIATRIC	25915	18712	3558675		4549669	25915	25915	31
33 NURSERY	2468	9637	2197774		2699993	2468	2468	33
ANCILLARY SERVICE COST CENTERS								
37 OPERATING ROOM	20909	506179	5549962		11479997	20909	20909	37
39 DELIVERY ROOM & LABOR ROOM	8123	47142	2501840		3381308	8123	8123	39
40 ANESTHESIOLOGY	1495	160305	428771		1135873	1495	1495	40
41 RADIOLOGY--DIAGNOSTIC	22101	640927	1624186		4494495	22101	22101	41
43 RADIOISOTOPE	1990	46248	136468		736151	1990	1990	43
43A C.A.T. SCAN	2732	54842	123258		246811	2732	2732	43A
44 LABORATORY	29022	340789	5275142		8880453	29022	29022	44
47 BLOOD STORING,PROCESS,TRANSFUS	9428	55699	1016284		3502926	9428	9428	47
49 RESPIRATORY THERAPY	728	94933	956064		1706509	728	728	49
50 PHYSICAL THERAPY	4383	17451	746761		984031	4383	4383	50
53 ELECTROCARDIOLOGY	11760	217516	991905		3639835	11760	11760	53

❖ **EXHIBIT 8A–3** *Continued*

PROVIDER NO.
PERIOD FROM 01/01/90 TO 12/31/90

EICR - EMPIRE BLUE CROSS AND BLUE SHIELD
IN LIEU OF FORM HCFA-2552-89 (12/89)

VERSION: 91.02
05/31/91

COST ALLOCATION - STATISTICAL BASIS

WORKSHEET B-1

	COST CENTER DESCRIPTION	LAUNDRY & LINEN SERVICE (POUNDS OF LAUNDRY) 7	HOUSE-KEEPING (HOURS OF SERVICE) 8	DIETARY RAW FOOD (MEALS SERVED) 9A	DIETARY OTHER (MEALS SERVED) 9B	CAFETERIA (AVG NO OF EMPLOYEES) 10	MAINT OF PERSONNEL (NUMBER HOUSED) 11	MEDICAL RECORDS & LIBRARY (% OF TIME SPENT) 15	SOCIAL SERVICE (TIME SPENT) 16	
	GENERAL SERVICE COST CENTERS									
1	CAP-REL COSTS-BLDGS & FIXTURES									1
2	CAP-REL COSTS-MOVABLE EQUIPMENT									2
3	EMPLOYEE BENEFITS									3
4	ADMINISTRATIVE AND GENERAL		42250			4393	18			4
5	MAINTENANCE AND REPAIRS									5
6	OPERATION OF PLANT									6
7	LAUNDRY AND LINEN SERVICES	4600657								7
8	HOUSEKEEPING	3000	182150							8
9A	DIETARY - RAW FOOD			974351						9A
9B	DIETARY - OTHER	7933			974351					9B
10	CAFETERIA			203971	203971	22995				10
11	MAINTENANCE OF PERSONNEL						443			11
15	MEDICAL RECORDS AND LIBRARY					615		10000		15
16	SOCIAL SERVICE					254			10000	16
17A	MEDICAL SUPPLIES AND EXPENSE									17A
17B	CENTRAL SERVICES & SUPPLY					210				17B
17C	PHARMACY					735				17C
17D	NURSING ADMINISTRATION	46518	650			686				17D
17E	INTENSIVE NURSING CARE									17E
17F	GENERAL NURSING SERVICE									17F
18	VISUAL AIDS									18
19	NON-PHYSICIAN ANESTHETISTS									19
21	INT-RES-SAL & FRINGES (APPVD)		3900			2654	121			21
21A	SUPERVISING MDS - TEACHING									21A
22	INT-RES-OTHER PGM COSTS (APPVD)									22
22A	SUPERVISING PHYSICIANS									22A
	INPATIENT ROUTINE SERV COST CENTERS									
25	ADULTS & PEDIATRICS	2499317	87900	598562	598562	6596	256	4553	7268	25
26	INTENSIVE CARE UNIT	430061	9750	18766	18766	491	17	517	15	26
27	CORONARY CARE UNIT	69626		8890	8890	237		304	15	27
28	SURGICAL ICU	232961	1950	8207	8207	276	4	376	15	28
28D	NEO-NATAL INTENSIVE CARE UNIT	119902	3900			388		225	372	28D
31	SUBPROVIDER I-PSYCHIATRIC	76650	14720	73650	73650	864		459		31
33	NURSERY	256038	3900			446		254		33
	ANCILLARY SERVICE COST CENTERS									
37	OPERATING ROOM	641853	5850			1285	3			37
39	DELIVERY ROOM & LABOR ROOM		7800			577				39
40	ANESTHESIOLOGY					150	12			40
41	RADIOLOGY--DIAGNOSTIC	49275	4875			612	6			41
43	RADIOISOTOPE					34				43
43A	C.A.T. SCAN					30				43A
44	LABORATORY	15715	2925			1561	6			44
47	BLOOD STORING,PROCESS,TRANSFUS					311	6			47
49	RESPIRATORY THERAPY					282				49
50	PHYSICAL THERAPY	17446				194	6			50
53	ELECTROCARDIOLOGY	9816				378				53

❖ **EXHIBIT 8A–3** *Continued*

```
PROVIDER NO.                                    EICR - EMPIRE BLUE CROSS AND BLUE SHIELD   VERSION: 91.02
PERIOD. FROM  01/01/90  TO  12/31/90               IN LIEU OF FORM HCFA-2552-89 (12/89)          05/31/91

        COST ALLOCATION - STATISTICAL BASIS                                               WORKSHEET B-1
```

	COST CENTER DESCRIPTION	MEDICAL SUPPLIES & EXPENSE (COSTED REQSTNS) 17A	CENTRAL SERVICES & SUPPLY (COSTED REQSTNS) 17B	PHARMACY (COSTED REQSTNS) 17C	NURSING ADMINI-STRATION (SPVSN OF NRS TIME) 17D	VISUAL AIDS (VISUAL AIDS) 18	NON PHYSI-CIAN ANES-THETISTS (ASSIGNED TIME) 19	I/R-APPRVD SALS & FR BENEFITS (ASSIGNED TIME) 21	SUPERVIS-ING PHY-SICIANS SALARIES RENDERED) 21A	
	GENERAL SERVICE COST CENTERS									
1	CAP-REL COSTS-BLDGS & FIXTURES									1
2	CAP-REL COSTS-MOVABLE EQUIPMENT									2
3	EMPLOYEE BENEFITS									3
4	ADMINISTRATIVE AND GENERAL							261974		4
5	MAINTENANCE AND REPAIRS									5
6	OPERATION OF PLANT									6
7	LAUNDRY AND LINEN SERVICES									7
8	HOUSEKEEPING									8
9A	DIETARY - RAW FOOD									9A
9B	DIETARY - OTHER									9B
10	CAFETERIA									10
11	MAINTENANCE OF PERSONNEL									11
15	MEDICAL RECORDS AND LIBRARY									15
16	SOCIAL SERVICE									16
17A	MEDICAL SUPPLIES AND EXPENSE	6837655								17A
17B	CENTRAL SERVICES & SUPPLY		448681							17B
17C	PHARMACY			7265140						17C
17D	NURSING ADMINISTRATION				10000					17D
17E	INTENSIVE NURSING CARE									17E
17F	GENERAL NURSING SERVICE									17F
18	VISUAL AIDS					10000				18
19	NON-PHYSICIAN ANESTHETISTS						10000			19
21	INT-RES-SAL & FRINGES (APPVD)			953				11444		21
21A	SUPERVISING MDS - TEACHING								2839477	21A
22	INT-RES-OTHER PGM COSTS (APPVD)									22
22A	SUPERVISING PHYSICIANS									22A
	INPATIENT ROUTINE SERV COST CENTERS									
25	ADULTS & PEDIATRICS	3684735	293580	5955182	4934	10000	8348	5306	1052211	25
26	INTENSIVE CARE UNIT	347926	35044	229242	291			616		26
27	CORONARY CARE UNIT	121381	20572	21784	287			308		27
28	SURGICAL ICU	278636	21120	211423	290			148		28
28D	NEO-NATAL INTENSIVE CARE UNIT	121873	16124	13127	232			497		28D
31	SUBPROVIDER I-PSYCHIATRIC	186691		81404	2552			367	75508	31
33	NURSERY	21132		4615				168		33
	ANCILLARY SERVICE COST CENTERS									
37	OPERATING ROOM	932719	5650	16842	950					37
39	DELIVERY ROOM & LABOR ROOM	323849	2038	7804	464			434		39
40	ANESTHESIOLOGY	144970		62214				640	50838	40
41	RADIOLOGY--DIAGNOSTIC	19658	5053	42286				320		41
43	RADIOISOTOPE									43
43A	C.A.T. SCAN									43A
44	LABORATORY	55038		49				360	181369	44
47	BLOOD·STORING,PROCESS,TRANSFUS	15726		11					16190	47
49	RESPIRATORY THERAPY	36367								49
50	PHYSICAL THERAPY	491								50
53	ELECTROCARDIOLOGY	23591	5094	1017						53

CHAPTER

9

Costs and Other Issues Related to Recruiting and Retaining Staff

CHAPTER GOALS

The goals of this chapter are to:

- ◆ Describe the relationship between the availability of nursing staff and budgeting

- ◆ Explain how to plan for variations in the availability of nursing staff

- ◆ Discuss retention as a strategy to maintain cost-effective nursing staff

- ◆ Analyze the costs of retention programs

- ◆ Discuss recruitment as a strategy to maintain cost-effective nursing staff

- ◆ Identify some alternative solutions when nursing staff are in short supply

- ◆ Examine the use of computers to improve recruitment and retention

INTRODUCTION

The largest part of most operating budgets for nursing units and departments consists of *personnel* costs. Justifying the need for a given level of staff requires careful calculations and a lucid argument. However, in the preparation of an operating budget, it is often assumed that hiring the amount of labor approved in the final budget is not a problem. That is not necessarily the case in nursing. Nursing shortages have occurred on and off in the 1960s, 1970s, and 1980s and persist into the 1990s. To staff adequately in the face of a shortage substantially increases the costs of recruiting and retaining nurses. Even when there is no shortage these costs are significant. Nurse managers must be aware of the substantial resources that should be devoted to this area.

Recruitment of staff is a critical element in the overall management process. If vacant positions are left unstaffed throughout the year, two potentially serious side effects occur. The first is that the nurses working on a unit begin to suffer burnout from being overburdened. Shortages of staff lead to overwork, poor morale, increased sick leave, and other stress-related problems. This in turn tends to lead to loss of staff, exacerbating the shortage on the unit.

The second side effect is that the health care organization starts to assume that less money will be spent than has been put into the budget. Positions are approved with the expectation that they will never be filled. Eventually, if staff is finally available to be hired, the organization may resist filling the positions because it has made its overall plans based on the expectation that the money allocated for those positions would never be spent. The approved but vacant positions provide top management with a cushion to ease the impact of other unexpected financial problems throughout the year. Essentially, the budgeted but unfilled positions may be permanently lost. This effectively lowers the nursing care hours per patient day on a permanent basis.

The costs of these two side effects on the quality of patient care and on staff satisfaction are almost never measured and rarely considered. However, their existence stresses the importance of attempting to understand and explicitly measure the costs of staff recruitment and retention.

Furthermore, an attempt must be made to make financial decisions based on the expected *actual* staffing pattern. If twelve FTEs are authorized in a budget, the dollars in the budget should be based on the best expectation of how those twelve FTEs will be staffed. Suppose that due to recruitment difficulties, the most likely event is that the unit will be able to have eleven FTEs filled with regular full-time or part-time employees. The twelfth position will be filled with overtime or agency staff. In that case, the excess cost of overtime or an agency nurse as compared to a full-time employee is a cost related to retention and recruitment.

Another approach to the problem of retention and recruitment is to revise the manner in which nursing care is offered to use fewer professional staff. Nursing units can be reorganized to make greater use of alternative types of workers. Or computers could be acquired in an effort to reduce the number of nursing hours needed for documentation. It is likely that attempts to introduce shared governance, case management, alternative workers, or computers will have an impact on the actual staffing of a nursing unit. These expected changes and their costs are in a sense costs related to retention and recruitment in that they represent money spent to achieve and maintain an appropriate staffing level.

This chapter will confine itself to the actions that individual nurse managers can take, or should be aware of, in their management of recruitment and retention of nursing staff within their organizations. When shortages occur, a given organization may be relatively helpless when it comes to overcoming the entire national or regional shortage in the supply of nurses. However, organizations have a great degree of control over recruitment and retention for their own organizations. Recruitment and retention are important management concerns regardless of whether there is a shortage.

RETAINING STAFF

Although some degree of *turnover* will keep an organization "healthy" by bringing new blood into the organization, the most effective personnel strategy a health care organization can take is to work at retaining the staff it already has. It is often the case that every nurse you hire must be hired away from somebody else or recruited from nonworking nurses. Therefore, it should be clear that recruiting nurses may require a costly level of competition. Major efforts should be made in an attempt to reduce turnover. Both individual characteristics and organizational factors are postulated to be related to nurse *retention*. One key to staff retention is to have a high level of nurse satisfaction.

Nurse Satisfaction

Surprisingly, very little is definitively known about what leads to nurse satisfaction. Many factors are believed to be relevant to keeping a nursing staff happy. Studies have not consistently shown any one factor or any unique set of factors that are always present in satisfied staffs, or whose absence will necessarily lead to a dissatisfied staff. Nevertheless, a number of elements are generally accepted as being related to nursing satisfaction. These elements are discussed here.

One primary element of nursing satisfaction is the development of professionalism in the delivery of health care services through a combination of increased autonomy and the availability of resource personnel for consultation. Nurses must feel like professionals and be treated like professionals to be satisfied in their employment. Time cards, for example, are often thought to be demeaning for nurses and can lead to dissatisfaction. Similarly, working as hourly workers does not generally result in the same level of satisfaction as working as salaried employees.

A positive attitude toward nursing and professional treatment by the physician staff and the administration can be critical factors in having a satisfied staff. Negative attitudes by these groups can cause significant unhappiness on the part of the staff. This ties in with the overall issue of nursing image. The institution has little control over the national image of nursing. However, it can take strides toward creating a positive image internally. The way nurses are treated and the way nursing is presented to patients can make a substantial difference in the attitudes of nurses as well as the rest of the organization's staff. Image building begins with actions taken by nursing to create a positive image. Programs with physicians and administration can be suggested by nursing administration, if they are not forthcoming otherwise.

The issue of financial payment is, of course, relevant. Nurses report that pay is important to them in determining their level of satisfaction. High salaries and good benefits will help keep staff from wanting to look elsewhere. This also requires that there be ample opportunity for advancement, either into management or on a clinical track.

Flexible hours have also become a key to retaining staff. A wide variety of alternative working hours have been developed by organizations attempting to recruit new nurses. These flexible arrangements must be made available to existing staff as well, or they may become dissatisfied and move to an organization that will offer such hours.

From a budgeting perspective, this can become quite complex. The use of four ten-hour shifts to create a four-day work week is not a major budgeting problem. Although it may create a complicated staffing pattern for coverage, it still results in forty hours of pay for forty hours of work, the same as five days, eight hours each. On the other hand, innovations such as three twelve-hour shifts, or two twelve-hour weekend shifts, for forty hours of pay can create a variety of budgeting complications. Clear decisions must be made concerning whether a full-time equivalent (FTE) employee represents forty hours of work or forty hours of pay. (See Chapter 12 for further discussion.)

Fringe Benefits

Clearly, one element of nursing satisfaction will be related to the organization's employee benefits, commonly referred to as *fringe benefits*. How many weeks of vacation do staff get each year? How many paid holidays are there? Is free life insurance provided to employees? Those are several of the most obvious employee benefits. Some benefits are required by law. For example, the employer must pay for "FICA," a tax for Social Security, which will eventually provide the employee with a Social Security pension. Most benefits, however, are voluntary or else the result of labor negotiations.

Other critical benefits concern the quality of the health insurance package offered to employees. At the time this book was written health insurance rates for group plans were rising nearly 25% per year. Do nurses have to contribute to the cost of their health insurance? If so, how much? Are their family members covered? If so, is there additional cost to the nurse? Are staff members subject to *coinsurance* and *deductibles* on their health insurance? Coinsurance means that the insurer bears a portion of the cost (often 80%) and the employee bears the remainder (usually 20%). A deductible means that 100% of some amount must first be paid by the employee before there are any health benefits (often $500 or $200 per year).

Most employers also offer a variety of other benefits that are somewhat less obvious and are more responsible for the term "fringe benefits" as opposed to employee benefits. For example, if the CEO belongs to a golf club and the membership is paid for by the organization, that is a fringe benefit. If the CEO drives a hospital-owned car, that is another example of fringe benefits.

In terms of the budget, the fringe benefits referred to above really represent several different types of cost. The vacation and holiday time for each employee is already built into the annual salary cost for that individual. There is no need to budget for that fringe benefit, except for making sure that there is adequate staff coverage for all days off. That is accounted for by budgeting additional personnel (see Chapter 12). On the other hand, the cost of life insurance, pension payments, Social Security taxes, health insurance, and other fringe benefits that require cash outlays must be budgeted for explicitly.

In most organizations the specific costs of the fringe benefits are calculated by the finance office and are assigned to departments based on salaries, usually as a percentage. For example, a nursing unit might be charged 22% for fringe benefits for every dollar of salary paid to any staff member. Certainly, not all employees have the same cost to the organization per dollar of salary. That is simply an average. Is it fair? It might well be that certain fringe benefits are worth more to members of some departments than employees of other departments. However, over the years it has been decided that it is not worth the effort to get a more refined measure of costs. Therefore budgeting for fringe benefits generally requires only the addition of a set percentage (provided by the finance office) to the budgeted salary amounts.

Many organizations are now offering a *cafeteria* approach to fringe benefits. The organization determines the amount of money it will contribute to fringe benefits. The cost of each fringe benefit is determined and employees choose from the list, much as food is chosen in a cafeteria. This costs the organization slightly more in administrative expense but no more in total fringe benefit costs. Employee wants for fringe benefits vary. The young new graduate might not care about life insurance but might prefer a low deductible on health insurance. The young mother might prefer child care and have no need for health insurance because her spouse has family coverage from his employer.

Retention Programs

The problem of turnover is significant enough to warrant specific attention and direct programs aimed at staff retention. This should go beyond the basic notions of having competent managers, physicians who work on a collegial professional basis with nurses, autonomy in work, and the other elements of nurse satisfaction. Such programs should work toward making the institution one that shows caring for its staff and creates a loyalty bond that is hard to break. Some such programs involve significant financial investment, while others take relatively little. Prior to the development of a retention program, the manager should determine the desired retention goal and the actual retention level at the organization.

The first step in a retention program is to determine the retention level goal for an organization or unit. Most organizations would be unhappy with 100% retention. Unless the organization expands, this level of retention would leave no room for new staff. New staff are desired both because they provide new ideas to an organization and because new staff nurses are generally paid a lower wage than experienced nurses. On the other hand, most managers would agree that 70% retention is perhaps too low. Orienting 30% of the staff each year is likely to be too costly and disruptive.

The second step is to determine the historical level of retention. Most nurse managers determine turnover. This is defined as the number of employees terminating during a period of time. The converse of turnover is then considered retention. If 10% of the staff terminate each year, retention is considered 90%. However, this approach tells the manager little about the retention pattern of the nursing staff. Do most people leave within the first three months? Is there an even distribution among staff with all levels of tenure? Using a "life tables" approach actual retention rates can be determined.[1]

Using this method actual patterns of retention are determined. All staff are identified, and measurement is made about how long staff stay. For example, how many of the staff stay more than six months, more than three years, more than ten years? If 50% of the staff leave within the first year and less than 5% of those who have been there more than five years leave, efforts can be directed at the former group, rather than the nurses who have been at the institution for more than five years. It could also be the case that nurses who have been

---

[1]See M. Beth Benedict, Jay H. Glasser, and Eun Sul Lee, "Assessing Hospital Nursing Staff Retention and Turnover: A Life Table Approach," *Evaluation & The Health Professions*, Vol. 12, No. 1, March 1989, pp. 73–96, for a more detailed description of this process.

at the organization for over five years are now leaving because the organization raised salaries of entry level staff, whereas a competing organization instituted a policy for increases in salary for every year of service. After determining the organization's retention goal and the historical retention rate, a retention program can be developed.

First of all, employees should have a way of being recognized. There should be a formal mechanism that allows a pattern of exemplary work, or even one good deed, to gain recognition. There are a variety of ways that employee behavior can be recognized. The first is in the form of performance evaluations with interviews. Such evaluations are a two-edged sword. They need to be firm enough to make clear that poor performance will not be ignored or rewarded. However, there should be a strong focus on positive aspects. This may be in terms of recognizing good performance, or even in terms of offering training in areas where performance should be improved. Rather than dwelling on poor past performance, a greater amount of time should be spent on discussing ways to accomplish more and to improve future performance.

Performance evaluation meetings are often uncomfortable for both the evaluator and the one being evaluated. However, such meetings should not be given short shrift. Employees should leave the meeting with a feeling that they understand what is expected of them, with a sense that their individual efforts make a difference in the overall performance of the unit, and with a clear sense that their positive contributions have been noted and specifically recognized by the organization.

Another key element of performance conferences should be to elicit input. What is going on that the employee likes, and what is going on that the employee objects to? Open lines of communication—with honest follow-up on suggestions and complaints—are likely to win over support and loyalty. A refusal to budge from the way things are is more likely to result in resentment and, in some cases, resignations.

In addition to meetings, specific actions may warrant letters of commendation. Such letters could be the result of favorable patient comments on a form supplied to patients for that purpose. Or they could be based on recommendations from other staff. Commendations should be presented in appropriate ceremonies and noted in organizational newsletters, so that as many people as possible are made aware of them. This provides further psychic benefit to the recipient and perhaps serves notice to other workers of the possibility of gaining such recognition. Achievement of such recognition should be within the reach of most staff members.

In providing motivation, the carrot or the stick can be used. Some schools of thought argue that the stick is more appropriate than the carrot. Poor performance is unacceptable and that fact should be conveyed to workers. Other schools of thought argue that in the long run the carrot will have more positive results. Accentuating the positive and decentuating the negative results in a happier and psychologically healthier work environment. In many cases a combination of the carrot and the stick is probably optimal.

Another program for retention involves financial remuneration. Money is not a solution to all problems. One study has shown that having adequate numbers of staff, nursing management support, alternate weekends off, support of administration, and permanent shift assignments all rank ahead of benefits and salary in terms of importance to nurses. On the other hand, benefits and salary ranked ahead of general staffing patterns, support of physicians, opportunity for advancement, location, and staff development programs.[2] Nursing departments should attempt to deal with all these factors. However, while money is not the solution to all problems, financial incentives have become a major competitive factor.

Higher wages are one type of financial incentive. They can be very costly to health care organizations. Other types of financial incentives can be achieved without substantially higher cost to the institution. One example is annual salaries instead of hourly wages. This approach may make nurses feel better about themselves and their institutions. Another financial approach is bonuses. Bonuses generally are paid only out of cost savings. Thus, the institution can afford to pay for them because the payment is only part of a larger amount that would otherwise have been spent anyway. Bonuses had little use just a decade ago but are becoming more and more widespread.

Innovative employee benefits are another area that can be used to help retain nurses. For example, child-care centers at the health care organization (perhaps with discounted or subsidized rates) can help retention significantly. Additionally, such centers have the capacity to reduce sick leave substantially. Much sick leave is the result of a nurse staying home to take care of a sick child. Sick leave can therefore be reduced if the child-care center has facilities for mildly ill children.

The above approaches to retention are already in the nursing literature. However, to be truly competitive an organization must be innovative. For example, suppose that a nurses' dramatics group were formed and each six months it staged a dramatic or musical play with performances for the staff and patients. A club of that type provides an excellent release from the routine work pressures. In that way it reduces the burnout syndrome. Over the years such a "club" develops intense loyalties. Nurses might not leave the organization because they don't want to be left out of the show. Bridge clubs and other organization-sponsored activities (annual picnics and trips to the ballpark) result in the development of a sense of family and community rather than strictly a workplace. And when times get tough, families and communities hang together.

Clinical Ladders

A frequent complaint of staff nurses is that there is little room for advancement within the clinical ranks. Nurses can go into management. However, if they choose to pursue a bedside hands-on clinical career, there is little difference in reward for a nurse with thirty years of experience compared to one with five years. The concept of clinical ladders is one suggestion for overcoming that deterrent to nurse retention.

There are a wide variety of clinical ladder models. Some are completely distinct from administrative career paths. Others allow for branching off from a clinical ladder into an administrative path after a certain point. Some clinical ladders require simple on-the-job experience for promotions, while others require additional education including advanced degrees. In some models moving up the ladder requires community and/or professional service and publi-

---

[2]"What Nurses Want Most from a Job," *Nursing 88,* Springhouse Corp., Vol. 18, No. 2, February 1988, p. 38.

cations. Another distinction among models is the amount of additional responsibility that must be assumed as one moves up the ladder.

There is a widespread belief that clinical ladders do improve nurse retention. Such an approach improves the professional identity of the nurse and generates loyalty. Another perspective is that if nurses with more experience with a given institution earn substantially more than those with fewer years at the specific organization, it becomes more costly to move. It becomes expensive to give up seniority. If that is the case, then retention of the more experienced/expensive personnel becomes easier, but higher turnover rates may occur among the nurses at the lower (and less expensive) rungs of the ladder. Over time this may lead to an organization with a large proportion of its staff near the higher end of the ladder.

The Hawthorne Effect

With all attempts to improve retention, it is necessary to be wary of the Hawthorne effect, which is widely discussed in the general management literature. The Hawthorne effect is based on a study in which a number of changes were made in a factory to examine their impact on worker productivity. With each change, productivity improved. However, it turned out that the specific changes were not directly responsible for the improvement. Improvement occurred as a result of the attention the workers were receiving.

Consider researchers making factory lighting brighter to see if more light improves worker productivity. Productivity in fact increases after the lighting is changed. Then the researchers add music, and productivity goes up again. If the lighting and music are responsible, then taking them away should reduce productivity to the earlier levels. However, removing the better lighting and the music causes productivity to go up even further. The *attention* rather than the lighting or the music makes productivity improve.

All the efforts to improve nurse retention risk falling subject to the Hawthorne effect. Put a clinical ladder in place and turnover decreases. Have joint awareness seminars with nurses, administrators, and physicians; institute a bonus system; have performance evaluations twice a year; declare a new era of nursing autonomy. After each change, turnover decreases. The one thing not known about any of the changes is whether it is the specific nature of the change that is significant or simply the response of nurses in recognition of the fact that the organization finally seems to care about them.

This does not mean that the changes in themselves have no impact. There has been enough literature reporting results to indicate that certain factors are in fact likely to improve nurse satisfaction and hopefully retention. Open communication, greater participation in decision making, being salaried, and clinical ladders do likely make a difference. However, the very element of change itself should not be underplayed.

Putting a clinical ladder in place and then assuming retention will take care of itself is not likely to work satisfactorily in the long run. The organization must adopt an attitude of making changes each year to improve the lot of its nurses. It may well not be possible to improve all areas that affect nurse satisfaction in any one year. But a constant attitude of working toward improvement is needed. This may mean new major innovations each year or it may mean modifications to past innovations. Some years changes may be financial, while other years they may relate to nursing image. A constant approach that each year looks to see what improvements can be added is more likely to have a lasting positive impact than a dramatic one-shot change. Nursing staff should be able to see that the organization has a commitment to the improvement of the lot of nurses each and every year.

Determining the Cost

What does it cost to retain staff? As with any decision in a health organization, the cost-benefit ratio of a retention program should be estimated in advance and also evaluated after the program has been implemented. Having accurate data on current retention patterns and knowing the organization's goal provide the first step in determining the costs of the program. Although it is often difficult to associate a particular retention program with overall retention, some estimates can be made. If a new program such as free parking is instituted, the cost of that can easily be determined. Often, however, new programs have several goals and potential benefits. A bedside computer system is installed to retain nurses who want to work in a "high tech" environment where charting is easier. However, the computer system is also expected to improve the quality of patient care and to decrease the time nurses spend on documentation. Other programs aimed at improving retention may have additional benefits as well. Shared governance may be instituted to improve retention, but it may improve patient care and have that benefit as well. Increasing salaries may retain staff in the short run, but as soon as the hospital across town increases its salaries, the benefits of such a program may disappear.

Determining the costs of turnover and therefore the benefits of decreasing turnover is somewhat more straightforward. What is important to remember is that the costs of turnover do not include just the costs of advertising for staff and the nurse recruiter's salary. Costs include the effect short staffing has on the remaining staff and the decreased productivity of new staff. Jones describes a detailed approach to determine the costs of turnover. She suggests that the following costs be included:

- Advertising/recruiting
- Costs of unfilled positions
- Hiring costs
- Termination costs
- Orientation/training
- Decreased new RN productivity[3]

For the hospitals studied by Jones the mean cost per RN turnover was $10,198 (range $6,886–$15,152).

Blaufuss, Maynard, and Schollars present an alternative approach to evaluating turnover costs in response to a specific incentive.[4] They do not include general advertising and recruiting costs in their calculations. This is because they argue that hospitals must advertise regardless of turnover rates, since there will naturally be some turnover in all organizations.

---

[3]See Cheryl Bland Jones, "Staff Nurse Turnover Costs: Part II, Measurements and Results," *Journal of Nursing Administration*, Vol. 20, No. 4, May 1990, pp. 27–31, for a complete description of this approach.

[4]Judy Blaufuss, Jan Maynard, and Gail Schollars, "Methods of Evaluating Turnover Costs," *Nursing Management*, Vol. 23, No. 5, May 1992, pp. 52–61.

They include interviewing, preparing for orientation, the orientation itself, and a learning period. Using a zero-base approach, they identify the individual cost of hiring each new staff member. In addition, they include estimated revenue enhancements as an offset to the recruiting cost. This is particularly important when increases in staff can lead to opening more beds or in some other way increasing the number of patients cared for. Essentially, if you look at the cost of attracting new staff, you must also consider the extra revenue the organization will earn if it has those new staff members.

RECRUITING STAFF

No matter how effectively an organization works to retain its existing staff, some turnover must be expected. Some staff members will retire; others will move to different parts of the country. Some replacement of staff will always be occurring. Concurrent with the nursing department setting retention goals and working toward achieving them, a *recruitment* effort should occur. Recruitment is an ongoing process, not something that is done just at a time of staff shortage. Recruitment strategies may change during shortages, but the successful organization continually works on recruitment.

Identifying the existing level of recruitment is the first step in developing a recruitment strategy. What is the current level of recruitment? Is this acceptable? Do you anticipate any changes in the organization (e.g., the addition of a new unit) that will require changes in that level or an improvement in retention due to new initiatives in the organization?

The second step is to assess the external environment. What changes are occurring that will impact on the level of recruiting? Are enrollments increasing in nursing schools, thus making recruitment easier? Is the increase likely to continue? What specific factors in the environment may impact on the organization's ability to recruit? Have there been salary increases in competing organizations? After assessing the external environment and determining a desired level of recruitment, a specific recruitment plan can be developed.

Marketing

A key element of recruiting is an effective marketing strategy. As long as a limited supply of talented nurses exists, there will be a winner and a loser in the effort to recruit qualified personnel. Therefore a plan must be developed for addressing the recruiting issue.

The essence of marketing is that the needs and desires of a group are determined on the basis of market research and then an effort is made to satisfy them. Notice that this definition does not revolve around advertising, which may or may not be part of a marketing effort. The first step is to find out what nurses want from their employment. Next, efforts must be made to ensure that the hospital meets those needs to the extent possible. Finally, it is necessary to be able to convey the fact that the needs have been met.

In performing market research, a decision should first be made concerning whom the organization wants to recruit. New nurses, right out of school? Experienced nurses? Nurse managers? Specialists? Local nurses? Out-of-state nurses? In trying to determine what the potential employee wants and needs, it is critically important to correctly evaluate the group that is to be the target of the marketing effort.

Since most health care organizations already have some staff, there must be some attractive characteristics of the organization. In relative terms, all existing organizations have some strengths. Therefore, there should not be a hopeless attitude of "how can we compete with the rich research-oriented medical center in town?" Perhaps many nurses would prefer to provide care in a patient-oriented rather than research-oriented setting. It is important to identify the existing strengths of the organization so that the information can be conveyed to a target group.

At the same time, weaknesses must be identified and a long-term plan designed to overcome as many of them as possible. Perhaps lack of convenient parking is the one overwhelming negative the organization has. In that case, replacing expensive advertising with a major fund-raising campaign to allow for the building of an enclosed parking garage may be an appropriate marketing strategy. That is an example of a one-shot, expensive solution to a recruiting problem.

In other cases solutions may be less expensive but require ongoing efforts. For example, a hospital could distinguish itself through a concerted effort to develop a system of shared governance. Such efforts are not necessarily expensive. They do, however, require tremendous cooperation and commitment. The potential result is that expensive newspaper ads can be replaced with free news stories on the change at the hospital. Nursing schools can be encouraged to have the organization's staff give lectures on the shared governance approach employed by the organization. If the new system really provides something that nurses value, the word will eventually get out, even without advertising. Advertising may be employed to speed the communication process if desired.

Note, however, that marketing does not start with advertising. It starts with the identification of the need or desire and the filling of that need or desire. These elements must precede the advertising. Only then can a specific plan be developed regarding the communication of what strengths the organization has to offer. Advertising in newspapers, television, radio, or direct mail is one approach to that communication. Another is college visits. Bonuses to existing employees who bring in new employees is another.

Each of these approaches often results in inquiries by potential employees. The package of material that the organization develops to respond to those inquiries is a critical element of the overall marketing strategy. The marketing strategy should take into account all the steps in the recruiting process. Generating inquiries without a strategy to follow up effectively is one critical mistake often made by those who view marketing only in terms of advertising. If a strategy is likely to generate inquiries, the organization should not appear unorganized or uncaring when it receives them. That is the point when the organization has the chance to reaffirm the feeling that caused the nurse to inquire about the position.

Suppose a hospital runs a newspaper ad that says "Join the nursing staff at ABC Hospital, where nurses work in an environment of shared governance and shared commitment to the highest level of patient care." Some carefully planned literature must be available for the person who asks for more information about the shared governance program. Its history, how it works, and the hospital's commitment should be included.

If the response to the inquiry leads to an interview, the interviewer should be aware that the candidate has inquired about the hospital's shared governance program. The interview should include at least some specific discussion that emphasizes or highlights the shared governance system.

Marketing is a critical element of recruiting. That does not mean that the organization has to sell someone something that he or she doesn't want or need. Rather, having researched the wants and needs of a targeted nursing group, marketing should allow the hospital to effectively convey to the target group the extent to which the organization has made efforts to meet those desires and needs.

Although advertising is not the first part of a marketing plan, in many instances it is an effective mechanism for speeding the word-of-mouth process. Targeted advertising can reach a potential group of employees very effectively. This is particularly important in a competitive marketplace. If competing organizations are effectively communicating what they have to offer, your organization must be prepared to get its message to that group of potential employees as well.

One important element of advertising is that only a part of current advertising should be aimed at current recruitment. Another part, equally substantial, should be aimed at long-term image building. Often people associate with an organization because of its "well-known" reputation. Such reputations are built over a period of years. They are built through an effort of getting the message out year in and year out. When there is a staffing shortage the institution advertises why it is a good place to work. It should also do so when there is no shortage of personnel. Image building is not a short-term response to shortages. By laying the groundwork over a long period of time, when the need for personnel occurs, the organization will have a head start over its competition.

In budgeting for a marketing plan, it is necessary to include the costs of advertising. However, any other costs related to the overall marketing plan should also be included in the budget. These might include consulting costs and the costs of doing market research.

Determining the Cost

Recruitment and replacement of staff is inherently costly. The costs of replacing staff include:

+ Overtime and agency nurse costs while the position is vacant
+ Advertising
+ Interviewing potential employees
+ Travel for recruiters
+ Entertainment
+ Moving
+ Administrative processing
+ New employee training

Depending on the specific institution, these costs may be shared by the unit with the vacancy and the personnel department, or they may all be borne by the unit with the vacancy. For example, if ads are run to replace a staff member for one unit, the cost of the ad may be charged back directly to the unit with the vacancy. If ads are run to attract candidates for a number of different units, the cost may be divided and a share may be allocated among the various units. Alternatively, the price of advertisements may be borne solely by a department responsible for recruiting, such as the personnel or nurse recruitment departments. If units share the cost of advertising, then the operating budget should contain an estimate of the number of vacancies and the cost of advertisements for the year.

Other costs related to the replacement of personnel should also be budgeted. The average length of the vacancies should be anticipated, and the extra cost of overtime and agency nurses should be included in the coming year's operating budget. Newly hired employees are often less productive than experienced staff. This may require extra hours of nursing care per patient day, often in the form of overtime. An effort should be made to anticipate turnover and to anticipate the costs related to turnover. Sufficient nursing care hours should be budgeted to allow for the lower productivity of new staff. If relocation costs are charged directly to the unit, those costs should be included in the budget as well.

ALTERNATIVE MANPOWER

Despite the efforts of organizations to retain nurses, nurse retention will be unable to solve all health care organizations' nursing needs. Recruitment more often results in shifting the staff from one organization to another rather than increasing the overall supply. Thus, despite the best efforts to retain and recruit nurses, there will probably be at least some organizations with inadequate staffing. Decreasing the demand for nurses will decrease the need to both retain and recruit staff. One suggested approach to solving this shortage is the use of alternative manpower.

Alternative manpower comes in a variety of forms. One is foreign nurses. This approach attempts to retain the concept of using RNs to the extent possible. It comes to grips with the national nursing shortage by looking outside the United States. A very different approach is to use non-RNs to perform activities that in the past had been performed by RNs.

Foreign Nurse Recruitment

Foreign nurses are one possible alternative for staffing a health care institution. However, this solution involves a number of difficulties ranging from regulatory to language barriers. On the other hand, many foreign nurses welcome the chance to come to the United States on either a temporary or permanent basis, and this approach can be used to fill a large gap in the nursing staff.

Because of language problems, most foreign recruitment takes place in English-speaking countries such as Canada, the British Isles, and Australia. The Philippines and India are also common places for recruitment. Northern states may be able to recruit in Canada relatively easily, compared to other alternatives. For recruiting outside the continent, expenses of travel and relocation can become substantial. An alternative to an organization doing it all by itself is to use an agency and pay a flat fee for each nurse hired. The more nurses hired, the more likely it is to be cost effective to undertake the entire recruiting project yourself.

If a strategy of foreign recruiting is chosen, careful budgeting becomes essential. The choice between using a recruiting agency and doing it yourself can have a dramatic financial impact. A budget allows considering the costs of each alternative. For example, suppose that an agency charges one month's salary for recruiting an individual plus one month's salary for relocation expenses. It could easily cost $6,000 or $7,000 for each nurse recruited.

There are other recruiting costs as well. One cost of recruiting foreign nurses is the time between their arrival and the time when they have completed all examinations and other requirements necessary to practice as an RN. During this period they are being paid but are not fully productive. Other costs include providing convenient housing and helping the nurses settle in. Another cost is related to loss of recruits between their recruitment and their arrival. Since a fairly lengthy period is required to meet various visa and other requirements, there is a dropout rate.

Each state has its own laws concerning the licensing and practice of RNs. Additionally, there are federal limitations on how long a foreigner can work in this country. Immigrant status can allow the nurse to stay permanently, but it is much harder to obtain and can take substantially longer than a temporary visa.

Alternative Care Givers

A drastically different approach to the use of foreign nurses is the alteration of the pattern of care within a health care organization to assign more activities to non-RNs. While this is a movement away from the goal of all-RN staffs, it is based on recognition of the realities of the 1990s. There simply are not enough RNs to meet the goal of having all-RN staffs in most organizations.

There are many types of alternate care givers. These include, but are not limited to, the traditional alternate providers: LPNs, nurses' aides, and technicians. A variety of new positions such as hosts or hostesses are also being developed to help organizations cope. Such a person would introduce patients to the unit and respond to many of the nonclinical needs and questions of patients and their families. There is little controversy about the use of alternative care givers to perform nonnursing functions such as transport and clerical activities.

There is some controversy about using non-RN staff to perform nursing activities. In terms of clinical alternative care givers, many approaches are being tried at different health care organizations around the country. In some cases, the RN is placed in a position of greater direct supervision of other types of staff who provide more of the care. In other cases "partnerships" are developed between nursing and nonnursing staff members. In many cases the ultimate impact of the use of alternate care givers is less bedside time for the RN and more supervisory responsibility.

At the time of the writing of this book, no single approach had emerged as the dominant path for providing nursing care in the future. There is little information about the costs of these alternative models. The main conflict seems to be between a model that would have RNs serving as supervisors of non-RNs and a model in which nursing activities are divided into an RN subset and a non-RN subset. In the case of the former, RNs have a decreasing bedside role but greater authority and responsibility for patient care. In the latter alternative RNs may spend as much time in bedside care but perform only activities that require the clinical skills of an RN.

There is no question that the 1990s will see a great deal of experimentation in search of a model that works well. The result may be several different models, each of which works well and each of which attracts nurses with a preference for that approach. There is little question, however, that the organization of nursing services in the year 2000 will be substantially different from that observed at the start of this decade.

THE USE OF COMPUTERS

Changing how nursing care is provided because of a staff shortage is a less than ideal way for a profession to evolve. The changes are not the result primarily of an impetus to find better ways to give care. Rather they represent recognition of personnel availability constraints. If nursing shortages could be permanently eliminated, the approach to the delivery of nursing care might be substantially different. The computerization of nursing units has been put forth as a potential solution.

If computerization of patient documentation could live up to its billing, nursing shortages could be eliminated overnight. Some claims have been made that up to half of all nursing time is spent on documentation and that bedside computer terminals could save half that time. If true, that would mean that up to one-quarter of all required nursing time could be eliminated without taking away any time from nursing care provided to patients.

Although highly touted for their timesaving potential throughout the 1980s, computer systems have yet to live up to that glowing potential. The *hardware* (equipment) capacity exists. Technological advances have reached a point at which terminals by each bedside are quite feasible. In fact, it would be surprising to see a new hospital without computer wiring to each room as part of the electrical blueprints. Gaining nurse acceptance for the use of unit or bedside computers has not turned out to be the problem that many predicted. On the other hand, developing the *software* (computer programs) has been a complicated process.

Each health care institution tends to be unique in its procedures. This lack of industry standardization creates difficulties in the development of software. Furthermore, the process of recording the activities surrounding patient care and integrating patient care clinical and financial information with those activities is highly complicated.

Whether the claims of 25% savings in staff time will ever be realized is uncertain. It is likely, however, that computer software advances will be made and that computer usage by staff nurses will become commonplace in most health care organizations. In the long run this will likely increase the quality of patient care due to more accurate and timely information, while at the same time creating at least some efficiencies in the use of nursing time. This should allow more RN time to be available for patient care. To the extent that computers reduce time spent on documentation relative to time spent in providing patient care, computerization should work both to reduce nursing shortages and to increase nursing satisfaction.

IMPLICATIONS FOR NURSE MANAGERS

Recruitment and retention have been the topic of much research in the last few years. One example of a demonstration project in this area was the New

Jersey Nursing Incentives Reimbursement Awards program (NIRA).[5] NIRA was an $18 million state effort to improve retention and recruitment at thirty-seven hospitals. These hospitals implemented a variety of approaches including bedside computers, case management, shared governance, reorganization, and educational programs directed at management skills and team building. In some cases, although the purpose was improved recruitment and retention, the outcome was a decrease in the number of professional nurses needed to provide care. As we write this book, final results about the impact of these innovations on recruitment and retention are not available.

The authors of this book were members of the evaluation team for the NIRA study. In some hospitals the number of nurses recruited each quarter decreased after the NIRA initiative. Although the first impression may be to see that as a negative, it may not be. Recruitment may go down because retention has gone up and fewer new staff are needed. Recruitment may go down due to a reorganization in the way care is delivered, which incorporates less skilled workers to assist the nurse and requires fewer professional nurses.

In the NIRA study how little we really know about factors associated with recruitment and retention became apparent. In the New Jersey sample, nurses indicated that pay was the most important factor in determining their satisfaction with work. Our academic colleagues suggested that wasn't possible, since "it wasn't consistent with theory." It is, however, what nurses from New Jersey said. We anticipate that the literature on this subject will expand rapidly over the next ten years and urge the reader of this book to read it.

Retention and recruitment of staff will be ongoing issues for organizations that employ nurses. A certain amount of turnover is expected and is in fact healthy for an organization. Historically there have been national and local shortages of nurses. This cyclical pattern will likely continue. Organizations should be concerned with recruitment and retention regardless of shortages.

The issue of retention and recruitment of staff members—whether RNs, LPNs, aides, or other staff—is significant. There should be careful enumeration of all the costs related to recruitment and retention. These include market research, consulting, advertising, travel, and relocation. They also include the costs necessary to make an organization attractive, such as training costs related to implementing a system of shared governance.

One fundamental point in this process is that for a specific organization to have an adequate staff, it must recognize a need to change over time. The environment of health care organizations is in a constant state of change. Other career opportunities exist for potential staff. If a hospital job is not adequately attractive, a nurse can go into home health care or work in a physician's office. It is important to remain current in understanding what nurses desire from their employment in addition to a salary.

Successful organizations will be aware of the desires of the work force, respond to those desires, and effectively communicate to potential employees the ways in which they meet those needs and desires.

---

[5]James Knickman, Christine Kovner, Gerry Hendrikson, et al., *An Evaluation of the New Jersey Nursing Incentive Reimbursement Awards Program: Annual Report*, Health Research Program, New York University, New York, September 1991.

KEY CONCEPTS ❖

Retention Continued employment of personnel. This is often measured as the converse of turnover or staff leaving an organization.

Fringe benefits Compensation in addition to wages; also called employee benefits. This usually includes such things as health insurance, life insurance, and disability insurance. Some organizations provide child care, free parking, and other benefits as a way to recruit and retain staff. Fringe benefits often cost as much as 25% of a worker's wages.

Cafeteria plan Method of providing fringe benefits in which the employee chooses from a variety of options those fringe benefits which the employee wants.

Retention programs Variety of approaches used by organizations to retain staff. These include clinical ladders, reorganization of the way care is provided, and a variety of compensation plans.

Clinical ladders Approach to promotion and compensation based on clinical excellence.

Hawthorne effect Based on a study in which a number of changes were made in a factory to examine their impact on worker productivity. With each change, productivity improved. However, it turned out that the specific changes were not directly responsible for the improvement. Paying attention to the workers was responsible.

Recruitment Effort directed at getting potential employees to become employees. This process should be ongoing and not just developed in times of shortages of key workers.

Alternative manpower Use of manpower not traditionally used to provide care. This includes foreign nurses and workers who are less skilled than professional nurses but who may be able to assume some activities traditionally performed by RNs.

SUGGESTED READINGS ❖

Adams, Gregory A., "Computer Technology: Its Impact on Nursing Practice," *Nursing Administration Quarterly*, Vol. 10, No. 2, Winter 1986, pp. 21–33.

Aiken, Linda H., and Connie Flynt Mullinix, "The Nurse Shortage: Myth or Reality?" *The New England Journal of Medicine*, Vol. 317, No. 10, September 3, 1987, pp. 641–645.

Albarado, Rosalind S., Virginia McCall, and Judith M. Thrane, "Computerized Nursing Documentation," *Nursing Management*, Vol. 21, No. 7, July 1990, pp. 64–67.

Allen, David, Joy Calkin, and Marlys Peterson, "Making Shared Governance Work: A Conceptual Model," *Journal of Nursing Administration*, Vol. 18, No. 1, January 1988, pp. 37–44.

Ames, Adrienne, Sharon Adkins, Dana Rutledge, et al., "Assessing Work Retention Issues," *Journal of Nursing Administration*, Vol. 22, No. 4, April 1992, pp. 37–41.

Andersen, Sharon L., "The Nurse Advocate Project: A Strategy to Retain New Graduates," *Journal of Nursing Administration*, Vol. 19, No. 12, December 1989, pp. 22–26.

Barigar, Denise L., and Marian L. Sheafor, "Recruiting Staff Nurses: A Marketing Approach," *Nursing Management*, Vol. 21, No. 1, January 1990, pp. 27–29.

Benedict, M. Beth, Jay H. Glasser, and Eun Sul Lee, "Assessing Hospital Nursing Staff Retention and Turnover: A Life Table Approach," *Evaluation of the Health Professions*, Vol. 12, No. 1, March 1989, pp. 73–96.

Beyers, Marjorie, and Joseph Damore, "Nursing Shortage Requires Lasting Solution, Not a Quick Fix," *Health Progress*, Vol. 68, No. 4, May 1987, pp. 33 + .

Blaufuss, Judy, Jan Maynard, and Gail Schollars, "Methods of Evaluating Turnover Costs," *Nursing Management*, Vol. 23, No. 5, May 1992, pp. 52–61.

Bloom, Joan, Jeffrey Alexander, and Sylvia Flatt, "Organization Turnover Among Registered Nurses: An Exploratory Model," *Health Services Management Research*, Vol. 1, No. 3, November 1988, pp. 156–167.

Butler, Joan, and Robert J. Parsons, "Hospital Perceptions of Job Satisfaction," *Nursing Management*, Vol. 20, No. 8, August 1989, pp. 45–48.

Cahill, Cheryl A., and Mary H. Palmer, "Individual Professionalism: Part of the Solution to the Nursing Shortage Crisis," *Nursing Forum*, Vol. 24, No. 1, January 1989, pp. 27–31.

Corcoran, Nora M., Lesley A. Meyer, and Bonnie L. Magliaro, "Retention: The Key to the 21st Century for Health Care Institutions," *Nursing Administration Quarterly*, Vol. 14, No. 4, Summer 1990, pp. 23–31.

Curren, Connie R., Ann Minnick, and Joan Moss, "Who Needs Nurses?" *American Journal of Nursing*, Vol. 87, No. 4, April 1987, pp. 444–447.

Curry, James P., Douglas S. Wakefield, James L. Price, et al., "Determinants of Turnover Among Nursing Department Employees," *Research in Nursing and Health*, Vol. 8, No. 4, December 1985, pp. 397–411.

DeCrosta, Anthony A., "Meeting the Nurse Retention Challenge," *Nursing 89*, Vol. 19, No. 5, May 1989, pp. 170–171.

del Bueno, Dorothy J., "Warning: Retention May Be Dangerous to Your Organization's Health," *Nursing Economics*, Vol. 8, No. 4, July/August 1990, pp. 239–243.

Findling, Patricia, R. Edward Howell, and Cecelia Golightly, "Alternative Care Providers: Are They the Answer?" in *Managing the Nursing Shortage*, edited by Terence F. Moore and Earl A. Simendinger, Aspen Publishers, Rockville, MD, 1989, pp. 243–251.

Ford, Joan, "Computers and Nursing: Possibilities for Transforming Nursing," *Computers in Nursing*, Vol. 8, No. 4, July/August 1990, pp. 160–164.

Garre, Patricia Pierce, "A Computerized Recruitment Program," *Journal of Nursing Administration*, Vol. 20, No. 1, January 1990, pp. 24–27.

Gillies, Dee Ann, Martha Franklin, and David A. Child, "Relationship Between Organizational Climate and Job Satisfaction of Nursing Personnel," *Nursing Administration Quarterly*, Vol. 14, No. 4, Summer 1990, pp. 15–22.

Hancock, Walton M., Patricia L. Flynn, Sharon DeRosa, et al., "A Cost and Staffing Comparison of an All-RN Staff and Team Nursing," *Nursing Administration Quarterly*, Vol, 8, No. 2, Winter 1984, pp. 45–55.

Helmer, F. Theodore, and Patricia McKnight, "Management Strategies to Minimize Nursing Turnover," *Health Care Management Review*, Vol. 14, No. 1, 1989, pp. 73–80.

Hendrikson, Gerry, and Christine T. Kovner, "Effects of Computers on Nursing Resource Use: Do Computers Save Nurses Time?" *Computers in Nursing*, Vol. 8, No. 1, January/February 1990, pp. 16–22.

Hendrikson, Gerry, Theresa M. Doddato, and Christine T. Kovner, "How Do Nurses Use Their Time?" *Journal of Nursing Administration*, Vol. 20, No. 3, March 1990, pp. 31–37.

Herrick, Linda, Diane Newman, Julianne Hass, et al., "Job Satisfaction in the Head Nurse Role," *Nursing Management*, Vol. 23, No. 3, March 1992, pp. 27–29.

Hesterly, Sandra C., and Margaret Robinson, "Alternative Caregivers: Cost-Effective Utilization of RN's," *Nursing Administration Quarterly*, Vol. 14, No. 3, Spring 1990, pp. 18–23.

Hinshaw, Ada Sue, Carolyn Smeltzer, and Jan R. Atwood, "Innovative Retention Strategies for Nursing Staff," *Journal of Nursing Administration*, Vol. 17, No. 6, June 1987, pp. 8–16.

Hinshaw, Ada Sue, and Jan R. Atwood, "Nursing Staff Turnover, Stress, and Satisfaction: Models, Measures, and Management," *Annual Review of Nursing Research*, Vol. 1, 1983, pp. 133–153.

Hutto, Christine Bowers, and Linda Lindsey Davis, "12 Hour Shifts: A Panacea or Problems," *Nursing Management*, Vol. 20, No. 8, August 1989, pp. 56A, D, F, H.

Joel, Lucille, "Reshaping Nursing Practice," *American Journal of Nursing*, Vol. 87, No. 6, June 1987, pp. 793–795.

Jolma, Dena Jones, and Deborah E. Weller, "An Evaluation of Nurse Recruitment Methods," *Journal of Nursing Administration*, Vol. 19, No. 4, April 1989, pp. 20–24.

Jones, Cheryl Bland, "Staff Nurse Turnover Costs: Part I, A Conceptual Model," *Journal of Nursing Administration*, Vol. 20, No. 4, April 1990, pp. 18–23.

Jones, Cheryl Bland, "Staff Nurse Turnover Costs: Part II, Measurements and Results," *Journal of Nursing Administration*, Vol. 20, No. 5, May 1990, pp. 27–32.

Kersten, Joanne, and Jeanne Johnson, "Recruitment: What Are the New Grads Looking For?" *Nursing Management*, Vol. 23, No. 3, March 1992, pp. 44–48.

Kotler, Philip, *Marketing Management, Analysis, Planning and Control*, 3rd edition, Prentice-Hall, Englewood Cliffs, NJ, 1976.

Landstrom, Gay L., Diana Biordi, and Dee Ann Gillies, "The Emotional and Behavioral Process of Staff Nurse Turnover," *Journal of Nursing Administration*, Vol. 19, No. 9, September 1989, pp. 23–28.

Larson, Elaine, Pat Chikamoto, Marie Annette Brown, et al., "Job Satisfaction: Assumptions and Complexities," *Journal of Nursing Administration*, Vol. 14, No. 1, January 1984, pp. 31–38.

Loveridge, Catherine E., "Contingency Theory: Explaining Staff Nurse Retention," *Journal of Nursing Administration*, Vol. 18, No. 6, June 1988, pp. 22–25.

Mann, Everett E., and Kunkan J. Jefferson, "Retaining Staff: Using Turnover Indices and Surveys," *Journal of Nursing Administration*, Vol. 18, No. 7 and 8, July/August 1988, pp. 17–23.

Marquess, Roxanne, and Barbara Petit, "An Analysis of the Effect of Percent of RN Staff on Nursing Costs by DRG," *Nursing Management*, Vol. 18, No. 5, May 1987, pp. 33–36.

Marquis, Bessie, "Attrition: The Effectiveness of Retention Activities," *Journal of Nursing Administration*, Vol. 18, No. 3, March 1988, pp. 25–29.

Martin, Elaine G., Amy M. Harris, Robin Kimberly, et al., "Retention Strategies That Work," *Nursing Management*, Vol. 20, No. 6, June 1989, pp. 72I, L, M, P.

McClure, Margaret, Muriel A. Poulin, Margaret D. Sovie, et al., *Magnet Hospitals: Attraction and Retention of Professional Nurses*, ANA Publishing, Kansas City, KS, 1983.

Moore, Terence F., and Earl A. Simendinger, eds., *Managing the Nursing Shortage*, Aspen Publishers, Rockville, MD, 1989.

Morse, Gwen Goetz, "Resurgence of Nurse Assistants in Acute Care," *Nursing Management*, Vol. 21, No. 3, March 1990, pp. 34–36.

Mottaz, Clifford J., "Work Satisfaction Among Hospital Nurses," in *Health Services Management: Readings and Commentary*, Anthony R. Kovner and Duncan Neuhauser, eds., Health Administration Press, Ann Arbor, MI, 1990, pp. 298–315.

Mueller, Charles W., and Joanne Comi McCloskey, "Nurses; Job Satisfaction: A Proposed Measure," *Nursing Research*, Vol. 39, No. 2, March/April 1990, pp. 113–117.

Neathawk, Roger D., Susan E. Dubuque, and Carolyn A. Kronk, "Nurses' Evaluation of Recruitment and Retention," *Nursing Management*, Vol. 19, No. 12, December 1988, pp. 38–45.

Office of the Inspector General, "Hospital Best Practices in Nurse Recruitment and Retention," *Nursing Economics*, Vol. 7, No. 2, March/April 1989, pp. 98–106.

Pattan, John, "Developing a Nurse Recruitment Plan," *Journal of Nursing Administration*, Vol. 22, No. 1, January 1992, pp. 33–39.

Pooyan, Abdullah, Bruce J. Eberhardt, and Elvira Szigeti, "Work-related Variables and Turnover Intention among Registered Nurses," *Nursing and Health Care*, Vol. 11, No. 5, May 1990, pp. 255–258.

Porter, Rosemary T., Michael J. Porter, and Mary S. Lower, "Enhancing the Image of Nursing," *Journal of Nursing Administration*, Vol. 19, No. 2, February 1989, pp. 36–42.

Porter-O'Grady, Timothy, and Sharon Finnigan, *Shared Governance*, Aspen Publishers, Rockville, MD, 1984.

Powers, Patricia Harrison, and Carol A. Dickey, "Evaluation an RN/Co-Worker Model," *Journal of Nursing Administration*, Vol. 20, No. 3, March 1990, pp. 11–15.

Prescott, Patricia A., and Sally A. Bowen, "Controlling Nursing Turnover," *Nursing Management*, Vol. 18, No. 6, June 1987, pp. 60–66.

Prescott, Patricia, "Forecasting Requirements for Health Care Personnel," *Nursing Economics*, Vol. 9, No. 1, January-February 1991, pp. 18–24.

Sanford, Rhea, "Clinical Ladders: Do They Serve Their Purpose?" *Journal of Nursing Administration*, Vol. 17, No. 5, May 1987, pp. 34–37.

Sanger, Eldine, Jamie Richardson, and Elaine Larson, "What Satisfies Nurses Enough to Keep Them?" *Nursing Management*, Vol. 16, No. 9, September 1985, pp. 43–46.

Sheedy, Susan, "Responding to Patients: The Unit Hostess," *Journal of Nursing Administration*, Vol. 19, No. 4, April 1989, pp. 31–34.

Shockey, Barbara, "Foreign Nurse Recruitment and Authorization for Employment in the United States," in *Managing the Nursing Shortage*, Terence F. Moore and Earl A. Simendinger, eds., Aspen Publishers, Rockville, MD, 1989, pp. 252–263.

Sigmon, Paula, "Clinical Ladders and Primary Nursing: The Wedding of the Two," *Nursing Administration Quarterly*, Vol. 5, No. 3, Spring 1981, pp. 63–67.

Spitzer-Lehmann, Roxanne, "Recruitment and Retention of Our Greatest Asset," *Nursing Administration Quarterly*, Vol. 14, No. 4, Summer 1990, pp. 66–69.

Stewart-Dedmon, Mary, "Job Satisfaction of New Graduates," *Western Journal of Nursing Research*, Vol. 10, No. 1, February 1988, pp. 66–72.

Stillwaggon, Carol A., "Financial Management: The Impact of Nurse Managed Care on the Cost of Nurse Practice and Nurse Satisfaction," *Journal of Nursing Administration*, Vol. 19, No. 11, November 1989, pp. 21–23.

Stukalin, Terry, "Institutional Approach to Preventing Nurse Burnout," in *Managing the Nursing Shortage*, Terrence F. Moore and Earl A. Simendinger, eds., Aspen Publishers, Rockville, MD, 1989, pp. 33–49.

Taunton, Roma Lee, Sydney D. Krampitz, and Cynthia Q. Woods, "Manager Impact on Retention of Hospital Staff: Part 1," *Journal of Nursing Administration*, Vol. 19, No. 3, March 1989, pp. 14–19.

Taunton, Roma Lee, Sydney D. Krampitz, and Cynthia Q. Woods, "Manager Impact on Retention of Hospital Staff: Part 2," *Journal of Nursing Administration*, Vol. 19, No. 4, April 1989, pp. 15–19.

Taunton, Roma Lee, Sydney D. Krampitz, and Cynthia Q. Woods, "Absenteeism-Retention Links," *Journal of Nursing Administration*, Vol. 19, No. 6, June 1989, pp. 13–21.

Taylor, Betty Ann, and Patricia Salome, "Mt. Sinai's Four-Track Career Ladder Program," *Nursing Administrative Quarterly*, Vol. 9, No. 1, Fall 1984, pp. 73–81.

Tonges, Mary Crabtree, "Redesigning Hospital Nursing Practice: The Professionally Advanced Care Team (ProACT) Model, Part 1," *Journal of Nursing Administration*, Vol. 19, No. 8, July/August 1989, pp. 31–38.

Tonges, Mary Crabtree, "Redesigning Hospital Nursing Practice: The Professionally Advanced Care Team (ProACT) Model, Part 2," *Journal of Nursing Administration*, Vol. 19, No. 9, September 1989, pp. 19–22.

Wall, L. Louise, "Plan Development for a Nurse Recruitment-Retention Program," *Journal of Nursing Administration*, Vol. 18, No. 2, February 1988, pp. 20–27.

Warren, Margaret Townsend, "SUN Program: An Approach to the Health Care Personnel Shortage," *Nurse Educator*, Vol. 15, No. 4, July/August 1990, pp. 38–39.

Whaley, Barbara A., Wendy B. Young, Constance J. Adams, et al., "Targeting Recruitment Efforts for Increased Retention," *Journal of Nursing Administration*, Vol. 19, No. 4, April 1989, pp. 35–38.

Wolmering, Carolyn, "Incentive Programs: A Way to Cost Containment," *Nursing Management*, September 1987, pp. 49–51.

IV

PLANNING AND CONTROL

Planning and *control* are central elements to the success of any organization. Planning helps the organization know where it wants to go and develop a plan to get there. Control helps to ensure that the adopted plan is carried out.

A long-standing definition of planning is "an analytical process which involves an assessment of the future, the determination of desired objectives in the context of that future, the development of alternative courses of action to achieve such objectives and the selection of a course (or courses) of action from among those alternatives."[1] Control has been defined as a "process that involves measurement and evaluation of the performance of organizational units, the identification of deviations from planned performance, the initiation of appropriate responses to these deviations, and the monitoring of remedial actions, all done with the intent of ensuring that managers' decisions and actions are consistent with planned organizational objectives."[2] Planning and control together have developed into a strategic management process for the organization, operational budgeting, and control of the activities of an organization, department, or unit.

Strategic management is an emerging field that is an outgrowth of the *long-range planning* of the 1950s. However, it goes beyond long-range planning, integrating strategic thought throughout the management process. Organizational success largely depends on the care with which the organization acts strategically. Knowing its strengths and weaknesses and being aware of its opportunities and threats are the critical elements upon which the field of strategic management has developed.

Strategic management is discussed in Chapter 10. How are strategic plans defined? Why are they prepared? What benefits can the organization hope to achieve from strategic management? The chapter also discusses

---

[1]Brian Scott, "Some Aspects of Long-range Planning in American Corporations with Special Attention to Strategic Planning," Ph.D. dissertation, Harvard University, 1963, p. 8.
[2]John Camillus, *Strategic Planning and Management Control*, Lexington Books, Lexington, MA, 1986, p. 11.

some specific elements of strategic management, namely, long-range plans, program budgets, and business plans.

The budgeting aspect of planning is explored in the middle two chapters of this part of the book. Chapter 11 provides an overview of the various types of organizational budgets and of the budget process. Chapter 12 provides greater depth on the preparation of the operating budget.

Plans are of only limited usefulness unless actions are taken to ensure that the plans are followed to the extent possible. Chapter 13 discusses the issue of control. That discussion includes the provision of specific tools of variance analysis, which are used to help managers to discover variations from the original plan and to keep outcomes as close to the plan as possible. ❖

CHAPTER

10

Strategic Management

CHAPTER GOALS

The goals of this chapter are to:

♦ Define strategic management, its importance to health care organizations, and the benefits of the strategic planning process

♦ Describe the evolution of strategic management from long-range planning to strategic planning to strategic management

♦ Distinguish between broad, long-term goals and time-oriented, specific, measurable objectives

♦ Introduce the concepts of total quality management and continuous quality improvement

♦ Discuss each element of a strategic plan, including a mission statement or nursing philosophy, a statement of long-term goals, a statement of competitive strategy, a statement of organizational policies, a statement of needed resources, and a statement of key assumptions

♦ Stress the importance of strategic thought by all managers in carrying out all elements of their managerial responsibilities

♦ Explain the role of the long-range budget and strategic plan in the planning process

♦ Define program budgeting and discuss the zero-base budgeting technique, stressing the importance of examining alternatives

♦ Outline the elements of a business plan

♦ Introduce the concept of pro forma financial statements

❖

INTRODUCTION

Strategic management is the process of setting the *goals* and *objectives* of the organization, determining the resources to be allocated to achieving those goals and objectives, and establishing policies concerning getting and using those resources.[3] This process includes an environmental assessment and depends heavily on data concerning the organization's external environment. The strategic management process is critical to the organization's success. Managers and their staffs must not only do the things they do well but also carefully decide what must be done.

One planning text quotes Henry Thoreau: "It is not enough to be busy— the question is, what are we busy about?"[4] This simple question should cause nurse managers to pause and consider their role in the management process. Day-to-day routine activities often cause nurse managers to become overloaded. Managers become so busy that they have little time to plan for the future or to introduce innovations. It is important for all managers to structure their jobs so that planning does not become pushed aside by the pressing day-in and day-out issues.

Planning theory indicates that the higher a manager is in the organization's chain of command, the greater the portion of time that should be spent on planning. That planning should not simply be a rote repetitive process each year. It should focus on change. It should focus on improvement. For CEOs it has been suggested that at least two-thirds of their time be spent on planning and one-third or less on day-to-day operations.[5] Chief nurse executives should probably spend between half and two-thirds of their time on planning and innovation. The proportion of time spent on planning decreases as one continues to move down through the ranks of nursing management, but it should never become an insignificant amount.

Strategy applied in managing organizations is still a developing field. In the middle of the twentieth century, businesses began to place a growing reliance on *long-range planning*. Long-range plans focus on general objectives to be achieved by the organization over a period of typically three to five years. By the 1960s the term *strategy* became commonplace, and long-range planning started being referred to as *strategic planning*. It was contrasted with operational planning—the development of a detailed plan for the coming year.

When strategic planning was introduced, the concept of strategy was that operational planning is tactical, whereas long-range planning is strategic. Under strategic or long-range planning an organization prepares a set of goals, then a strategy is developed for accomplishing them. That strategy is formalized into a plan of action generally covering a horizon of three to five years.

In the late 1980s and early 1990s experts in the area started to use the more generic term *strategic management* to better define the role of strategic thought in organizations.[6] Such experts argue for a broad view of strategic planning. The primary focus remains the identification of broad, long-term goals and the creation of plans to achieve them. However, the current view of strategic management or strategic planning relies on the use of strategic thought in guiding

---

[3]John C. Camillus, *Strategic Planning and Management Control*, Lexington Books, Lexington, MA, 1986, p. 18.

[4]Darryl J. Ellis and Peter P. Pekar, Jr., *Planning for Nonplanners*, Amacom, New York, 1980, p. 24.

[5]Ibid. p. 25.

[6]Jack Koteen, *Strategic Management in Public and Nonprofit Organizations*, Praeger, New York, 1989, pp. 19–21.

all plans and actions in an organization. This relates to short-term operational plans as well as long-range plans.

Strategic planning is no longer simply long-range planning with a new name, as it was in the 1960s, 1970s, and into the 1980s. Strategic management "stresses three points: that the strategic planner is clearly the advisor and facilitator to line management decision-makers; that the program executive, not the strategic planner, is the key strategist; and that strategic planning is always integrated with other functions of the program management process—program design, organizing, budgeting, staffing, controlling, and evaluating."[7] Long-range planning is still a part of strategic planning, but it is no longer the only feature.

The current philosophy is that thinking strategically should not be the sole domain of the strategic planners of the organization. Planning by planners is important but insufficient. Strategic thought should be an element of the job description of all managers throughout the organization. Nurse managers have a central role in strategic planning in this new philosophical approach. The way a nursing unit is organized to provide care, the way it establishes patterns of staff to provide care, and the financial budgets it develops to gain authorization of needed resources to provide care should all be outcomes of a strategic process managed at the unit level. The principal change from earlier views of strategic planning is the emphasis on bringing all managers into the direct process of working to achieve the organization's primary goals instead of focusing narrowly on specific short-term objectives.

This chapter first discusses the definition, aims, and benefits of strategic planning and strategic thought. It then focuses on several specific aspects of strategic management, namely, long-range plans, program budgets, and business plans.

TOTAL QUALITY MANAGEMENT

A theme for the provision of health services in the 1990s has become total quality management (TQM) and continuous quality improvement (CQI). These represent philosophies concerning the production of an organization's goods and services. Arikian notes that "TQM emphasizes a preventive approach to management, one that addresses problems before they arise, and handles concerns with a studied, long-term commitment to continuous improvement in product and service."[8] From a strategic management perspective, production in America has been dominated by an attitude of getting it done and then fixing it if it is wrong. Observations of the Japanese production process, however, have taught us that if more time is spent on planning, less will be done wrong and less will have to be fixed.

Many American corporations learned this lesson throughout the 1980s as they lost some of their competitive edge. To regain that edge corporations have adopted procedures that focus on avoiding the costs associated with poor quality. Examples of the change in attitude are apparent in the slogans adopted

---

[7]Ibid. p. 21.
[8]Veronica Arikian, "Total Quality Management: Applications to Nursing Service," *Journal of Nursing Administration*, Vol. 21, No. 6, June 1991, p. 46.

by corporations. For example, Ethicon, a manufacturer of sutures, adopted the policy, "Get it right the first time, every time."

Quality costs money. However, so does lack of quality. TQM focuses on the issue of being responsive to the needs of customers, while at the same time reducing waste. Kirk notes in examinations of Japanese firms: "The most significant discovery related to their determination to *build quality into the product (or service)* rather than to inspect for errors and assume that error removal would lead to quality. Many Japanese managers bought into the concept of planning and followed through on it—unlike many American managers who avoid this concept like the plague, in preference to the ready-fire-aim approach. 'We don't have time to plan,' some American managers say. Contrarily, many Japanese businessmen say 'We don't have time *not* to plan.' "[9]

Various authors have identified different elements of TQM and CQI. Deming, the pathbreaker in the field, established fourteen points related to TQM.[10] These include such factors as a focus on education and training of employees, viewing employees not only as providers but also as customers, quality insurance, and a constant focus on finding ways to continuously improve quality.

TQM and CQI are not financial management tools per se. We will not go into a detailed analysis of the methods here.[11] However, TQM and CQI have tremendous financial implications. Historically, health care organizations have minimized planning and maximized control over day-to-day operations. The lesson of TQM and CQI is that managers will be more likely to achieve their objectives if they can redesign their work to allow much more time for planning and innovating. Such activities are not occasional but rather should be viewed as a major element of the management function. We must learn to focus on improving the service we provide rather than simply making sure we get it provided. In the long run increased focus on improvement of quality may well lead to more satisfied staff and patients, higher quality of care, and lower costs.

STRATEGIC PLANNING

As noted earlier, strategic management calls for setting objectives, allocating resources, and establishing policies concerning those resources. Under this strategic planning approach, all managers become involved in this process.

To establish and achieve goals, strategic planners have found it useful for the managers of an organization to focus on a series of key questions. The following questions are the most essential an organization must consider:

♦ Why does the organization exist?
♦ What is the organization currently?
♦ What would it like to be?
♦ How can we make the transformation to what it wants to be?
♦ How will it know when it is done?

[9]Roey Kirk, "The Big Picture: Total Quality Management and Continuous Quality Improvement," *Journal of Nursing Administration*, Vol. 22, No. 4, April 1992, p. 24.
[10]T. Gillem, "Deming's 14 Points and Hospital Quality: Responding to the Consumer's Demand for the Best Value in Health Care," *Nursing Quality Assurance*, Vol. 2, No. 3, 1988, p. 70.
[11]The interested reader is referred to the readings on the topic listed at the end of this chapter.

These questions in turn lead to a large number of other questions. What are the organization's strengths? Its weaknesses? Its opportunities? Its threats? Who are the organization's primary customers? Are they being well served? Does the organization learn from its mistakes? Does the organization have a vision for the future? These questions are related to the organization as a whole, but they also relate to each department and unit within the organization.

Managers need to step aside from the current day-to-day activities and assess the nature of the existing organization. Has the organization over the years lost track of its reason for existence? Is the current status of the organization the desired one? If not, then the organization needs to formally address the issue of how it can change things to become the type of organization it believes it should be. Again, this is true for departments and units as well as for entire organizations.

Strategic planning asserts that the way to become the type of organization you want to be is to establish a set of clear goals and objectives and then a plan for achieving them. Goals are defined as the broad aims of the organization, while objectives are specific targets to be achieved to attain those goals.[12]

Once goals and objectives are identified, then specific tactics can be designed to move the organization toward those goals. Tactical plans require resources. Often in the segregation of strategic planning as the long-range plan vs. operational planning for the short run, operating resource allocations fail to match the allocation needed to reach strategic goals. That is one reason that strategic management now takes a more global perspective.

In developing a short-term operating budget for the coming year, the unit manager must decide whether to place more emphasis on short-run profits or long-term growth. Spending extra money on quality improvements now will generate expenses not offset by revenues. But the reputation for quality will generate more revenues in the future. The dichotomizing of strategic plans and operating budgets forces managers with responsibility for operating expenses to focus on reducing short-run expenses. That tends to be exactly counter to the long-run strategic goals of the organization as designed by preparers of the strategic plan. Therefore managers must balance the short-term objectives of their units or departments with a long-range vision for the organization.

It is not clear if any organization will ever get where it wants to be. The target goals tend to be modified over time in reaction to changes both inside and outside the organization. However, to make progress toward the goals, the organization should constantly be attempting to answer the various questions stated earlier and to take necessary actions based on the answers to the questions.

The Elements of a Strategic Plan

Strategic plans must be adapted to specific situations. The elements of a plan for one organization may not be perfectly suited to another. Flexibility is

---

[12]The planning literature is inconsistent in the definition of goals and objectives. In some instances the definition used here for goals is assigned to objectives, and vice versa.

a positive attribute in the strategic planning process. For most organizations, however, the basic elements of a strategic plan would include:

♦ Mission statement or philosophy
♦ Statement of long-term goals
♦ Statement of competitive strategy
♦ Statement of organizational policies
♦ Statement of needed resources
♦ Statement of key assumptions

The Mission Statement or Philosophy

The first step in strategic management is the development of a *mission statement* for the organization, department, or unit. What is the purpose of the organization or unit? An organization cannot begin to plan goals effectively and allocate resources sensibly until it first clearly determines its reason for existence. Strategic planners refer to an organization-wide statement of purpose or focus as the mission statement. In the department of nursing this is often referred to as the philosophical statement.

A great deal of care should be taken in developing a mission statement. The mission statement of the organization should focus the organization by defining what it does. Some health care organizations set their mission statement either too broadly or too narrowly. At one extreme they wind up running restaurants or other nonhealth facilities that sap time and energy and often fail because the organization lacks expertise in that area. At the other extreme, growth and change are not encouraged by the statement, and the organization stagnates.

Some degree of limitation in the mission statement is beneficial, forcing the organization to concentrate on what it knows how to do. At the same time, the mission statement should allow growth and diversification. The mission statement should be defined in such a way as to prevent the organization from exceeding its manageable boundaries, but encouraging exploration within those boundaries. Camillus notes that a

> health care organization engaged in providing eye-care services can describe itself as fulfilling the mission of examining eyes and writing prescriptions for corrective lenses or the mission of protecting and improving human vision. The first statement is essentially a description of activities in which the organization is engaged. The second statement, in contrast, identifies consequences rather than activities and thus leads to the identification of such possibilities as opening clinics where eye surgery is carried out, engaging in the development and possibly the manufacture of devices for rectifying faulty vision, and running programs for educating the public about the proper care of eyes.[13]

The key to designing the mission statement is to focus not on what the organization does right now as much as think about the range of possible types of activities one would see as a logical extension for the organization over time. Several examples of mission statements are shown in Exhibits 10–1 to 10–4.

Statement of Long-term Goals

Goal setting is the organization's attempt to set the direction for itself as it tries to meet its mission. Often an organization will have both quantitative and

---

[13]John Camillus, *op. cit.*, p. 47.

❖ **EXHIBIT 10–1**
Examples of Simplified Mission Statements

Hospital
Narrowly defined mission To provide short-term acute hospital care to the community in the area immediately surrounding the hospital.
Broadly defined mission To improve the health of members of the community.
Overly broadly defined mission To provide health care and other services and products to all potential patients and customers.

Hospital Nursing Department
Narrowly defined mission To deliver high-quality care to the hospital's patients.
Broadly defined mission To deliver high-quality nursing care at a reasonable cost to the citizens of this community.
Overly broadly defined mission To promote the well-being of the organization by undertaking such activities as might be in the organization's interests.

---

qualitative goals. Quantitative goals may relate to financial outcomes, such as rates of growth in the number of patients served and in revenues. Qualitative goals may relate to patient satisfaction and general reputation.

In developing the long-term goals of the organization, their timeless nature should be kept in mind. Objectives are intended to be attained within a specific time frame. Goals tend to stay in force over long periods. Providing the needs of an increasing percentage of the community's citizens is a long-term goal. Increasing the number of patients by 8% in the coming year is a specific measurable objective.

While statements of objectives are necessary, the statement of goals is of greater concern in strategic management. As managers attempt to respond in their operations to specific, time-oriented objectives, they should bear in mind the overriding goals that the organization wants to achieve. Innovations that allow the organization to make major steps forward toward achieving its long-run goals should constantly be sought by all managers.

❖ **EXHIBIT 10–2**
Actual Mission Statement of Beth Israel Medical Center

MISSION
Since its founding, over 100 years ago as a medical dispensary to serve the Jewish community of the Lower East Side, Beth Israel Medical Center has been committed to serving and caring for the health and well-being of persons of all races, religions and creeds. Now a major health care provider of specialized, tertiary services, the Medical Center remains proud of its heritage and reaffirms the original mission of Beth Israel Hospital: to provide the highest quality patient care, with compassion and with concern for patient well-being.

To this end, we pledge all our available resources. We will continue to maintain the highest standards of professionalism and dedication. Through our training of physicians, nurses and other health care professionals, as well as our clinical and research programs, we remain committed to attracting and retaining outstanding staff at all levels. We will also continue to seek innovative and cost effective ways to deliver the finest and highest quality of health care services possible.

Reprinted with the Permission of Beth Israel Medical Center, New York, New York.

❖ EXHIBIT 10–3
Actual Mission Statement of Lutheran Medical Center

LUTHERAN MEDICAL CENTER
Board of Trustees
Statement of Mission
Adopted October 24, 1990

Preface
Lutheran Medical Center, founded in 1883 by a Norwegian Lutheran Deaconess-nurse, Sister Elisabeth Fedde, gratefully affirms both its Christian heritage exemplified by her Christ-like compassion and dedicated care for struggling new immigrants and its contemporary call to enhance the health and well being of its neighbors throughout a diverse urban area. For 80 years Lutheran Medical Center grew and declined with other neighborhood institutions as a function of an economy based on the Brooklyn waterfront. In recent decades, however, Lutheran Medical Center aggressively volunteered to be the corporate stimulus for community renewal, the catalyst for constructive change, and the advocate for the health and well being of an entire urban area.

Principles and Point of View
Lutheran Medical Center has no reason for being of its own; it exists only to serve the needs of its neighbors.
Lutheran Medical Center defines health as the total well being of the community and its residents. Beyond the absence of individual physical illness, this includes, at least, decent housing, the ability to speak English, employment and educational opportunities, and civic participation.
Lutheran Medical Center understands a hospital not as a collection of buildings, machines and beds, but a staff of talented, creative and committed people who serve the community as they are needed.
Lutheran Medical Center works in partnership with its neighbors, each relying on the other as friends who care about and assist each other.

Program
Guided by these principles, Lutheran Medical Center serves the communities of Bay Ridge, Sunset Park and Park Slope and adjacent areas of southwest Brooklyn. As an acute general community hospital Lutheran Medical Center endeavors to bring the benefits of scientific research and academic medicine to the people of southwest Brooklyn. Through its Family Health Center, Lutheran Medical Center operates an extensive ambulatory care network to provide primary care for the ethnically and economically diverse population of southwest Brooklyn. Lutheran Medical Center also provides home care and other innovative programs for the frail and elderly as well as other educational and human services in response to specific current needs within the community. In addition to its total reimbursement income Lutheran Medical Center devotes other financial resources and seeks major grants to sustain its comprehensive spectrum of health and human services.
Motivated to serve by its own history within the biblical tradition of faith and teaching, and organized as a not-for-profit organization according to the uniquely American heritage of democratic voluntary associations, Lutheran Medical Center's purpose is to serve as the corporate vehicle for its trustees, medical and dental staff, nurses, employees, volunteers and others to care for the needs of our neighbors.

❖ **EXHIBIT 10–4**
Actual Mission Statement for Family Home Care Services

MISSION
The mission of *Family Home Care* is to be an excellent provider of home care services to clients with a commitment to improving their quality of life.
Family Home Care will enable clients to be cared for safely and with dignity;
Family Home Care will respond to changing health care needs;
Family Home Care will provide an atmosphere of mutual respect and growth for every employee; and
Family Home Care will ensure long-term financial viability for the Agency in order to continue to provide quality services in the future.

Reprinted with permission of Family Home Care Services, Brooklyn, New York.

Statement of Competitive Strategy

The organization's competitive strategy is its plan for achieving its goals, specifically, what services will be provided and to whom. The development of this strategy relies to a great extent on a thorough internal and external review. What are the organization's strengths and weaknesses, its opportunities and threats?

Competitive strategy is the planning of what care will be provided and to whom. To develop such a plan the organization must consider what competitors are or are not doing and what expertise the organization does or does not possess. Based on that information the organization can decide where it should expand and perhaps where it should contract.

Essentially the organization must evaluate its mission and goals in light of its particular strengths and weaknesses and in light of the demand for services and competition in the external environment. Based on that evaluation it can make a plan that will take advantage of opportunities that present themselves and plan a reaction to the threats that exist.

Statement of Organizational Policies

The role of policies is to specify what are and are not acceptable practices by the organization. The establishment of a mission and objectives incorporates a set of values. It integrates the values of the organization's founders, the values of its management and staff, and the values of the community. Those values should be incorporated in the decisions made by the organization.

In most organizations no single person can review each and every decision and decide if it is appropriate. A set of policies that clearly indicates what actions are appropriate and what actions are not removes an unreasonable burden from managers throughout the organization. It removes the necessity for guesswork by individual managers in many specific situations.

Policy statements are substantially different from mission statements, statements of goals, and statements of competitive strategy. In each of those earlier statements there is a need to encourage creativity. Each one leaves room for the organization to innovate or grow. In contrast, policy statements are generally limiting. They provide the constraints that the organization wants to place on managerial discretion.

Surprisingly, such constraints can ultimately enhance organizational growth. Without specific policies, managers may find that they are chastised for specific actions without any rhyme or reason. They become uncertain as to when it is okay to take initiative and make changes and when higher levels of management want things done just the way they always have been done. This high degree of uncertainty will lead managers over time to become reluctant to innovate in any respect. The availability of specific procedures clearly delineates where innovation is not allowed. However, that also provides the manager a sense of where innovation is allowed and welcomed.

Statement of Needed Resources

Strategic planning cannot be held apart from the reality of the resources needed to carry out the plan. These include resources in terms of personnel, the facilities for the personnel to work in and with, and the other requirements for accomplishing the goals of the organization. Without linkage between the plan and the resources to carry it out, there can be little hope of achieving the organization's goals.

Statement of Key Assumptions

Part of the planning process is development of a statement of key assumptions. Since strategic management calls for a decentralization of the planning process, there must be a set of guidelines that all managers use in common. If management expects new competitors, that will affect the entire organization. The same assumption about such new competition should be used consistently by all managers. This will make plans consistent and will also improve coordination of plans throughout the organization. It will also help in determining whether variations from the plan are due to carrying out the plan or the accuracy of the underlying assumptions.

Benefits of the Strategic Planning Process

One can think of a number of benefits that result from having a strategic planning system. One of the most predominant benefits is that it forces the organization to determine its long-run goals and come up with an approach to accomplish them. Establishing long-run goals forces managers to decide what the organization's purpose is and to formalize that purpose. Many health care organizations were established long before any of the current employees worked for the organization. The original goals of the organization can easily become lost among the personal needs and desires of the current management and staff. The process of establishing a formalized mission and goals gives a sense of direction to the organization.

A strategic planning system also promotes efficiency. Managers working toward clear goals are less likely to be inefficient. When everyone clearly knows what the organization is trying to achieve, there is a likelihood that less effort will be spent on unnecessary activities.

The strategic planning process provides a means of communication among the various hierarchical levels of the organization. In large organizations (and sometimes even in relatively small ones) communication between organizational levels becomes difficult. The managers on the lower rungs may know that things are not being done efficiently. The managers at the upper rungs may believe that the systems they have in place do generate efficiency. Inadequate channels exist for moving information up or down through the ranks. Innovation in such cases is expected to be dictated from the higher levels of the organization. In fact, often the need for and opportunities for improvements are most visible at the lower levels. A strategic management process should allow new ideas to flow smoothly down or up.

Lower-level managers will learn more about why changes are taking place if they share the strategic plan and can see how changes relate to achieving the plan's goals. Higher-level managers will receive better information if lower-level managers focus some of their attention on factors that affect the organization's long-run goals.

The strategic planning process develops management skills at levels throughout the organization. Management skills are developed primarily by giving managers the opportunity to make decisions and to handle things that are not part of the routine. Out-of-the-ordinary activity requires skilled management even more than repetitive tasks. By working at the planning process managers develop some skills needed to deal with change and with unusual events.

The strategic planning process provides managers with an improved sense of the needs of the organization and of its environmental constraints. It has often been found that a partnership approach to management works better than a dictatorial approach. Managers who are told that they must live within constraints resist them. Managers who are asked to become part of the team to solve the problem of constraints learn to understand the difficulty in the constraints and are more willing to work cooperatively instead of adversarially.

The strategic planning process increases the level of organizational creativity in addressing problems. Successful organizations encourage rather than resist change. Things are done very differently now than they were twenty years ago. Change, however, doesn't occur at some arbitrary point every twenty years. It occurs gradually in an evolutionary process. The fact that most organizations do things a certain way now that they didn't do twenty years ago indicates that someone tried a new approach and found it superior. Who is that someone? Is it the lucky one who accidentally fell upon an improved approach?

Generally, this is one area where organizations make their own luck. Creativity cannot be forced upon people. One cannot tell employees to be creative and to develop innovative improvements. However, creativity can be either fostered or stifled. A strong commitment to strategic management throughout the organization will convey the organization's view of creativity as a positive rather than a negative element.

One can summarize strategic management as the process that adds creative vision to all the other processes of the organization. Strasen defines vision as "the ability to set goals that are not limited to what is presently inevitable. In order to be meaningful, goals must stretch the imagination and efforts of the individual or organization setting them. If goals are inevitable occurrences in the future, they are set too low and are no real measure of progress or accomplishment."[14] Once the vision of the future is in place and is clearly communicated, the organization's managers will creatively work on changes that can bring that vision to fruition.

---

[14]Leann Strasen, *Key Business Skills for Nurses*, J. B. Lippincott, Philadelphia, 1987, p. 208.

Implementing a Strategic Management Process

This chapter has alternatively referred to the strategic plan and to the strategic planning or management process.

The specific development of a strategic plan will be discussed in the next section of this chapter. However, strategic management relies not just on a plan but on a broad planning process. That process is one of making managers aware of the need to think strategically as they carry out all their management activities. In developing the long-range plan, managers must relate the plan to the mission. In designing specific program budgets or business plans, the manager must consider how the program will help the organization achieve its goals. In developing the specific details of the operating budget, again the manager should be trying to link the details with how they help the organization reach its long-term aims.

The remainder of this chapter focuses on several of the long-range elements of strategic planning. Specifically, long-range planning, program budgets, and business plans are addressed. As the reader proceeds to the remaining three chapters in Part IV of this book, the notion of trying to link operational activities with strategic thought should be kept in mind.

LONG-RANGE PLANNING

In developing the long-range budget the organization begins the process of translating its general goals and objectives into a specific action plan. Long-range budgets or long-range plans are often referred to as the organization's strategic plan. Such plans generally cover a period of three to five years.

Given a strategic management process that calls upon managers to focus on the organization's goals, is a strategic plan essential? The answer is clearly yes. Long-range planning is critical to the vitality of an organization. For organizations to thrive, they must move forward rather than being stagnant. The staff of an organization should be able to look back and see the progress that has been made over an extended period. Budgeting for one year at a time does not allow for the major types of changes that would take years to plan and implement. Yet that lengthy process is needed for the efforts that will substantially move the organization forward.

For example, suppose that one goal of the organization is to move from being a primary care community hospital to a regional tertiary care center. This cannot be accomplished by having each department attempt to modify its operating budget. An overall organizational plan is needed. Which of the new tertiary services can or should be added in the next five years? Which programs already exist but need to be expanded in the next five years to accommodate the changing role of the organization? These questions are specifically addressed in the strategic plan or long-range budget.

Nursing should be involved in this planning process. The success of the plan will depend on how well it is carried out. If the plan does not have adequate nursing input when it is prepared, it is unlikely that the nursing staff will fully support it. Nurses must push their organizations to incorporate nursing leadership into the planning process not only for the good of nurses and nursing but also for the ultimate success of the organization.

The strategic plan may lay the groundwork for a fund-raising campaign to precede and parallel expansion of services. Or the plan may indicate that each year for five years growth in specified existing profitable areas must be undertaken to offset the start-up losses on the introduction of major new programs. Specific dollar amounts of additional revenue and new program cost may be projected only in terms of an extremely rough estimate. Although quite general, such a plan does give the organization enough specific information about the implications and requirements for the expansion into a tertiary care center to allow for the development of specific programs to move the organization toward that ultimate goal.

The strategic plan may be somewhat more detailed, showing projections of the dollar amounts expected to be available (and their sources) as well as which specific programs will be adopted and what their approximate costs will be. Since a strategic or long-range plan projects at least three, and up to ten, years into the future, it is unlikely that revenue and cost estimates will be highly accurate. Therefore while rough estimates are often included in such plans, they are generally not overly detailed or refined.

The plan should not focus only on major program additions. The services and programs that already exist are equally important to an organization. Expanding a service, contracting one, or even deleting a program or service requires the same consideration and planning as the addition of a program or service. A part of the planning process should be to explicitly address whether those services and programs which make up the majority of operations of the organization are being retained at a steady-state level or whether they are to be contracted or expanded in scope.

One serious potential problem arises if this issue is ignored in preparing strategic plans. If existing programs are implicitly assumed to continue unchanged, a plan that includes a number of new programs may appear feasible. However, it may not be feasible when technological and other changing factors are explicitly considered for the ongoing operations of the organization. Therefore, expectations regarding existing programs should be explicitly reviewed and included as part of the plan.

Once the plan has been finalized and formalized, it serves as a guide for a number of years. Long-range plans are typically prepared only once every three or five years. Creating a new plan each year would only lead to constant changes in the organization's direction. This would lead to wasted efforts and frustrated managers. However, such plans should be reviewed each year. Assumptions may turn out to be wrong. A cure for AIDS could change patient volume. The external environment can change dramatically. An influx of refugees could change the demand for services. Annual reviews allow the organization to adjust the strategic plan to react to current events.

Each year elements of the plan are brought into the current activities of the organization. To make the transition from the plan into operations, many proposed additions or changes require a thorough evaluation. This may be accomplished through the development of a program budget.

PROGRAM BUDGETING AND ZBB

Program budgeting is the part of the overall strategic planning process that focuses on all the costs and benefits associated with a specific program. The program may be an existing one that the organization is considering expanding, contracting, or eliminating, or it may be a new program that the organization is thinking of adding. Program budgeting examines alternative programs to meet the organization's objectives and examines feasible alternative ways to accomplish each given program.

Some program budgeting is done within a nursing unit or department. Often, however, the program changes generated by a strategic plan have interdepartmental impacts. Such program changes are much more complicated because of the need for coordination between departments. It is vital that nursing participate fully in such interdepartmental planning. Working on key committees is essential not only to protect the interests of nursing but also, as noted earlier, to ensure that any plans developed make sense from a nursing perspective and can be supported by the nursing staff.

In most cases program budgets relate directly to the strategic planning of the organization. The projects being evaluated are under consideration because they relate directly to moving the organization toward the achievement of its long-term goals.

Program budgets are substantially different from other types of budgets. Long-range budgets or strategic plans look in general terms at the entire organization over a period of years. Their information is based on rough approximations rather than being highly detailed. Operating and cash budgets look in great detail, but only at the coming year. A program budget combines a great amount of detailed information for a long period for one specific program. Further, while most budgets focus on a given department's revenues and costs, program budgets compare revenues and expenses for an entire program, cutting across departments or cost centers.

A program budget compares all its costs and benefits to evaluate the entire program's effect on the organization over its lifetime. In doing this the program budgeting methods identify costs and benefits of different programs aimed at the same purpose or of different approaches to one program. Because resources are not unlimited, program budgeting often focuses on trade-offs. That is, program budgeting considers the extra benefit to be gained by spending additional money on a program. Alternatively, program budgeting considers how much of the benefit of a program would be lost if less money were spent on the program.

Zero-base Budgeting (ZBB)

Zero-base budgeting is a popular program budgeting technique that gained fame for its strong push toward analysis of all costs. All costs from a base of zero must be justified. Until the introduction of ZBB, it was common for budget negotiations to revolve around the appropriate amount of the increase in a budget. How much more should be spent next year than was spent in the current year? Implicitly, such an approach assumes that all current-year spending continues to be reasonable and justified for the next year. Only the amount of the increment is subject to examination and discussion.

In reality, as technology and diseases change, some departments have growing financial needs, while other departments could get by with decreasing resources. The concept of requiring a zero-base evaluation is attractive because it means that budgets would not be allowed to become "fat" over time. Many organizations use ZBB analysis to see exactly how money is being spent within a unit or department. Such an approach requires existing programs to justify their continued existence. Rather than basing the future budget on the past budget, all expenditures in the proposed budget must demonstrate why they are needed.

Additionally, the ZBB approach pays great attention to the alternative ways that any one given program can be offered. ZBB collects information regarding a program into a *decision package*. A decision package contains documentation in support of the program and summaries of the analyses performed. In that sense, the decision package is just a mechanism to ensure a formal, systematic review of each budget.

Each package (see Fig. 10–1) contains a statement of the purpose of the program, the consequences of not performing the program, and the ways that the costs and benefits of the program can be measured. More interestingly, the package also includes statements of alternatives. These statements are the heart of ZBB.

ZBB provides a great degree of sophistication in the analysis of alternatives. Not only may different programs with separate decision packages be compared, but ZBB also compares three major types of alternatives within the decision package for each individual program. The first alternative involves ways to produce the treatment, service, or other output. The second set of alternatives relates to the quantity of treatments, service, or output to be provided. The third set of alternatives considers varying levels of quality.

For many nurses, considering trade-offs such as these is counter to their traditional education. Nurses, as health care professionals, are trained to provide the best possible care to each patient. At the larger level of organizational planning, however, it must be acknowledged that no health care provider can provide everything to everyone. There simply are limited resources. ZBB forces recognition of the need to determine the greatest overall good that can be provided to the entire population served by an organization, in contrast to the view of providing care to a specific individual.

Perhaps the best way to understand how these alternatives are examined is to work through a potential program budget problem.

ZBB Case Study—Hemodialysis

Suppose that the hypothetical Wagner Hospital has decided on the basis of its environmental review that there is a pressing need for additional hemodialysis services in the community. In Wagner's long-range plan the introduction of a hemodialysis program has been included, although the plan does not include much in the way of specifics other than to note that within the next five years some form of hemodialysis program should be fully instituted. This program was highly placed when priorities were established, although it would have to vie for funds with several other important new programs that were also included in the long-range plan, such as a new burn care center.

Figure 10–1. Elements of a ZBB decision package.

Wagner has compiled a decision package for the hemodialysis program. The formal documentation in the package first notes the name of the program (hemodialysis) and the sponsoring department within the hospital (internal medicine). The stated purpose of the program is to reduce levels of mortality and morbidity currently experienced in the community due to insufficient hemodialysis facilities. The resources needed for the program are stated in general terms. They include dialysis machines, physicians, nurses, technicians, supplies, and overhead items such as electrical power and physical space.

If Wagner were not a user of ZBB, it is likely that the renal specialists in the hospital would have designed a first-class hemodialysis center, perhaps as a new hospital wing, with five machines to satisfy all community needs. The proposal would have been a take-it-or-leave-it package, with strong political emphasis on its acceptance.

There is nothing wrong with wanting everything to be first class. It is not wasteful to provide top-quality care. However, that does not mean that an organization can afford to provide that care. Having a first-class hemodialysis center may mean that there will not be enough resources left for adequate cancer treatment.

Because Wagner Hospital uses ZBB, the hemodialysis plan cannot be approved until an analysis is performed that examines a number of alternatives. The first issue concerns the level of output. How much treatment will be provided? Suppose that five machines would take care of the entire community demand now and for the foreseeable future. Suppose that the estimated annual cost of this alternative were $2 million including depreciation, supplies, personnel, overhead, maintenance, and so on. A second alternative may be to purchase only four machines. Suppose that at this level it would still be possible to eliminate all mortality and morbidity, but some of the machines might have to operate two or three shifts per day, causing some inconvenience for nurses and physicians.

Four machines might cost a total of $1,700,000. Note that while the number of machines would fall 20%, from five to four, the costs would fall only 15%. That would be quite possible because some costs associated with the program are likely to be fixed. As discussed in Chapter 7, fixed costs do not change in total as the output level increases. Does this mean that five machines would be better than four, since the hospital would get 20% more machines for only 15% more cost? Not necessarily. That is the wrong comparison. The goal is to provide cost-effective, high-quality health care to the community. The goal is not to buy unnecessary equipment to minimize the cost per machine.

The alternative of four machines instead of five would save $300,000. Although there would be some inconvenience, the reduced cost would not result in any extra mortality or morbidity. The extra convenience gained by having five machines must be compared to the benefits available by spending $300,000 for some other program. Would the extra machine generate any additional revenue, or would it solely impact on scheduling?

Other alternative levels of output might be the use of three machines, which would eliminate all mortality and 50% of the morbidity for a cost of $1,400,000; two machines, which would eliminate only 80% of the mortality at a cost of $1,100,000; and one machine, which would eliminate only 40% of the mortality at a cost of $800,000.

Itemizing the costs and benefits of the alternative output levels is very informative. Unlike the usual all-or-nothing presentation for a new program, either five machines or no program at all ("We don't practice second-class medicine here!"), the choice is not that dramatic. In fact, in a constrained environment it may well be that upon seeing all the alternatives, the choice will focus between either three machines or four machines. Less than three may be considered inadequate to accomplish the long-run objectives; more than four may raise questions of priorities.

It is not only the amount of output that is a question here. The ZBB system requires that alternative ways to produce the output also be considered. Is there a choice? Isn't it hemodialysis machines or nothing? Perhaps the answer is yes, but one of the major roles of ZBB is to ask questions such as that. The next question might be, does hemodialysis have to be performed in the hospital? The answer is no. While one alternative would be to perform all dialysis in the hospital, another alternative would be to perform all dialysis in one clinic location. Another alternative would be to have a series of external locations spread throughout the community, one location for each machine. It is also possible to use one mobile van for each machine, allowing dialysis to be performed at many locations. Each of these alternatives would be matched with one, two, three, four, and five machines.

Other alternative options must also be considered. Can the patient be on the machine for a shorter period, thus increasing the number of people who have access to it? Can money be saved by buying machines with fewer accessories? Such questions almost certainly hit upon issues of quality. However, the trade-offs between quality and cost must be examined.

Trade-offs are always made, and they sometimes impact on the quality of care. If one person dies of heart disease, it may be because not enough resources were devoted to having the very latest open heart surgery equipment. That person suffered from a lack of high-quality care. More resources devoted to heart surgery equipment might have saved that individual. Perhaps the hospital should cut back in another area and pursue the very best heart surgery. In the vast majority of cases, that would simply result in other people dying in the other area. The program budgeting system must attempt to select a set of projects that are carried out in a way that minimizes the overall negative impact on quality. That may mean undertaking two new services, each at less than the optimal level of care, rather than totally sacrificing the existence of either service so the remaining one could be run on an optimal basis. Table 10-1 provides a summary of the hemodialysis decision package and its focus on trade-offs in this hypothetical example.

The difficult part of the analysis is to explicitly and creatively seek and examine trade-offs from alternatives. Specifically, it is necessary to ask whether more lives could be saved by the organization if it spent $300,000 less on hemodialysis and got four machines instead of five. Could even more lives be saved in some other program if dialysis was cut to three machines and $600,000 less was spent on this? Three machines might mean less care and lower quality care—less time on the machine for each noncritical patient. What could $600,000 do elsewhere in the organization? Would $600,000 spent elsewhere provide enough benefit to justify less care and lower-quality care in this area?

Suppose that in addition to hemodialysis, a burn care center has also been proposed. A first-class burn care center might cost $1 million per year (the numbers here are hypothetical). This burn center would eliminate all mortality

❖ TABLE 10–1
ZBB Decision Package—Hemodialysis

1. Name of program: Hemodialysis
2. Department: Internal Medicine
3. Purpose: Reduce mortality and morbidity due to lack of hemodialysis facilities
4. Resources required: Dialysis machines, physicians, nurses, technicians, supplies, overhead
5. Quantity or level of output alternatives

Level	Medical Implications	Cost
Five machines	Eliminates all mortality and morbidity; no inconvenience to staff	$2,000,000
Four machines	Eliminates all mortality and morbidity; some inconvenience to staff	1,700,000
Three machines	Eliminates all mortality and 50% of all morbidity	1,400,000
Two machines	Eliminates 80% of mortality	1,100,000
One machine	Eliminates 40% of mortality	800,000

6. Alternative ways to produce the output: This section should consider the various approaches to providing the product and the cost of each. For instance, it should consider providing the care in the hospital, in clinics, or in mobile vans. For each way of providing the output, each output level (i.e., one machine, two machines, etc.) should be considered.
7. Alternative levels of quality of care: This should consider the cost of using different types of machines and/or changing the amount of time each patient is on the machine for each way of producing the output and for each level of output in terms of numbers of machines.

that a burn center possibly can and also all morbidity associated with burns to the extent medically possible. However, a ZBB review of burn care indicates that for $600,000, a burn care stabilization unit could be established. All preventable mortality would still be eliminated, but some morbidity would remain, and patients would have to be transferred to a regional burn center after being stabilized.

Due to the large capital investment, the Wagner Hospital does not have sufficient cash to establish both a burn care center and a hemodialysis service at the ideal first-class levels. It is highly likely that without a zero-base review, the hospital might well select either hemodialysis or burn care—and the choice would likely depend largely on politics. The well-being of the community can get lost in the struggle between vested interest groups within the organization.

There might, however, be enough resources to provide both hemodialysis and burn care at slightly reduced levels of care. The result might well be elimination of all avoidable mortality in both these areas. The hospital could add three dialysis machines and a burn care stabilization unit.

The zero-base review forces the examination of alternatives. It forces recognition of the fact that more lives would be saved by scaling back the size of hemodialysis and burn care and then providing both services. Given the explicit information contained in the ZBB reviews, both vested interest groups are likely to be more willing to accept the resulting compromise.

Ranking Decision Packages

Since the resources of the organization are always limited, it is rare that all proposed packages can be accepted. Therefore ZBB requires each manager to rank the alternative decision packages. The best alternative would be ranked number 1.

During the process of budget review and negotiation, managers at higher levels of the organization will receive ranked decision packages from a number of subordinate managers. For example, a nurse manager with responsibility for a number of units might receive packages from each unit nurse manager. The packages from all these different units must be ranked in order of importance by the manager responsible for the group of units. Then the packages will continue up through the organization. The CNE and her administrative staff will rank all the packages received from all the different nursing areas.

In large organizations the ranking process can become quite tedious. However, it is a necessary evil if the goal of the program budgeting process is to compare all the alternatives available to the organization and to ultimately allocate the organization's resources to those projects which best lead to attainment of the organization's goals.

BUSINESS PLANS

One approach to program budgeting that first became widely used in the 1980s is the business plan. This technique, widely used in industry, became popular in health care as it became clear that health care organizations would have to take a more business-like approach to providing their services in an ever more difficult financial environment. It is a method that is still gaining support in all types of health care organizations.

What Is a Business Plan?

A *business plan* is a detailed plan for a proposed program, project, or service including information to be used to assess the venture's financial feasibility. Often the plan is used as a sales document that makes the case for undertaking a new project. However, despite its advocacy role, the plan should provide an honest appraisal of the project. If in fact the proposed project is not good for the organization, that should be determined at the planning stage rather than after a large financial investment has been made to implement it.

The first step in planning a new program should be to understand which goals of the organization the program promotes. Does the proposed project fit with the organization's mission statement? In developing the plan, sufficient information must be gathered to indicate whether the proposed program will move the organization closer to its goals. In evaluating the plan, it is important not to lose sight of the original organizational goal to which the project relates.

For example, one business plan might relate to the development of a community education program for diabetics, while another plan focuses on providing home health care. Both of these new programs might fit nicely within a mission of providing health care services to the community. It is possible, however, that the former program on community education would not be expected to be financially self-sufficient. It fits into the element of mission that concerns providing important services on a charitable basis. On the other hand, the home care plan may be based on the notion of earning profits to be used to subsidize the charitable elements of the organization's mission. The organization cannot provide some services at a loss unless it provides some at a profit.

Even the program aimed at the charitable mission would require a business plan. The fact that it is not expected to earn a profit does not remove the need to understand just how much of a subsidy it might require. At the same time, if home care is being proposed to earn profits to subsidize the other operations of the organization, we should not lose sight of that fact during the planning process.

The plan should define the tactics that are being taken to accomplish the organization's goal. It should clearly state the objectives of the proposed project and provide a linkage that shows how the plan's objectives will lead to accomplishment of the organization's goal.

The plan must clearly communicate the concept of the project. It must also communicate the organization's ability to carry out the project. One can think of a business plan as a document that answers the questions one should ask before investing money in a project:

- What exactly is the proposed project?
- To what extent does the organization have the capabilities to undertake the project?
- Where will the organization acquire the capabilities that it lacks?
- Will the project make or lose money?
- How much?
- Does the organization have the financial resources to undertake the project?
- If not, where can those resources be obtained?
- How will the new product or service be marketed?
- What alternative approaches have been considered?
- Why is the proposed approach considered better than the alternatives?

The Steps in Developing a Business Plan
Project Proposal

The first step in developing a business plan is the proposal of a new product or service or an expansion of an old one. Nursing is often involved in new products and services, either in a support role or as the principal proponent. For example, the addition of a new type of laser surgery would clearly have implications for nursing. Changes would likely occur in the operating room as well as the med/surg units. The project might be proposed by the surgeons, with the nursing department providing valuable assistance in developing the business plan. On the other hand, the decision to add an outpatient surgery unit might be suggested by the nursing director of the operating room. As such, it would be primarily a nursing business plan. Nurses can become involved in developing a variety of different programs and innovative services. Developing a new home care agency or additional home care services for an existing agency, developing a nursing agency, and developing an educational or counseling clinic are just a few examples.

Product Definition

Once a program has been proposed, the product or service must be carefully defined. What is the specific product; what are the ways it can be provided; what are the resources needed to provide it? Are the patients homogeneous or mixed in terms of diagnoses; in terms of acuity? Are the required resources limited to labor and other operating items, or are capital investments needed as well? How long will it take to get the program up and running? Are there economic or technological trends that could impact on patient demand in the future?

Market Analysis

Having defined the product, the next step is a market analysis. Are there people who want that product and are willing to pay for it? How many potential buyers are there, and how many other organizations offer the product or service? What *market share* can this organization get? Market share refers to a percentage of the total demand or volume for the product or service. For example, if there are 10,000 patients in your community who will be treated and your organization gains a 10% market share, it will expect to treat 1,000 patients. The organization must be convinced that there will be sufficient demand to justify the investment in this project as opposed to some other project.

As part of the market study, it is necessary to consider change. Is the market likely to grow? That is, will there be a growing number of patients? Will competition grow? Will there be more and more providers competing for the patients? If so, will this organization's market share fall?

The issue of competition is critical. Is there competition? Is there the potential for competition? What will competition do when they see this organization's new program or project? What are the strengths and weaknesses of the competition?

The market analysis must consider who the patients will be and who the payers will be. Is the population largely insured; largely indigent? Having enough patients is the first step. Equally important, however, is knowing the mix of patients.

Mix of patients refers to different types of ailments and different types of payers. The types of ailments must be known so that the expected costs can be calculated. The mix of payers is also important. What percentage are Medicare patients, Medicaid, Blue Cross, other insurance? The program's revenue can vary dramatically based on who will ultimately be responsible for paying the organization's charges. The charges represent gross revenues. Generally, however, only a portion of total charges is collected because of government-mandated rates or special discount arrangements or because the patients are uninsured and unable to pay. The ultimate cash receipts must be known in addition to the volume of patients.

If the market analysis shows little demand or excessive competition, the planning process for this specific program may be discontinued. If it appears that there is demand for the product or service and a reasonable potential market share for the organization, the planning can continue.

Rough Financial Plan

After the market analysis is completed indicating a demand exists for the product, a rough financial plan can be developed. The purpose of this rough plan is to determine whether the project warrants further attention. The rough financial plan revolves around an operating budget.

The operating budget includes rough estimates of both revenues and expenses. The revenues can be calculated based on the demand projections from the market analysis. The expenses can be based on rough approximations of the types and amounts of various resources needed.

The results of a rough financial plan are imprecise. The purpose of the plan is to arrive at one of three findings. The first possible finding is that the cost of the program will far exceed the revenues under any reasonable set of assumptions. In that case, managers should save their time by discontinuing the planning process if the project is being evaluated solely on financial merit. A second finding is that the program looks as if it will definitely be profitable. In that case the manager can proceed with the substantial time investment required to develop a fully detailed plan. A third finding is that it is unclear whether the project will be profitable.

The third result creates some difficulty for managers. A major potential danger in program planning is that the manager working on the data collection will begin to push harder and harder for the project, the more time has been invested in the analysis. The more time managers invest, the greater their psychological need to justify that investment by having the plan indicate that the project is favorable. This could result in a bias in the collection and interpretation of data concerning project feasibility.

Given the unknowns that one encounters in putting any new program into place, there should be a healthy degree of skepticism about any new project. "If it's such a good project, why isn't someone else already doing it" is a reasonable thought. Therefore, one should always continue with analysis cautiously. Plans should be discontinued unless factors lead the manager to believe that a more detailed analysis may in fact produce information in the project's favor.

Detailed Operations Plan

Assuming that planning for the project is still continuing after the rough financial plan, the next step would be to develop a detailed operations plan. The essence of this plan is to consider the entire impact that the new project will have on the existing operations of the organization.

The first element of the plan is to consider the physical location and structure required by the program or project. Next one must consider the specific human resources required. Equipment and supplies must also be taken into account. These are all direct costs of the project. It is possible, however, that the project will also cause indirect costs to vary. For instance, the admitting department may need more personnel. The marketing department may have to make a substantial effort to get the new service off the ground. The engineering department may have to devote many personnel hours to the project. It is necessary to account for the impact of the program on all the organizational overhead components.

Detailed Financial Plan

Once a thorough analysis has been made concerning the various impacts of the proposed plan on the operations of the organization, a detailed and thorough financial plan can be developed. This financial plan incorporates all the information from the operations plan, considering the financial impact of the resources to be used. This information will ultimately be used to determine whether it is possible to go ahead with the new program.

The financial plan has three critical elements: a break-even analysis, a cash-flow analysis, and the development of a set of *pro forma* financial statements. Pro forma financial statements present a prediction of what the financial statements for the project or program will look like at some point in the future.

The break-even analysis provides information on the minimum volume of patients that must be achieved for the new program not to lose money. Many new programs or projects start with low volume and gradually attract more patients. The pattern of growth in the volume of patients is predicted as part of the market analysis. Break-even analysis is valuable because combined with the volume projection it can help give the organization a sense of how long it will take before the new program stops losing money. The techniques of break-even analysis were discussed in Chapter 7.

The cash-flow analysis provides information on how much cash the program or project will spend each year and how much cash will be received. This information is not available from the operating budget for the program. That budget will focus on revenues and expenses. However, revenues are generally received some time after the patients are treated. In many cases it takes payers (including Medicare, Medicaid, Blue Cross, and others) weeks or months to pay for the services provided. On the other hand, cash outlays at the beginning of the project may be substantial. In addition to paying salaries on a current basis, the organization will need to acquire supplies, equipment, and, in some cases, buildings.

In the case of salaries and supplies, the time between cash payment and ultimate cash receipt may be a matter of months. In the case of buildings and equipment, substantial amounts of money may be needed to start the program, while the receipt of cash from the use of the buildings and equipment may stretch out over a period of years. Therefore it is quite important for the organization to know the amount of cash required. That information will allow the organization to decide if it has sufficient cash available to undertake the project. Cash budgeting is discussed further in Chapters 11 and 14.

Pro forma financial statements present a more comprehensive summary of the financial implications of the plan than is provided by the operating budget developed as part of the rough financial plan.

Pro Forma Financial Statements

Every organization has a set of financial statements that are financial summaries used to indicate the financial position of the organization at a point in time, as well as the financial results of its activities for a period of time. Often financial statements are used to indicate the organization's financial position at the end of its fiscal year and its revenues and expenses and cash receipts and payments for an entire fiscal year. The most typically used financial statements are the balance sheet (also called the statement of financial position), the statement of revenues and expenses (also called the activity statement or the income statement), and the statement of cash flows (or the cash flow statement). (See Chapters 5 and 6 for a discussion of financial statements.)

When a business plan is prepared, an operating budget is developed. The operating budget provides some basic information used for developing the pro forma statements. Using the planned operating budget and the various projections and assumptions about the proposed program or project, the key financial statements are projected for each year into the future, usually for a period of three to five years. Any predictions beyond five years are generally considered unreliable. Any predictions fewer than three years fail to give a picture of what the financial impact of the program is likely to be once it is fully up and running.

Pro forma statements allow the user to determine some basic financial information about the proposed program or project. The pro forma balance sheets will indicate for each future year what the year-end obligations are likely to be relative to the resources. One would want to always have sufficient resources to be able to pay obligations as they become due. The pro forma statements of revenues and expenses will tell the project's expected profitability for each future year. The pro forma cash flow statements provide a summary of the information from the cash-flow analysis discussed above.

Forecasting and Capital Budgeting

The detailed financial plan, as noted above, includes a break-even analysis, a cash-flow analysis, and a set of pro forma financial statements. To get the information needed for these elements, the business plan relies heavily on several aspects of budgeting. Two critical areas of budgeting are forecasting and capital budgeting.

To prepare a cash-flow analysis and to generate pro forma financial statements, a great number of items must be forecast. These include, but are not limited to, inflation, regulation, revenues, wage rates, availability of personnel, detailed expenses, cash flows, and patient volumes. To make these forecasts, the techniques discussed in Chapter 17 are employed.

Program budgets frequently require the acquisition of capital assets. Such assets, however, require special attention because of their multiyear life and frequently high costs. The techniques of capital budgeting, which will be discussed in Chapter 11, must be taken into account in preparing this part of the business plan.

Sensitivity Analysis

In developing the detailed financial plan, a helpful technique is sensitivity analysis. Sensitivity analysis is concerned with the fact that often a number of assumptions and predictions are made in calculating the financial aspects of a business plan. The number of expected patients used to develop pro forma financial statements is the result of a forecast, which may not be exactly correct. The revenues are based on a stated average charge, which is an assumption. The actual rates charged may be higher or lower. Sensitivity analysis is a process whereby the financial results are recalculated under a series of varying assumptions and predictions. This is often referred to as "what-if" analysis.

Suppose that the pro forma financial statements lead one to believe that the proposed project will be a reasonable financial success. Using sensitivity analysis, one could then say, "What if there are 5% fewer patients than expected? 10% fewer? What if there are 5% more patients than expected? 10% more? What if the average amount charged is raised by 10%? What if the number of staff nurses needed is three FTEs greater than anticipated? What if the construction costs are $30,000 more than expected?

Essentially, sensitivity analysis provides recognition of uncertainty. Uncertainty creates risk. Before a final business plan is put together and accepted, one needs to have some idea of the magnitude of risk involved. By going through the what-if analysis, one can get a sense of how unfavorable the financial results would be if some things do not occur just as hoped for or expected. If a project can show an expected favorable financial result over a range of what-if questions, it can provide an extra degree of assurance. If that is not the case, then one must carefully question whether the potential benefits are worth the risk that must be undertaken.

Examination of Alternatives

A final consideration in the development of a detailed financial plan is the examination of alternatives. There is often more than one way to do a new program. The alternatives relate to factors such as the capacity of the program, the approach to providing the service, and the quality of the program. The business plan should be based on having selected one specific approach after having considered a wide variety of potential alternatives. Calculations regarding the costs and benefits of the various alternatives that have been considered become part of the final business plan package.

The Elements of a Business Plan Package

With business plans, as with great cooking, presentation of the finished product is an essential component of the process. Business plan development requires a significant amount of time and effort. The finished result is often a very long document. Unless carefully presented in a final package, the benefits of much of the work may be lost.

The first and most critical element is a concise executive summary. The executive summary should be brief. Ideally it is no more than one paragraph or one page. It may be two or three pages if absolutely necessary. The summary should convey what the project is, why it is being proposed, and what the projected most likely results are. This should be able to be done in just a few brief sentences. If the information in the summary indicates that the project is worth pursuing, the reader will read further.

The next part of a business plan should be a detailed abstract. Such an abstract is generally about twenty or thirty pages long. This should provide a much greater amount of detail than the executive summary. However, it still is a summary or abstract. It does not include all the specific documentation for the calculations that underlie the plan.

The abstract should describe the mission of the organization and the way that the proposed program fits in with the mission. It should provide a description of both the product or service and its potential consumer. The abstract should explain how the new product fits in with the organization's existing services. It should explain why there is a belief that the organization has a competitive edge for this product or service that will allow it to gain and maintain a certain level of market share. The profitability of the program should be discussed in greater detail than that provided in the executive summary. The pro forma financial statements should be included.

It is essential that the abstract discuss potential risks. Regulation and other elements that would impede the project should be discussed as well. Finally, the abstract should include some estimate of the requirement for management time needed to implement the program and a statement of commitment by the manager who will bear primary responsibility for the implementation of the program.

The final part of the business plan package is the detailed analysis of each element. At this point all remaining data are included: detailed descriptions of the product and service, a detailed market research plan indicating market potential and competition, a detailed time line for implementation of the plan, a detailed marketing plan for attracting patients, and a detailed financial plan including the analyses used to develop the pro forma statements. Some of the data may be organized into appendixes to the detailed analysis.

By grouping the business plan into these three sections—executive summary, detailed abstract, and full detailed analysis—the manager allows other managers less familiar with the project to understand it. This will allow the project to get a fair examination and should lead to a reasoned final decision on whether to implement the proposed program.

IMPLICATIONS FOR NURSE MANAGERS

Often nurse managers at all levels of the organization have insights that can result in significant operational changes that will move the organization closer to its strategic goals. That is why strategic management takes the view that strategic planning is not limited to the development of the long-range plan and program budgets. Strategic management must exhibit itself through strategic thought by managers throughout the organization. All nurse managers should make themselves aware of their organization's mission and goals as well as its specific objectives and policies. Knowing the philosophical statement of the nursing department alone is too narrow a view.

The organization-wide goals developed in the strategic management process are used as a point of reference in assessing where the organization has been, where it is going, and what it hopes to accomplish in the coming years.

Strategic management requires a significant effort from managers at all levels. However, that effort is rewarded. Careful planning reduces the extent to which managers move from crisis to crisis. It promotes the efficient use of resources and the financial health of the organization. It results in goal setting and the establishment of a vision for the organization. Strategic planning helps ensure that managers will identify opportunities and take reasonable risks to take advantage of those opportunities. Strategic management promotes organizational change within a stable framework of constant mission and goals.

The strategic plan or long-range budget indicates which programs are to remain at a steady state, which are to be reduced in size or eliminated entirely, which are to be expanded, and which are to be added. This gives impetus to specific program budgets in which a unit, department, or program undergoes a complete assessment.

Using a method such as ZBB, the organization's managers can systematically examine all the implications of a program over its lifetime. The program can be compared to others that would achieve the same end. The program can also be assessed in terms of alternative ways to produce the output, alternative levels of quality, and alternative levels of quantity of output.

Program budget analyses can uncover unneeded costs in existing programs. There is waste in health care organizations as in virtually all organizations. Further, program budgeting can help the organization to make effective choices of how to best use limited resources. Trade-offs among various alternatives can be more clearly assessed with the increased information program budgets provide about the impact of different available options.

The organization can settle for a less-than-first-class bedside computer system but can also have new unit-based video cassette recorders (VCRs) for patient education. Alternatively, it can have a new first-rate bedside computer system and forgo having unit-based VCRs. This book cannot say which of the choices would be best. However, there should be an awareness that the alternatives do exist. The organization should not blindly get a first-rate bedside computer system because of internal political pressure and then simply accede to the fact that there is no money for VCRs. The alternatives should be considered and an explicit choice made.

Program budgeting techniques are equally effective for reviewing the operations of an ongoing unit as they are for evaluating a new program. The way a nursing unit performs its tasks may go unchanged from year to year. A ZBB review, however, can force the manager to consider whether there are alternative ways or levels of effort that could be used to accomplish the unit's goals.

Performing a zero-base review for a nursing unit is expensive. It takes a substantial amount of time to evaluate all the cost elements of a budget. It is much simpler to simply indicate the next year's operating budget will be 5% more than the current year's. However, the chances of making a significant positive gain for the organization are much higher when a thorough justification of each and every expenditure is undertaken. Managers tend to accept the status quo. Instead, managers should spend less time on day-in and day-out routine activities and more time on being innovative. Examining all aspects of a unit's operations can result in significant and lasting benefits for the unit and the entire organization.

Business plans are documents that are becoming essential for the introduction of new programs. Such plans help managers to complete a comprehensive examination of a proposed program. By making such a thorough review, the manager and the organization gain an in-depth understanding of the program as well as its financial implications for the organization.

Strategic management has broader implications than just for use in specific areas such as zero-base reviews or business plans. Managers should be creative in their applications. For example, there are many models for the delivery of nursing services. Each one has financial, quality, and other implications. A nurse manager who understands strategic management can apply its principles when the organization makes choices among alternative delivery care models.

In this way the choice made will reflect consideration of the wide range of factors that relate to that decision.

KEY CONCEPTS

Strategic management   Process of setting the goals and objectives of the organization, determining the resources to be allocated to achieving those goals and objectives, and establishing policies concerning getting and using those resources. The current view of strategic management or strategic planning relies on the use of strategic thought by all managers in guiding all plans and actions of an organization. Strategic thought requires managers to balance the short-term objectives of their units or departments with a long-range vision for the organization. Nurse managers have a central role in strategic management under this new planning philosophy.

Goals and objectives   Goals are the broad, timeless ends of the organization meant to aid the organization in accomplishing its mission, while objectives are specific targets to be achieved to attain goals. Planning calls on each organization to establish a set of clear goals and objectives and then a plan for achieving them.

Elements of a strategic plan   Basic elements of a strategic plan include:
 ◆ Mission statement
 ◆ Statement of long-term goals
 ◆ Statement of competitive strategy
 ◆ Statement of organizational policies
 ◆ Statement of needed resources
 ◆ Statement of key assumptions

Mission statement   Statement of the unit's, department's, or organization's purpose or reason for existence. The mission statement should be defined in such a way as to prevent the organization from exceeding its manageable boundaries but encouraging exploration within those boundaries.

Competitive strategy   Organization's plan for achieving its goals, specifically, what services will be provided and to whom. The development of this strategy relies to a great extent on a thorough internal and external review. What are the organization's strengths and weaknesses, its opportunities and threats?

Policy statements   Limiting statements indicating what managers can or cannot do as they work to carry out the organization's mission by the attainment of goals and objectives.

Benefits of strategic planning
 ◆ forces the organization to determine its long-run goals and come up with an approach to accomplish them;
 ◆ promotes efficiency;
 ◆ provides a means of communication among the various hierarchical levels of the organization;
 ◆ develops management skills at levels throughout the organization;
 ◆ provides managers with an improved sense of the needs of the organization and of its environmental constraints;

- increases the level of organizational creativity in addressing its problems;
- reduces the extent to which managers move from crisis to crisis;
- promotes the efficient use of resources and the financial health of the organization;
- results in goal setting and the establishment of a vision for the organization;
- helps ensure that managers identify opportunities and take reasonable risks to take advantage of those opportunities;
- promotes organizational change within a stable framework of constant mission and goals.

Long-range budgets (or long-range plans)   Often referred to as the organization's strategic plan. Such plans generally cover a period of three to five years.

Program budgeting   Part of the overall strategic planning process that focuses on all the costs and benefits associated with a specific program. A program budget combines a great amount of detailed information, cutting across departments, for a long-term period.

Zero-base budgeting (ZBB)   Popular program budgeting technique that gained fame for its analysis and justification of all costs. From a program budgeting perspective ZBB is especially useful because of its strong focus on an examination of alternatives.

Business plan   Detailed plan for a proposed program, project, or service, including information to be used to assess the venture's financial feasibility. The plan should clearly state the objectives of the proposed project and provide a linkage that shows how the plan's objectives will lead to accomplishment of the organization's goal.

SUGGESTED READINGS ──────────────────────────

Arikian, Veronica, "Total Quality Management: Applications to Nursing Service," *Journal of Nursing Administration*, Vol. 21, No. 6, June 1991, pp. 46–50.

Bandrowski, James F., *Corporate Imagination Plus*, The Free Press, New York, 1990.

Camillus, John C., *Strategic Planning and Management Control*, Lexington Books, Lexington, MA, 1986.

Carroll, Glenn R., and David Vogel, eds., *Organizational Approaches to Strategy*, Ballinger Publishing Company, Cambridge, MA, 1987.

Casalou, R., "Total Quality Management in Healthcare," *Hospital & Health Services Administration*, Vol. 36, No. 1, 1991, pp. 134–146.

Crego, Edwin T., Brian Deaton, and Peter Schiffrin, *How to Write a Business Plan*, 2nd edition, American Management Association, New York, 1986.

Day, George, *Marketing Research*, John Wiley and Sons, New York, 1983.

Dillon, Ray, *Zero-Base Budgeting for Health Care Institutions*, Aspen Systems Corporation, Germantown, MD, 1979.

Ellis, Jeffrey R., *Managing Strategy in the Real World*, Lexington Books, Lexington, MA, 1988.

Ellis, Darryl J., and Peter P. Pekar, Jr., *Planning for Nonplanners*, Amacom, New York, 1980.

Finkler, Steven A., "Developing a Business Plan," *Hospital Cost Accounting Advisor*, Vol. 3, No. 10, March 1988, pp. 1–6.

Fredrickson, James W., ed., *Perspectives on Strategic Management*, Harper Business, New York, 1990.

Gillem, T., "Deming's 14 Points and Hospital Quality: Responding to the Consumer's Demand for the Best Value in Health Care," *Nursing Quality Assurance*, Vol. 2, No. 3, 1988, pp. 70–78.

Gitlow, H., and S. Gitlow, *The Deming Guide to Quality and Competitive Position*, Prentice-Hall, Englewood Cliffs, NJ, 1987.

Goodspeed, Scott, "How to Write a Business Plan for a New Venture," *Health Care Strategic Management*, May 1986, pp. 11–14.

Harris, John, "Selling Your Concept: How to Prepare and Market an Effective Business Plan," *Topics in Health Care Financing*, Winter 1986, Vol. 13, No. 2, pp. 32–34.

Hax, Arnoldo, and Nicolas Majluf, *The Strategy Concept and Process*, Prentice-Hall, Englewood Cliffs, NJ, 1991.

Holloway, Clark, *Strategic Planning*, Nelson Hall, Chicago, 1986.

Johnson, Joyce E., *The Nurse Executive's Business Plan Manual*, Aspen Publishers, Rockville, MD, 1988.

Jones, Katherine R., "Strategic Planning in Hospitals: Applications to Nursing Administration," *Nursing Administration Quarterly*, Vol. 13, No. 1, Fall 1988, pp. 1–10.

Kirk, Roey, "The Big Picture: Total Quality Management and Continuous Quality Improvement," *Journal of Nursing Administration*, Vol. 22, No. 4, April 1992, pp. 24–31.

Koteen, Jack, *Strategic Management in Public and Nonprofit Organizations*, Praeger, New York, 1989.

Lynch, Thomas D., *Public Budgeting in America*, 3rd edition, Prentice-Hall, Englewood Cliffs, NJ, 1990.

Nash, Mary G., and Barbara C. Opperwall, "Strategic Planning: The Practical Vision," *Journal of Nursing Administration*, Vol. 18, No. 4, April 1988, pp. 12–18.

Omachonu, Vincent K., *Total Quality and Productivity Management in Health Care Organizations*, Industrial Engineering and Management Press, Institute of Industrial Engineers, Norcross, GA, 1991.

Phelan, Grace, "Zero Base Budgeting," *Hospital Cost Management and Accounting*, Vol. 1, No. 9, December 1989, pp. 1–6.

Pyhrr, P.A., *Zero-Base Budgeting: A Practical Management Tool for Evaluating Expenses*, Wiley-Interscience, New York, 1973.

Shortell, Stephen M., Ellen M. Morrison, and Bernard Friedman, *Strategic Choices for America's Hospitals*, Jossey-Bass Publishers, San Francisco, 1990.

Smeltzer, Carolyn G., and Timothy Vicario, "Changing Roles of Nurse Managers Through Strategic Planning," *Nursing Management*, Vol. 19, No. 11, November 1988, pp. 68–71.

Strasen, Leann, *Key Business Skills for Nurse Managers*, J.B. Lippincott, Philadelphia, 1987.

Suver, James D., and Ray L. Brown, "Where Does Zero Base Budgeting Work?" *Harvard Business Review*, Vol. 55, No. 6, November/December, 1977, pp. 76–84.

CHAPTER

11

Budgeting Concepts

CHAPTER GOALS

The goals of this chapter are to:

- ◆ Define budgeting and control
- ◆ Describe some benefits of budgeting
- ◆ Introduce and describe the various types of budgets including master, operating, capital, long-range, program, and cash
- ◆ Discuss the generation, justification, and evaluation of capital budget proposals
- ◆ Introduce the concepts of the time value of money, discounting, net present value, and internal rate of return
- ◆ Distinguish between revenue and expense and between cash inflows and outflows
- ◆ Outline the steps in cash budget preparation and provide a cash budget example
- ◆ Describe the budgeting process
- ◆ Provide an example of a budget timetable
- ◆ Discuss specific steps in the budgeting process
- ◆ In a technical appendix the chapter also discusses technical aspects of time-value-of-money computations.

❖

INTRODUCTION

A *budget* is a plan. The plan is formalized (written down) and quantified (e.g., stated in dollar terms). It represents management's intentions or expectations. In financial terms, an organization-wide budget generally compares expected revenues to expected expenses to ascertain the organization's expected excess of revenues over expenses (i.e., net income or loss) for the coming year.

Preparation of a budget forces the organization's managers to plan ahead.

Management experience has shown that, in general, actively managed organizations will do better than those which just let things happen. A budget forces managers to establish goals. Without goals, organizations tend to wander aimlessly, rarely improving the results of their operations or the services they offer.

By requiring managers to prepare a budget at least annually, organizations compel their management to forecast the future. Changes in nursing and medical practice, technology, and *demographics* can be anticipated and their impact predicted. This allows managers to anticipate changes that will affect the organization and to plan actions accordingly. When one responds to changes after the fact, alternatives may be quite limited. By looking at the impact of changes during the planning phase, the broadest possible range of alternative actions can be considered. Often the result of careful planning is that more cost-effective approaches can be found and put into place.

In the budget process, after plans are made an effort is made to meet or exceed the goals of the plans. This latter effort is referred to as the *control* process. Control of costs requires a concerted effort by both managers and staff. Control techniques such as variance analysis (discussed in Chapter 13) uncover problems that may have a negative financial impact on the organization and allow actions to be taken to correct those problems at an early stage.

Budgets can be used to provide both managers and staff with the motivation to work positively for the organization. They can also show how well both management and units or departments are performing. However, budgeting requires effort and commitment from all levels of management. Often a budget committee (which should include the chief nurse executive) is formed to ensure maximum cooperation and coordination throughout the budget process.

Many organizations produce a "budget calendar," which indicates the various specific activities to be carried out in the budget process, identifies the responsible individuals (e.g., finance office, unit or department managers, board of trustees), and provides deadlines for completion of each budget activity. Larger organizations have budget manuals. These manuals include uniform instructions and forms to be used throughout the organization, a copy of the budget calendar, and a statement of organizational mission. They also generally include a variety of other pieces of information relevant to the process of budget preparation. For instance, inflation rates, specific measurable goals, and an environmental statement would often be included. Budget manuals or packages are institution specific, differing substantially from one organization to another.

The budgeting process in any organization will depend as much on the specific individuals working in that organization as it will on the formalized mechanical steps involved in budget preparation and use. The role of individual human beings in the budget process cannot be overemphasized. Not only do organizations have their own forms and procedures but they also tend to have specific philosophies of fiscal affairs. The amount of participation that any individual manager has in the budget process depends on the approach or philosophy of the organization's top management. Some organizations are top-down—allowing unit managers very limited control over their budget. Other organizations delegate substantially all budget preparation and control duties to the unit level.

Teachers of budgeting often stress the importance of participation in the budget process by individuals at all levels in the organization. If the budget is expected to be a useful tool for managing, it must be realistic. It is often not possible for top-level managers to be aware of all the specific circumstances and conditions that exist in the day-to-day operations throughout the organization. Unit managers have experience, judgment, and specific information about their units that lets them provide valuable input to the budget.

TYPES OF BUDGETS

Many managers tend to think of the budget as simply a cap on expenses that instructs them regarding how much they may spend. This is a very limited view of just the *operating budget*. The operating budget, in turn, is only a small part of the overall budget of the organization. A well-managed organization will have a *master budget*. The master budget is a set of all the major budgets in the organization. It will generally include the *operating budget*, a *long-range budget, program budgets*, a *capital budget*, and a *cash budget*. Many organizations are also starting to use *product-line* budgets. From time to time the organization will also need to budget for some additional special project that is not part of the organization's normal activities. In those cases it will prepare a *special purpose budget*.

An operating budget typically plans for the revenues and expenses of the organization for the coming year. A long-range budget covers a period of three to five years. Program budgets look at specific programs that cut across a number of departments. Such budgets take a multiyear perspective. Capital budgets look at proposed equipment and building acquisitions that will be used by the organization for more than one year. Cash budgets look specifically at the organization's cash inflows and cash outflows. Product-line budgets focus on groupings of specific types of patients rather than focusing on budgets for cost centers. Special purpose budgets are used to develop a plan for any specific special purpose not covered by one of the other types of budgets.

Operating Budget

The operating budget is the plan for day-in and day-out operating revenues and expenses for the organization. It generally covers a period of one year. If the budget shows an excess of revenues over expenses, it means that the organization expects to make a *profit* from its activities for the year. If the organization is a *for-profit* company, some of the profits can be paid to the owners of the company in the form of a *dividend*. Even not-for-profit hospitals need to earn profits. These profits can be used to replace worn-out equipment and old buildings or to expand the services available to the community. If any health care organization, for-profit or not-for-profit, consistently fails to earn profits, it will not be able to add new technologies and continue to provide high-quality care. Chapter 12 provides a detailed discussion of the operating budget and its preparation.

Long-range Budgets

Budgets help managers plan for the future. Operating budgets give a very detailed plan but just for the coming year. Many changes in an organization require a long lead time and take a number of years to be fully implemented. To avoid suffering from shortsightedness, many organizations employ a long-range plan or budget. Such a budget is often referred to as a strategic plan (strategic plans were defined and discussed in Chapter 10). Such three-, five-, or even ten-year plans allow management to temporarily ignore the trees and focus on the whole forest. Where is the organization relative to its peer group? What improvements can be made over the next three, five, or ten years? What must be done each year to move toward those goals?

In many organizations, managers tend to look at the current year, then add an increase for inflation and produce a budget for the next year. The problem with this approach is that it contains no vision. There is no way to make a major leap forward because what has been done in the past is simply being projected into the future. If one would like to be able to look back five years from now and say, "Look at how far we have come," it is necessary to have a way to make major strides forward. Otherwise five years from now the organization will have made little, if any, advancement.

That is where long-range or strategic plans are helpful. Their focus is not on how to get through next year but rather on the overriding organization goals and on the major changes that ought to be made over the coming years to achieve those goals. Long-range plans help to give the organization a sense of commitment to the future. Such plans serve a vital function in allowing the organization to prepare each year's detailed operating budget on the basis of an overall sense of purpose and direction. The operating budget becomes more than just next year's survival plan; it becomes a link between where the organization has been and where it is going. Long-range budgets were discussed as part of strategic management in Chapter 10.

Program Budgets

Program budgets are special budgeting efforts analyzing specific programs. Generally the orientation is toward evaluating a planned new program or closely examining an existing program rather than merely planning the revenues and expenses for the program for the coming year. Often the program involved is in some way optional. The purpose of the program budget is to make a decision. Should the new program be undertaken or not?

Often program budgets are developed for specific programs as a result of the long-range budgeting process. The long-range budget or strategic plan may determine that three tertiary care services should be added over the next five years. Because new services often require a year to plan and sometimes more than a year to implement once the planning phase is complete, one result of the long-range plan may be to immediately select one new service to be added. Frequently new services involve labor and equipment from numerous departments. By setting up a program budget process for the new service, all the information related to the addition of that service can be considered and evaluated.

Since program budgets often cut across departments, they generally must be developed with committee input from at least the major departments that will be impacted upon by the service. Program budgets also cut across years. The financial impact of the service needs to be assessed not just in the coming year but over a reasonably long period. Since the operating budget is a one-year budget, this is another reason for special budget treatment for new programs or services.

In recent years business plans have become a vital tool for program budgeting. The elements of such plans were discussed along with long-range budgets and other aspects of program budgeting in Chapter 10.

Capital Budgets

A capital budget is a plan for the acquisition of long-term investments. These investments can range from investments as small as acquiring a new IV pole to projects as large as completely rebuilding a hospital at a new location. The key element in capital budgeting is that the building or piece of equipment being acquired has a lifetime that extends beyond the year of purchase. Capital budget items are often referred to as *capital assets, long-term investments, capital investments,* or *capital acquisitions.* The money used to purchase long-term investments is often referred to as "capital."

These assets are treated separately from operating budget expenses because of their multiyear nature. They are only partly used up in any one year, and in any one year the organization earns only part of the revenues that the capital assets generate over their useful lifetimes. If these assets were included in the operating budget, their entire acquisition cost would be compared to revenues only in the year the asset was purchased. Many capital assets that are good financial investments over their entire useful lifetime would appear to lose money when only one year's worth of revenues is considered. By having a separate capital budget, multiyear assets can be evaluated based on their implications for the organization over their entire useful life.

Capital assets generally are purchased to replace older items of a similar nature, to improve productivity (substituting equipment for more expensive labor), to improve quality of care (often addition of newer technology), or to provide needed equipment for a new service or expansion of an existing service. A variety of other reasons to acquire capital assets will also arise from time to time, such as for equipment that will improve employee safety.

Capital assets are often quite expensive. However, high cost is not a required element for an asset to be classified and treated as a capital asset. The only requirement is that the capital asset must be able to provide useful service beyond the year it is first put into use. For pragmatic purposes, most organizations set a minimum dollar limit for inclusion in the capital budget. It is not worth the extra effort to analyze and track relatively inexpensive items over a period of years. Items that have a low cost will be treated as part of the operating budget even if they have a multiyear life. Most health care organizations have a minimum cost requirement of anywhere from $300 to $1,000 for an item to be included in the capital budget.

Generation of Capital Budget Proposals

The starting point in the capital budgeting process is the generation of proposed investments. The nurse manager in a home health agency may propose the acquisition of several company cars to reduce travel time between patients (assuming public transportation is currently being used). The nurse manager in the coronary care unit or the operating room of a hospital may suggest the acquisition of a particular piece of equipment.

Exhibit 11–1 presents an example of the type of worksheet a nurse manager would use to list capital proposals. The first column represents the manager's priority ranking for the request. The most important acquisition would be ranked number 1. The second column indicates the type of capital item being

❖ EXHIBIT 11–1
Capital Budget Worksheet

CAPITAL BUDGET WORKSHEET

FY____

COST CENTER ____

PRIOR. #	TYPE CR/RE/RU AS/AN	EQUIP. QTY	DESCRIPTION	UNIT COST	EXTENDED COST	COMMENTS

requested. These include construction or remodeling (CR), replacement of an existing item (RE), replacement and upgrading of an existing item (RU), an item that is an addition to similar existing items and adds to their capacity (AS), or an additional item that is not currently available in the unit (AN).

In proposing a capital acquisition, the manager must provide financial information with respect to the asset. A required piece of information is the likely cost of the asset. Additionally, to the extent possible, information must be collected about how much cash will be spent or received each year over the life of the investment or project. The difference between the cash received and the cash spent in any given year is referred to as the *net cash flow* for that year.

The nurse manager can generally seek the aid of financial managers of the organization for the specific estimates of annual cash inflows and outflows. Cash inflows can be particularly difficult, since the entire billing process is often handled outside the control of the nurse manager. On the other hand, with respect to estimating costs, the nurse manager is more likely than any financial manager to be able to estimate what resources will be needed and when. The payroll and purchasing departments will be a great aid in converting the raw resource information into dollars based on projected salaries and prices. This estimating process should be done separately for each year that the capital asset is expected to provide useful service. Having information on the annual cash flows as well as the acquisition cost will make it easier for the organization's managers to make a decision about whether to acquire the asset.

Justification of Capital Requests

Sufficient resources are not usually available to allow an organization to acquire all the items it desires. The capital budget facilitates choices that have to be made in deciding how to spend the organization's limited resources. In describing proposed capital expenditures the nurse manager provides a priority ranking. It is also appropriate to justify each requested purchase by giving a description of the item, its cost, its impact on operating expenses and revenues, and the justification for acquiring it. See Exhibit 11–2 for an example of a justification form for a capital asset acquisition.

The justification should be thorough and should specifically indicate the consequences if funding for the item is not made available. Equipment costs include not only the purchase price but also shipping and installation. Construction costs should be reviewed by the planning and engineering departments. In all cases vendor estimates or proposals should be included if possible. The impact on operating costs should include salaries, fringe benefit costs, maintenance costs or maintenance contracts, utilities, supplies, and any interdepartmental impacts. Incremental revenue to be generated by the capital asset, if any, should be described and estimated to the extent possible.

Evaluation of Capital Budget Proposals

The capital budgets for all departments are evaluated in light of available cash. An investment that seems to make a lot of sense to a clinical department manager may have to be deferred for one year, or indefinitely, simply because the organization does not have enough cash to make the purchase.

Even if sufficient cash is available to make a capital acquisition, the organization may choose not to acquire the item because of its financial evaluation

❖ **EXHIBIT 11–2**
   Capital Justification Form

CAPITAL JUSTIFICATION FORM

FY_____

COST CENTER_____   PRIORITY ITEM #_____

Description of item or project:

Justification:

Construction Costs:		Equipment Costs:	
Fees	_____	Purchase Price	_____
Construction	_____	Installation	_____
Contingency	_____		
Total	_____		

Date of Estimate_____ By_____

Impact on Operational Expenses:

Impact on Revenues:

of the asset. In recent years the financial analysis of capital assets has been growing more sophisticated. Organizations have been starting to adopt investment analysis techniques used in other industries.

One widely used approach is the payback method. The payback approach calculates how many years it takes for the profits from a capital expenditure to repay the initial cash outlay. The less time it takes to recover the initial investment, the better the project.

The payback method does have some severe weaknesses. First, it ignores what happens after the payback period is over. Thus, one might fail to select a very profitable project that does not earn substantial profits until after the payback period in favor of a less profitable project with a shorter payback period. Second, it ignores the timing of cash flows within the payback period. Two projects would be considered equal if they both have a three-year payback period. However, if one pays the bulk of the investment back in the second year and the other pays back the bulk of the invested cash in the third year, they are not equally good.

The payback method is often used for a first appraisal of the project. If a proposed investment cannot pay back its cost within a reasonable period, it should be rejected. If an investment passes the payback test, more sophisticated evaluation is still needed to determine if a specific proposal is acceptable.

The more sophisticated methods used to overcome the problems of the payback method are called discounted cash flow methods. These methods consider the cash flow over the full life of the capital asset rather than just the payback period. They also consider the timing of cash flows or the time value of money. The time value of money is a concept based on the fact that money paid or received at different points in time is not equally valuable. One would always prefer to receive money sooner and to pay it later. By receiving money sooner, one can use the money for current needs or can invest it and earn interest.

When a nurse manager looks at alternative investment opportunities, there must be consideration of not only how much the organization will put in and how much it will get out but also of *when* money will be spent and received. Financial managers can calculate the economic viability of a project by using discounted cash flow techniques. *Discounting* is the reverse of compounding interest. One hundred dollars today would be worth $121 in two years with 10% compound interest. In the first year, $10 of interest is earned on the $100 investment (i.e., 10% of $100 = $10). In the second year the $10 of interest earned in the first year itself earns interest. Therefore the original $100 plus the $10 of interest earned in the first year equals a total of $110. Ten percent interest in the second year would be $11 (i.e., $110 × $10%). The $110 plus the $11 would total $121. When interest earns interest, it is referred to as compound interest. In just the reverse process, $121 received two years from now would be worth just $100 today if one were to *discount* the interest earned in the two intervening years.

Discounted cash flow techniques are designed to take future receipts and discount the interest to find out what those receipts would be worth today. The receipts can then be compared to current cash outlays to determine if a project is financially worthwhile. The two most common discounted cash flow models are *net present value* and *internal rate of return*.

The net present value approach requires the manager to indicate a specific interest rate, called the discount rate. It is sometimes called the required rate of return. Under this method the cash outlay to acquire an asset must be recovered, plus a return at least equal to the discount rate. The discount rate is usually set at the rate that the bank would charge the organization if it borrowed money. Thus the capital asset must recover not only its cost but also the interest the organization would have to pay the bank if it borrowed the money necessary to buy the asset. If the project earns a positive net present value, it is earning at more than its cost plus interest. Therefore it is profitable. If the net present value is negative, the project does not even recover the investment plus the interest cost, so it is unprofitable.

The internal rate of return method does not require the manager to indicate a specific discount rate. Instead, the method looks at how much cash is required to acquire the capital asset and how much cash will be received and determines the rate of return (called the internal rate of return, or IRR) the asset earns. If that rate is higher than the organization's discount rate, the asset should be acquired. The technical details of calculating net present value and internal rate of return are discussed in the appendix to this chapter.

Many times health care organizations acquire capital assets that cannot be clearly connected to specific inflows of cash. Replacing old monitors on the ICU with a newer type may improve quality of care rather than increasing revenues. The use of formalized, quantitative approaches to capital investment evaluation should not and does not rule out the acquisition of assets that cannot be evaluated on a profit basis, or even those which seem to result in losses. The evaluation of capital budget requests should consider both the quantitative and qualitative benefits that any asset provides the organization and its community.

Product-line Budgets

A product line is a group of patients with some commonality that allows them to be grouped together, such as a common diagnosis. Budgeting in health care organizations is largely focused on departments and units. In all hospitals, for example, radiology has a budget; dietary has a budget; nursing has a budget. It is less common for there to be a budget for heart attack patients.

The national introduction of *diagnosis related groups* (DRGs) by Medicare in 1983 has substantially reoriented the attention of hospital managers. Since the DRG system has a fixed payment for each group of patients, it becomes of great managerial interest to be able to budget for the planned revenues and expenses of specific patient groups. Such an approach has the potential to reveal the profitability of different types of patients.

The move toward product-line budgeting has also gained impetus from the active pressure by health maintenance organizations (HMOs) and preferred provider organizations (PPOs) in negotiating with hospitals for discounted rates for specific groups of patients. It is difficult to negotiate sensible revenue rates unless the related costs of the patients are known.

Health care organizations have therefore been moving in a product-line budgeting direction, while not abandoning department budgets. However, the process is difficult. Measurement of the cost of nursing care by patients in any one DRG is more complicated. Yet to determine a budget for all the costs of patients in each DRG such information is essential. Product-line costing was discussed in Chapter 8.

Cash Budgets

Cash is the lifeblood of any organization. Survival depends on the ability to maintain an adequate supply of cash to meet monetary obligations of the organization as they become due. Operating budgets focus on the revenues and expenses of the organization. If the organization is expected to lose money, that will be reflected in the operating budget. It is possible, however, for the organization to have a cash crisis even if it is not losing money. Many expenses an organization incurs are paid currently. Wages are typically paid at least monthly and frequently biweekly or weekly. However, revenues may take several months to collect because of the internal lags in processing patient bills and the external lags before organizations such as Blue Cross or Medicare make payment. Thus an organization can literally run out of cash even though it is making a profit!

Another cash problem relates to major capital expenses. Suppose the organization budgets to add a wing for $10 million and it is expected to have a twenty-year life. The full $10 million will not be an operating budget expense in the budget year. However, the entire $10 million will have to be paid in cash in the coming year.

For these reasons, a cash budget is prepared. Cash budgets plan for the monthly receipt of cash and disbursement of cash from the organization. If a shortage is predicted for any given month, appropriate plans can be made for short-term bank financing or longer-term bond financing (see Chapters 14 and 15).

Cash budgeting is as vital as program, capital, and operating budgets to the survival and well-being of the organization. The nurse manager should have a reasonable understanding of cash budgets and the cash budgeting process for this reason. Additionally, often cash budget constraints force a need for modifications in the budgets nurse managers prepare. While the organization's managers should try to pursue various ways to get the cash for worthwhile investments—whether they are worthwhile because they are profitable or simply because they are good for the patients—there is a responsibility to the well-being of the organization not to spend the money until it is first determined that there will be sufficient cash available.

Cash Budget Preparation

In health care organizations the cash budget is generally prepared for the entire coming year on a monthly basis. Each month begins with a starting cash balance. The expected cash receipts for the month are added to this. These receipts may be broken down into categories such as inpatient, outpatient, other operating, and nonoperating or by payer (e.g., Medicare, Medicaid, Blue Cross, other insurers, self-pay patients, donations, and cafeteria sales). The starting cash balance is added to the total receipts to get a subtotal of available cash.

Expected cash payments are subtracted from the available cash. The principal categories of payments include salaries, payments to suppliers, payments for capital acquisitions, and payments on loans. The result of subtracting total payments from the available cash is a tentative cash balance. This balance is considered tentative because the organization will generally have a minimum desired cash balance at the end of each month. That minimum balance is used for cash payments at the beginning of the next month and also serves as a safety net for any required but unexpected cash outlays.

If the tentative balance exceeds the minimum desired balance, the excess can be invested. If the tentative cash balance is less than the minimum desired balance, the organization will borrow funds to meet the minimum level, if its credit is good enough. The final cash balance is the tentative cash balance less any amounts invested or plus any amount borrowed. The ending cash balance for one month becomes the starting balance for the next month.

Cash Budget Example

An example of a cash budget for the first quarter of a year is presented in Table 11–1.

In the example, the beginning cash balance for January is $20,000. With the $385,000 expected in receipts during January, there is $405,000 available in cash. With expected disbursements of $375,000, the tentative cash balance is $30,000. Assuming that $20,000 is desired as a safety cushion, there is $10,000 available to invest. In February, cash payments have risen by $25,000 to a total of $400,000, but cash receipts have risen even more. The result is that an additional $18,000 is available for short-term investment.

In March cash receipts are down and cash payments are up. What could logically cause this result? Does it indicate a serious problem? Very possibly not. It is reasonable to assume that during December, substantially fewer elective procedures were done because of the Christmas holiday season. The March cash receipts from Medicaid, Medicare, and Blue Cross are likely to be influenced by what happened in December. On the other hand, because January, February, and March may have colder weather, they are quite possibly very busy months with high salary payments for overtime and per diem agency

❖ **TABLE 11–1**
Cash Budget for One Quarter

	January	February	March
Starting cash balance	$ 20,000	$ 20,000	$ 20,000
Expected receipts			
Medicare	$120,000	$140,000	$115,000
Medicaid	80,000	90,000	75,000
Blue Cross	90,000	90,000	85,000
Other insurers	42,000	40,000	45,000
Self-pay	40,000	38,000	41,000
Philanthropy	5,000	10,000	8,000
Other	8,000	10,000	9,000
Total receipts	$385,000	$418,000	$378,000
Available cash	$405,000	$438,000	$398,000
Less expected payments			
Labor costs	$170,000	$180,000	$190,000
Suppliers	25,000	30,000	40,000
Capital acquisitions	0	10,000	15,000
Payments on loans	180,000	180,000	180,000
Total payments	$375,000	$400,000	$425,000
Tentative cash balance	$ 30,000	$ 38,000	$ (27,000)
Less amount invested	(10,000)	(18,000)	28,000
Plus amount borrowed			19,000
Final cash balance	$ 20,000	$ 20,000	$ 20,000

nurses. Thus it is not surprising to see lower cash receipts in a given month and at the same time see cash payments that are rising during that month. Frequently hospitals find that in any given month their payments are influenced by that month's activity, but their receipts are more influenced by what happened in earlier months.

The March tentative balance indicates a cash deficit of $27,000. Additionally, there is a desired $20,000 ending balance. The organization needs $47,000 of additional cash for March. This need can be met in several ways. The organization could simply borrow $47,000. A more likely result is that the $10,000 invested in January and the $18,000 invested in February will be used to reduce the amount needed to $19,000. Then the $19,000 will be borrowed. In Table 11–1 the $28,000 in March in the "less amount invested" row indicates a use of money previously invested.

Planning for necessary borrowing should take place well in advance. The plan developed should also include a projection of when it will be possible to repay the loan. Bankers are much more receptive to an organization's needs if it has specific plans and projections than if it simply tries to borrow money when an immediate cash shortage becomes apparent. From the bank's perspective, an organization that can plan reasonably well is more likely to be able to repay a loan than one that does not even know several months in advance that a cash shortage is likely.

Special Purpose Budgets

A budget is a plan. There is not a great deal of rigidity in the definition of a budget. Therefore, there is also not a great limitation placed on the types of possible budgets. Any health care organization can prepare a budget for any activity for which it desires a plan.

In recent years a number of health care organizations have offered screening for high cholesterol, colon cancer, diabetes, and AIDS. In some cases these screenings have been free, and in others there has been a charge. What will it cost to provide the service for free (i.e., to help the community and at the same time get some favorable press)? How much would you have to charge to just cover the costs of such a program?

Often these programs are not part of the yearly operating budget. They are special programs, put together on the spur of the moment as a public relations effort or in response to a current need. A special purpose budget can be prepared any time a plan is needed for some activity that is not already budgeted as part of one of the ongoing budget processes. The budget does not have to have any formal system or set of forms. It is desirable, however, to know the impact on staffing and on the morale of the staff. One would want to know if a profit, loss, or neither is anticipated. The key to development of a special purpose budget is to try to rationally consider all the human and financial consequences of the proposed activity.

THE BUDGET PROCESS

Although a budget is simply a plan, the budgeting process in health care organizations has become quite complex. To compile all the information necessary for the organization to complete a master budget, most organizations require completion of a number of complicated documents. Often a budget timetable is developed that outlines the deadlines for completion of various parts of the budget process.

Throughout the budget process it is important to consider the fact that the budget is carried out by all employees of the organization. Therefore it is essential to involve the nursing staff in all aspects of budgeting. Their input should be solicited as the budget is prepared, as it is implemented and carried out, and after the fact as well.

One of the first steps that must be taken in the annual budgeting process is the establishment of the foundations for budget preparation. The foundations of the budgeting process consist of a statement of environmental position; a statement of general goals, objectives, and policies; a list of organization-wide assumptions; specification of program priorities; and a set of specific, measurable operating objectives. The information developed in these foundations provides the direction needed by unit and department managers in preparing their own budgets. Additionally, strategic plans and program budgets must be developed early in the process to provide further input needed by managers in completing budgets for specific parts of the organization.

Once that information is available, unit and department managers prepare budgets for their individual areas. That information in turn is used to compile a cash budget. After the initial round of budget preparation, it is often found that budget requests exceed resources available to the organization. Negotiation and revisions follow in an attempt to arrive at an acceptable budget. Once a budget is approved, the organization must work to control results and keep to the plan as closely as possible.

Budget Timetable

It is important to have a plan for the planning process itself. Managers should have a road map that tells them what steps must be taken in the planning process and when they should be undertaken. Table 11–2 presents a sample budget calendar or timetable. Each organization will have its own timetable. In small organizations the entire process described by the timetable may take only several months. In large hospitals the budgeting process often takes more than six months from start to finish.

Just as the length of time to complete the budget process varies from organization to organization, so do the specific elements of the budget timetable. Table 11–2 assumes a budget process for an organization with a July 1 through June 30 fiscal year. As one reviews this sample timetable, it becomes clear why budgeting is a complex task and one constantly subject to deadlines.

The first step is the appointment of the supervisory budget committee. This committee is usually selected by the CEO but may be appointed by the board. It is especially important for the CNE to be a member of this committee. This selection process should take place as early as feasible, and the committee should meet promptly. In this example it is assumed that the committee first meets no later than January, a full six months before the next fiscal year. The committee must ensure that department heads will have the information needed to prepare their budgets. In this example, two months are allowed for that process.

During the month of March the strategic plan must be reviewed and specific programs considered. The decisions regarding these programs must be known

❖ TABLE 11–2
Sample Budget Timetable

Activity	Responsibility	Deadlines
1. Appointment of budget committee	CEO	December
2. First meeting of budget committee	Budget committee chair	January
3. Complete budget foundations activities and communicate to department heads	Budget committee	February 28
4. Complete long-range and program budgets	Budget committee and subcommittees	March 31
5. Unit capital and operating budgets	Unit managers	April 15
6. Negotiation between nursing units and nursing administration	Chief nurse executive	April 22
7. Compilation of all nursing unit budgets	Chief nurse executive	April 30
8. Development of cash budget	Chief financial officer	May 15
9. Negotiation and revision process	All managers	June 15
10. Approval and implementation	Board of trustees; all managers	June 16

early in the budget process so that each department head can take the impact of new programs or of program changes into account in preparing their operating and capital budgets. In actuality, the strategic plan and new programs are generally considered at some length even before the budget process begins. The month of March in this example is used to finalize decisions based on months of consideration and data collection and analysis.

Unit managers will have started preparing their budgets in early March. However, the revisions to the strategic plan and the new program budgets may result in some changes. This leaves just a two-week period for unit nurse managers to finish preparing a first draft of their unit's budget. This is followed by a brief but intense period of negotiation between the nursing administration and its units. In this example, only one week is available for this negotiation process. If this period of time can be expanded, there would be less likelihood of an atmosphere of crisis and more time for reasoned discussions.

The nursing department has one week in this timetable to compile all the unit budgets into a final nursing department budget. Finance has two weeks to take the information from all the hospital budgets and develop a cash budget. One month is then allowed for organization-wide negotiation and budget revision. If all goes well, the budget can be approved by the board at its June meeting so that it can be put into effect July 1. Even with this seven-month process, delays would not be unusual (especially in negotiation and revision), which prevent developing an acceptable budget by July 1. To avoid such a situation, the process could be started earlier. However, to start the process any earlier would mean that the information collected at the very start of the budget process would be outdated by the start of the year.

Since many aspects of the budgeting process cannot be undertaken without information generated by one of the previous activities, the budget timetable becomes a crucial guide in the budget process. Failure to meet one deadline may impact on all the remaining deadlines.

Statement of Environmental Position

No organization exists in a vacuum. The community, its economy, shifting demographics, inflation, the roll of a key employer, the socioeconomic setting, and other external factors play a vital role in the organization's success or failure. Each organization must understand its position within the community and its relative strengths and weaknesses. Based on knowledge of the needs of the community, the characteristics of the population, the existing competition, and other similar factors, the organization can determine its relative strengths and weaknesses and set its overall goals and objectives.

The lessons of strategic management (Chapter 10) tell us that it is inadequate to review the environment only when the strategic plan is being formulated once every three to five years. Each year the external environment must be evaluated, and changes in the environment must be factored into the planning process.

What data can a nurse manager collect to contribute to the organization's environmental review? Although much of the demographic data will be collected by the marketing and other nonclinical staff, nurse managers can contribute some critical information. For example, they can get a sense about changing physician attitudes toward the use of the organization's facilities as opposed to a competitor's. Based on their industry contacts, they may be aware of changes taking place at other organizations that will affect the competitiveness of their facilities. These types of information form part of the overall picture that the organization requires to correctly assess its position in the community.

The annual environmental analysis serves as a good review of where the organization is and where it is feasible for it to go. Having done that review, it is more likely the budgets prepared by its managers will merge the organization's desired long-term direction with its range of reasonable possible actions. The result should be a plan that is within the organization's capabilities and strives to achieve the organization's strategic goals.

General Goals, Objectives, and Policies

Once the organization's position in the environment is understood, the overall goals of the organization can be established. These goals are broad, long-term objectives, reassessed in light of the organization's strengths and weaknesses. It is not likely that goals will change annually. Over time, however, factors may arise that would cause goals to change.

For example, based on the environmental review, a home health agency may decide that the adjacent communities are underserved and that it is consistent with its mission to initiate a five-year period of geographic expansion. A nursing home may set a goal of establishing a life-care community. A hospital may decide to phase out its maternity service.

The key to long-run goal setting is that it is basically more of a qualitative direction-setting process than a quantitative exercise with specific numerical objectives. The detailed numbers can be worked out later. First, the overall direction must be set. The overall goals, objectives, and policies of the organization may not change each year. They should be reviewed annually, however, if only to place in the minds of budget preparers the picture of the forest before they start to plan for the individual trees.

Organization-wide Assumptions

Throughout the budget process it will be necessary for all managers to work on the basis of some explicit assumptions. How large will salary increases be during the next year? What will the impact of inflation be on the purchase price of supplies? Will the government change its policies with respect to reimbursement of Medicare and Medicaid patients? Probably the most crucial assumptions concern workload. What will the occupancy or patient volume be in the coming year? These assumptions must be prepared annually.

Specification of Program Priorities

The next step is to establish a set of priorities for the entire organization. It is not unusual for the strategic plan, program budget, and capital budget to contain proposed spending for more things than the organization will be able to afford. There is a tendency to want to achieve all elements of a long-range plan immediately. When it becomes clear that the organization cannot do everything, a choice must be made between what is done and what is postponed.

It is advisable to try to set a generalized hierarchy of priorities at an early stage before detailed program budgets are developed. When it is necessary to make choices, top management can use the formalized guidelines that have been developed from the perspective of long-term growth and development, as opposed to letting power politics rule the budgeting process. Prioritization should be designed so that resources are allocated to areas that best promote the organization's long-term goals.

Specific, Measurable Operating Objectives

One of the most frustrating elements of budgeting for unit and department managers is the process whereby they develop a budget, totally unaided by any communicated guidelines, and then find the budget rejected because it does not provide for adequate achievement of objectives such as improved efficiency or reduced cost per patient day.

Organizations should provide a set of specific, measurable objectives that the budget should accomplish. This set of objectives should be communicated before the units and departments prepare their budgets. Managers can then attempt to prepare a budget that achieves those objectives. If the objectives are unattainable, managers can be prepared to explain why they feel that is the case.

The established objectives should be consistent with the overall general policies and goals of the organization, but they should be much more specific. For example, staffing reductions of 5% or ceilings on spending increases of 3% provide firm, specific objectives.

Budget Preparation

Once the above foundations have been laid, the organization can establish its various budgets. Strategic plans and program budgets must be completed first. Decisions made about new programs or changes in existing programs will have specific impacts on the capital and operating costs of the various departments throughout the institution. Once that information is available, the next step in the budget process is preparation of unit and departmental budgets. The operating and capital budgets are generally prepared at the same time. Decisions concerning one budget are also likely to impact upon the other. For example, if the capital budget includes computer equipment for the nursing station, there may be some impact on staffing.

Having completed an operating and capital budget, the next step in the budget process is preparation of a cash budget by the finance office. This is followed by budget negotiation and revision.

Budget Negotiation and Revision

As a result of limitations on the resources available to health care organizations, budgets often cannot be accepted as submitted. Some needs will be so critical that certain departments will have to receive larger-than-average increases. However, such increases may necessitate cuts in other departments. This results in a series of negotiations, with managers having to defend why their proposed budgets should not be cut. This creates substantial complexity because most of the budgets that constitute the organization's master budget are interrelated. Changes in one type of budget can have direct ramifications on the other budgets of the organization.

For example, the capital budget for the various units and departments of the organization cannot be finalized until all program budgets have been prepared. This is because a new program may require departments to purchase additional capital items. The operating budget, in turn, must contain revenues and expenses related to capital items to be purchased during the coming year. And the cash budget cannot be prepared until after the operating budget is established.

The cash budget may show an unacceptable deficit. This will necessitate a reevaluation of which programs and capital budget items provide the most benefit and which can be postponed or disapproved. These changes may result in an acceptable set of budgets that constitute the master budget. On the other hand, there may be so many vital capital expenditures that it is preferable to go back and increase revenues or cut the operating budget expenses. Or perhaps more borrowing will be planned.

Eventually, negotiation with all departments, followed by budget revisions, will result in a budget that top management feels is acceptable. Such a budget may be far from optimal. However, it represents the overall management attempt to accomplish organizational goals to the extent possible, given the limited resources available to the organization. The completed budget is sent to the board for review and approval.

Control and Feedback

The last steps in the budget process are control and feedback. Control relates to actions taken to help the organization follow its plan. Feedback relates to using actual results to improve the accuracy and usefulness of future budgets.

The control process is one in which managers attempt to keep the organization operating in an efficient manner. Much of the control process centers around variance analysis, which is discussed in Chapter 13. Variances compare actual results to the budget. The underlying causes of differences between actual results and the budget are determined. If the cause is something managers can control, then actions are taken to eliminate the variance in the coming months. If the causes are beyond the control of managers, then that information goes into the feedback process.

Any information about actual results that is used to improve future plans is called feedback. During the year many things will not happen according to budgeted plans. Some variations from the budget will be due to random uncontrollable events that establish no pattern. Those items should be discounted when the next budget is prepared. Other actual results will indicate that certain factors were not adequately considered in making the current budget. Those factors must be given more weight in the preparation of the next budget. Other elements will simply change from past patterns. Those changes will also have to be accounted for in future budgets.

IMPLICATIONS FOR NURSE MANAGERS

Budgeting consists of planning and controlling. The planning phase of the budget process requires that managers think ahead, anticipate changes, establish goals, forecast the future, examine alternatives, communicate goals, and coordinate plans. The controlling phase of budgeting requires that managers work to keep actual results close to the plan, motivate employees, evaluate performance of staff and units, alert the organization to major variances, take corrective actions, and provide feedback for future planning.

Each organization has its own approach to budgeting and its own philosophies regarding the budget process. Some health care organizations treat budgeting as a highly centralized process. That approach tends to generate frustration by the managers asked to carry out the budget. Other organizations call for more participation by managers throughout the organization. Such budgets tend to gain more support by the staff and are more likely to result in targets that are achieved.

The actual budgeting process requires that the organization consider its environment, define goals and policies, make assumptions for use throughout the organization, specify priorities, and define specific, measurable objectives. Each of the various types of budgets in the master budget must be prepared, and they are generally not approved without a process of review, justification, and revision. Finally, once budgets have been approved and are in place, a system must be created to control the results of operations.

Often the approved budget will be more constrained than one would like. However, it is necessary to balance the long-term financial needs of the organization with the short-term quality-of-care needs for patients and the needs of the organization's employees. The final budget is a result of a compromise of these and other factors that affect the organization.

KEY CONCEPTS ———————————————————————

Budget plan The plan is formalized (written down) and quantified (e.g., stated in dollar terms). It represents management's intentions or expectations.

Control Effort to meet or exceed the goals of the plans.

Operating budget   Plan for day-in and day-out operating revenues and expenses for the organization. It generally covers one year.

Long-range budget or strategic plan   Covers a period of three, five, or ten years. Serves a vital function as a link between where the organization has been and where it is going.

Program budgets   Special budgeting efforts analyzing specific programs. They cut across departments and look at programs over their expected lifetime rather than one year.

Capital budget   Plan for the acquisition of investments that will be used by the organization beyond the year they are acquired. Such assets are excluded from the operating budget because of their multiyear nature.

Time value of money   Any specific amount of money is worth more today than the same amount in the future. Capital assets often require large cash outlays in the budget year. To assess the financial impact of those outlays, one must consider the time value of money.

Discounted cash-flow techniques   Capital investment analysis techniques that incorporate the time value of money. The two most common are net present value and internal rate of return.

Net present value   Method that determines whether a proposed investment earns at least a predetermined rate of return.

Internal rate of return   Method that determines the specific rate of return earned by a proposed investment.

Qualitative analysis   Evaluation of capital budget requests should consider the qualitative benefits that the asset provides the organization and its community.

Product-line budget   Budget for a group of patients with some commonality that allows them to be grouped together, such as a common diagnosis.

Cash budgets   Budget for the cash receipts and cash payments of the organization. Since capital expenditures require large cash outlays and revenues often are received in cash after expenses are paid, it is vital for the organization to have a plan for its cash flows.

Budget process   Organization develops a statement of environmental position, a statement of general goals, objectives, and policies, a list of organization-wide assumptions, specification of program priorities, and a set of specific, measurable operating objectives. Then long-range and program budgets are prepared. Next, unit and departmental budgets are compiled. Based on those budgets, a cash budget is prepared. Based on information from all these elements, a process of negotiation and revision generally precedes budget approval. A final essential element of the budget process is control of actual results and feedback.

SUGGESTED READINGS

Anthony, Robert N., and David Young, *Management Control in Nonprofit Organizations*, 4th edition, Richard D. Irwin, Inc., Homewood, IL, 1988.

Barenbaum, Lester, and Thomas Monahan, "Developing a Planning Model to Estimate Future Cash Flows," *Healthcare Financial Management*, Vol. 42, No. 3, March 1988, pp. 50–56.

Berman, Howard J., Lewis E. Weeks, and Steven F. Kukla, *The Financial Management of Hospitals*, 7th edition, Health Administration Press, Ann Arbor, MI, 1990.

Bockow, Lester D., "A New Approach to Reviewing Proposed Capital Projects," *Hospital Topics*, Vol. 63, No. 6, November/December, 1985, pp. 49 + .

Carroll, John J., and Gerald D. Newbould, "NPV vs. IRR: With Capital Budgeting Which Do You Choose?" *Healthcare Financial Management*, Vol. 40, No. 11, November 1986, pp. 62–68.

Esmond, Truman H., Jr., *Budgeting Procedures for Hospitals*, American Hospital Association, Chicago, 1982.

Finkler, Steven A., *Budgeting Concepts for Nurse Managers*, 2nd edition, W.B. Saunders, Philadelphia, 1992.

Greenfield, James, and William McGinly, "Where Does Philanthropy Fit in Fiscal Imperatives," *Healthcare Financial Management*, Vol. 42, No. 1, January 1988, pp. 66–70.

Herkimer, Allen G., Jr., *Understanding Health Care Budgeting*, Aspen Systems Corp., Rockville, MD, 1988.

Hoffman, Francis M., "The Capital Budget: Developing a Capital Expenditure Proposal," *Association of Operating Room Nurses Journal*, Vol 44, No. 4, October 1986, pp. 604, 606–607, 610.

McAlvanah, M., "Fiscal Planning—The Capital Budget," *Pediatric Nursing*, Vol. 15, No. 1, January/February 1989, pp. 70–75.

McGrail, George R., "Budgets: An Underused Resource," *Journal of Nursing Administration*, Vol. 18, No. 11, November 1988, pp. 25–31.

Neumann, Bruce R., James D. Suver, and William N. Zelman, *Financial Management: Concepts and Applications for Health Care Providers*, 2nd edition, National Health Publishing, USA, 1990.

Pelfrey, Sandra, "Financial Techniques for Evaluating Equipment Acquisitions," *Journal of Nursing Administration*, Vol. 21, No. 3, March 1991, pp. 15–20.

Stevens, Barbara J., "What Is the Executive's Role in Budgeting for Her Department?" *Journal of Nursing Administration*, Vol. 11, No. 7, July 1981, pp. 22–24.

Swansburg, Russell, Philip Swansburg, and Richard Swansburg, *The Nurse Manager's Guide to Financial Management*, Aspen Publishing, Rockville, MD, 1988.

Willson, James D., *Budgeting and Profit Planning Manual*, 2nd edition, Warren, Gorham, and Lamont, Boston, MA, 1989.

Capital Budget Evaluation

INTRODUCTION

The concept of the time value of money requires sophisticated analysis to calculate the profitability of a proposed investment. The critical issue is that money received at different points in time has a different value. One would much rather have $100 today than one year from now. At the very least the $100 could be put in a bank and earn interest.

Suppose that two investments are being considered. One investment requires an outlay of $10,000 today, while another requires an outlay of only $7,500. Over the life of the investment, the operating costs will be $3,000 each year for five years for the first alternative but $3,600 per year for the second alternative over the same five years.

	Alternative 1	Alternative 2
Initial Outlay	$10,000	$ 7,500
Year 1	3,000	3,600
Year 2	3,000	3,600
Year 3	3,000	3,600
Year 4	3,000	3,600
Year 5	3,000	3,600
Total Cost	$25,000	$25,500

Which alternative is less expensive?

Note that there is no revenue in this example. Often in health care the focus is on cost-efficient ways to accomplish an objective. Suppose different types of air conditioners are being compared. Over the five-year life of the air conditioners, the organization will have spent $25,000 for the first alternative. The second type of air conditioner is less expensive but not as fuel efficient. It will cost a total of $25,500. Which alternative is cheaper? The first project requires the organization to spend $500 less over its lifetime. But it does require spending $2,500 more at the beginning. That $2,500 could have been earning interest, thus offsetting some of the extra operating costs.

A way is needed to compare dollars spent at different points in time. Then one would be able to consider not just how much cash is involved but also when it is received or spent. Rather than solve the problem of the air conditioners now, put it aside for the time being. Let us focus attention on the methodology for dealing with cash flows at different points in time. Then it will be possible to solve the problem of the air conditioner investment later in this appendix.

TIME-VALUE-OF-MONEY CALCULATION MECHANICS

In time-value-of-money calculations, the amount of money spent or received today is referred to as the present value (PV). The interest rate is referred to as i%. The number of interest compounding periods is referred to as N. There are several time-value-of-money calculation formulas. The most funda-mental is:

$$FV = PV (1 + i\%)^N$$

This formula allows a one-step determination of the future value (FV) of some amount of money invested today (PV) at an interest rate (i%) for a period of time equal to N. Many modern hand-held business calculators have this and other time-value-of-money formulas built in. Calculators are relatively simple to use for this process. One should be sure to coordinate N and i%. If N is years, then i% is the annual interest rate. If N is months, then the annual interest rate must be divided by twelve to get a monthly i%.

So far this discussion has focused on finding out how much an amount of money held today would grow to in the future. Discounting requires that one be able to take an amount of money to be received in the future and determine what it would be worth today. That requires reversal of the compounding process. The interest rate used in the calculation is called the *discount rate*.

What if it is expected that some money will be received or spent every year rather than all at one time in the future? For instance, what is the value today of receiving $100 every year for the next three years? One way to solve this problem would be to take the PV of $100 to be received one year from now, plus the PV of $100 to be received two years from now, plus the PV of $100 to be received three years from now.

Obviously this has the potential to be a rather tedious process. Anytime payments are to be made or received and the payments are exactly the same in amount and evenly spaced in time, those payments are referred to as an annuity payment (PMT). To calculate the PV of $100 received every year for three years, the PMT = $100, N = 3, and i% = 10. A calculator could be used to determine the PV, which is $248.69. Note that FV does not enter into this calculation because there is not one single future value but rather a series of payments, all considered by the term PMT.

THE PRESENT COST APPROACH

To return to the problem raised earlier, recall that there are two potential air conditioners. One will cost $10,000 and will have operating costs of $3,000 per year for five years. The other will cost $7,500 and will have operating costs of $3,600 per year for five years. The problem of choosing one or the other concerns the fact that the total cost of the first alternative is $25,000, while the second alternative costs $25,500, but the one with the lower total cost has the higher initial cash outlay.

In today's dollars, the first alternative is $10,000 plus the present value of an annuity of $3,000 per year for five years. The second alternative is $7,500 plus the present value of $3,600 per year for five years. Assume that the discount rate is 10%. At N = 5, i% = 10, and PMT = $3,000, the PV is $11,372. When the PMT = $3,600, the PV is $13,647. Combined with the initial outlays, the PV of the first alternative is $21,372 and for the second alternative it is $21,147. Therefore, other things being equal, the second alternative would be chosen because it is less expensive when one considers the time value of money.

This method is the present-cost approach. It considers the present value of the costs of alternative projects accomplishing the same end. Assuming that both projects are just as effective in terms of accomplishing the desired outcome, the alternative with the lower cost in present value is superior.

THE NET PRESENT VALUE APPROACH

The net present value (NPV) method of analysis determines whether a project earns more or less than a stated desired rate of return, which is used as the discount rate in the calculations.

It is reasonable to assume that any investment that can earn more than the rate for borrowing money should be accepted, assuming the organization has a good enough credit rating to be able to borrow the necessary funds. Therefore the interest rate that the organization would pay on a loan is often used as the discount rate.[1]

The NPV method can be used to assess whether a project is acceptable. The NPV method compares the present value of a project's cash inflows to the present value of its cash outflows, as calculated at a particular hurdle rate. If the present value of the money coming in exceeds the present value of the money going out, then the project is earning a rate of return greater than the hurdle rate. In equation form NPV can be defined as follows:

$$NPV = PV\ inflows - PV\ outflows$$

If the NPV is greater than zero, the inflows are greater than the outflows when evaluated at the hurdle rate. If the NPV is less than zero, then the organization is spending more than it is receiving. If the NPV is exactly zero, the inflows are equal to the outflows, and the project is earning exactly the hurdle rate. In most cases financial managers rather than nurse managers will perform the actual calculations. Nevertheless, nurse managers should understand the evaluation process capital projects are subjected to prior to approval.

To find the NPV, first sum the PVs of the cash received in each year. Then find the sum of the PVs of the cash spent each year. Then compare the sum of the PVs of the inflows to the sum of the PVs of the outflows.

For example, suppose that a hospital is considering adding a new wing. There is an initial cash outflow of $10 million. Assume that the money for the wing could be borrowed at 10%. Suppose that the operating cash expenses (including information about the costs relating to nursing, which you have contributed to the analysis) and the cash revenues for each of the twenty years of the useful life of the wing are as shown in Table 11A–1. Without considering the timing of the cash flows, a total of $16,570,000 is being spent and $35,435,192 is being received. The project appears to be very profitable. Note, however, that a large amount of money is spent at the beginning of the project, while revenues are earned gradually over the twenty years.

By using present value methodology, the present value of each cash flow can be calculated, then the present values of the inflows and the outflows can be summed. The result is that the total PV of the inflows is $12,622,639, while

---

[1]In addition, assets that earn less than the rate for borrowing money should be acquired if they have strong social merit and there are sufficient donated funds available to the organization to acquire the asset.

❖ TABLE 11A–1
An Example of Project Cash Flows and Present Values

	Cash Flow		Present Value (PV)	
	Cash Expenses	Cash Revenues	Cash Expenses	Cash Revenues
Start	$10,000,000		$10,000,000	
Year 1	200,000	$ 1,000,000	181,818	$ 909,091
2	230,000	1,020,000	190,083	842,975
3	250,000	1,081,200	187,829	812,322
4	270,000	1,146,072	184,414	782,783
5	270,000	1,214,836	167,649	754,318
6	280,000	1,287,726	158,053	726,888
7	290,000	1,364,990	148,816	700,456
8	310,000	1,446,889	144,617	674,985
9	310,000	1,533,703	131,470	650,440
10	320,000	1,625,725	123,374	626,787
11	330,000	1,723,269	115,663	603,995
12	345,000	1,826,665	109,928	582,032
13	355,000	1,936,265	102,831	560,866
14	370,000	2,052,440	97,433	540,472
15	380,000	2,175,587	90,969	520,818
16	390,000	2,306,122	84,875	501,879
17	400,000	2,444,489	79,137	483,628
18	410,000	2,591,159	73,742	466,043
19	420,000	2,746,628	68,673	449,096
20	440,000	2,911,426	65,403	432,765
Totals	$16,570,000	$35,435,192	$12,506,777	$12,622,639

the PV of the outflows is $12,506,777. The NPV, equal to the PV of the inflows less the PV of the outflows, is $115,862. Since this is greater than zero, the project is earning more than 10% and is acceptable. However, it is not nearly so profitable as it appeared at first glance.

THE INTERNAL RATE OF RETURN APPROACH

The principal objection to the net present value approach is that it does not indicate the specific rate of return that a project is earning. This creates problems if several capital assets exceed the hurdle rate and the projects conflict, or if there are insufficient funds to undertake all the projects with a positive NPV. The internal rate of return (IRR) method is a mathematical formulation that sets the present value of the inflows equal to the present value of the outflows. That equation is true only at the exact interest rate that a project is earning. If the equation is solved for the interest rate that makes it hold true, then that is the rate of return that the project is earning.

The mathematics for calculating the IRR are complex. This is particularly true when the cash flows are not the same from year to year (see Table 11A–1 for example). However, business calculators can be used to solve for the IRR with variable cash flows.

The IRRs calculated can be used to rank projects by profitability. The IRR method tells the specific interest rate that each project is expected to return. Even if the organization is not-for-profit, it must consider the fact that the projects with the highest return on investment, or rate of return, will provide the largest amount of cash coming into the organization in the future. That cash can in turn be used to allow for additional projects to be undertaken. By listing projects in order from the highest rate of return to the lowest, this ranking makes the project selection process far easier.

SUMMARY

Discounted cash flow techniques—including net present cost, net present value, and internal rate of return—account for the time value of money. The present-cost approach is useful for comparing alternative ways to accomplish the same goal. The method does not evaluate revenues. Both the net present value and internal rate of return methods determine whether the cash inflows are adequate to justify the cash outflow from a strictly economic point of view. The internal rate of return method additionally allows for a ranking of projects by rate of return on investment.

KEY CONCEPTS _____

Time-value-of-money calculation mechanics   Amount of money spent or received today is the present value (PV), interest rate is i%, number of interest compounding periods is N, and

$$FV = PV \, (1 \, + \, i\%)^N$$

where FV is the future value (FV).

Net present value approach   Comparing the present value of a project's cash inflows to the present value of its cash outflows, as calculated at a particular hurdle rate, determines whether a project earns more or less than a stated desired rate of return.

Internal rate of return approach   Method sets the present value of the inflows equal to the present value of the outflows and solves for the interest rate at which that is true.

12

Operating Budgets

CHAPTER GOALS

The goals of this chapter are to:

- ◆ Explain the various factors related to preparation of an operating budget
- ◆ Define the elements of workload
- ◆ Provide a technique for calculating personnel service requirements and costs
- ◆ Provide a technique for calculating other-than-personnel service requirements and costs
- ◆ Discuss the revenue element of the operating budget
- ◆ Describe the process of budget submission, negotiation, and approval
- ◆ Consider issues related to the implementation of the operating budget

INTRODUCTION

The operating budget is a plan for the organization's revenues and expenses. It generally covers a period of one year. Preparation and control of the operating budget is probably the single most time-consuming aspect of most nurse managers' involvement with financial management.

In most organizations the manager of each cost center becomes directly involved in the preparation of the operating budget. The finance office of the organization provides support as needed throughout the budget process. The budgets for the costs centers are consolidated, and the executive management of the organization makes final decisions on a budget to be submitted to the board for approval.

For nurse managers to begin the process of preparing operating budgets for their cost centers, they need a variety of information. Much of this information is generated by the budgeting foundations process that was discussed in Chapter 11. Specifically, the information generated by the organization's environmental review and by its development of general goals, objectives, policies, organization-wide assumptions, program priorities, and specific measurable objectives is essential to the manager in preparing a budget.

That information will accomplish two primary objectives: It will enable the manager to understand the forest before becoming immersed in the trees, and it will provide specific budget preparation guidance. The environmental review and the general goals, objectives, and policies allow the manager to understand what the organization wants to accomplish and what it believes it will be able to accomplish. Program priorities provide the manager with information about the level of importance that will likely be assigned to various types of budget requests. These pieces of background information will help the manager focus on what the specific cost center should be trying to accomplish.

The organization-wide assumptions and specific measurable objectives then provide the manager with information needed to start preparing the specific details of the budget. Inflation rates and likely changes in patient volume and mix are examples of assumptions that are critical for the manager in determining likely resource requirements and costs. Measurable objectives such as an overall 3% maximum increase in unit costs provide a target to aim for in the budget development process. They also serve notice to the manager that it will be necessary to justify any proposed budget expenses that exceed those specified in the objectives or revenue categories that fall short of stated objectives.

Within nursing administration additional background data are needed before nurse managers can commence cost center budget preparation. Specifically, the organization's approach to delivering nursing care must be clearly understood by all nurse managers. To what extent does the organization rely on LPNs as opposed to RNs? What is the role of aides? What proportion of staff works on each of the three shifts of the day, and what variations are there between weekday and weekend shifts? Is the mix of staff different on different shifts and, if so, how? The answer to these questions may vary from unit to unit. Once resolved, these guidelines may remain unchanged for a number of years (although they should be reviewed annually for needed changes).

Information from long-range and program budgets (discussed in Chapter 11) should also be available to unit managers as they begin their budgeting process. The addition of new services or programs will have a direct bearing on the planning of the budget for each cost center affected, even if only indirectly. For example, the addition of certain types of esoteric surgery may result in increased demands upon the recovery room, postsurgical ICUs, or even upon the general medical/surgical (med/surg) units.

Similarly, if other units or departments of the organization are planning changes in procedures, that information must be communicated to all relevant cost centers. For example, if pharmacy plans to ask nursing units to reconstitute more drugs on the unit, this will save money in the pharmacy but will likely increase nurse staffing needs on the units. Coordination, cooperation, and communication are vital to arriving at an operational plan that is best for the organization as a whole and allows all cost centers to plan their budgets according to their work requirements.

Once the background information required to commence the budget process is available, nurse managers can move forward to prepare the three primary elements of the operating budget: the expense budget for personnel, the expense budget for costs other than personnel services, and the revenue budget. All nursing cost centers have expense responsibility. Many nursing units are not required to prepare revenue budgets. However, some cost centers managed by nurses, such as the operating room (OR), do have revenue responsibility. The role of nursing with respect to revenue is growing and will be discussed in this chapter. After the budget is prepared, it must be submitted and possibly negotiated prior to approval. Once it is approved, it must be implemented and controlled.

The development of the operating budget discussed in this chapter is one possible approach to calculating the elements of the budget. Various institutions will have specific forms and specific step-by-step procedures. Therefore, the forms used in this chapter and the order of the steps taken in developing the budget should not be viewed as the focal points. Rather, one should try to understand the elements of the budget—what items must be included and why. A conceptual understanding of the operating budget will allow the reader to adapt to a wide variety of types of organizations and to the specific procedures of any organization.

WORKLOAD BUDGET

To prepare the revenue or expense portions of the operating budget, the first step is to ascertain the volume of work for the coming year. The amount of work performed by a unit is referred to as its *workload*. Workload is often measured in terms of *units of service*. A unit of service is the measurement of the work performed by the cost center. Workload may be measured in a variety of ways, such as the number of patients, patient days, deliveries, visits, treatments, or procedures. Each cost center must determine the measure that is most appropriate for its unit of service.

Units of service can provide a meaningful basis for both revenue and expense calculations. For example, a patient may be charged based on the number of hours an operation takes. Hours of operations represent the unit of service. That measure may also be used as a starting point in developing the staffing needs for the OR.

Once a cost center defines its key unit or units of service, it must predict the number of units of service that will be provided in the coming year. This will allow development of the operating budget. In some organizations nurse managers may be told a specific number of units of service to use in their budget. In many cases, however, the nurse manager will have to forecast that number. In fact, given the specific knowledge a unit manager has about that specific cost center, probably the individual nurse manager is in the best position to forecast units of service for the cost center. (See Chapter 17 for specific forecasting techniques.)

In addition to units of service, it may be necessary to forecast things such as the average length of stay or the mix of patients by DRG or severity of illness. Once these forecasts are made, the nurse manager will translate the work that must be done into a set of personnel and other-than-personnel resource requirements.

Activity Report

One aid in forecasting the coming year budgeted workload is the *activity report*. This report measures key statistics concerning current activity. It centers on both the number of units of service and the relative proportion of the organization's capacity that is being used. For example, in a hospital or nursing home the most common measure of capacity is the number of beds available for patients in total. The *census* represents the number of these beds occupied each day at a certain point in time (usually midnight). The occupancy rate is the percentage of total beds filled. For example, if a nursing home has 120 beds and on average 108 of them are occupied, it has a 90% occupancy rate (i.e., 108 filled beds divided by 120 total beds × 100%).

Two other statistics commonly found in an activity report are the *average daily census* (ADC) and the *average length of stay* (ALOS). The average daily census is the number of patients cared for per day on average over a period of time. One patient cared for, for one day, is a patient day. The ADC is found by dividing the number of patient days over the time period by the number of days in the period. The average length of stay is the average number of days that each patient is in the hospital or nursing home. It is found by dividing the total number of patient days by the total number of admissions.

The activity report is very valuable, but it must be used with care. Patients tend not to be *homogeneous*. Knowing the number of patient days is inadequate for planning purposes. A more useful budget for a med/surg unit would be developed if the manager knew the type of patients and their severity of illness rather than just the number of patient days. An operating room needs to know the types of different procedures rather than simply the number of hours of operations. The same total number of patients in two different years can have widely differing nursing care costs if they represent a different mix of patients. The unit of service often needs adjustment for patient mix in the budget process.

Adjusting Units of Service

As a consequence of the heterogeneity of patients, whenever possible budgeting should be based on adjusted units of service. For example, in the case of a hospital, the number of med/surg patient days for a nursing unit can be adjusted using a system for classifying patients based on the resources they are expected to use; this is often referred to as the patient's acuity.

The most general approach to using patient classification is to determine workload based on required hours of nursing care. Suppose that a med/surg unit expects to have 9,000 patient days for the coming year. Rather than trying to determine a budget based solely on the number of patient days, an estimate can be made based on the acuity level of the 9,000 patient days. For example, assume that a unit classifies patients into one of five categories from 1 to 5. The 9,000 patient days might be expected to be as follows:

Patient Classification	Number of Patient Days
1	1,500
2	3,700
3	2,400
4	900
5	500
Total	9,000

Segregating the 9,000 patients into the five classifications allows the operating budget to be developed based on the resource requirements of the specific mix of patients expected for the unit.

Calculating Workload

For the separation of patient days by classification level to be valuable for budgeting, there must be a way to differentiate resource consumption by patients in each category. Patient classification systems generally provide information on the average required care hours per patient day per twenty-four hours for each level. The number of hours of care are based on a specific staff mix. If the staff mix changes, the required hours of care at any patient classification level would also change.

Using expected patient classification information, it is possible to determine the number of care hours that these 9,000 patient days would need. For example, assume the average care hours are as shown in Table 12–1.

In this case the total care hours required for the year, based on the organization's patient classification system, are 60,820 for this unit. Based on 9,000 patient days, the care hours per patient day on average are 6.76 (60,820 care hours divided by 9,000 patient days).[1] This 6.76 care hours per patient day can be thought of as a measure of average patient acuity.

Note, however, that one cannot assume based on the above that for this particular nursing unit 6.76 care hours per patient day is a permanent standard. The 6.76 care hours result is very sensitive to the expected mix of patients each year. Suppose, for instance, that the original mix of patients had been:

Patient Classification	Number of Patient Days
1	1,100
2	3,000
3	2,600
4	1,400
5	900
Total	9,000

In that case the total work load is 7.98 care hours per patient day, calculated as in Table 12–2.

The total care hours of 71,830 divided by 9,000 patient days is 7.98 care hours per patient day. Without the total number of patient days having changed at all, the change in the mix of patients calls for an increase in nursing care

---

[1]An alternative approach to measuring workload is to use a relative value unit (RVU) system. In such an approach a specific level of patient classification is chosen to be assigned an acuity index value of 1. All other levels are assigned relative value units based on the amount of hours of care they require relative to the index level. For example, if classification level 2 were set to a relative value index of 1, and if classification level 5 required four times as many care hours as level 2, then level 5 would be assigned a relative value of 4. The advantage of the relative value unit scale over the average required hours scale is that the former describes the patient population, while the latter focuses on the resources required to treat the population. For a further discussion of using RVUs for acuity and staffing see Christina Graf, "The Operating Budget," in Steven A. Finkler, *Budgeting Concepts for Nurse Managers*, 2nd edition, W.B. Saunders, Philadelphia, 1992, Chapter 8.

❖ TABLE 12–1
Required Patient Care Hours

Patient Classification	Number of Patient Days	×	Average Care Hours per 24-hr Period	=	Total Unit Workload
1	1,500		2.5		3,750
2	3,700		4.7		17,390
3	2,400		8.0		19,200
4	900		12.2		10,980
5	500		19.0		9,500
Total	9,000				60,820

hours of 18%, from 6.76 to 7.98! On average, patient resource requirements have risen from 6.76 hours of care per patient day to 7.98 hours. To accurately budget for expenses it is essential that the anticipated workload be specified as accurately as possible. That is the purpose of adjusting units of service for the specific anticipated mix of patients.

EXPENSE BUDGET—PERSONNEL SERVICES

Once the manager has a workload forecast, the next step is to start the process of determining the staff requirements for the unit. These requirements include all personnel under the manager's direction. This will usually include RNs, LPNs, aides, and clerical staff. Additionally, many other types of employees may be part of the unit, such as technicians, orderlies, and unit hostesses.

There are no universally accepted standards for staffing levels. Each institution has unique physical plant characteristics, a unique mix of services offered and types of patients, and its own philosophy concerning the appropriate provision of care. Therefore the mix of staff and standard care hours deemed appropriate will vary from one health care organization to another. The patient classification system in place provides the institution's assessment of the care hours required per patient by classification level. It often does not address the mix of staff, which will be discussed below.

Calculation of staffing requires more than simply knowing the total number of hours of care to be provided per patient day on average. To explain how staffing needs can be determined, we will use an example. Assume that the

❖ TABLE 12–2
Required Patient Care Hours for Revised Patient Mix

Patient Classification	Number of Patient Days	×	Average Care Hours per 24-hour Period	=	Total Unit Workload
1	1,100		2.5		2,750
2	3,000		4.7		14,100
3	2,600		8.0		20,800
4	1,400		12.2		17,080
5	900		19.0		17,100
Total	9,000				71,830

number of hours of care needed by a thirty-bed med/surg unit is 71,830. This number was calculated earlier for an expected workload of 9,000 patient days, spread across five different patient-classification levels.

Average Daily Census and Occupancy Rate

Assuming that the unit is open 365 days of the year, we can start by calculating the average daily census (ADC) and the occupancy rate.

$$\text{ADC} = 9{,}000 \text{ patient days}/365 \text{ days per year}$$
$$= 24.7 \text{ patients per day}$$

$$\text{Occupancy} = 24.7 \text{ patients per day}/30 \text{ beds} \times 100\%$$
$$= 82\%$$

This information is important to managers because it indicates the capacity of the unit to expand its service. Recall from Chapter 7 that since some costs are fixed and some are variable, volume is critical. As volume rises, revenues tend to rise in direct proportion. Costs also rise but less than proportionately. That means that increases in patient volume are especially profitable. The 82% occupancy rate seen here indicates that there is still substantial physical capacity for expansion of the services provided by this unit.

Staffing Requirements and FTEs

Next, we need to consider staffing requirements for the number of expected hours. In this case, as noted, 71,830 hours of care are required. How many staff members will be needed to provide that care? Some people work full-time. Others are part-time employees. We need a way to distinguish between those who are full-time workers and those who are not. The approach that has been developed is to distinguish between *positions* and *full-time equivalent* (FTE) employees. One person working for the organization for any number of hours per week occupies a position. One person who works full-time is a full-time employee. Any number of positions that combine to provide the hours of work of a full-time employee is a full-time equivalent.

Thus, one employee working full-time is one full-time equivalent. So are two employees each working half-time. They occupy two positions but generate only one FTE of work. Staffing calculations must first determine how many FTEs are required. Then those FTEs can be provided by filling any number of positions that add up to that amount of FTEs.

One FTE gets paid for full-time work. That is most commonly pay for eight hours per day for five days per week, fifty-two weeks per year, or a total of 2,080 hours per year.[2] However, the staff needed to provide the 71,830 required care hours cannot be determined by dividing 71,830 by 2,080. That would assume that all 2,080 paid hours per FTE were productive hours. The 2,080 paid hours include "nonproductive" time. Vacations, sick leave, holidays, and any other nonworked time are nonproductive hours. The organization may also count time worked, but away from the nurse's unit, to be nonproductive.

---

[2]In some geographic areas it is common for employees to work a 7.5 hour day. This totals to 37.5 hours per week or 1,950 paid hours per year per FTE. Some organizations use seven ten-hours shifts per two-week period for an FTE. That adds up to 1,820 paid hours per year. Each organization can set its own standard number of paid hours per FTE.

For example, this would include things such as time spent at educational seminars. Since the 71,830 hours represent needed care hours, we must relate them to productive hours rather than paid hours.

Productive vs. Nonproductive Hours

How can one distinguish between productive hours and nonproductive hours? This information is generally available from reports that payroll provides to each unit. The report will show the total paid hours as well as the number of nonworked hours or worked but nonproductive hours in each category. Based on paid and worked hours over the last twelve months, the nurse manager should determine an average number of productive hours per FTE. This requires dividing total worked hours by total paid hours and multiplying by 100% to arrive at a percentage of paid hours that are productive. For example, assume that for this unit for the previous twelve months:

$$\begin{array}{ll}\text{Productive hours:} & 75,480 \\ \text{Paid hours:} & 94,350 \\ (75,480/94,350) \times 100\% = 80.0\% \end{array}$$

This means that 80% of paid hours are productive. There are .8 productive hours for every paid hour.

Using a standard 2,080 paid hours per FTE, we could then determine how many productive hours one would expect from each FTE:

2,080 paid hours × 80.0% = 1,664 worked or productive hours per FTE

The total care hours—71,830—can be divided by the 1,664 productive hours per FTE to find the number of FTEs needed.[3] In this example, the result of that division is 43.17 FTEs. Based on decisions made by the organization, that FTE total will be separated into different types of staff members (RN, LPN, aide) and assigned to different shifts. Those 43.17 FTEs will be responsible for providing direct and indirect care twenty-four hours per day, seven days per week, all year long.

Assignment of Staff by Type and Shift

One should not assume that there will be 43.17 staff members working each day. The 43.17 FTEs represent an adequate number to provide care seven days per week, every week. On any given day some people are sick or on vacation, taking a holiday, or taking one of their "weekend" days (not necessarily on the weekend). How many staff members will actually be working each day? The total hours of care required were 71,830 over a period of one year. Dividing the 71,830 by 365 days in a year produces the required care hours per day on average.

71,830 care hours/365 days per year = 197 hours of care per day

---

[3]As noted in Footnote 2, not all organizations use 2,080 paid hours for one standard FTE. Regardless of the number of paid hours per FTE for a specific organization, if the percentage of productive paid hours is determined, it can be multiplied by the total paid hours per FTE to find how many productive hours are provided per FTE. That can be divided into the total hours of care needed to determine the number of FTEs needed.

   Assuming that employees work eight-hour shifts, that results in 24.6 person-shifts per day (197 hours per day divided by eight hours per shift = 24.6 shifts).[4] These 24.6 person-shifts per twenty-four hours must be allocated by shift and by type of employee. Suppose that this med/surg unit has a pre-determined pattern that requires approximately 65% RN staff, 25% LPN, and 10% aides. Assume further that the scheduling standard is 45% days, 35% evenings, and 20% nights. These numbers, like the others in this chapter, are hypothetical. In practice, these standards must be established by the nursing department based on its decisions about the most appropriate division of staff for this specific unit.

   Table 12–3 spreads the available 24.6 person-shifts across the various staff categories and shifts. First, the total number is calculated for each type of staff. Since 65% of shifts are to be covered by staff nurses, 65% of the 24.6 is allocated to the staff nurse category, generating the 16.0 in the total column for the staff nurse row. Then 25% and 10% are used to allocate 6.1 total LPNs and 2.5 total aides.

   The next step is to take 45% of the total for each type of staff and allocate that to the 7–3 shift. Of 16.0 staff nurses, 45% is 7.2, so there will be 7.2 staff nurses on the 7–3 shift each day. Continuing, 45% of 6.1 is 2.7, and 45% of 2.5 is 1.1. This step is repeated for the 3–11 shift and 11–7 shift using 35% and 20%, respectively. The results of these calculations fill in the numbers of staff on each shift, by type of staff, as shown in Table 12–3.

   This provides a basic guideline for the manager. However, the manager will next want to make some minor modifications to determine the actual number of people to be on duty on each shift (see Table 12–4). In this case, the manager might decide to decrease the number of staff nurses on the 7–3 day shift to an even 7.0, instead of using the exact 7.2 that had been calculated. The number of RNs (staff nurses) on the 3–11 shift was increased to 6.0, while the number on the 11–7 shift was decreased to 3.0. This leaves the total of staff nurses at

---

[4]Alternately, 197 divided by 10 equals 19.7 ten-hour shifts per day. Use of ten- or twelve-hour shifts instead of eight-hour shifts does not create a problem for finding the number of persons needed on duty each day. However, if the length of shift creates overlapping shifts (the second shift comes on duty before the first shift goes off duty), then the manager must plan work activities with care to ensure that patients receive all required care and productivity levels are maintained.

❖ TABLE 12–3
Allocation of Staff by Type and Shift

Staff Type	Staff Allocation	7–3 Shift	3–11 Shift	11–7 Shift	Total
	100%	45%	35%	20%	
Staff nurse	65%	7.2	5.6	3.2	16.0
LPN	25%	2.7	2.2	1.2	6.1
Aide	10%	1.1	.9	.5	2.5
Total		11.0	8.7	4.9	24.6

❖ TABLE 12–4
Final Allocation of Staff by Type and Shift

Staff Type	Staff Allocation	7–3 Shift	3–11 Shift	11–7 Shift	Total
	100.0%	44.9%	36.7%	18.4%	
Staff nurse	65.3%	7.0	6.0	3.0	16.0
LPN	24.5%	3.0	2.0	1.0	6.0
Aide	10.2%	1.0	1.0	.5	2.5
Total		11.0	9.0	4.5	24.5

16.0 per day. The LPN category, on the other hand, is increased somewhat on the day shift and reduced on the other two shifts. The total coverage has also been reduced by .1. Similar changes are made in the aide category. The total number of shifts per day has been reduced from 24.6 to 24.5.

After the manager modified the categories, the percentages are recalculated. This allows the manager to see how far from the guidelines the actual proposed staffing pattern has varied as a result of the adjustments. The new total for each shift is divided by the new total shifts, and the new total for each type of staff is divided by the new total for all shifts to get the updated percentages. For example, in Table 12–4 there are now 4.5 total employees on the night shift. Dividing 4.5 by 24.5 total shifts gives 18.4%, as compared to the guideline of 20%. Most of the percentage changes for both shift and staff type were reasonably small in this example. Large variations from the guidelines would require specific justifications.

It is important to bear in mind that the required total staffing hours are based on the hours needed per patient at differing patient classification levels. However, the hours per patient are established based on a specific staff mix. If the staff mix changes substantially, then the required hours might change as well. In this example, the changes in actual staff mix from that pre-established are minor and would not require any adjustment.

The patterns developed here also assume that staffing is the same through-out the week. If some days are particularly busy or slow, it would be possible to have a daily staffing guide. In that case the total number of shifts per week would be kept at approximately the target level, i.e., 24.6 shifts per day × 7 days per week = 170.2 shifts per week. However, these 170.2 shifts per week could be allocated so that there would be more than 24.6 shifts on some days of the week and less on others.

Fixed Staff

In addition to the staff calculated above, there are employees who do not vary with the patient volume. This includes the unit manager, perhaps clinical specialists, and clerical staff. Such staff members are budgeted in addition to the staff retained to directly fill the 71,830 required hours of care. Often such staff members are not replaced when they are out sick or on vacation. In those cases there is no need to calculate sufficient hours to provide coverage when they are out, as was done with the staff FTEs.

Table 12–5 adds fixed staff to the patient care staff in the example. In the table a nurse manager, a clinical specialist, three secretaries (one per shift), and one clerk have been added. Note that it is assumed that there is only one manager, with no coverage when that manager is not present on the unit. This clearly represents fixed staffing. On the other hand, a secretary is required all three shifts, every day. Therefore, enough FTEs will have to be hired to ensure that the secretarial position is filled every single day. Nevertheless, the secretaries are still fixed staff because they do not vary with the number of patients. Were the expected 9,000 patient days to increase or decrease by 5, 10 or 15%, the unit would not employ more or fewer secretaries.

Converting Staff and FTEs to Positions

At this point the number of shifts per day and the number of FTEs needed have been calculated. The next step is to convert this information into the specific positions that will be needed to provide that care. Specifically it is necessary to determine how many full-time and part-time employees will be needed, how much overtime, and how much per diem agency time.

Calculating FTEs by Type and Shift

To establish staff positions, it is necessary to calculate the relationship between shifts per day and FTEs. If the manager divides the 43.17 required FTEs by the 24.5 daily staff shifts, it turns out that each person-shift calls for employing 1.76 FTEs. Recall that one FTE will provide coverage one shift per day, five days per week, fifty-two weeks per year, less vacations, holidays, and other nonproductive time. An adequate number of FTEs are needed to provide for the other two days out of seven per week plus the vacations, holidays, and so on. It is important to note that the staff hired to fill in two days per week, plus vacation, holidays, etc., will *themselves* be taking vacations, holidays, and so on. Therefore, it is not unreasonable to find that coverage of one shift 365 days per year would require the organization to employ 1.76 FTEs.

❖ **TABLE 12–5**
Staff by Type and Shift (Including Fixed Staff)

Staff Type	7–3 Shift	3–11 Shift	11–7 Shift	Total
Fixed Staff				
Nurse manager	1.0			1.0
Clinical specialist	1.0			1.0
Clerk	1.0			1.0
Secretary	1.0	1.0	1.0	3.0
Subtotal	4.0	1.0	1.0	6.0
Variable Staff				
Staff nurse	7.0	6.0	3.0	16.0
LPN	3.0	2.0	1.0	6.0
Aide	1.0	1.0	.5	2.5
Subtotal	11.0	9.0	4.5	24.5
Total	15.0	10.0	5.5	30.5

❖ TABLE 12–6
FTEs by Type and Shift (Including Fixed Staff)

Staff Type	7–3 Shift	3–11 Shift	11–7 Shift	Total
Fixed Staff				
Nurse manager	1.0			1.0
Clinical specialist	1.0			1.0
Clerk	1.0			1.0
Secretary	1.8	1.8	1.8	5.4
Subtotal	4.8	1.8	1.8	8.4
Variable Staff				
Staff nurse	12.3	10.6	5.3	28.2
LPN	5.3	3.5	1.8	10.6
Aide	1.8	1.8	.9	4.5
Subtotal	19.4	15.9	8.0	43.3
Total	24.2	17.7	9.8	51.7

Table 12–6 converts the number of staff needed to the number of FTEs to be employed. For those employees for whom coverage is not provided when they are on vacation, etc., the number of person-shifts from Table 12–5 is identical to the number of FTEs in Table 12–6. For example, the one nurse manager shown in Table 12–5 remains as one FTE in Table 12–6.

For each position that must be covered 365 days per year, the number of person-shifts from Table 12–5 is multiplied by 1.76.[5] For example, the 7.0 person-shifts for staff nurses from 7 AM to 3 PM (see Table 12–5) when multiplied by 1.76 becomes 12.3. This procedure is carried out for each type of staff member for each shift.

Establishing Positions

The 12.3 FTE staff nurses could be provided by hiring twelve full-time staff nurses and having those twelve nurses additionally share a total of .3 FTEs of overtime. Or it could be staffed with twenty-four half-time nurses and .3 FTEs of per diem agency nurses. Or it could be staffed by any of a wide variety of other combinations.

Once the manager knows how many FTEs are needed for each shift for each type of employee, the next step is to divide the FTEs into straight time (ST) and overtime (OT), as is shown in Table 12–7. This division will depend on organizational policy and on practical realities. In this example the policy of the organization is to never use overtime for more than one-half FTE for any type of employee on any shift. It is assumed that if more than one-half FTE is needed, it can be supplied by hiring a half-time employee who would be less

---

[5]Note that 1.76 is not an industry standard. It depends on the portion of paid time that is productive at a specific institution. In this example we want to cover each position eight hours a day for 365 days per year. That means we need 2,920 productive hours (365 × 8). On the basis of our productive/total paid time ratio of .8, we determined that we get 1,664 productive hours/FTE (2,080 paid hours/FTE × .8). If we divide 2,920 required hours by 1,664 productive hours/FTE, we find that we need 1.76 FTEs for each position covered one shift for 365 days per year.

❖ TABLE 12–7
FTEs Divided by Straight Time (ST) and Overtime (OT)

Staff Type	7–3 Shift			3–11 Shift			11–7 Shift			Total		
	ST	OT	Total	ST	OT	Total	ST	OT	Total	ST	OT	Total
Fixed Staff												
Nurse manager	1.0		1.0							1.0		1.0
Clinical specialist	1.0		1.0							1.0		1.0
Clerk	1.0		1.0							1.0		1.0
Secretary	1.8	—	1.8	1.8	—	1.8	1.8	—	1.8	5.4	—	5.4
Subtotal	4.8	—	4.8	1.8	—	1.8	1.8	—	1.8	8.4	—	8.4
Variable Staff												
Staff nurse	12.0	.3	12.3	10.5	.1	10.6	5.0	.3	5.3	27.5	.7	28.2
LPN	5.0	.3	5.3	3.5	—	3.5	1.5	.3	1.8	10.0	.6	10.6
Aide	1.8	—	1.8	1.8	—	1.8	.9	—	.9	4.5	—	4.5
Subtotal	18.8	.6	17.6	15.8	.1	15.9	7.4	.6	8.0	42.0	1.3	43.3
Total	23.6	.6	22.4	17.6	.1	17.7	9.2	.6	9.8	50.4	1.3	51.7

costly than paying an overtime premium to full-time employees. For example, a total of 1.8 FTEs are needed for LPNs on the 11–7 shift. It is assumed that 1.5 FTEs will be filled at straight time, probably by using one full-time employee and one half-time employee. The remaining .3 FTEs will be filled by overtime.

In some cases, it is assumed that there is even more flexibility that allows overtime to be avoided. For example, 1.8 FTEs are needed for secretaries on each shift. However, the straight-time vs. overtime breakdown differs from that used for the LPN on the 11–7 shift. It is assumed by the organization in this example that secretaries are easier to hire on a part-time basis than clinical staff. Therefore, no overtime is planned. It must be expected that the organization can hire secretaries who will work part of an FTE as needed by the organization. A similar assumption is made about aides.

Once the separation of straight time and overtime is made, the FTEs shown in Table 12–7 can be converted into specific numbers of positions, as shown in Table 12–8. This budget is a link between resources required to care for patients and the cost of the resources. By converting FTEs into the specific number of full-time and part-time positions, the manager can start to assign specific individuals to positions to provide patient care. By determining the number of hours that each position will be paid for at straight time and overtime, the manager is beginning to develop the specific information that will be needed to determine the cost of the personnel resources. Often the current-year positions budget is used as a guide in preparing the positions budget for the coming year.

Table 12–8 is derived by taking the information from Table 12–7 that indicates the number of FTEs needed on each shift by type of employee. The FTEs are split between full-time and part-time employees according to the manager's perception of staffing needs. In some cases full-time employees are desired for continuity of care. In other instances part-time employees are desired because they allow the manager greater flexibility in filling in for vacations, holidays, and other nonproductive time.

According to the number of positions column of Table 12–8, a total of fifty-nine individuals will be hired by the unit. In many instances the employees hired are either full-time or half-time. However, that is not always the case. A variety of staffing patterns are observed. For example, under fixed staff in Table 12–8, note that it is assumed that one secretary can be hired to work .8 FTEs on the 7–3 shift. On the 3–11 shift, it is expected that two part-time employees will split .8 FTEs, and on the 11–7 shift four employees will make up .8 FTEs. Under variable staff it is noted that even though twelve full-time staff nurses could have been hired for the 7–3 shift, two half-time positions are used. This may provide a greater degree of staffing flexibility for the manager.

Calculating Labor Cost

Once the positions have been identified, the next step is to determine the labor cost. This will include straight-time hours, overtime hours, differentials, premiums, and benefits.

Straight-time and Overtime Salaries

Table 12–8 indicates the paid hours related to the positions. These hours are calculated based on the number of FTEs for each position at a rate of 2,080 paid hours per FTE. For example, two part-time aide positions have been

Text continued on page 332

❖ TABLE 12–8
Positions and Hours Budget

Position Title	Shift	Number of Positions	ST FTEs	ST Hours	OT FTEs	OT Hours	Total FTEs	Total Hours
Fixed Staff								
Nurse manager	7–3	1	1.0	2,080	.0	0	1.0	2,080
Clinical specialist	7–3	1	1.0	2,080	.0	0	1.0	2,080
Clerk	7–3	1	1.0	2,080	.0	0	1.0	2,080
Secretary: full-time	7–3	1	1.0	2,080	.0	0	1.0	2,080
Secretary: part-time	7–3	1	.8	1,664	.0	0	.8	1,664
Secretary: full-time	3–11	1	1.0	2,080	.0	0	1.0	2,080
Secretary: part-time	3–11	2	.8	1,664	.0	0	.8	1,664
Secretary: full-time	11–7	1	1.0	2,080	.0	0	1.0	2,080
Secretary: part-time	11–7	4	.8	1,664	.0	0	.8	1,664
Subtotal		13	8.4	17,472	.0	0	8.4	17,472
Variable Staff								
Staff nurse: full-time	7–3	11	11.0	22,880	.3	624	11.2	23,296
Staff nurse: part-time	7–3	2	1.0	2,080	.0	0	1.1	2,288
Staff nurse: full-time	3–11	10	10.0	20,800	.1	208	10.1	21,008
Staff nurse: part-time	3–11	1	.5	1,040	.0	0	.5	1,040
Staff nurse: full-time	11–7	5	5.0	10,400	.3	624	5.3	11,024
Staff nurse: part-time	11–7	0	.0	0	.0	0	.0	0
LPN: full-time	7–3	5	5.0	10,400	.3	624	5.3	11,024
LPN: part-time	7–3	0	.0	0	.0	0	.0	0
LPN: full-time	3–11	3	3.0	6,240	.0	0	3.0	6,240
LPN: part-time	3–11	1	.5	1,040	.0	0	.5	1,040
LPN: full-time	11–7	1	1.0	2,080	.3	624	1.2	2,496
LPN: part-time	11–7	1	.5	1,040	.0	0	.6	1,248
Aide: full-time	7–3	1	1.0	2,080	.0	0	1.0	2,080
Aide: part-time	7–3	1	.8	1,664	.0	0	.8	1,664
Aide: full-time	3–11	1	1.0	2,080	.0	0	1.0	2,080
Aide: part-time	3–11	1	.8	1,664	.0	0	.8	1,664
Aide: full-time	11–7	0	.0	0	.0	0	.0	0
Aide: part-time	11–7	2	.9	1,872	.0	0	.9	1,872
Subtotal		46	42.0	87,360	1.3	2,704	43.3	90,064
Total		59	50.4	104,832	1.3	2,704	51.7	107,536

established on the 11–7 shift. Those two positions total .9 FTEs. Multiplying .9 by 2,080 hours results in a total of 1,872 paid straight-time hours for that employee type. It is important to know the paid hours for overtime separately from total paid hours because overtime is generally paid at a higher rate.

As a check in the process, it would be appropriate to determine if the number of care hours budgeted is approximately the number that had earlier been calculated as being required. Recall that for these 9,000 patients, it was determined that 71,830 care hours were needed. From Table 12–8 it is noted that the variable staff subtotal for total hours is 90,064. These represent paid hours. Since 80% of paid hours are productive, according to the earlier calculations, 80% of 90,064 is the budgeted number of care hours. Multiplying 80% by 90,064, the result is 72,051. This is almost exactly the required care hours.[6]

On the basis of hours by type of employee, a cost budget can be prepared. This can be done either by using an average wage rate by category or by listing each of the individuals who will fill the positions and specifying their exact pay rate. The latter approach is more time-consuming but also more accurate.[7] In Table 12–9 the straight-time (ST) and overtime (OT) hours are taken from Table 12–8, and an average wage is used for each class of employee for each shift. That average would generally be based on the manager's knowledge of the specific individuals making up each category.

The rates used in the budget should be based on the anticipated rates for the coming year. That rate includes any raises over current rates. In some cases raises are an across-the-board percentage. In other cases raises may differ by type of employee or even employee by employee.

In some cases, top management may change the amount of raises built into the operating budget. They may either raise or lower the amount of raises calculated in the initial preparation of the budget. This may require recalculation of the entire budget. It is advisable to prepare all budgets on computers, using a spreadsheet program such as the widely used LOTUS 1-2-3.[8] If such a program is used, hourly rates used in the budget preparation could be changed and a new budget generated without the manager's having to manually recompute the entire budget. Such a computerized approach is also advisable because it will ease the process of budget revision caused by any other changes in the budget as well.

Note that the wage rates for the same type of employee do tend to vary by shift and by whether the employee is full-time or part-time. Since part-time employees may not receive the same benefits as full-time employees (perhaps no pension, life-insurance, etc.), it may be necessary to pay a higher hourly wage to attract sufficient numbers of part-time employees. In some cases the less desirable shifts may be staffed by less senior staff, and therefore their base rate is lower than for those working on the day shift.

Such rate differences tend to be highly idiosyncratic. For instance, in this

---

[6]The difference of 221 care hours over the course of the year is a rounding error. We had originally expected to need 43.2 FTEs. The actual plan resulted in 43.3 FTEs, a minor difference.
[7]See Christina Graf, "The Operating Budget," in Steven A. Finkler, *Budgeting Concepts for Nurse Managers*, 2nd edition, W.B. Saunders, Philadelphia, 1992, p. 192, for an example of that detailed approach.
[8]LOTUS 1-2-3 is a registered trademark of the LOTUS Development Corp.

example the base pay rate for aides is the same on all shifts for both full-time and part-time. Part-time secretaries receive a lower hourly base wage than full-time. Part-time RNs and LPNs receive a higher hourly wage.

If positions are vacant, care must be exercised in selecting an appropriate pay rate. Will those positions most likely be filled by entry-level employees at the lowest wage rates or by experienced employees at higher pay levels? Managers should try to assess who will be hired to keep the budget as accurate as possible.

That assumes that vacancies are filled. In some cases, positions may remain open for some time. According to Graf, "If float, per diem or agency staff are used only rarely to cover temporarily vacant positions, then the dollars allocated to the vacant positions can be assumed to cover the alternate staff and the nurse manager can be authorized to hire into all positions.[9]

If it is known that a fair amount of per diem agency time will be used even if positions are not vacant, then those hours should be converted to FTEs and budgeted for in addition to the staffing shown in Table 12–8.

Differentials and Premiums

Table 12–9 provides a calculation of personnel cost based on average wage rates. Average rates can be obtained from the personnel or payroll offices or by simply averaging the specific rates paid to current staff members. It is common for health care organizations to provide a higher wage for evening and night shifts and sometimes for weekend shifts. There are two common approaches for including these costs in the budget. One is to calculate the total lump-sum cost of the differentials to the unit. The other approach is to adjust the hourly wage of employees to include the differential.

To calculate differentials on a lump-sum basis it would be necessary to calculate the number of evening and night hours by class of employee for all the days per year and multiply that by the differential for that class of employee. For example, in the shift premium column in Table 12–9 we note that secretaries on the night shift receive a $2 per hour differential. There are 2,080 and 1,664 total night hours scheduled for full-time and part-time secretaries, respectively. That adds up to 3,744 hours for the year. At $2 per hour differential, the night secretary differential will be $7,488 (i.e., $2 per hour multiplied by 3,744 hours). That amount and the differential for each other class of employee must be added into the total personnel cost. The lump-sum approach is especially useful if differentials are stated by the organization on an annual basis per FTE rather than on an hourly basis.

The alternative approach is to calculate the differentials as shown in Table 12–9. This figure specifically adjusts the straight-time hourly wage of each class of employee (column B) based on the appropriate shift differential (column C). This adjustment results in a total straight-time rate (column D) including the differential (i.e., column B + column C = column D).

In this example some differentials are a flat dollar amount and some are based on a percentage of base salary. In the case of secretaries, there is a $1 per hour premium for working the 3–11 shift and a $2 per hour premium for working the 11–7 shift. The clinical staff in this example receive a 10% differential for the 3–11 shift and a 15% differential for the 11–7 shift. For example,

---

[9]Graf, op. cit., p. 187.

Text continued on page 334

❖ TABLE 12–9
Personnel Cost Budget

Column:		A	B	C	D	E	F	G	H	I
Position Title	Shift	ST Hours	Average Rate	Shift Premium	Total ST Rate (B + C)	Total ST $ (A × D)	OT Hours	OT Rate (D × 1.5)	Total OT $ (F × G)	Total $ (E + H)
Fixed Staff										
Nurse manager	7–3	2,080	$28.00	$0.00	$28.00	$ 58,240	0	$ N/A	$ 0	$ 58,240
Clinical specialist	7–3	2,080	24.50	0.00	24.50	50,960	0	N/A	0	50,960
Clerk	7–3	2,080	6.50	0.00	6.50	13,520	0	9.75	0	13,520
Secretary: FT	7–3	2,080	11.00	0.00	11.00	22,880	0	16.50	0	22,880
Secretary: PT	7–3	1,664	10.00	0.00	10.00	16,640	0	15.00	0	16,640
Secretary: FT	3–11	2,080	11.00	1.00	12.00	24,960	0	18.00	0	24,960
Secretary: PT	3–11	1,664	10.00	1.00	11.00	18,304	0	16.50	0	18,304
Secretary: FT	11–7	2,080	11.00	2.00	13.00	27,040	0	19.50	0	27,040
Secretary: PT	11–7	1,664	10.00	2.00	12.00	19,968	0	18.00	0	19,968
Subtotal		17,472				$252,512	0		$ 0	$252,512

Variable Staff

	Shift									
Staff nurse: FT	7–3	22,880	$21.50	$0.00	$21.50	$ 491,920	624	$32.25	$20,124	$ 512,044
Staff nurse: PT	7–3	2,080	24.00	0.00	24.00	49,920	0	36.00	0	49,920
Staff nurse: FT	3–11	20,800	20.00	2.00	22.00	457,600	208	33.00	6,864	464,464
Staff nurse: PT	3–11	1,040	22.00	2.20	24.20	25,168	0	36.30	0	25,168
Staff nurse: FT	11–7	10,400	18.50	2.78	21.28	221,260	624	31.91	19,913	241,173
Staff nurse: PT	11–7	0	20.00	3.00	23.00	0	0	34.50	0	0
LPN: full-time	7–3	10,400	14.00	0.00	14.00	145,600	624	21.00	13,104	158,704
LPN: part-time	7–3	0	15.00	0.00	15.00	0	0	22.50	0	0
LPN: full-time	3–11	6,240	13.50	1.35	14.85	92,664	0	22.28	0	92,664
LPN: part-time	3–11	1,040	14.00	1.40	15.40	16,016	0	23.10	0	16,016
LPN: full-time	11–7	2,080	13.00	1.95	14.95	31,096	624	22.43	13,993	45,089
LPN: part-time	11–7	1,040	14.00	2.10	16.10	16,744	0	24.15	0	16,744
Aide: full-time	7–3	2,080	8.00	0.00	8.00	16,640	0	12.00	0	16,640
Aide: part-time	7–3	1,664	8.00	0.00	8.00	13,312	0	12.00	0	13,312
Aide: full-time	3–11	2,080	8.00	.80	8.80	18,304	0	13.20	0	18,304
Aide: part-time	3–11	1,664	8.00	.80	8.80	14,643	0	13.20	0	14,643
Aide: full-time	11–7	0	8.00	1.20	9.20	0	0	13.80	0	0
Aide: part-time	11–7	1,872	8.00	1.20	9.20	17,222	0	13.80	0	17,222
Subtotal		87,360				$1,628,110	2,704		$73,999	$1,702,108
Total		104,832				$1,880,622	2,704		$73,999	$1,954,620

note in column C of Table 12–9 that a full-time 3–11 shift LPN, paid a base wage of $13.50, earns a shift differential of 10%, or $1.35 per hour, while a full-time 11–7 shift LPN, paid a base wage of $13.00, earns a shift differential of 15%, or $1.95 per hour. The ST rate from column D, which includes the differential, is multiplied by the straight-time hours from column A (taken from Table 12–8) to find the cost of straight-time wages (column E).

An overtime rate is calculated in column G by multiplying the column D straight-time rate by 1.5. The resulting overtime rate is multiplied by the column F overtime hours, which came from Table 12–8, to find total overtime dollars (column H). The column I combination of straight-time and overtime wages gives the total of these two cost elements.

Overtime in this example was calculated at time and a half. In some organizations the straight-time salary is increased by 50% for overtime, and then the shift differential is added. If the differential is added to the straight-time salary and then the rate was increased by 50%, the resulting wage is higher than if the differentials are added after the salary has been multiplied by 150%.

Weekend differentials, holiday premiums, and on-call premiums create additional complexities in the calculations of personnel cost. A complete budget will consider all factors that affect the total salary received by each employee in each position. The specific approach to calculating these premiums differs from organization to organization. Effectively, however, the manager must determine the hourly differential or premium; the number of weekend, holiday, and on-call shifts per year; the number of employees on each of those shifts; and the total cost of those differentials. That total cost must be added into the budget for the unit.

Fringe Benefits

An additional element of personnel cost is fringe benefits. Fringe benefits are costs of employees in addition to their salary. Fringes typically include health and life insurance, pension costs, Social Security (FICA) payments, and other employee benefits. Generally, an average fringe benefit rate is calculated and applied on a uniform basis to payroll costs. The calculation of the fringe benefit rate itself is generally performed by the finance or payroll departments. In some organizations those departments adjust the budgets of each department or unit to include fringes. In other cases they communicate the rate, and the unit or department managers increase their budgets by the amount of the fringe benefits.

For example, Table 12–10 shows the addition of fringes to personnel cost in our example. In this organization, two different fringe benefits rates are used, one for full-time and one for part-time personnel. Frequently, part-time employees receive substantially fewer benefits than full-time employees. By calculating two rates to be used, the manager realizes the financial impact on the organization of the decision of using full-time vs. part-time personnel to provide the needed FTEs. Keep in mind, however, that there is a trade-off, as noted earlier. While part-time employees have a lower fringe benefit cost to the organization, they may have a higher hourly base salary.

In Table 12–10, the total personnel costs before fringe benefits (column A) is from the last column in Table 12–9 (column I). Those costs (column A, Table 12–10) are multiplied by the appropriate fringe benefit rate to find fringe benefit costs (column C). The cost before fringe benefits (column A) plus the fringe benefit cost (column C) is the total personnel cost (column D).

Special Situations

A variety of specific situations may cause the manager to need to make additional calculations. An important element of the budget process is for the manager to think about various additional costs that are incurred every year but not included or accounted for in the budget. Such hidden costs can result in a failure to meet the budget. However, the failure is not the result of poor control of operations but rather poor planning. To avoid such problems it is essential that managers understand how their staff uses its time and whether any factors are not adequately accounted for in the existing budget formulation.

EXPENSE BUDGET—OTHER-THAN-PERSONNEL SERVICES

The personnel budget is often by far the largest part of the operating budget for a nursing unit or department. However, a complete budget also requires inclusion of a budget for expenses for other-than-personnel services. The nurse manager should exercise care in this portion of the budget, even if it is substantially smaller than the personnel budget. Miscalculations made in this element of the budget may lead to a need to cut back costs during the year. Often such cutbacks can only be made in the area of personnel. Thus, an underestimated budget for clinical supplies may negatively impact on a nursing unit's ability to provide high-quality care.

The nonpersonnel portion of the operating budget, often called the OTPS budget (other-than-personnel services), includes a wide variety of items, such as clinical supplies, office supplies, minor equipment (noncapital budget items), seminars, books, and a variety of *overhead* items. Overhead are indirect costs charged to the unit or department from other departments. Some overhead is at least partly controllable by the unit, such as the cost of laundry. The more laundry used by a department, the higher the overhead charge for laundry. Other elements of overhead are completely outside the unit manager's control, such as administrative salary or building depreciation charges.

OTPS expenses may be either fixed or variable items. Clinical supplies, for example, are variable. Their cost should be determined based on the expected number and mix of patients. Publications for the nursing department are a fixed cost. Assuming that publications (such as management journals or newsletters) are ordered by the organization only for the use of managers, then the number of patients would have no effect on that cost. Managers must determine a budgeted amount for publications on a somewhat more subjective basis.

Table 12–11 provides a budget worksheet for OTPS costs. This worksheet is generally a summary of detailed supporting schedules providing calculations for each of the lines in the worksheet. The worksheet provides information on actual costs incurred to date, the budget for the current year, a projection of total costs for the current year, and the proposed budget for the coming year.

The projection for the current year can be done in one of two ways. The simpler approach is to divide the current year-to-date actual result by the number of months it covers to get an average monthly amount. That amount could then be multiplied by twelve to get an annual projection. A more accurate

Text continued on page 339

❖ TABLE 12–10
Personnel Cost Budget (Including Fringes)

Position Title	Shift	A Total Cost before Fringes	B Fringe Rate	C Fringe $ (A × B)	D Total Personnel Cost (A + C)
Column:					
Fixed Staff					
Nurse manager	7–3	$ 58,240	23.5%	$ 13,686	$ 71,926
Clinical specialist	7–3	50,960	23.5	11,976	62,936
Clerk	7–3	13,520	23.5	3,177	16,697
Secretary: FT	7–3	22,880	23.5	5,377	28,257
Secretary: PT	7–3	16,640	14.3	2,380	19,020
Secretary: FT	3–11	24,960	23.5	5,866	30,826
Secretary: PT	3–11	18,304	14.3	2,617	20,921
Secretary: FT	11–7	27,040	23.5	6,354	33,394
Secretary: PT	11–7	19,968	14.3	2,855	22,823
Subtotal		$ 252,512		$ 54,288	$ 306,800

Variable Staff

Staff nurse: FT	7–3	$ 512,044	23.5%	$120,330	$ 632,274
Staff nurse: PT	7–3	49,920	14.3	7,139	57,059
Staff nurse: FT	3–11	464,464	23.5	109,149	573,613
Staff nurse: PT	3–11	25,168	14.3	3,599	28,767
Staff nurse: FT	11–7	241,230	23.5	56,676	297,849
Staff nurse: PT	11–7	0	14.3	0	0
LPN: full-time	7–3	158,704	23.5	37,295	195,999
LPN: part-time	7–3	0	14.3	0	0
LPN: full-time	3–11	92,664	23.5	21,776	114,440
LPN: part-time	3–11	16,016	14.3	2,290	18,306
LPN: full-time	11–7	45,089	23.5	10,596	55,685
LPN: part-time	11–7	16,744	14.3	2,394	19,138
Aide: full-time	7–3	16,640	23.5	3,910	20,550
Aide: part-time	7–3	13,312	14.3	1,904	15,216
Aide: full-time	3–11	18,304	23.5	4,301	22,605
Aide: part-time	3–11	14,643	14.3	2,094	16,737
Aide: full-time	11–7	0	23.5	0	0
Aide: part-time	11–7	17,222	14.3	2,463	19,685
Subtotal		$1,702,108		$385,917	$2,088,025
Total		$1,954,620		$440,205	$2,394,826

TABLE 12–11
OTPS Costs

	Year-to-Date Actual	Current Year Budget	Current Year Projection	Proposed Budget
Direct Unit Expenses				
Med/surg supplies	$126,533	$187,546	$191,249	$216,237
Office supplies	8,348	12,493	13,021	15,027
Noncapital equipment	14,325	17,094	17,000	18,255
Seminars	23,450	28,000	27,655	30,000
Publications	1,788	2,000	2,000	2,100
Other	7,351	10,000	10,000	10,500
Total direct unit OTPS	$181,795	$257,133	$260,925	$292,119
Overhead Expenses				
Administration	$ 28,345	$ 42,517	$ 43,394	$ 45,234
Depreciation—buildings	34,592	51,888	51,888	51,888
Depreciation—equipment	18,492	27,738	27,738	29,956
Laundry	13,295	21,340	22,431	24,390
Pharmacy	8,391	12,309	13,125	14,150
Laboratory	11,090	14,398	15,232	16,342
Duplication	3,113	4,310	4,100	4,100
Communications	14,321	19,430	19,834	21,079
Other	8,310	12,321	12,500	12,857
Total overhead OTPS	$139,949	$206,251	$210,242	$207,139
Total OTPS	$321,744	$463,384	$471,167	$499,258

approach would be to assess whether the remaining months of the year are likely to be busier or slower than the year has averaged up to the current time. The projected annual totals could be estimated after adjusting for expected activity levels. These two approaches are primarily useful for variable costs.

For fixed costs, the manager must determine the typical expenditure patterns. If these costs are incurred reasonably evenly throughout the year, the average monthly approach is adequate. If all seminars and meetings take place during certain months of the year, then a specific calculation of remaining seminars will need to be made to project the current year total. Similarly, if publications and equipment are all purchased near the beginning of the year (to have their benefit throughout the year) or near the end of the year (after the manager has a feeling for whether spending cuts will be needed near year-end), then the manager will have to take those factors into account in making the current year projection.

Developing an accurate current year projection is worth a reasonable effort because it is an important starting point in planning the OTPS costs for the coming year. Much of that cost is based on an increase or decrease as compared to current-year spending. If the level of photocopying stays the same from year to year, then this year's actual duplication costs serve as a primary guide to developing next year's budget.

Costs for the coming year can be developed based on sophisticated forecasting techniques (see Chapter 17), which rely on historical and current information as well as the manager's knowledge and intuition. A simpler, although possibly less accurate, approach is to project next year's budgeted cost as being the current-year cost increased by a percentage for inflation.

In some instances the manager will be able to prepare a budget based on specific circumstances. If turnover is expected to be unusually high because of planned retirements and/or maternity leave, then a higher budget for training new staff may be necessary. The specific number of individuals who will need such training can be estimated and a budget developed. That number may not bear much relation to costs incurred currently or in the recent past. Rather, the costs will relate primarily to the number of new staff. As Graf points out:

> The key to budgeting nonsalary expenses . . . is to identify the most reasonable predictor . . . and to make expense projections based on that predictor. In some cases, more than one predictor may be needed. For example, assume that the delivery room's disposable linen account includes linen packs for . . . deliveries and . . . scrub clothes packs for fathers attending deliveries. The predictor for the linen packs is logically the number of deliveries. . . . The predictor for the scrub clothes packs, however, may be the attendance at prepared childbirth classes.[10]

The predictor approach will be quite useful for some OTPS accounts, but noncapital equipment typically requires a more direct approach. During the current year managers should accumulate lists of noncapital equipment needed for the unit. Any such items that cannot be accommodated during the current year within the existing budget would be explicitly included in the operating budget for the coming year. In addition, at budget preparation time the manager should consider and specify equipment needs. Therefore, this category is less

---

[10]Ibid., p. 196.

likely to be just a repeat of the prior year adjusted for patient volume and/or inflation, in contrast to a category such as med/surg supplies.

REVENUE BUDGET

Nursing is critical to the revenues of the organization. Without a nursing staff providing services, it is unlikely that hospitals, nursing homes, home care agencies, or a number of other kinds of health care organizations would be able to provide care and earn revenues. However, the association of revenues with nurses has been uneven. Some nurse managers have always had revenue responsibility—a few examples include the OR, outpatient surgery, and clinics managed by nurses. In other cases, nursing has little if any revenue responsibility.

Even in cases where nursing does not have to calculate revenue for the budget or control revenue results, it is important for nurse managers to learn about the key determinants of revenue in their organization. The revenue base is critical to the organization's survival and its ability to provide resources to the various departments.

In recent years revenue has become more and more of a direct concern for nurse managers. Patient classification systems have substantially increased the feasibility of variable billing for nursing services. Rather than simply including nursing as a part of the per diem charge, it is possible to charge patients for nursing each day at different amounts based on their classification for that day (see the discussion of variable billing in Chapter 8). As a result, organizations are starting to bill directly for nursing care, and nurse managers are becoming more involved in the revenue aspects of the budget.

Calculation of Budgeted Revenue

Gross patient revenue is the number of units of service times the price per unit. As discussed in Chapter 6, there are a variety of reasons for the net revenue received being less than gross patient revenues. Those reasons include contractual allowances, bad debts, and indigent care. Generally, nurse managers do not have to calculate reductions from gross revenues.

On the other hand, the units of service that are useful for estimating the expense portion of the budget are not necessarily appropriate for the revenue part of the budget. For example, the OR may calculate its expense budget by considering the number of each type of procedure it expects to have, with differing staffing and supplies costs for different types of procedures. However, patients are generally charged based on minutes or hours of operations. Therefore the OR would have to estimate both the total numbers of hours of operations (to get a revenue budget) and the total number of each type of procedure (to develop an expense budget).

In health care organizations, departments do not generally set prices. The prices the organization charges are set by the finance department based on a large number of factors, including government reimbursement regulations, prices of competitors, and a need to earn enough revenues in total to cover all costs and allow for desired expansions and improvements, if possible.

For example, the federal government sets the rates for Medicare hospital inpatients under the DRG system. Those rates cover the entire stay of the patient, and they are not broken out separately by unit or department. Similarly, state governments generally set rates for Medicaid patients. Health care organizations must estimate the amount that they expect to receive from those patients for whom they cannot set the price, such as Medicare and Medicaid patients. They then set prices for the remaining patients high enough to bring in remaining revenues needed by the organization to carry out its mission.

Even when revenues are per patient, such as DRG revenues, many health care organizations do have prices for the various services provided by many departments. Different services provided by a department will have different prices. In preparing a revenue budget it is necessary to get a price list from the finance office and apply it individually to each different type of patient. For example, there is likely to be a different standard charge for different types of outpatient surgery. Once the revenue for each type of service is determined, the revenue for all the different services can be summed to arrive at total budgeted department revenue.

Variable Billing

The increasingly widespread use of patient classification systems not only provides information for calculating staffing needs and personnel costs more accurately but also provides an ability to charge directly for nursing services. The main constraint most health care organizations face with respect to charging for nursing services (as opposed to lumping them in with per diem costs) is the fact that there is no ready way to determine the different nursing costs the organization incurs for different patients. Patient classification systems eliminate that problem.

When patients are charged for various types of health care services, there is generally an attempt to charge patients for the resources they consumed. If a patient does not have an operation, there is no surgery charge. A patient who has a more expensive operation than another is charged a higher amount. Patients are charged for the number and type of x-rays, lab tests, and drugs they consume. As long as patients consume different amounts of a resource and those differences can be measured, then patients can reasonably be charged for the resources they consume. If those requirements are not met, then costs are frequently lumped together in a catchall category such as the per diem charge.

It is clear that different patients consume different amounts of nursing care. Historically, however, there was not a reasonable method available to determine the differing nursing resources consumed by different patients. To track nursing resources consumed would have required extensive data-collection efforts at an extremely high cost.

Patient classification systems provide a solution to this problem. It is not necessary to measure the actual nursing costs of each individual patient. Instead, a special study establishes the average relative consumption of nursing resources by patients in each classification level. Suppose that a hospital's patient classification system indicates that level 2 patients consume 4.7 hours of care on average and level 4 patients consume three times as much care. A charging system can be established with patients being charged three times as much for each day that they are classed as level 4 as they are charged for each day that they are classed as level 2.

A number of hospitals have started to budget and charge for revenue based

❖ TABLE 12–12
Variable Billing Revenue Calculation

Patient Classification	Number of Patient Days	×	Charge per 24-hour Period	=	Budgeted Revenue
1	1,100		$ 150		$ 165,000
2	3,000		250		750,000
3	2,600		500		1,300,000
4	1,400		700		980,000
5	900		1,100		990,000
Total	9,000				$4,185,000

on variable billing tied to patient classification. The process is not complicated. Suppose that the hospital established nursing rates, based on an examination of nursing department costs, of $150 for a patient day at level 1, $250 for a patient day at level 2, $500 for level 3, $700 for level 4, and $1,100 for level 5, for a typical med/surg unit. Assuming the same mix of patients used in the example earlier in this chapter, budgeted revenue could be calculated as in Table 12–12.

BUDGET SUBMISSION, NEGOTIATION, AND APPROVAL

The three elements of the operating budget—personnel services expenses, other-than-personnel services, and revenues—must be compiled into a coherent total document for submission. The budget may not be accepted as submitted, in which case a period of negotiation and budget revision will take place. Finally the budget is approved.

The submitted budget should include an overview page that summarizes the revenues and expenses of the unit or department. In some cases, only expenses will be calculated at the unit or department level, and revenues will not be part of the operating budget process. In addition to the budget's overview or summary page there should be detailed schedules that support the requested amounts. Each number from the summary page should be easily traceable to its supporting documentation through titles on the supporting schedules and/or by a series of references.

The supporting schedules should contain not only numerical calculations, like those which appear in Tables 12–3 through 12–12, but also narrative support. The narrative would define the unit of service used for the budget, the sources of projections for the coming year, and explanations of why the requested amounts are needed. It should also discuss the ramifications of denying the full requested amounts.

Negotiation of the budget will usually follow its submission. Because health care organizations' resources are limited, requests for funds are often in excess of the amount available. The subsequent reductions in the budget requests should be done in a way that best allows the organization to accomplish its goals and objectives. The budget negotiation process was discussed in Chapter 11.

Once the budget has completed the negotiation and revision process, it will be approved by top management and the board. If they do not approve the submitted budget, it must be further revised until it is approved. The manager must then implement the approved budget.

IMPLEMENTING THE APPROVED BUDGET

The development of the operating budget and its ultimate approval are in many ways just the beginning of the budget management process. The manager must convert the approved resources into a working document that can guide specific staffing decisions throughout the year.

The manager must address a number of specific problems. First, a staffing schedule must be developed to allow the number of positions approved to be used to fill the daily staffing need. Recall that in the example there was a need for 30.5 shifts per day on average (including fixed staff [see Table 12–5]) and a total of fifty-nine staff positions to fill those shifts. It is necessary to determine when those fifty-nine individuals will be working.

That is a complicated task. Not only must there be coverage seven days per week, but holiday and vacation coverage must also be planned. Further, there must be flexibility to deal with sick leave, which does not occur on a planned basis. If turnover is expected, the manager must also be able to deal with low productivity of new workers during their orientation period.

An additional complicating factor is the seasonal nature of many health care organizations. There are busy periods and slow periods. Adequate staff must be available to work the busier periods; that requires maintaining a lower staffing level during slower periods. Sometimes that problem can be somewhat offset by using float pools, which allow for "borrowing" nurses from other units during busy periods and "loaning" nurses to other units during slow periods. That, however, requires a commitment on the part of the nursing department and the nursing staff to cross training.

Finally, a key element of the implementation process is control. An attempt must be made to keep as close to the approved plan as possible. Control aspects of budgeting are discussed in the next chapter.

IMPLICATIONS FOR NURSE MANAGERS

The operating budget often consumes more of a nurse manager's time than any other aspect of financial management. For that reason it is worthy of special attention. The three aspects of operating budgets are revenues, personnel expenses, and other-than-personnel expenses.

Revenue is becoming more important to nurse managers. For many years health care organizations received revenues as a reimbursement for costs. Governments and large third-party payers such as Blue Cross based the amount paid to health care organizations directly on the costs those organizations incurred. Recent years have seen a movement away from cost reimbursement. As a result, revenues must be managed to a greater extent. Over time, this will likely lead to more nursing involvement in the area of organizational revenues. At a minimum, nurse managers should prepare operating budgets with an understanding of the implications of the budgets for revenue.

Some proposed changes in operating budgets will lead to changes in revenues, and other changes will not. It is vital for nurse managers to consider whether a proposed change impacts on both costs and revenues or solely on costs. Cutting costs may seem to promote organizational efficiency, but one must consider whether the expense reduction will impact on the organization's revenues.

For example, suppose that hours per patient day of care were decreased to reduce costs. This might lead to a longer length of stay. The extra days would be costly in themselves. Furthermore, if the hospital had high occupancy, the increased length of stay would reduce the number of possible admissions. That would have a direct negative impact on revenues.

Increasing expenses may seem to jeopardize the organization's finances, but once again the short-run and long-run impact on revenues must be considered. Spending money to increase quality of care, for example, may improve the organization's reputation, leading ultimately to more patients and more revenues. Spending money to provide more nursing care hours per day may shorten average length of stay, allowing for more patients and therefore more revenues.

In placing a growing focus on revenues, the nurse manager must not reduce the effort spent on budgeting unit or departmental expenses. Nursing departments have the largest budget in many health care organizations. The amounts spent by nursing can have a dramatic impact on the organization. A 5% change, either up or down, in the costs of the nursing department will affect the organization by a greater total dollar amount than a 5% change in any other area. As a result, nurses have an obligation equal to that of other managers throughout the organization to carefully consider the resources needed by their units or departments to provide patient care.

The largest element of nursing operating budgets usually is labor. Personnel costs dominate, largely because the clinical care provided by the nurse is essential to the process of providing health care services. To account for labor costs as carefully as is warranted requires a lengthy and complicated budgeting process. A work-load budget must be developed specifying care hours needed. The work-load estimate must be as accurate as possible, adjusting for patient mix whenever possible. Care hours are converted to FTEs and positions. FTEs and positions are converted to dollar costs.

The process as described in this chapter is laborious for the manager. However, it is essential. Two critical things are at stake in the proper preparation of the personnel budget for nursing. One is the ability of the organization to survive; the other is the ability of the organization to provide patients with high-quality care.

Budgets not prepared with the greatest measure of care may lead to wasted resources. Overstaffing on one shift or one unit is a mistake that may lead to understaffing elsewhere due to inadequate total resources. The budgeting process attempts to allocate the organization's scarce resources to the areas where they are most needed to achieve the organization's objectives. Any resources allocated to a unit where they are not essential represent a failure to allocate those resources to parts of the organization where patients had a greater need for them.

The goal of budgeting is neither to maximize nor to minimize a budget. It is important for managers to overcome the adversarial impulse that naturally arises in the budgeting process. The goal of budgeting is to develop a plan that places the organization's available resources in the appropriate places where the sum total accomplishment of the organization goal's will be the greatest.

KEY CONCEPTS —————————————————————————

Workload budget   Budget that indicates the amount of work performed by a unit or department, measured in terms of units of service. This information is used to prepare expense budgets.

Activity report   Measures key statistics concerning current activity. It centers on the number of units of service and the relative proportion of the organization's capacity being used.

> **Average daily census (ADC)**   Number of patients cared for per day on average over a period of time.

> **Average length of stay (ALOS)**   Average number of days that each patient is in a hospital or nursing home.

Adjusted units of service   Whenever possible budgeting should be based on expected workload units of service adjusted for the specific mix of patients expected.

Care hours calculation   Determination of the average required care hours per patient per twenty-four hours for each classification level and the total required care hours for all patients.

Expense budget—personnel services   Budget for all personnel under the manager's direction.

> **Variable staff**   Staff needed to provide the required number of care hours, calculated as follows:
>
> 1. Determine the number of paid hours per FTE.
> 2. Determine the percentage of productive hours to total paid hours.
> 3. Multiply the number of paid hours per FTE by the percentage of productive hours to find the number of productive hours per FTE.
> 4. Divide required care hours by productive hours per FTE to find the required number of FTEs.
> 5. Divide the required care hours by the number of days per year that the unit has patients to find care hours per day. Divide that result by hours per shift to find the number of person shifts needed per working day.
> 6. Assign staff by employee type and among required shifts per day.

> **Fixed staff**   In addition to the staff calculated above, there are employees who do not vary with the patient volume.

> **Establishing positions**   Number of staff required per day can be filled by a variety of full-time and part-time positions that total to the required number of FTEs. The breakdown between full-time and part-time is at the manager's discretion.

> **Calculating labor cost**   Each position's hours must then be converted to a dollar basis considering the straight-time salary, overtime rate, differentials, raises, and fringe benefit costs for each employee type.

Expense budget—other-than-personnel services Budget for all expenses for other-than-personnel services, including both direct unit or department expenses and indirect overhead expenses.

Revenue budget Plan for the unit's or department's revenues for the budget year. Variable billing is leading to an increased role of revenues in nursing budgets.

Budget submission Revenue and expense portions of the budget must be summarized and submitted for review together with detailed supporting calculations and narrative justification. Budget revisions may be required as the result of a series of negotiations over the submitted budget.

Budget implementation Managers must address a number of issues in implementing an approved budget, including development of a staffing plan that provides coverage for staff weekends, holidays, vacations, and sick leave as well as busy and slow periods.

SUGGESTED READINGS

Beck, Donald F., *Basic Hospital Financial Management*, Aspen Systems Corp., Rockville, MD, 1980.

Berman, Howard J., Lewis E. Weeks, and Steven F. Kukla, *The Financial Management of Hospitals*, 7th edition, Health Administration Press, Ann Arbor, MI, 1990.

Bryans, William, "Budgeting for Beginners: Checking Your Budget," *Nursing Times*, Vol. 82, No. 14, April 2–8, 1986, pp. 60–61.

Bryans, William, "Budgeting for Beginners: Finance for Managers," *Nursing Times*, Vol. 81, No. 37, September 11–17, 1985, pp. 28–29.

Covaleski, Mark A., and Mark W. Dirsmith, "Building Tents for Nursing Services Through Budgeting Negotiation Skills," *Nursing Administration Quarterly.* Vol. 8, No. 2, Winter 1984, pp 1–11.

Denies, E., *Staffing for DRG's: Unit-Specific Approach for Nurse Managers*, Grune & Stratton, Orlando, 1983.

Dominiak, Geraldine F., and Joseph G. Louderback, *Managerial Accounting*, 5th edition, PWS-Kent Publishing Co., Boston, 1988.

Esmond, Truman H., Jr., *Budgeting Procedures for Hospitals*, American Hospital Association, Chicago, 1982.

Etheridge, Phyllis, "The Case For Billing by Patient Acuity," *Nursing Management*, Vol. 16, No. 8, August 1985, pp. 38–41.

Finkler, Steven A., *Budgeting Concepts for Nurse Managers*, 2nd edition, W.B. Saunders, Philadelphia, 1992.

Finkler, Steven A., "Electronic Spreadsheets and Budgeting: A Case Study," *Nursing Economics*, Vol. 2, No. 3, May/June 1984, pp. 166–174.

Herkimer, Allen G., *Understanding Health Care Budgeting*, Aspen Publishers, Rockville, MD, 1988.

Hutto, Christine Bowers, and Linda Lindsey Davis, "12 Hour Shifts: A Panacea or Problems," *Nursing Management*, Vol. 20, No. 8, August 1989, pp. 56A,D,F,H.

Kirby, Karen, and L. Wiczai, "Budgeting and Variable Staffing," *Nursing Economics*, Vol. 3, No. 3, May/June 1985, pp. 160–166.

Kirk, Roey, *Nurse Staffing and Budgeting: Practical Management Tools*, Aspen Publishers, Rockville, MD, 1986.

Kirk, Roey, "Using Workload Analysis and Acuity Systems to Facilitate Quality and Productivity," *Journal of Nursing Administration*, Vol. 30, No. 3, March 1990, pp. 21–30.

McCabe, J.P., and J.L.P. Hartnack, "FTE Reports and Fiscal Management," *Nursing Management*, November 1989, Vol. 20, No. 11, pp. 46–48.

McGrail, G., "Budgets: An Underused Resource," *Journal of Nursing Administration*, Vol. 18, No. 11, November 1988, pp. 25–31.

Stevens, Barbara J., "What Is the Executive's Role in Budgeting for Her Department?" *Journal of Nursing Administration*, Vol. 11, No. 7, July 1981, pp. 22–24.

Villemaire, Mary, and Charlotte Lane-McGraw, "Nursing Personnel Budgets: A Step-by-Step Guide," *Nursing Management*, Vol. 17, No. 11, November 1986, pp. 28–32.

Wanat, John, *Introduction to Budgeting*, Brooks/Cole Publishing Co., Monterey, CA, 1978.

13

Controlling Operating Results

CHAPTER GOALS

The goals of this chapter are to:

- ♦ Introduce the concept of management control systems
- ♦ Explain the role of employee motivation in control
- ♦ Explore alternative incentive systems, including their strengths and weaknesses
- ♦ Consider the negative implications of unrealistic expectations
- ♦ Discuss the role of communication in the control process
- ♦ Clarify the importance of interim evaluation
- ♦ Define variance analysis and explain the reasons for doing variance analysis
- ♦ Discuss traditional variance analysis
- ♦ Outline some possible causes of variances
- ♦ Explain flexible budgeting
- ♦ Introduce flexible budget variance analysis notation
- ♦ Define volume, quantity, and price variances
- ♦ Provide variance analysis tools and examples
- ♦ Provide insight into the problems encountered when variance information is aggregated
- ♦ Introduce the concept of exception reports and explain their benefits
- ♦ Discuss revenue variances

INTRODUCTION

Organizations exercise control over operations through the use of a *management control system*. Such a system is a complete set of policies and procedures designed to keep operations going according to plan. Furthermore, a management control system detects any variations from plan and provides managers with information needed to take corrective actions when necessary.

The focus of health care management control systems is on *responsibility accounting*. Responsibility accounting is the assignment of the responsibility for keeping to the plan and carrying out the elements of the management control system. Such responsibility is generally assigned to managers of cost centers. This chapter discusses a variety of elements of the management control system, with a special emphasis on a system for motivating managers and staff and on variance analysis techniques.

THE BUDGET AS A TOOL FOR MOTIVATION

The budgeting process primarily concerns individuals, not numbers. If the employees of an organization do not work to make the organization succeed, the numbers constituting a budget will have little relevance. Motivation of staff and managers cannot be overemphasized. If *people* are not motivated to carry out the budget, it is likely to fail. That is why budgets arbitrarily imposed from above without fair consideration of input from those expected to carry them out tend to do so poorly. It is why such a sense of frustration exists when managers are denied the needed authority to go along with their responsibility. It is why budget flexibility is needed in the face of changing realities. Motivation is the critical underlying key to budget success.

Control is complicated by the fact that individuals act in their own self-interest. The primary goal of the nursing staff may be to help patients. However, they will have other goals as well. It is the basic nature of individuals for their own personal goals to be different from the goals of the organization they work for (see Fig. 13–1). This does not mean that human nature is bad but only that there is such a thing as human nature and one is foolish to refuse to recognize it as such.

For example, other things being equal, most employees of a hospital would prefer a salary substantially larger than they are currently receiving. There is nothing particularly wrong in their wanting more money. In fact, ambition is probably a desirable trait among staff. Most nurse managers would like more staff to carry out their existing functions. However, all organizations must make choices concerning how to spend their limited resources.

Health care organizations will not provide employees with 100% raises because they lack the revenues to pay for those raises. While the nursing staff is not wrong to desire the raises, the organization is not wrong to deny them.

Thus the fact must be faced that even where morale is generally excellent and is not considered a problem, an underlying tension will naturally exist. Even though the employees may want to achieve the mission of the organization in providing care, their personal desires will be for things the organization will choose not to provide. This is referred to as *goal divergence*.

Figure 13–1. Divergent goals.

The organization must bring together the interests of the individual and its own interests so that they can work together. In the budgeting process there must be some motivation for the people involved to want to control costs. Bringing the individuals' and organization's wants and desires together is referred to as *goal congruence* (Fig. 13–2). To be sure that the human beings will in fact want to control organizational costs, managers need to make sure that it is somehow in their direct best interests for costs to be controlled. Organizations generally achieve such congruence by setting up a system of incentives that make employees want to work toward the best interests of the organization.

MOTIVATION AND INCENTIVES

Although nurses are motivated by factors other than money, it would be foolish to ignore the potential of monetary rewards to influence behavior. As health care organizations search for the proper mix of incentives that will motivate managers and staff to control costs, financial incentives are frequently

CONGRUENT GOALS

Organization   Individual

INCENTIVE EFFECT

Figure 13–2.   Congruent goals.

employed. The most basic financial incentives are the ability to retain a job and to get a good raise.

Another motivating tool is a bonus system. Since managers have many desires that relate to spending more money (e.g., larger offices, fancier furniture, larger staffs), formalized approaches need to be developed that will provide incentives to spend less money. For example, one can tell a nurse manager that last year the manager's department spent $2 million and that next year its budget is $2,080,000 (a 4% increase). However, for any amount that the department spends below $2,080,000, the manager and the staff can keep 10% of the savings. If spending is below the budgeted $2,080,000, the nurses benefit and the organization benefits. In this case goal congruence is likely to be achieved.

Many health care organizations have added bonus systems. These have both positives and negatives. The positives relate primarily to the strong motivation employees have to reduce hospital costs. The negatives relate to the potential detriment to quality of patient care and to the potential negative effect on employee morale.

When an incentive is given to accomplish one end, sometimes the responses to that incentive are unexpected. Bonus systems may give a nurse manager an incentive to provide less staff nurse time per patient day. Health care organizations must be concerned about the impact their incentives will have on the quality of patient care. A strong internal quality assurance program is essential.

Further, bonuses are not necessarily the solution to all motivational problems. If everyone gets a bonus, then no one feels that individual actions have much impact. As long as everyone else holds costs in check, all individuals may feel that they do not have to work particularly hard to reap the benefits of the bonus. On the other hand, bonuses given only to some employees may create jealousy and discontent. This may create a competitive environment in a situation in which teamwork is needed to provide high-quality care.

There are incentive alternatives to bonuses. For example, one underused managerial tool is a letter from supervisor to subordinate. All individuals responsible for controlling costs should be explicitly evaluated with respect to how well they do in fact control costs. That evaluation should be communicated in writing. This approach, which is both the carrot and the stick, costs little to implement but can have a dramatic impact.

Telling managers that they did a good job and that their boss knows that they did a good job can be an effective way to get the manager to try to do a good job the next year. In the real world praise is cheap and in many cases effective. On the other hand, criticism, especially in writing, can have a stinging effect that managers and staff will work hard to avoid in the future.

MOTIVATION AND UNREALISTIC EXPECTATIONS

While motivational devices can work wonders at getting an organization's staff to work hard for the organization and its goals, they can also backfire and have negative results. This occurs primarily when expectations are placed at unreasonably high levels.

A target that requires hard work and stretching but is achievable can be a useful motivating tool. If the target is reached, there might be a bonus, or there should be at least some formal recognition of the achievement, such as a letter. At a minimum, the worker will have the self-satisfaction of having worked hard and reached the target.

But all those positive outcomes can occur only if the target is reachable. Some health care organizations have adopted the philosophy that if a high target makes people work hard, a higher target will make them work harder. This may not be the case. If targets are placed out of reach, this will probably *not* result in people reaching to their utmost limits to come as close to the target as possible.

It may seem as if the organization is shortchanging itself whenever someone achieves a target. The manager may think, "We set the target too low. Perhaps if the target were higher, this person would have achieved the higher target. Since the target we set was achieved, we haven't yet realized all of their potential." There are risks associated with that logic.

If people fail to meet a target because they are not very competent or because they do not work very hard, the signal of failure sent is warranted. In fact, repeated failure may be grounds for replacement of that individual in that job. But if a manager is both competent and hard working, failure is not a message that should be sent. Even though it is desirable to encourage the individual to achieve even more, the signal of failure will be discouraging. When people work extremely hard and fail, they often question why they bothered to work so hard. If hard work results in failure to achieve the target, then why not ease off. Managers must be extremely judicious to ensure that all goals assigned are reasonable.

COMMUNICATION AND CONTROL

Communication is an essential part of a management control system. Communication should be an ongoing process. When a manager has a once-a-year meeting with the staff concerning the budget, it is quickly forgotten. To reinforce that meeting, a short weekly or monthly meeting should be held to discuss the budget. It is adequate to discuss just one or several items, such as bandage tape, diapers, chest tubes, disposable gloves, or sponges, at each meeting. It does not even have to be a separate meeting; it can be two minutes of any regularly scheduled meeting. The key is to make the staff aware of specific, definite, attainable goals that they can work toward. Further, by having the budget mentioned often, an awareness is created and it becomes second nature to conserve the organization's resources.

If the manager does not mention the budget until a month of excessive use has occurred, a strong admonition at that time will tend to create budget antagonism rather than cost control. When a nurse manager conveys specific, measurable goals in a routine manner, then cost control can become a routine part of the way nurses function.

USING BUDGETS FOR INTERIM EVALUATION

Interim evaluations are of particular importance in controlling operational results. If the manager simply prepares a budget, tells everyone what it is, and then puts it in a drawer until it is needed to help prepare next year's budget, an important element of motivation and control is lost. The budget has not been used to evaluate how well the unit, staff, and manager are doing and where improvements are possible. The role of evaluation should be primarily to focus on learning from past results to improve future outcomes.

Each month there should be comparisons between what was expected and what has been accomplished. First, this will allow the manager to give feedback to the staff nurses and to the manager's supervisor as to whether the budget's goals are being attained. Telling the staff the unit's goals without giving timely reports on whether they are being attained will weaken their motivation. Second, these monthly evaluations help to bring any unanticipated results to the manager's attention. Then the manager may be able to adjust staffing or take other corrective actions so that the budget will be met in the future months.

Monthly information also allows a manager to provide early notice to a superior if a problem outside the manager's control exists. If the problem is controllable elsewhere in the organization (e.g., by the purchasing department), appropriate action can then be taken. In evaluating any individual in an organization, one primary rule must be followed: *Responsibility should equal control.* If managers are held responsible for things they have no control over, the organization will reward and punish the wrong individuals. The result is invariably demoralization of managers and staff. Using budgets for control can help locate the cause of inefficiency and help avoid waste. In addition, in the hands of a skilled manager, budgeting can also help establish a defense for not meeting the budget (if there are valid reasons for spending in excess of budget, such as increases in noncontrollable costs).

We now turn our attention to the topic of variance analysis, one of the most widely used tools for interim evaluation.

VARIANCE ANALYSIS

Variance analysis is the aspect of budgeting in which actual results are compared to budgeted expectations. The difference between the actual results and the planned results represents a *variance*, i.e., the amount by which the results *vary* from the budget. Variances are calculated for three principal reasons. One reason is to aid in preparing the budget for the coming year. By understanding why results were not as expected, the budget process can be improved and be more accurate in future planning. The second reason is to aid in controlling results throughout the current year. By understanding why variances are occurring, actions can be taken to eliminate some of the unfavorable variances over the coming months. The third reason for variance analysis is to evaluate the performance of units or departments and their managers.

For variance reports to be an effective tool, managers must be able to understand the causes of the variances. This requires investigation of the variances. Such investigation in turn requires the knowledge, judgment, and experience of nurse managers. Variances can be calculated by financial managers. However, those finance personnel do not have the specific knowledge to explain why the variances are occurring. Without such explanation the reports are not useful managerial aids.

Causes of Variances

It is important to be aware of the fact that variance analysis is only a tool to point the manager in the direction to begin investigation. Variances can highlight an actual cost in excess of budget but cannot indicate whether it resulted from quality-of-care improvements or longer coffee breaks. The nurse manager must investigate and make the final determination of what caused a variance.

Variances may be caused by factors internal or external to the organization. Some common internal causes of variances include shifts in quality of care provided; changes in technology, in the efficiency of the nurses, and in organization policy; or simply incorrect standards. External causes of variances commonly include price changes for supplies, volume changes in workload, and unexpected shifts in the availability of staff.

Justification of Variances

Variance reports are given by finance to nurse managers for *justification*. The word justification, which is often used, is unduly confrontational. It focuses attention on the evaluation role of variance analysis instead of on the planning and control roles. The goal of the investigation process is to arrive at an explanation of why the variances arose. In the majority of cases, the variance report is being used to understand what is happening and to control future results to the extent possible. The focus should not be on a defensive justification of what was spent.

If variances arose as a result of inefficiency (e.g., long coffee breaks), then the process of providing cost-effective care is out of control. By discovering that inefficiency, actions can be taken to eliminate it and to bring the process back under control. In that case, future costs will be lower because of the investigation of the variance. The improvement comes, however, not from placing blame on who failed to control past results but from using the information to improve control of future results.

TRADITIONAL VARIANCE ANALYSIS

At the end of a given time period, the organization compares its actual results to the budget. Suppose that the organization does this monthly. Several weeks after each month ends, the accountants gather all the cost information and report the actual totals for the month.

The simplest approach is to then compare the total costs that the entire organization has incurred with the budgeted costs for the entire organization. For example, suppose that the Wagner Hospital had a total budget for the month of March of $4,800,000. The actual costs were $5,200,000. Wagner spent $400,000 more than it had budgeted. The difference between the amount budgeted and the amount actually incurred is the total hospital variance. This variance will be referred to as an *unfavorable variance* because the organization spent more than had been budgeted. Accountants use the term *favorable variance* to indicate spending less than expected.

Assuming that the Wagner Hospital begins its fiscal year on January 1, its variance could appear in a format somewhat like the following:

This Month

Actual: $ 5,200,000   Budget: $ 4,800,000   Variance: $400,000 U

Year-to-Date

Actual: $15,150,000   Budget: $14,876,000   Variance: $274,000 U

In future examples the *year-to-date* information will be dispensed with for simplicity. The focus will be on the current month under review. In health organizations, nurse managers are generally provided with information for the year-to-date as well as the current month. The capital U following the variance refers to the fact that the variance is unfavorable. If the variance were favorable, it would be followed by a capital F.[1]

Why has Wagner had a $400,000 unfavorable variance for the month of March? If variance analysis is to be used to evaluate results, it is necessary to be able to determine not simply that the organization was $400,000 over budget but why that occurred. Given this simple total for the entire organization, the CEO has no idea of what caused the variance. The CEO does not even know which managers to ask about the variance, since all that is known is a total for the entire organization.

To use budgets for control, it must be possible to assign responsibility for

---

[1] An alternative presentation to using U and F would be to use a negative number for an unfavorable variance and a positive number for a favorable variance. Alternatively, parentheses are placed around unfavorable variances and no parentheses around favorable ones. Exercise caution in interpreting variance notation. Any systematic approach can be used to indicate favorable vs. unfavorable variances. It would not be wrong to use parentheses or negative numbers for favorable variances and no parentheses or positive numbers for unfavorable variances, as long as the use is consistent throughout the organization.

variances to individual managers. Those managers can investigate the causes of the variances and attempt to eliminate the variances in the future. The key is that it must be possible to hold individual managers accountable for the variance. This leads to the necessity of determining variances by unit and department.

Unit and Department Variances

The overall Wagner variance of $400,000 is an aggregation of variances from a number of departments. Focus on the results for the nursing department.

THE WAGNER HOSPITAL
Department of Nursing Services
March Variance Report

Actual	Budget	Variance
$2,400,000	$2,200,000	$200,000 U

Apparently, half the variance for the Wagner Hospital for March occurred in the nursing services area. Now there is more information than there was previously. Previously it was known that there was an excess expenditure of $400,000 but it was not known how that excess came about. Now it is known that half of it occurred in the nursing area. The chief nurse executive (CNE) can be asked to explain why the $200,000 variance occurred.

Unfortunately, at this point the CNE has not been given much to go on. She simply knows that $200,000 was spent that was not budgeted. Most hospitals would take this total cost for the nursing department and break it down into the various nursing units. Each nursing unit that has a nurse manager who is responsible for running that unit should have both a budget for the unit and a variance report that shows the unit's performance in comparison to the budget.

The variance for one particular nursing unit might appear as follows:

THE WAGNER HOSPITAL
Department of Nursing Services
Med/Surg 6th Floor West
March Variance Report

Actual	Budget	Variance
$120,000	$110,000	$10,000 U

Line-item Variances

Even once the total nursing department variance has been divided among the various nursing units, more information is still needed as a guide. Is the variance the result of unexpectedly high costs for nursing salaries? Does it relate to usage of supplies? To have any real chance to control costs, there must be variance information for individual line items within a unit or department. For example:

THE WAGNER HOSPITAL
Department of Nursing Services
Med/Surg 6th Floor West
March Variance Report

	Actual	Budget	Variance
Salary	$108,000	$100,000	$ 8,000 U
Supplies	12,000	10,000	2,000 U
Total	$120,000	$110,000	$10,000 U

This obviously is a great simplification. There should be line items for each line in the unit's budget.

Understanding Variances

The objective in doing variance analysis is to determine why the variances arose. Nothing can be done with respect to the goal of controlling costs until the nurse manager knows where the unit or department is deviating from the plan and why.

Once the variance for each line item for each unit has been calculated, there must be a determination of whether to investigate the variance. It must be kept in mind that budgets are "guesstimates" of the future. They cannot be expected to come out exactly on target. Small variances can generally be ignored. Hopefully, over the course of a year, the small unfavorable variances will be balanced out by small favorable variances. One of the most difficult aspects of variance analysis is determining when a variance is large enough to warrant investigation. Should a manager investigate $5, $50, $100, or $1,000 variances? How big a variance is too big to tolerate without investigation?

Unfortunately, there is no set answer. The solution favored by these authors is as follows: When managers look at a variance, they should assume that it will occur in the same amount month after month until the end of the year. For instance, suppose that a $500 unfavorable variance was found for January for nurses' aides salaries. If that variance occurred every month, it would total $6,000 for the year. If $6,000 is an unreasonably high variance, investigate the $500 January variance as soon as possible. Managers should also investigate variances that appear to be growing from month to month.

The key to controlling variances is to be timely, to correct behavior if necessary, and to use the information from variances to correct rates promptly. If variances are not investigated promptly after each month's variance report is received, then the budget will only serve as a planning tool and not a tool to help the organization control its operation. Information about last month's performance should be used to improve the performance for the remaining months of the year.

In some cases it will be found that the variances are simply out of the unit or manager's control. A shortage of a key raw material may drive the price of supplies up. If there appears to be a protracted change that is outside the control of the manager and will result in continuing unfavorable variances, it is important to bring this to the attention of the organization's rate-setting personnel. The sooner this is known and the rates are corrected upward, the better it is for the financial stability of the organization.

Traditional variance analysis requires that the nurse manager proceed to use the unit line-item variance information to attempt to discover the underlying causes of the variances. Consider the $8,000 variance for salaries. Why was $8,000 more than budgeted spent on salaries? At this point we really do not know what caused the variance. Expenditure for staff in excess of the budgeted amount could have a number of possible causes. Without more information, corrective action cannot be taken.

One potential cause of the $8,000 salary variance is that the unit manager did not do a very good job in controlling the usage of staff. As a result, more hours of nursing care per patient were paid for than had been expected. Another possibility is that the patients were sicker than anticipated, and the higher average acuity level caused more nursing hours to be used per patient. Another possible cause is that the hourly rate for nurses increased. Still another possible cause of the variance is that there were more patients and the additional patients caused more consumption of nursing hours.

The most serious problem of traditional variance analysis is that it compares the predicted cost for a predicted number of patients to the actual cost for the actual patient volume. Unless the actual workload is exactly as predicted, there is very little chance that a unit will achieve exactly the budgeted expectations because some costs are variable. Such costs will rise or fall if volume is greater or less than the budgeted level.

Many health care organizations are now starting to use a more sophisticated variance approach based on a flexible budget. The main goal of that approach is to allow for changed expectations as the number of patients changes.

FLEXIBLE BUDGET VARIANCE ANALYSIS

Flexible budgeting is a system that requires more work than traditional variance analysis but can provide nurse managers with substantially more information. The key concept of flexible budgeting is that the amount of resources consumed varies with the volume of patients. Suppose that the following was the variance report for nursing department salaries:

THE WAGNER HOSPITAL
Department of Nursing Services
March Variance Report

	Actual	Budget	Variance
Salary	$1,000,000	$1,000,000	$ 0

It looks as if the department came in right on budget. Suppose, however, that the budget of $1 million for nursing salaries was based on an assumption of 25,000 patient days, but there actually were only 20,000 patient days. The department should have spent less than $1 million if any of the salary costs are variable. The original budget ignores that fact. The flexible budget is a restatement of the budget based on the volume actually attained. The flexible budget shows what a line item should have cost, given the volume level that actually occurred.

The flexible budget is prepared after the fact. The actual volume must be known to prepare the flexible budget for that volume.[2] Keep in mind that because some costs are fixed and some are variable, total costs do not change in direct proportion with volume. One would normally expect that a 10% increase in patient days would be accompanied by less than a 10% increase in costs, since only some costs are variable and increase as census does. On the other hand, a 10% reduction in workload would only be expected to be accompanied by a less than 10% reduction in cost because the fixed costs would not decline.

Use of the flexible budget technique allows the variance for any line item to be subdivided to get additional information. The variance is divided into three pieces: a *volume variance*, a *price variance*, and a *quantity variance*.

The Volume Variance

The *volume variance* will be defined as the amount of the variance caused simply by the fact that the patient volume has changed. For example, if the budget calls for 25,000 patient days but actually there were 30,000 patient days, then it would be expected that it would be necessary to spend more. The additional cost of the resources needed for an extra 5,000 patient days constitutes a volume variance. Volume variances are generally outside the control of the nurse manager. Note that unfavorable volume variances are often accompanied by higher than budgeted revenue.

Many hospitals have adopted use of this aspect of flexible budgeting. Unit managers are then asked to explain the differences between the actual amounts spent and the amounts that should be spent according to the flexible budget. Thus the noncontrollable volume variance is excluded from the variance that the manager is expected to justify or explain. While this is a major step in the direction of making variance analysis more relevant and useful, it does not yield all the potential benefits of flexible budget variance analysis.

The Price or Rate Variance

The *price* or *rate variance* is the portion of the total variance caused by spending more or less per unit for some resource than had been anticipated. For example, if the average wage rate for nurses is more per hour than had been expected, that would give rise to this type of variance. When the variance is used to measure labor resources, it is generally called a *rate variance* because the average hourly rate has varied from expectations. When considering the price of supplies, such as the cost per package of sutures, it is called a *price variance* because the purchase price has varied. The terms price and rate are often used interchangeably in practice.

The price or rate variance may or may not be under the control of the nurse manager. If the purchasing department predicts all prices used for supplies and then winds up paying a higher price than predicted, it should be possible to measure the price variance so that the responsibility can be placed with the purchasing department. If the nursing department bears the responsibility for price variances on supplies, the purchasing department will have no incentive

---

[2]As part of the budget preparation process, some organizations prospectively prepare flexible budgets. This provides the organization with a sense of what costs are likely to be at differing levels of workload.

to try to find the best prices. On the other hand, if the nurse manager hires temporary nurses directly from the agency, then the responsibility for the rate variance may lie with the nurse manager. Were overqualified people hired? Was an attempt made to seek out an agency that would give the best rate? The manager who can exercise some control over the outcome should be the manager held accountable for the outcome.

The Quantity or Use Variance

The third general type of variance under the flexible budgeting scheme is the *quantity* or *use variance*. This is the portion of the overall variance for a particular line item that results from using more of a resource than was expected for a given work-load level. For example, if more supplies were used per patient day than expected, that would give rise to a quantity variance because the quantity of supplies used per patient day exceeded expectations.

This variance is also frequently referred to as a *use variance* because it focuses on how much of the resource has been used. For example, if one-half roll of bandage tape was used per patient day, while the expected usage was only one-quarter roll, there would be a use variance. The terms "quantity" and "use" are often used interchangeably.

THE MECHANICS OF FLEXIBLE BUDGET VARIANCE ANALYSIS

The first step in flexible budgeting is to establish the flexible budget for the actual patient volume. Given the actual cost for a particular line item and the original budgeted amount, it must be determined what that line item should have cost given the actual patient volume.

For example, consider the supplies budgeted for and used by the Med/Surg 6th Floor West nursing unit at the Wagner Hospital in March:

THE WAGNER HOSPITAL
Department of Nursing Services
Med/Surg 6th Floor West
March Variance Report

	Actual	**Budget**	**Variance**
Supplies	$12,000	$10,000	$2,000 U

The actual consumption was $12,000. The budgeted consumption was $10,000. Suppose that the budget assumed that there would be 500 patient days for this unit for March, but there actually turned out to be 600 patient days.[3] Assuming that the consumption of supplies would normally be expected to vary in direct

---

[3]It is assumed in this example that the average patient classification or acuity is unchanged. If average acuity is different from the expected level, then it is logical that resource consumption in terms of nursing requirements will also differ from the budgeted amount. Acuity can be built into variance analysis through the flexible budget model. The portion of the variance resulting from changes in acuity can be separated and specified. See the reprinted article on this topic in the appendix at the end of this chapter for further discussion of the variance due to patient acuity.

proportion to patient days, then the planned consumption was apparently $20 per patient day (the $10,000 supplies budget divided by the 500 expected patient days).

For 600 patient days at $20 per patient day, $12,000 would have been budgeted for supplies. This is the flexible budget. It is the amount the department would have expected to spend had the actual number of patient days been known. Notice that in this case the flexible budget and the actual amount spent are identical:

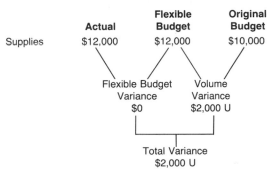

The difference between the original budget and the actual amount spent is the total variance. That is still $2,000 unfavorable. The difference between the original budget and the new flexible budget is the volume variance. In this case the difference is $2,000 U. Note that this volume variance is considered unfavorable because the flexible budget requires more spending than was expected. The increased number of patient days may represent more patients and more revenues. That may be a favorable event for the organization, but the accountant always refers to cost in excess of the original budget as being an unfavorable variance. Unfavorable variances are not necessarily bad.

The difference between the flexible budget and the actual amount spent can be referred to as a flexible budget variance. Here the flexible budget variance is zero. The entire variance in supplies has been explained by the fact that there was a different volume of patients than had been anticipated.

What about the nursing salaries for the unit? Recall the variance report for nursing salaries:

THE WAGNER HOSPITAL
Department of Nursing Services
Med/Surg 6th Floor West
March Variance Report

	Actual	Budget	Variance
Salary	$108,000	$100,000	$ 8,000 U

To keep the discussion relatively simple at this point, assume that nursing salary costs should vary in direct proportion to the number of patient days. In other words, assume that nursing salary costs are variable.[4]

Nursing salaries had been budgeted at $100,000 with an expectation of 500 patient days. That is a cost of $200 per patient day. Assuming nursing salary costs are variable, had it been known that there would be 600 patient days, $120,000 would have been budgeted. The variance report can be restated as follows:

THE WAGNER HOSPITAL
Department of Nursing Services
Med/Surg 6th Floor West
March Variance Report

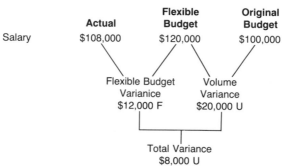

	Actual	Flexible Budget	Original Budget
Salary	$108,000	$120,000	$100,000

Flexible Budget
Varianice
$12,000 F

Volume
Variance
$20,000 U

Total Variance
$8,000 U

Subtracting the original budget from the flexible budget, the volume variance is found to be $20,000 U. When the flexible budget is subtracted from the actual cost, it turns out that the flexible budget variance is $12,000 F. Note that the volume variance is unfavorable because the extra patients require more spending. However, the actual amount spent was less than the flexible budget.

If the volume and flexible budget variances for salaries are combined, there is an unfavorable total variance of $8,000. (Note that since one of the variances is favorable and one is unfavorable, the smaller one must be subtracted from the larger one to get a combined total variance. The total variance will have the same label [i.e., favorable or unfavorable] as the larger of the two variances. Hence, $20,000 U − $12,000 F = $8,000 U).

At this point in the analysis, there is not yet sufficient information to determine the causes of the flexible budget variance. Suppose that the CNE of

---

[4]This may assume more flexibility of nurse staffing than most organizations have. Hospitals may have some flexibility to transfer nurses from one shift to another or from a unit with a temporarily low occupancy to one with a higher occupancy, or per diem agency nurses can be used. In some cases, however, such flexibility may be quite limited. This is particularly so at unionized hospitals with strong work rules. Nurse staffing tends to be variable only if there are substantial patient volume changes in such cases. Flexible budget variance analysis can still be used. However, the process is more complicated. See Steven A. Finkler, *Budgeting Concepts for Nurse Managers*, 2nd edition, W.B. Saunders, Philadelphia, 1992, pp. 289–291, for the mechanics and an example. Bear in mind, however, that it is only significant variances that require investigation. And significant variances are generally not the result of a minor shift in the number of patient days. Over major shifts in volume, staffing is likely to be reasonably variable.

the organization had come to the unit manager in the middle of April and complained about a total lack of cost control on the unit. The unit had a $2,000 unfavorable supplies variance and an $8,000 unfavorable salary variance. Based on traditional variance analysis (without using a flexible budget), there would be no way the unit manager could determine the cause of the problem.

Certainly the unit manager is aware of increased patient volume and would argue that extra patient days were a major factor. But how major? By using a flexible budget, it is possible to find out exactly what dollar impact the extra patient days should have had. In the example, flexible budgeting has shown that the entire variance in supplies is attributable to the extra patient days. The volume variance for supplies was $2,000 U, the same as the amount of the total supply variance. Furthermore, the volume variance was $20,000 U for salaries. The department manager should have expected to spend $20,000 more on nursing salaries than was in the original budget, given the 100 extra patient days. In fact, only $8,000 was spent above the original salary budget. Rather than being blamed for having gone over budget, the manager can now show that given the actual number of patient days, the unit actually spent $12,000 less than should have been expected!

Flexible Budget Notation

The next step in the process is to try to determine what caused the flexible budget variance. To do that it is necessary to formalize the flexible budgeting process by introducing some notation. The letter A will be used to refer to an actual amount. The letter B will be used to refer to a budgeted amount. The letter P will stand for a price or rate, and the letter Q will stand for a quantity. The letter i will be used to stand for an input and the letter o to stand for an output.

Inputs are the resources used to generate outputs. If one is considering how much was spent on nursing salaries, then the input is nursing time. If one is considering the cost of bandage tape, then the input is rolls of bandage tape. *Outputs* are a measure of what is being produced. Since improved health cannot readily be measured, proxies will be used to measure how much output is produced. Frequently used output measures include patients, patient days, visits, treatments, and procedures.

The notation is combined to form six key variables. Pi stands for the *price* of the *input,* such as $1 per roll of bandage tape or $25 per hour for nursing salary. Qo stands for the total *quantity* of *output.* Qi stands for the *quantity* of *input* needed to produce one unit of output. The definitions of the notation can be formalized as follows:

- BPi: *b*udgeted *p*rice per unit of *i*nput
- BQi: *b*udgeted *q*uantity of *i*nput for each unit of output
- BQo: *b*udgeted *q*uantity of *o*utput
- APi: *a*ctual *p*rice paid per unit of *i*nput
- AQi: *a*ctual *q*uantity of *i*nput for each unit of output produced
- AQo: *a*ctual *q*uantity of *o*utput

The notation can best be understood in an example.

An Example of Volume, Price, and Quantity Variances

Suppose that Wagner Hospital had the following line item in its variance report for a nursing unit for the prior month:

	Actual	Budget	Variance
Nursing labor	$34,038	$28,800	$5,238 U

The unit manager wants to find out what caused the variance, so the following information is gathered:

♦ BPi: $24.00 per hour budgeted nursing rate
♦ BQi: 3.0 hours of budgeted nursing time per patient day
♦ BQo: 400 budgeted patient days
♦ APi: $24.40 actual average nursing rate per hour
♦ AQi: 3.1 hours of actual nursing time per patient day
♦ AQo: 450 actual patient days

Before proceeding to use these data, consider what is involved in obtaining the information. Information is only worthwhile if it is more valuable than the cost to collect it. All three budgeted items are already known. It would not have been possible to prepare an operating budget without a forecast of patient days, the average rate for nurses, and the budgeted hours per patient day (or the total budgeted nursing hours, which can be divided by the expected patient days to get the budgeted nursing hours per patient day). What about the actual information? The actual number of patient days is readily available. The actual wage rate and the amount of actual paid nursing time is available from the payroll department. Given the actual nursing time and the actual number of patient days, one can divide to get the nursing time per patient day. Therefore, all the data needed for flexible budget variance analysis are readily available.

The first step in utilizing these data is calculating the original budget in terms of the notation. The original budget is simply the expected cost per patient day multiplied by the expected number of patient days. In this case the expectation is that nurses will be paid $24.00 per hour; the department will pay for an average of 3.0 hours per patient day. Therefore, the expected cost is $72 per patient day. For the month, 400 patient days are expected, so the budget is $28,800 ($24.00 × 3.0 hours × 400 patient days). In terms of the notation, this can be shown as follows:

Original Budget

$$BQi \times BPi \times BQo$$
$$3.0 \times \$24.00 \times 400$$
$$\$28,800$$

That is, BQi, the budgeted quantity of input per patient day, is 3.0 hours; BPi, the budgeted price per hour of nursing time, is $24.00; and BQo, the budgeted quantity of patient days, is 400. If these three numbers are multiplied together, the result is the originally budgeted amount for nursing labor.

The next step is to find the flexible budget. Keep in mind that the flexible budget is the amount that one would have expected to spend if the actual number of patient days had been known in advance. Therefore, leave the BQi at the budgeted 3.0 hours per patient day and the BPi at the budgeted $24.00 per hour. The only change is from a BQo of 400 patient days to a new AQo of 450 patient days. The flexible budget can then be calculated as follows:

Flexible Budget

BQi × BPi × AQo

3.0 × $24.00 × 450

$32,400

Note that the difference between the original budget and the flexible budget is caused by a difference in the number of patient days. Other than that, the calculations are the same. The originally budgeted amount of $28,800 can be compared with the flexible budget amount of $32,400 to determine the volume variance of $3,600 U. Since patient days are higher than expected, cost will be higher than expected. That will give rise to an unfavorable variance. The comparison between the original budget and the flexible budget can be shown as follows:

Flexible Budget	**Original Budget**
BQi × BPi × AQo	BQi × BPi × BQo
3.0 × $24.00 × 450	3.0 × $24.00 × 400
$32,400	$28,800

Volume
Variance
$3,600 U

At this point the flexible budget can be compared to the actual results to find the flexible budget variance. First, restate the actual costs in terms of the notation:

Actual

AQi × APi × AQo

3.1 × $24.40 × 450

$34,038

Note that for the actual cost, the actual paid time per patient day, the actual price paid per hour, and the actual number of patient days are used. If desired, the flexible budget can be compared to the actual results to determine a *flexible budget variance:*

Actual	**Flexible Budget**
AQi × APi × AQo	BQi × BPi × AQo
3.1 × $24.40 × 450	3.0 × $24.00 × 450
$34,038	$32,400

Flexible Budget
Variance
$1,638 U

The flexible budget variance is $1,638 U. Since the total variance is simply being broken into its component parts, it should be possible to combine the volume variance and the flexible budget variance and come out with the total variance. The difference between the original budget and the actual result is $5,238 (i.e., $34,038 − $28,800). Consider all the information available so far in notation form:

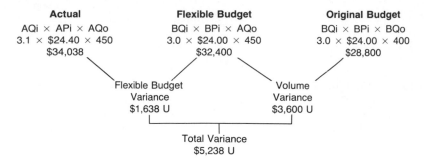

Actual
AQi × APi × AQo
3.1 × \$24.40 × 450
\$34,038

Flexible Budget
BQi × BPi × AQo
3.0 × \$24.00 × 450
\$32,400

Original Budget
BQi × BPi × BQo
3.0 × \$24.00 × 400
\$28,800

Flexible Budget
Variance
\$1,638 U

Volume
Variance
\$3,600 U

Total Variance
\$5,238 U

As can be seen, the total variance still is \$5,238, but it has now been separated into a flexible budget variance and a volume variance. If the \$1,638 U flexible budget variance is added to the \$3,600 U volume variance, the result is the \$5,238 total variance. The flexible budget variance is of greater concern to the nurse manager than is the volume variance. The volume variance is usually outside the nurse manager's control. The flexible budget variance is caused by the difference between the budgeted and actual price per hour for nursing services and by differences in the amount of nursing time per patient day. If possible, more should be found out about what makes up this variance.

To find out this extra information, it is necessary to derive something called a *subcategory*. This subcategory is simply a device to allow for separation of the flexible budget variance into two pieces—the price variance and the quantity variance. The subcategory is defined as the actual quantity of input per unit of output, multiplied by the budgeted price of the input, times the actual output level. In terms of the notation the subcategory can be calculated as follows:

Subcategory
AQi × BPi × AQo
3.1 × \$24.00 × 450
\$33,480

If the subcategory calculation is compared to the actual costs, the price variance can be determined:

Actual
AQi × APi × AQo
3.1 × \$24.40 × 450
\$34,038

Subcategory
AQi × BQi × AQo
3.1 × \$24.00 × 450
\$33,480

Price Variance
\$558 U

The only difference between the actual and the subcategory is in the hourly rate (Pi). The price variance of \$558 U results from the fact that on average \$24.40 was paid per hour for nursing time instead of the budgeted \$24.00. It is possible that this occurs because of poor scheduling, which results in unnecessary overtime. Perhaps it is the result of a larger raise for nursing personnel than the nurse manager had been told to put into the budget. Perhaps the extra patient volume resulted in extra overtime or the addition of high-priced per diem agency nurses. All these possibilities should be investigated by the nurse manager.

What effect will added patient load have on the quantity of nursing time per patient? The quantity variance addresses that question. That variance is calculated by comparing the difference between the subcategory and the flexible budget. The only difference between those two numbers is a result of the nursing time (Qi) per patient.

Subcategory	Flexible Budget
AQi × BPi × AQo	BQi × BPi × AQo
3.1 × $24.00 × 450	3.0 × $24.00 × 450
$33,480	$32,400

Quantity Variance
$1,080 U

The quantity variance of $1,080 U can be explained in a number of ways. It is possible that because of the substantial increase in patient days above expectations, many part-time nurses were hired. These nurses were unfamiliar with the institution and therefore were not as efficient as the regular nurses. Another possibility is that the population was sicker than anticipated and required more care. An approach to measuring the part of the variance due to patient acuity is discussed in the article reprinted in the Appendix at the end of this chapter. Of course, there is also the possibility that supervision was lax and that time was simply being wasted. Again, variance information can only point out the direction; the manager must make the final determination regarding why the variance occurred and how to avoid it in the future.

To use flexible budgeting, one should have an idea of how the pieces fit together. Review the price and quantity variances, looking at how they together comprise the flexible budget variance:

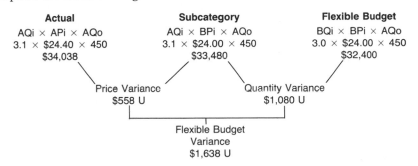

Actual	Subcategory	Flexible Budget
AQi × APi × AQo	AQi × BPi × AQo	BQi × BPi × AQo
3.1 × $24.40 × 450	3.1 × $24.00 × 450	3.0 × $24.00 × 450
$34,038	$33,480	$32,400

Price Variance
$558 U

Quantity Variance
$1,080 U

Flexible Budget
Variance
$1,638 U

Notice that adding the price variance of $558 U and the quantity variance of $1,080 U results in the flexible budget variance. Recall that the flexible budget variance and volume variance add up to the total variance. Exhibit 13–1 shows that the three individual variances—price, quantity, and volume—add up to the total variance for the line item.

Recall that without flexible budgets, the total variance for the line item would be the only piece of information available for analysis. There was an unfavorable variance of $5,238. Using Exhibit 13–1, it is possible to determine at the outset that of this total variance, $3,600 was caused by the increase in patient days. It is now also known that $558 of the variance was caused by having paid a higher average rate to the nurses than was anticipated and that $1,080 of the

Text continued on page 370

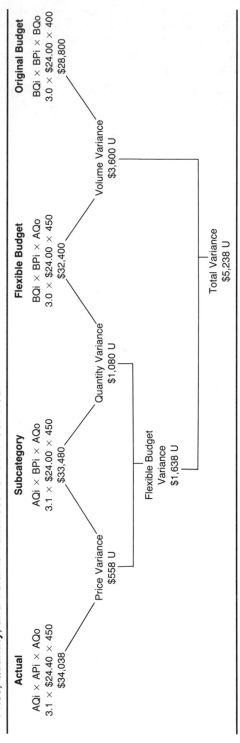

❖ **EXHIBIT 13–1**
Price, Quantity, and Volume Variances for 6th Floor West

Actual

AQi × APi × AQo
3.1 × $24.40 × 450
$34,038

Price Variance
$558 U

Subcategory

AQi × BPi × AQo
3.1 × $24.00 × 450
$33,480

Quantity Variance
$1,080 U

Flexible Budget
Variance
$1,638 U

Flexible Budget

BQi × BPi × AQo
3.0 × $24.00 × 450
$32,400

Volume Variance
$3,600 U

Original Budget

BQi × BPi × BQo
3.0 × $24.00 × 400
$28,800

Total Variance
$5,238 U

❖ **EXHIBIT 13–2**
Price, Quantity, and Volume Variances—A Generic Model

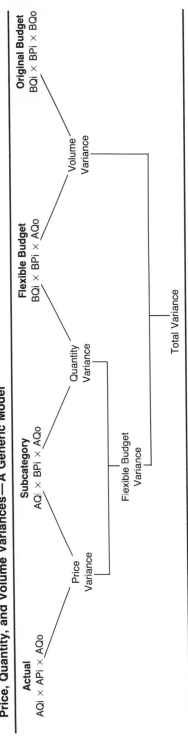

variance was caused by a longer average amount of nursing time per patient day than had been anticipated. Why these specific variances occurred is not known, but there is a much better focus on where the problem areas are.

A generic model for flexible budget variances is presented in Exhibit 13–2. In looking at this model, several things should be kept in mind. First of all, recall that basically all the necessary data are generally readily available. Second, these variances can be calculated on a computer system.[5]

It sometimes is not obvious whether a variance is favorable or unfavorable. Looking at Exhibit 13–2, an easy rule of thumb is that as one moves from the right side toward the left, larger numbers on the left indicate unfavorable variance. For example, if the flexible budget amount is larger than the originally budgeted amount, the volume variance is unfavorable. If the subcategory is greater than the flexible budget, the quantity variance is unfavorable. This is true because as one moves from the original budget toward the left, movement is toward the actual result. If the actual result is larger than the original budget, then more was spent than budgeted. The result is an unfavorable variance. Given the way this model is set up, this also holds true for each of the individual variances making up the total variance.

DETERMINATION OF THE CAUSES OF VARIANCES

What the nurse manager will not get from this analysis is the ultimate explanation of causes of the variances. The nurse manager will still have to investigate to find out *why* these variances have occurred. The analysis provides significant new information by pointing a finger in a specific direction instead of waving a hand in a vague direction.

For instance, if twice as much surgical supplies were used per patient day as expected, the nurse manager knows exactly what to investigate. The analysis does not tell why there was a variance, but it does tell where. Rather than simply saying that the operating room is over budget, it is known that the line item for surgical supplies is over budget. Furthermore, rather than simply noting that too much was spent for surgical supplies, it has been determined that the problem was not caused because there were extra procedures. Nor was it caused because the price of surgical supplies went up. It is specifically known that the problem lay in using more surgical supplies per procedure than had been budgeted. Managers must take over at this point and investigate why this occurred. Why were more surgical supplies used per procedure than expected? Was it sloppy use? Clear-cut waste? Was it pilferage? Was there a change in patient mix? Was there a major disaster that did not increase the number of procedures considerably but did bring in patients requiring a great amount of surgical supplies? Is the budget wrong and it is not really possible to get by with the budgeted amount of surgical supplies per procedure? Ultimately the nurse manager must find out the actual underlying cause of the variance.

---

[5]For more details on computerization of variances, see Steven A. Finkler, "Using Computers to Improve Variance Analysis," *Journal of Nursing Administration*, September 1991, reprinted in the appendix at the end of Chapter 16.

AGGREGATION PROBLEMS

One problem that requires caution on the part of nurse managers is caused by the aggregation of information. When variances are combined, there is a tendency to lose information. Some of the favorable and unfavorable variances may offset each other. A summary report for a number of departments may appear to have little if any variance either in total or for a particular line item such as salaries. However, one department might be well over budget and another well under budget. Both departments would warrant investigation.

The problem is not just at the interdepartmental level. The nursing department may appear to have little variance. However, two nursing units may have offsetting variances. Or it is possible that each nursing unit may appear to have little variance. However, within a nursing unit one line item may be offsetting another. For example, underspending in salaries could hide overspending in supplies.

Traditional variance analysis is adequate to disclose the types of aggregation problems discussed so far, if carefully used. By looking at each department and each unit individually and each line item rather than a summary for the department or unit, many aggregation problems are avoided. However, traditional variance analysis will not disclose a volume variance that offsets either a price or quantity variance. For example, if the number of patients is below budget, and staffing is unchanged from the budget, there will be a favorable volume variance and an unfavorable quantity variance. The staff salary line might well show no variance in total. The nursing unit might well show no variance in total.

In such a case the nurse manager of the unit is losing critical information. The volume variance is a strong signal. When volume is down, organizational revenues are probably down as well. The organization has a need to constrain costs. When the staffing is unchanged even though there are fewer patients, costs may be excessive compared to available revenues. However, unless flexible budget variance analysis is used to disclose the quantity and volume variances, the manager will lack this information. As a result, the manager may not be able to move as quickly and decisively as the situation warrants.

EXCEPTION REPORTING

Aggregation problems create substantial difficulty. The only way to be sure that one variance is not being offset by another variance is by examining every single price, quantity, and volume variance of every single line item of every single unit of every single cost center of the organization. This creates a potentially unmanageable burden. Should the CEO of a hospital have to examine every individual variance for the entire organization? Should the CNE have to examine every individual variance for all units of the nursing department? The time required would be enormous. A solution to this problem is the use of *exception reports.*

Assuming a computer prepares all the variances for each cost element, it is a simple process to have the computer prepare a list for the CEO of only those individual variances which exceed a certain limit. This is called an exception report. It only lists the variances that are large. How large depends on the desires of the individual CEO. When tight, centralized control is desired, smaller variances are of interest. For example, while some CEOs might be interested only in monthly or year-to-date variances that are greater than 20% of the budget or $50,000, a CEO running a more centralized operation might be interested in variances greater than 10% or $10,000.

This does not mean that variances less than $10,000 must go unnoticed. Department heads, such as the CNE, would get a report for their departments at a more detailed level, perhaps 5% or $1,000. Continuing the process, nurse managers would receive detailed exception reports for the variances in units under their supervision. Ultimately, the nurse manager who has direct control over a unit would want to review all variances for that unit. In all cases, if a nurse manager feels that a particular variance indicates a problem that is likely to grow worse in future months, the higher levels of nursing administration should be alerted to the problem rather than waiting until the variance is great enough to appear on the CNE's exception report.

REVENUE VARIANCES

The nurse manager's primary variance analysis effort focuses on expenses. This is predominantly because managers of health care organizations have a greater degree of control over expenses than they do over revenues. However, the information that can be yielded from revenue variance analysis is also quite important. For example, changes in revenue that result from changes in patient volume may be outside the control of the organization and its managers. Such changes, however, may require management actions or reactions to protect the organization's financial position.

Revenue variance methodology follows the same pattern as expense methodology. There is a traditional variance that tends to focus on the total revenue expected and actually achieved for a unit or department. There is also a flexible budget methodology that helps to identify the various underlying causes of variances. The total revenue variance for a unit, department, or organization can be broken down into a volume variance, a mix variance, and a price variance.

Consider an outpatient surgery department that has budgeted revenues of $1 million for the month just ended. Actual revenues were $850,000. Traditional variance analysis identifies a $150,000 unfavorable revenue variance. What caused the $150,000 shortfall?

The first step for flexible budget revenue variance analysis would be to identify the revenue per patient. Unlike costs, which may be fixed or variable, revenues are all variable. Therefore the total $1 million budget could be divided by the number of patients budgeted to get an average revenue per patient. This allows calculation of a volume variance. Suppose that 800 patients were expected for the month. In that case the average revenue per patient was expected to be $1,250 (i.e., the $1 million total revenue divided by 800 patients = $1,250 of revenue per patient).

If there were actually only 750 patients, then a flexible budget for revenue of $937,500 (i.e., 750 patients × $1,250 price) would be calculated. The revenue flexible budget indicates the amount of revenue that would have been budgeted if the number of patients had been forecast exactly correctly. The difference between the original budget for 800 patients and the flexible budget for 750 actual patients is an unfavorable volume variance of $62,500. Less revenue than expected is considered unfavorable.

The next calculation concerns the mix of patients. Not all patients would be expected to be charged $1,250. That figure represents an average. Assume that half the patients were expected to be type A patients charged $1,000 and half were expected to be type B patients charged $1,500. Any number of different types of patients with different prices is possible, but for this discussion we will limit it to just types A and B.

Suppose that of the 750 actual patients, 450 were type A and 300 were type B. Not only are there fewer than expected patients, but the mix of patients has changed as well. Less than half the patients are the more highly priced type B patients. Based on the actual number of patients and the actual mix, revenues would be expected to be $900,000 (i.e., 450 patients @ $1,000 + 300 patients @ $1,500). If we compare the flexible budget of $937,500 (what revenue would have been expected to be for 750 patients) to this new "subcategory" value based on the actual mix, the difference is $37,500. This is the mix variance, which is unfavorable. The variance is unfavorable because there is a greater proportion of lower-revenue patients.

This still leaves an unexplained variance of $50,000. This is a price variance. It is a result of charging a different price than expected. Although the outpatient surgery intended to charge $1,500 for type B patients, it is possible that because of government regulation or negotiated rates with insurance companies, the average price for type B patients was only $1,333.33. In that case actual revenue would be $850,000 (i.e., 450 patients @ $1,000 + 300 patients @ $1,333.33). The $50,000 difference between the $900,000 from the mix calculation is an unfavorable price variance. It is unfavorable because the price was less than budgeted.

The calculations for these variances can be seen in Exhibit 13–3. Note that in each case the number of patients is multiplied by the price per patient. For the budget and flexible budget the total number of patients and the budgeted average price per patient are used. For the subcategory, the mix of patients is used, splitting the total into the number of actual patients of each type. For the subcategory the budgeted price for each type of patient is used. For the actual costs the actual number of each type of patient and the actual prices charged for each type of patient are used.

Often revenue variances are calculated based on the contribution margin rather than the revenue. (See Chapter 7 for a discussion of contribution margin.) Revenue places too great a focus on the total charge for different types of patients rather than on the profit implications of each type patient. A patient with very high revenue could have even greater expenses. Another patient with only modest revenues could be quite profitable. Managers do not just need information about changes in revenues. They need to know whether the revenue changes are in profitable areas or unprofitable ones.

It is possible therefore to use the budgeted contribution margin rather than the revenue in all the calculations just discussed. There still would be a volume variance. Fewer patients would imply less overall contribution margin. There still would be a mix variance. However, whether the mix variance is favorable or unfavorable would depend on whether there is a greater or lesser proportion of the types of patients with higher contribution margins. The price variance would still depend on the actual price charged for each type of patient.

❖ **EXHIBIT 13–3**
Revenue Variances

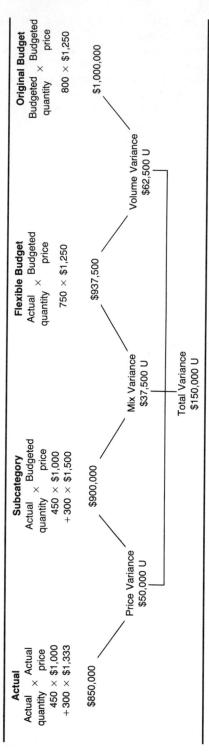

Knowing whether variances are caused by changes in prices, the mix of patients, or the volume of patients is important information that managers can use in taking actions to respond to increases or decreases in revenues. If the number of patients is falling, then steps should be taken to try to find out why and to make sure that there are corresponding reductions in organizational expenses. If the mix of patients is changing, it may be necessary to shift resources within the organization. If prices differed from budget, an effort must be made to understand why it occurred and its overall implications for the organization's finances.

IMPLICATIONS FOR NURSE MANAGERS

Controlling the results of operations is as important as developing a feasible plan. Organizations use management control systems to ensure that every attempt is made to carry out the organization's plans.

Budgets can help control costs if they are used to motivate all managers and staff members. This requires communication of specific, measurable goals on a regular, frequent basis. Such a process will improve results as individuals make a self-motivated effort to achieve specified, attainable goals.

One must try to understand what incentives are needed to cause individuals to work toward the overall well-being of the organization. When a health care organization asks nurses to accomplish something, it is necessary to be concerned with why they would want to do it. Perhaps they will do it to benefit patient care. But that motive provides little incentive for cost control. Perhaps they will control costs out of loyalty to the organization. Perhaps they will control costs out of fear of losing their jobs. Perhaps they will control costs in hopes of earning a promotion.

Getting an understanding of what people will want to do and what they will not want to do is important. And once managers know what they will not want to do, they should carefully attempt to develop some clear motivational device that will give them an incentive to do what the organization needs to have accomplished. The key issue to remember is that organizations do not control costs; people do.

The difference between the budget and what actually occurs is called a variance. Comparison of actual results to budgeted expectations and analysis of the resulting variances should generally be done monthly. This can allow for midstream corrections that will improve the year-end results. It also provides information for preparing the coming year's budget and for evaluating units', departments', and managers' performance.

Most health care organizations prepare variance reports by comparing the information in the original budget to the actual results. There are several problems with that type of comparison. First, it does not tell as much about the cause of the variance as one would like to know; for instance, traditional variance analysis does not indicate whether a variance is caused by more resource use per patient or by higher prices for resources used. Second, traditional variance analysis ignores the fact that resource consumption would be expected to vary with patient volume. Part of the variance will just be the result of changes in patient volume rather than being related to efficiency.

This has caused many health care organizations to start using a method called flexible budgeting. Flexible budgeting establishes an after-the-fact budget; that is, what it would have been expected to cost had the actual patient volume been known in advance. Using flexible budgets, it is possible to break a unit or department's line-item variances down into components caused by (1) changes in prices or salary rates from those expected; (2) changes in the amount of input used per unit of patient volume or output, such as the amount of nursing time per patient day; and (3) changes in the patient volume itself.

Efficient management requires investigation and evaluation of variances on a timely basis, followed by actions to correct variances whenever possible. Managerial expertise and judgment are needed to investigate and evaluate the variances. Flexible budget variance analysis can make the manager's job easier by segregating the variance into its component parts. This allows the manager to spend more time understanding and explaining why the variance occurred instead of trying to isolate the portion of the variance attributable to patient volume changes, the portion attributable to resource usage per patient, and the portion attributable to the prices of the various resources consumed.

In considering variances the nurse manager should attempt to put finances in perspective. The financial health and survival of the institution are essential. However, the quality of patient care provided is also critical. Performance should be measured using more than one set of criteria. Meeting the budget is one measure of performance. Quality of care, patient satisfaction, nurse satisfaction, and innovation are a few of the other things that nurse managers are trying to achieve. There should be a balance between evaluation of financial performance and evaluation of performance in nonfinancial areas.

This chapter has provided tools that can be used to identify the underlying causes of variances. Often this will allow the manager to explain a "poor" report. In some cases performance can be improved by using variance reports to learn where expenses are out of control. In other cases, spending over budget may mean that a trade-off was made. Some other desired objectives may have been achieved at the expense of financial goals. Which are more important? Each institution and its managers must make that decision in each specific case. Sometimes finances will be paramount. Sometimes they will not. If a nurse manager can meet the budget but fails to meet quality-of-care needs or can meet quality-of-care needs but fails to meet the budget, which choice is correct? Whichever choice is made, managers should be prepared to justify why they felt that it was the right choice.

Although expense variances often require great attention, managers should also consider whether revenue variances are creating situations that require management intervention.

KEY CONCEPTS ❖

Management control system Organizations exercise control over operations through the use of a complete set of policies and procedures called a management control system.

Responsibility accounting System of assigning responsibility for keeping to the organization's plan and carrying out the elements of the management control system. Responsibility is generally assigned to managers of cost centers.

Motivation The role of motivation of staff and managers in controlling operating results cannot be overemphasized. If people are not motivated to carry out the budget, it is not likely to be achieved. A variety of incentives such as bonuses can be used to help motivate staff and managers. If targets are set at unrealistically high levels, the negative motivational implications are likely to offset any hoped-for benefits.

Communication Both the budget and actual results compared to the budget must be communicated throughout the organization. This is an essential element of control and should be an ongoing process.

Responsibility should equal control If managers are held responsible for things they have no control over, the organization will reward and punish the wrong individuals. The result is invariably demoralization of managers and staff.

Interim evaluations These are of particular importance in controlling operational results. Each month there should be comparisons between what was expected and what has been accomplished.

Variance analysis Aspect of budgeting in which actual results are compared to budgeted expectations. Variances are used to improve future planning, allow for corrective actions to better control results in coming periods, and evaluate the performance of units or departments and their managers.

Traditional variance analysis Compares the budget with actual results for the most recent month and year to date for each line item in each cost center.

Flexible budget variance analysis Expands upon traditional variance analysis by dividing the total variance into a price, quantity, and volume variance.

Price or rate variance Part of the total difference between the budget and actual that results from a higher or lower hourly rate or purchase price than budgeted.

Quantity or use variance Part of the total difference between the budget and actual that results from the use of more or less resources per patient than budgeted.

Volume variance Part of the total difference between the budget and actual that results from a different volume of patients than budgeted.

Aggregation of variances Managers should be careful to avoid failing to identify variances because favorable variances and unfavorable variances offset each other when added together. Exception reports can be used to identify critical variances.

Revenue variances Can be calculated using either revenue or contribution margin to identify volume, mix, and price variances.

SUGGESTED READINGS _____

Felteau, Anne, "Budget Variance Analysis and Justification," *Nursing Management*, Vol. 23, No. 2, February 1992, pp. 40–41.
Finkler, Steven A., *Budgeting Concepts for Nurse Managers*, 2nd edition, W.B. Saunders, Philadelphia, 1992.

Finkler, Steven A., "Control Aspects of Financial Variance Analysis," in *Health Services Management: Readings and Commentary*, Anthony R. Kovner and Duncan Neuhauser, eds., Health Administration Press, Ann Arbor, MI, 1990, pp. 149–166.

Finkler, Steven A., "Variance Analysis: Extending Flexible Budget Variance Analysis to Acuity," *Journal of Nursing Administration*, Vol. 21, No. 7/8, July/August 1991, pp. 19–25.

Finkler, Steven A., "Using Computers to Improve Variance Analysis," *Journal of Nursing Administration*, Vol. 21, No. 9, September 1991, pp. 9–15.

Finkler, Steven A., "Variance Analysis: Future Directions: Part I: Conceptual Issues," *Hospital Cost Accounting Advisor*," Vol. 3, No. 8, January 1988, pp. 1–5.

Finkler, Steven A., "Variance Analysis: Future Directions: Part II: Calculations," *Hospital Cost Accounting Advisor*," Vol. 3, No. 9, February 1988, pp. 1–5.

Francisco, Perry D., "Flexible Budgeting and Variance Analysis," *Nursing Management*, Vol. 20, No. 11, November 1989, pp. 40–45.

Horngren, Charles T., *Cost Accounting: A Managerial Emphasis*, 7th edition, Prentice-Hall, Englewood Cliffs, NJ, 1990.

Kersey, James H. Jr., "Increasing the Nursing Manager's Fiscal Responsibility," *Nursing Management*, Vol. 19, No. 10, October 1988, pp. 30–32.

Norton, Virginia M., Karol Thorne, Cathy Bickerstaff et al., "Co$t Busters Fair: Increasing Staff Awareness of Cost Effective Practice," *Journal of Nursing Administration*, Vol. 18, No. 9, September 1988, pp. 16–19.

Robbins, Walter A., and Fred A. Jacobs, "Cost Variances in Health Care: When Should Managers Investigate," *Journal of Nursing Administration*, Vol. 15, No. 9, September 1985, pp. 36–40.

Spitzer, R., and W. Poate, "Effective Budgeting Variance Reporting," *in Nursing Productivity: The Hospital's Key to Survival and Profit*, R. Spitzer, ed., 5-N Pub. Inc., Chicago, 1986, pp. 21–25.

Vergara, Gail H., and Joan Bourke, "Reward Employees, Achieve Goals with Incentive Compensation," *Healthcare Financial Management*, Vol. 39, No. 8, August 1985, pp. 50–52.

Wellever, Anthony, "Variance Analysis: A Tool for Cost Control" *Journal of Nursing Administration*, Vol. 12, No. 7/8, July/August 1982, pp. 23–26.

Wilburn, Debbie, "Budget Response to Volume Variability," *Nursing Management*, Vol. 23, No. 2, February 1992, pp. 42–45.

Williams, Frank, "Employee Incentive Systems," from *Handbook of Health Care Accounting and Finance*, Volume I, William O. Cleverley, ed., Aspen Systems, Corp., Rockville, MD, 1982, pp. 395–412.

FINANCIAL MANAGEMENT SERIES

Variance Analysis

Part I, Extending Flexible Budget Variance Analysis to Acuity

Steven A. Finkler, PhD, CPA

The author reviews the concepts of flexible budget variance analysis, including the price, quantity, and volume variances generated by that technique. He also introduces the concept of acuity variance and provides direction on how such a variance measure can be calculated. Part II in this two-part series on variance analysis will look at how personal computers can be useful in the variance analysis process.

Recent years have seen a growing sophistication in the use of variance analysis by nursing departments. As cost containment has become more and more important to healthcare organizations, nurses have been among the leaders in pushing for techniques that can aid managers in controlling costs. Improved variance analysis—in particular, flexible budget variance analysis—is being adopted by an ever larger number of healthcare organizations.

Flexible budget variance analysis is based on the notion that budgets are prepared with a specific fixed volume of work in mind. When actual workload differs from budgeted expectations (which is more often than not the case), costs should be expected to change as well. That fact should be recognized in the variance analysis process. Flexible budget variance analysis explicitly recognizes this.

As healthcare organizations start taking workload *volume* into account in their variance analysis process, they should take the next major step in variance analysis. That step concerns the introduction of a technique for measuring the extent to which variances are caused by average patient

acuity levels that differ from budgeted expectations. Over the last decade, hospital lengths of stay have been decreasing, but average patient acuity has been rising. If the increase in patient acuity exceeds a nursing department's anticipations, the results are invariably understaffing or overspending. However, mechanical processes are available that can calculate the portion of a variance that is attributable to unexpected changes in acuity.

In this article, the concepts of flexible budget variance analysis, including the price, quantity, and volume variances generated by that technique, are reviewed. The concept of an *acuity variance* is also introduced, and direction on how such a variance measure can be calculated is provided. Part II in this two-part series on variance analysis will look at how personal computers can be useful in the variance analysis process.

Flexible Budget Variance Analysis

Variance is the difference between a budgeted value and an actual result. Most healthcare organizations have been using variance analysis for a number of years. Until recently, however, that analysis tended to be rather unsophisticated. Actual results for each line-item of a department or unit budget were compared with budgeted amounts for the month and year to date. Differences between the actual result and the budget value were investigated to the extent possible.

There are several limitations to such information. The first and most critical problem is that the budget is based on an anticipated workload volume, whereas the actual costs incurred are based on the actual workload encountered. Given the information contained in this basic type of variance report, there is no easy way to calculate how much of the variance is due to the change in workload and how much to other factors.

Steven A. Finkler, PhD, CPA, Professor of Health Administration, Accounting, and Financial Management, Robert F. Wagner Graduate School of Public Service, New York University, New York.

Reprinted from *Journal of Nursing Administration*, Vol. 21, No. 7/8, July/August 1991, pp. 19–25.

A flexible budget is a revised budget prepared after each month is over, estimating the cost that should have been incurred for the actual workload encountered. Use of such an ex-post budget allows the manager to determine the extent to which variances are simply a result of increased or decreased workload. Because the workload is rarely controllable by the manager, it is possible to focus the investigation on the remaining portion of the variances.

> ### Increased volume is often associated with increased revenues for the organization.

It should be noted that a flexible budget calculation is only appropriate for costs that are basically variable. For example, a 20% increase in patients on a unit would produce a 20% increase in supplies used. If the increase had been anticipated in advance, it is also likely that there would have been an increased level of staffing. On the other hand, the salary of head nurses and other nursing administrators is likely to be fixed. Costs that would not vary at all with changes in patient volume or acuity are not appropriate for flexible budget calculations.

Variance Components

The flexible budget approach allows any line-item for a variable cost to be divided into the portion caused by a change in the workload, called a *volume variance,* and a portion due to other causes. This latter portion, in turn, can be subdivided into a *quantity variance* and a *price variance.* The process involves taking the variance for a line-item for any unit or department, and subdividing it into several pieces or components. These individual pieces make it easier to track down the underlying causes of the line-item variances.

The volume variance is the change in resource consumption attributable to a change in workload volume. That volume might be measured in units such as patient days, admissions, hours of operating room time, emergency room treatments, or home care visits. In most cases, nursing has relatively little control over the volume of workload.

If hospital occupancy levels rise from 80 to 85% nursing is expected to handle the increased number of patients. From a management standpoint, it makes excellent sense to separate out the volume variance because of the fact that the number of patients is usually not controllable. Further, increased volume is often associated with increased revenues for the organization. It makes little sense for the organization to discourage departments from handling increased volume. By holding a unit or department's spending to the level in its original budget, even if volume (and revenues) have increased, one merely encourages the unit or department to set up roadblocks to future patient increases.

The quantity variance is the change in resource consumption attributable to a change in the amount of resources used for each unit of output. For example, if paid nursing hours per patient day rise, that would give rise to a quantity variance. Quantity variances can arise as a result of a number of different causes. Unexpectedly high sick leave may result in more paid hours for the same number of patients, and therefore a higher nursing cost per patient. Changes in staff efficiency (e.g., longer lunch hours on the negative side or greater staff effort on the positive side) may lead to increased or decreased nursing cost per patient. A quantity variance also occurs if the workload changes and there is no staffing adjustment (upward or downward) made in response to the changing workload.

The price variance is the change in resource consumption attributable to a change in the price of inputs. For example, payment of a higher average hourly pay rate would create a price variance. Price variances may be under the control of nurse managers (e.g., poor staffing leading to unnecessary overtime premiums), or may be beyond their control (poor estimates by the purchasing department for the unit cost of supplies).

The Acuity Variance

If we total the volume, price, and quantity variances, we arrive at the total variance for the particular line-item under investigation. It is possible, however, to subdivide the quantity variance even further. Part of the quantity variance may result from a change in patient acuity levels from those anticipated.

Although acuity may change systematically as average length of stay declines over time, it is also a random element. In any given month or year, average acuity for a unit may be unexpectedly high or low, depending on the specific mix of patients in the unit during that time period. Such fluctuations in acuity are clearly beyond the control of the nurse manager, but he or she may have to respond with changes in staffing.

Flexible budget variance analysis can allow the quantity variance to be split between the portion caused by a difference between actual and anticipated acuity levels, and the portion caused by other factors. Before the advent of patient classification systems, measurement of an acuity variance was not possible. For hospitals that actively use patient classification systems, such measurement is now feasible.

Calculating Variances

To subdivide the variance for any line-item into volume, quantity, acuity, and price variances, a number of pieces of information are needed. First, it is necessary to know the budgeted workload level, the budgeted price of the resources used, and the budgeted amount of resources used. For example, consider the line-item cost of staff RNs in a medical/surgical hospital unit. The unit's workload would be measured in terms of budgeted patient days. The price would be the budgeted average hourly rate for staff RNs on the unit. And the amount of resource used would be the total budgeted staff RN hours for the unit. Note that this automatically takes acuity into account in the variance analysis because the total budgeted labor hours are the hours allowed for the budgeted number of patient days at the expected acuity level.

Ideally, the advantages of more sophisticated analysis should not be offset by the disadvantage of high cost to obtain additional data. All of the information needed so far is readily available from the data used to compile the budget. Flexible budget variance analysis also requires the same three pieces of data for the actual outcome. That is, it is necessary to accumulate information on the actual number of patient days, actual average salary rate, and actual number of paid labor hours. To calculate the acuity variance in addition to the price, quantity, and volume variances, it will also be necessary to know the actual number of patient days at each patient classification level.

The first three pieces of information should be relatively easy to obtain. Hospitals already generally keep track of the actual number of patient days by unit, the actual salary rates paid to staff, and the actual total number of paid hours for staff by unit. However, calculation of the acuity variance would require that patient classification information be collected on an ongoing basis. Each nursing department must make its own decision regarding whether the use of such information for variance analysis combined with its other potential uses, such as for improved staffing, make such data collection worthwhile. The information needed for flexible budget variance analysis, including development of an acuity variance is summarized in Table 1, which also includes hypothetical data for use in an example.

The original budget consists of the average price for the resource in question (e.g., staff RNs) multiplied by the budgeted amount of resource. Using the data from Table 1, the original budgeted amount is $100,000 ($20/hour multiplied by 5,000 staff hours). In contrast, the actual cost would be the actual average price paid for the resource multiplied by the actual amount of the resource used. The actual cost is $136,500 ($21/hour multiplied by 6,500 staff hours). Traditional variance analysis would compare the budget with the actual and note that the unit spent $36,500 more than its budget ($100,000 budget vs. $136,500 actual). However, it would not indicate anything about the source of that $36,500 variance.

A flexible budget should be calculated to reflect changes in workload from original expectations. The flexible budget is a computation of the amount that would have been budgeted, had the true workload level been known. The flexible budget consists of the budgeted amount of re-

❖ **TABLE 1**
Data Needed for Flexible Budget Variance Analysis

Budget workload	1,000 patient days
Budgeted price of resource	$20 per hour
Budgeted amount of resource	5,000 hours
Actual workload	1,150 patient days
Actual price of resource	$21 per hour
Actual amount of resource used	6,500 hours
Actual acuity levels	200 at Level 1
	450 at Level 2
	300 at Level 3
	150 at Level 4
	50 at Level 5

source per unit of workload, multiplied by the budgeted price of the resource, multiplied by the actual workload level. In this case, the budgeted amount of resource is 5 hours per patient day (the budgeted total resource of 5,000 hours divided by the budgeted 1,000 patient days). Five hours per patient day, at $20 per hour, for 1,150 actual patient days yields a flexible budget value of $115,000 (5 × 20 × 1,150). Comparing the $115,000 flexible budget with the $100,000 original budget yields a difference of $15,000, which is an unfavorable volume variance. This would indicate that of the total $36,500 variance for the line-item, a portion equal to $15,000, is directly attributable to the fact that there were more patient days than expected. This portion of the variance would generally be considered beyond the control of the nurse manager.

In flexible budgeting, a calculation must be made to determine how much of a line-item variance results from changes in prices of the resources used. To make this calculation, the actual amount spent ($136,500 in this example) is compared with the amount that would have been spent had the actual price of the resource been as budgeted. In other words, using the actual amount of resources used but the budgeted price, how much would have been spent? In this case (Table 1), there are 6,500 actual staff RN hours. The budgeted price is $20. The product of those two number is $130,000. However, the actual cost for the nursing unit is $136,500 (6,500 hours × $21). The difference between the actual cost of $136,500 and the $130,000 cost using the budgeted price is $6,500. That is the price variance. It represents the portion of the total $36,500 variance attributable to the higher-than-expected hourly rate. Given the increased number of patient days, the use of either overtime or agency nurses might well be expected to drive up the average hourly wage, so this unfavorable price variance of $6,500 is not particularly surprising. However, it is large enough that it would probably warrant investigation to find its specific cause or causes.

The volume variance of $15,000 and the price variance of $6,500, combine to explain $21,500 of the total variance. However, the total variance for the line-item was $36,500. There is still $15,000 of variance that has not been explained. This is the quantity variance. It is caused by paying for more resource per unit of workload than expected. It is not attributable to more patients, but rather to the

amount used per patient. Without patient classification information, the nurse manager would have to investigate the $15,000 quantity variance and try to ascertain its causes.

Calculation of the price, quantity, and volume variances is summarized in Figure 1. This figure includes the actual amount spent at the extreme left, and the original budget at the extreme right. In between are two other headings. The flexible budget, as previously noted, represents the amount that would have been budgeted for the actual workload of patient days had that workload level been known in advance. This does not reflect acuity-adjusted workload, but rather looks only at changes in patient-day volume. The value that is compared with the actual results to determine the price variance is referred to as the Budgeted Cost of Actual Resources Used. When this is compared with the flexible budget, the result is the quantity variance.

If patient acuity information is available, the quantity variance can be divided into the portion due to acuity and that due to other factors. This will require inserting a value in between Budgeted Cost of Actual Resources and the Flexible Budget in Figure 1. The new value will be called an Acuity Category. The difference between the Acuity Category and the Flexible Budget is the acuity variance. The difference between the Budgeted Cost of Actual Resources and the Acuity Category is a new quantity variance. The new quantity variance will be the same as the old quantity variance, except that it will exclude the portion of the variance due to changes in acuity. The key to this calculation is the ability to determine the number of paid nursing care hours that would have been budgeted had the actual acuity been known. For example, suppose that the hypothetical patient classification system in place calls for the following paid nursing care hours per patient day:

Patient Classification Level	Paid Nursing Care Hours
1	3.5
2	5.0
3	6.2
4	7.8
5	9.0

In the example being used (Table 1), the actual patient days at each level can be combined with the above chart to generate the hours of nursing care that would have been budgeted, had the

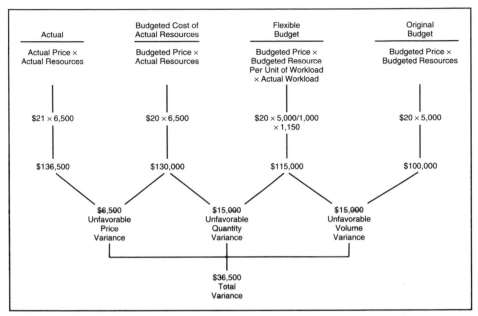

Figure 1. Calculation of price, quantity, and volume variances.

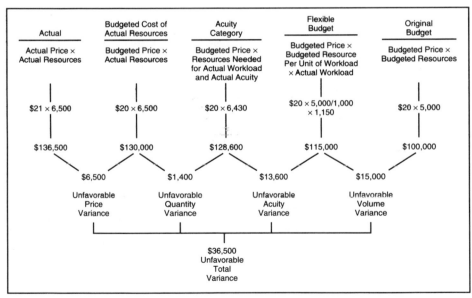

Figure 2. Calculation of price, quantity, volume, and acuity variances.

actual acuity level been known in advance. Essentially, the volume variance accounts for the fact that there were more or fewer patient days than expected. Similarly, the acuity variance will account for the fact that actual acuity differs from the level expected. The flexible budget asks the question, "how much should have been budgeted for the actual number of patients?," whereas the new Acuity Category (Fig. 2) asks, "how much should have been budgeted for the actual number of patients at the actual level of acuity?" Combining the patient classification scheme shown above with the data from Table 1, the number of nursing care hours that would have been budgeted, had the actual volume of patients and actual acuity levels been known, can be calculated as shown in Table 2.

Given that there would have been 6,430 budgeted nursing hours (Table 2) for the actual number of patient days and actual acuity, the acuity category can be calculated by multiplying the budgeted price of the resource, $20, by the 6,430 hours. The result is $128,600. When this is compared with the flexible budget value of $115,000 (Fig. 2), the difference is $13,600. That is the acuity variance. It is the result of actual acuity being higher than expected. When the $128,600 is compared with the Budgeted Cost for Actual Resources value of $130,000, the difference is $1,400. That is the new quantity variance. It represents the fact that more money was spent per patient, even after accounting for acuity. It could be caused by a wide variety of factors, and it could be investigated if the amount were considered large enough to warrant such an investigation.

It is important to note that although all variances in this example were "unfavorable," that does not mean that they were necessarily bad for the organization. Unfavorable simply means spent more than expected. If the extra patient days reflected more patients, revenue may have increased. Furthermore, if the increased acuity reflects a more complex mix of patients, the revenue per patient may be higher as well. Therefore, the unfavorable volume and acuity variances are not necessarily bad. A rule of thumb for determining whether a variance is favorable or unfavorable is that, moving from right to left in Figures 1 and 2, if the number on the left is larger, it indicates an unfavorable variance. However, managers must use thought, rather than rules of thumb, to determine if an unfavorable variance is good or bad.

Caveat

It is important to note one caveat regarding the development of the acuity variance. Budget line-items for nursing units and departments separate out each individual type of worker. Therefore it is appealing to determine the acuity variance for each line-item. However, patient classification systems do not usually isolate the amount of nursing care hours needed by class of care giver. When one calculates the number of nursing care hours needed for the actual acuity, it may be difficult to make that calculation for each separate type of employee. Therefore it may be necessary to aggregate some information in order to be able to calculate an acuity variance.

This is a less than ideal situation. Over time, patient classification systems may develop into more specific tools, looking at RNs, LPNs, and nurse's aides separately. In the meantime, however, the problem does create a complication for calculating acuity variances. Price, quantity, and volume variances are not affected by this problem.

❖ TABLE 2
Calculation of Required Paid Nursing Hours for Actual Number of Patient Days at Actual Acuity Levels

Patient Classification	Nursing Hours Per Patient Day		No. of Patient Days		Required Nursing Hours
Level					
1	3.5	×	200	=	700
2	5.0	×	450	=	2,250
3	6.2	×	300	=	1,860
4	7.8	×	150	=	1,170
5	9.0	×	50	=	450
Total			1,150		6,430

Conclusion

At a minimum, nurse managers should be receiving variance reports that in some way allow for the impact of changes in the workload volume. As the number of patients increases, nurses should not have to explain that more patients consume more resources. Some type of volume variance measure is a necessity. The introduction of price and quantity variance calculations can also be a great aid. They can help nurse managers focus their variance investigations in specific areas.

The introduction of an acuity variance is somewhat more complicated. For organizations that have patient classification systems in place and in use, however, it represents an opportunity to move into the cutting edge of healthcare management in the area of variance analysis. Although adoption of flexible budget variance analysis methodology requires some effort, once used on an ongoing basis, it can continue to pay dividends in the form of improved explanations of variance causes and reduced variance investigation effort by all nurse managers, month after month and years into the future.

In Part II of this series on variance analysis, there will be a discussion of how the variances discussed in this article can be generated within a nursing department by the use of a microcomputer and a spreadsheet software program. The upcoming article will also discuss the use of a variety of types of graphs to aid in the process of variance analysis and justification.

Suggested Readings

Alward RR. Patient classification systems: the ideal vs. reality. J Nurs Admin 1983;13(2):14–9.

Curtin L. Integrating acuity: the frugal road to safe care [Editorial]. Nurs Manage 1985;16(9):7–8.

Finkler SA. Budgeting concepts for nurse managers. 2nd ed. Philadelphia: WB Saunders, 1991.

Francisco PD. Flexible budgeting and variance analysis. Nurs Manage 1989;20(11):40–5.

Nagaprasann B. Patient classification systems: strategies for the 1990's. Nurs Manage 1988;19(3):105–106, 108, 112.

Robbins WA, Jacobs FA. Cost variances in health care: when should managers investigate. J Nurs Admin 1985; 15(9):36–40.

Spitzer R, Poate W. Effective budgeting variance reporting. In: Spitzer R, ed. Nursing productivity: the hospital's key to survival and profit. Chicago, 5-N Publishers, 1986:21–5.

Wellever A. Variance analysis: a tool for cost control. J Nurs Admin 1982;12(7/8):23–6.

PART

V

MANAGING FINANCIAL RESOURCES

All managers of health care organizations manage resources. Determining what personnel and other resources to use and how to use them is a managerial function. A subset within the realm of organizational resources is represented by financial resources. To the same extent that clinical resources must be carefully used, financial resources must be managed in an efficient manner.

Decisions concerning where and how to get financial resources—the source of financial resources—is one element of the management of financial resources. Some resources in proprietary organizations come from investments owners make in the organization. In not-for-profit organizations a common source of financial resources is charitable donations. Profits are a potential source of financial resources for all types of health care organizations. In this century it has become common for health care organizations to borrow much of their necessary financing.

Once the organization has financial resources, it must manage them efficiently. Decisions must be made concerning how much cash to have on hand. Management techniques must be employed to ensure that cash is received as promptly as possible. Managers must ensure that cash is available when needed for purposes such as employee payrolls or interest payments. This requirement to have control over the inflow and outflow of cash necessitates management of other assets and liabilities that impact directly on cash. As a result, receivables, inventories, marketable securities, payables, and leases all fall under the heading of management of financial resources.

While some managers perceive the management of financial resources as the strict domain of financial managers, that is not the case. For example, a financial manager can do little to control inventory levels. The nurse manager is in a much better position to make determinations regarding necessary inventory levels and to enforce policies established to avoid unnecessary stockpiling of inventory. Therefore the nurse manager and financial managers must work together in the management of financial resources to arrive at an optimal outcome for the organization.

Additionally, nurse managers should be aware of even those aspects of the management of financial resources which do not bear directly on their day-to-day activities. The decisions to borrow money or invest it have a direct bearing on the success of the organization and on the decisions it makes concerning the allocation of resources to various cost centers. Therefore it is beneficial for the nurse manager to be aware of the factors involved in the management of financial resources.

This part of the book is divided into two chapters. The first chapter focuses directly on the management of the short-term financial resources of the organization. The second chapter is concerned with the long-term financing of health care organizations.

Short-term relates to resources that appear in the current asset and current liability sections of the balance sheet. Such resources generally provide or require cash within a relatively short period, usually less than a year. These short-term resources and short-term sources of resources are referred to as the organization's working capital.

Long-term financing relates to the alternatives the organization has for acquiring financial resources that will not have to be repaid within a period of less than one year. To be able to acquire capital assets—buildings and equipment—the organization must know that it can acquire money that does not have to be repaid in a short period. The choices it makes regarding such long-term financing can have dramatic effects on the ability of the organization to provide health care services and to compete in the health care marketplace. ❖

14

Short-Term Financial Resources

CHAPTER GOALS

The goals of this chapter are to:

- ♦ Define working capital and working capital management
- ♦ Describe the role of cash in the organization
- ♦ Explain techniques for cash management
- ♦ Distinguish between cash flows and revenues and expenses
- ♦ Describe the cash budgeting process
- ♦ Provide a description of the elements of accounts receivable management
- ♦ Discuss factors related to efficient inventory management
- ♦ Define trade credit terms related to accounts payable
- ♦ Discuss elements of working capital management for other current liabilities

❖

INTRODUCTION

Working capital is the organization's current assets and current liabilities. *Net working capital* is the current assets less the current liabilities. The term *working capital management* refers to the management of the current assets and current liabilities of the organization. (A basic discussion of current assets and current liabilities was provided in Chapter 5.)

Working capital is sometimes referred to as "cash register money." When one opens a store for business, there must be some money in the cash register to make change for the first customer who makes a purchase. Additionally, some customers may charge their purchases. In those cases, the store will not receive any cash currently, but it still has to pay its suppliers for the items it has acquired for sale as well as paying its employees. There must be adequate cash for the store to use during the lag from the time when it must pay for its resources until it receives cash from its customers.

The cash resources of an organization are of concern to all its managers. Why should a nurse manager be concerned with issues such as cash flow and inventory levels? All organizations have limited resources. If ICU nurses stockpile IV fluids, the organization will pay out more cash now for inventory than is otherwise necessary. This in turn could mean that med/surg nurses will be told that there is no cash available to buy needed supplies. Nurses sometimes cope with this situation by stockpiling whenever they get a chance so they will have the supplies when they need them. This creates a vicious cycle. Since all nurses try to keep high levels of inventory to protect their patients, the overall inventories are maintained at too high a level. This means that money has been spent on inventory rather than being in a bank earning interest. The lost interest means that there is less total money available for purchases of supplies. A cooperative working relationship is needed throughout the organization to allow inventory levels to be maintained at adequate levels and money to be available for purchases when needed without unduly wasting resources by keeping high inventory levels.

One can envision a working capital cycle (Fig. 14–1) in which cash is used to buy inventory items such as clinical supplies. Then patients are treated, consuming inventory items and also using employees' services. Then the organization bills patients and waits to collect payment. Finally cash is received and the cycle starts over.

Working capital management is the role of the manager in ensuring that there is adequate cash on hand to meet the organization's needs and minimizing the cost of those resources. To do this, the manager must carefully control cash inflows and outflows. To be efficient, cash must not lie idle, so there should not be too much cash on hand. Cash not immediately needed should be invested, earning a return for the organization. Similarly, excess inventory should not be kept by the organization. The money spent to pay for inventory that is not needed could have been used by the organization for some other purpose.

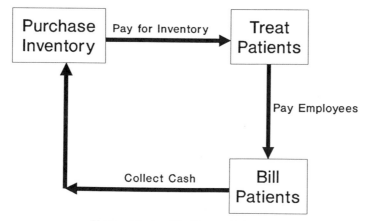

Figure 14–1. Working capital cycle.

Receivables from customers should be collected promptly so that the organization will have that cash available for its use.

By the same token, current liabilities must be managed carefully. The organization desires to have sufficient cash to pay its obligations when they are due. However, if the organization pays its bills before they are due, it will lose the interest it could have earned if it had invested its cash for a little longer rather than paying the obligation.

This chapter focuses on the management of all elements of working capital. The discussion will begin with current assets. Then we will turn our attention to issues related to current liabilities.

CURRENT ASSETS

A number of different current assets require careful management. The most essential financial resource is cash. Cash is what organizations must have to pay obligations as they come due. Cash is generally defined as both currency and balances available in bank accounts for withdrawal upon demand (such as checking accounts). Marketable securities provide managers with an outlet to invest idle resources while maintaining access to the resources when needed. In most health care organizations managers also focus a great deal of attention on accounts receivable. Such receivables often constitute the largest single element of working capital. Inventories also receive a great amount of attention because historically managers have had difficulty in managing them.

Cash and Marketable Securities

Organizations have cash requirements for three main purposes:
♦ Transactions
♦ Safety
♦ Investments

Transactions refers to having cash available for the day-in and day-out normal operating expenses of the organization such as staff payroll and supplies. As noted above, one cannot wait to receive patient payments before paying many of the organization's obligations; cash is needed for that purpose.

Safety is the second reason for holding cash. Managers are unable to anticipate all the organization's needs. Emergencies may require immediate, unexpected cash outlays. In some situations, managers may anticipate the likelihood of the event but not know when it is likely to occur. In other cases, the event may be totally unanticipated. Experience has proven that it is wise for the organization to have immediate access to cash just in case an unexpected need arises.

The third purpose for holding cash is to have cash available if a desirable investment opportunity arises. Such an opportunity may be the possibility of earning an attractive profit, or it may relate to the possibility of providing services to the community.

Given these reasons to hold cash, managers might desire to keep large amounts available, just to be safe. However, that is not necessarily an optimal approach. Cash does not generate a return for the organization. Often it sits in a non-interest-bearing checking account. Even if it is kept in a savings account, the rate of return is likely to be minimal. If the organization wants to be able to maximize the benefits from all its resources, it must minimize the extent to which it has unproductive assets.

Therefore, there is a conflict in cash management. The more cash on hand, the safer the organization, but the lower its return on invested money. The less cash the organization chooses to keep on hand, the better its financial profits, but the riskier it is. It has less protection against unexpected cash needs. Managers must walk a tightrope, attempting to determine a reasonable cash balance and keeping neither too much nor too little.

In a well-run organization, cash is actively managed. An initial projection is made regarding the timing of cash receipts from philanthropy, patients, the government, and insurance companies. A projection of the organization's required payments must also be prepared. The cash excess or shortfall is calculated for each period of time.

If there is a shortfall, it may be possible to go to a bank and arrange for a line of credit to be available at the time cash is projected to be needed. Before doing that, however, other approaches should be considered. Can the financial managers take actions to process patient billings more quickly so that payments will be received sooner? Will the extra cost of speedier invoicing be offset by the interest saved by borrowing less money from the bank? What if payments to the organization's suppliers are delayed by thirty days to avoid borrowing money? How angry will that make the organization's suppliers?

If a cash surplus is forecast, it can be invested to earn interest, used to repay loans, or used to provide more health care services. Financial managers must be careful to ensure that the organization will always have enough cash to meet obligations, but they should also be careful to ensure that the organization is not missing opportunities to provide additional health services because it is keeping too much cash in the bank. Either too little or too much cash leaves the organization in a less than optimal situation.

Short-term Cash Investment

Cash should rarely if ever be kept in non-interest-bearing accounts. In fact, even after checks are written, it is possible to invest the money drawn in the interim period until the check is cashed. That period is called the *float.* Many banks have arrangements that allow money to be automatically transferred into a checking account as checks are presented for payment. Until that point the money can remain in an interest-bearing account.

Managers should make great efforts to ensure that cash is deposited into interest-bearing accounts as quickly as possible and withdrawn only when actually needed. All organizations should have specific policies that result in cash and check receipts being processed and deposited promptly.

Interest-bearing bank accounts pay relatively low rates of interest. Many alternatives are available for health care managers to invest cash at a higher rate of return. In most cases, however, this requires reducing the organization's ability to get immediate access to the cash. Short-term investments include treasury bills, certificates of deposit (CDs), and *repurchase agreements.* Treasury bills are issued for thirteen weeks, twenty-six weeks, or fifty-two weeks. However, they are traded actively, making it quite easy to convert into cash when necessary. CDs generally tie up the organization's money for at least a month. However, they often pay interest rates higher than treasury bills. Repurchase agreements are flexible bank-related financial instruments. They can be for periods as short as one day. However, their interest rates are generally lower than those of treasury bills.

It is also possible for health care organizations to invest in other types of marketable securities such as corporate stocks and bonds. However, managers must exercise care in making such investments, since they are subject to market-rate fluctuations, i.e., their value might fall while they are invested. While that reduction in value may be recovered if the securities are held for a period of time, the organization may well suffer a loss if it must liquidate the investment to get the cash. In general, risk and return represent a trade-off in investments. To earn a higher return on invested money, one must be willing to take a greater risk with the initial principal investment.

Cash Flow vs. Revenue and Expense

Cash management concentrates on the inflows and outflows of cash. This is in contrast to the operating budget focus on revenues and expenses. Operating budgets consider overall profitability, but they do not consider when payments are made. Therefore the manager cannot use them to determine whether adequate cash will be available at any given point in time for the organization's needs.

At times cash management may cause the organization to make decisions that directly impact nurse managers and that seem to make no sense. For example, consider a request by nursing to buy bedside computers for nursing units at a total cost of $200,000. The computers are expected to have a useful lifetime of ten years and will improve the quality of documentation. This will result in improved care and will decrease overtime required for charting by $40,000 per year. The $400,000 of reduced overtime over the ten-year period is enough to make the initial investment of $200,000 financially sensible. Yet the financial officers may say that the organization cannot afford the computers. How can that decision make any sense?

Even though the computers are saving more money than their cost, it is not clear that the organization can afford to purchase them. The entire price of $200,000 for the computers will have to be paid in cash this year, even though the overtime savings are only expected to be $40,000 this year. Where will the cash for the initial $200,000 purchase come from?

The potential for reduced costs or for increased profits does not by itself provide the cash needed to make the investment. It might be wise to lease the asset rather than pay all the cash up front. Maybe the organization can borrow the money from a bank. Perhaps it can raise the money through contributions. While the organization's managers should try to pursue various ways to get the cash for worthwhile investments—whether they are worthwhile because they are profitable or simply because they are good for the patients—there is a responsibility to the well-being of the organization not to spend the money until it is first determined that there will be sufficient cash available to spend.

Financial officers must carefully consider the cash implications of the operating and capital budgets before they are approved. In effect, various departments submit their operating and capital budget requests. A *cash budget* is developed based on those requests. One reason that departmental budgets may be rejected is that the cash budget may show that the organization would simply run out of cash if it made all the requested payments. If an organization finds itself without cash to meet its obligations, it may be forced into bankruptcy. Even if the organization is making a profit, without careful management it may run out of cash and get into financial difficulty.

Cash Budgets

As a result of the importance of cash balances, health care organizations generally prepare a cash budget for the entire coming year on a monthly basis. The format of cash budgets is fairly standard. Each month begins with a starting cash balance. The expected cash receipts for the month are added to this. These receipts may be broken down into categories such as inpatient, outpatient, other operating, and nonoperating or by payer (e.g., Medicare, Medicaid, Blue Cross, other insurers, self-pay patients, donations, and cafeteria sales). The starting cash balance is added to the total receipts to get a subtotal of available cash. Then expected cash payments are subtracted. Cash budgeting was introduced in Chapter 11.

Accurate cash budgeting requires managers to estimate how much cash will be received by type of payer. Different types of payers have different bad-debt rates and pay on different schedules. For example, Blue Cross might pay an organization more promptly than Medicare but less promptly than other private insurance companies. Payer-mix information, combined with knowledge about the lags in payment by each type of payer, can then be used to project cash receipts for each month.

For example, suppose that a health care organization had revenues of $500,000 for January and that the payer mix is as in Table 14–1. The payment lags represent averages. Especially with respect to self-pay patients, there is likely to be a mix of faster and slower paying patients. Assuming that there are no bad debts, when would the $500,000 of revenue from January be received in cash? (See Table 14–2.) The payers with a one-month lag would pay in February, those with a two-month lag in March, those with a three-month lag in April, and those with a four-month lag in May. For example, a total of $225,000 from January revenues would be collected in April because both Medicare and self-pay patients pay with a three-month lag in this example.

If the expected cash balance for any month exceeds the minimum desired balance, the excess can be invested. This is true even if a surplus one month is followed by an expected shortfall the next. It may pay to invest the extra cash in a very short-term investment, such as a money market fund. In that way, the excess cash from one month can earn some interest and can still be available to meet the shortage the next month. Borrowing can thus be avoided or minimized.

❖ TABLE 14–1
Payment Lag by Payer

Payer	Percentage of Patients	Payment Lag
Medicare	30	3 months
Medicaid	20	4 months
Blue Cross	25	2 months
Other insurer	10	1 month
Self-pay	15	3 months

❖ **TABLE 14–2**
Timing of Cash Receipt of January Revenues

Payer	Percentage of Patients		Total Revenue		Revenue Share	Month Collected
Medicare	30	×	$500,000	=	$150,000	April
Medicaid	20	×	500,000	=	100,000	May
Blue Cross	25	×	500,000	=	125,000	March
Other insurers	10	×	500,000	=	50,000	February
Self-pay	15	×	500,000	=	75,000	April

Maintaining Security over Cash

Of all the assets the organization has, cash requires the greatest care to ensure that it is not misappropriated. Systems must be put into place that have checks and balances. Individuals who handle cash should be different from those who reconcile cash receipts. Controls should exist for both cash receipts and cash disbursements.

Disbursements are often easier to protect. Whenever possible, payments should be made by check. Large checks should require two signatures. All checks should be numbered. All checks should require an authorization by someone other than the one involved in drawing the checks.

Cash receipts should be handled by individuals who are bonded and reliable and take vacations. Bonding is an insurance procedure that protects the organization from cash theft by the insured individual. Reliable personnel are essential. The organization must have trustworthy individuals working in the cash area. Even with trustworthy individuals, it is a good practice to require individuals to take vacations. Knowing that someone else will be handling the function makes individuals less likely to do anything inappropriate that might be discovered in their absence.

Accounts Receivable

When an organization's customers do not pay for goods or services at the time they are provided, they are said to be buying the services "on account." An account is set up by both the buyer and seller to keep track of the amount owed. Providers of the service expect to ultimately receive payment, so they call the money owed to them an *account receivable*. Buyers will ultimately pay the amount owed, so they have an *account payable*.

Management of accounts receivable focuses on speed, accuracy, and communication. Managers must try to minimize the time between provision of care and ultimate receipt of payment. Accounts receivable earn no return for the organization. The sooner cash is collected, the sooner the organization can use that cash for its operations or else invest it. Also, efforts to collect cash quickly tend to reduce bad debts. For accounts to be collected on a timely basis, all documentation must be accurate and complete. Also, there should be great efforts to keep the lines of communication open between the organization and the payers.

The process of managing accounts receivable should start before a patient is even admitted to a health care institution. Preadmission data collection is one of the most important activities an organization can undertake to ensure efficient collection of its accounts. Another essential feature is the establishment of credit policies. Who is the organization willing to treat and under what circumstances? During a patient's course of treatment, there should be an ongoing data collection. When a patient is discharged, there should be a review to ensure comprehensive inclusion of charges, and a bill should be issued. Receivables management does not stop at this point. Receivables should be monitored while outstanding, using an aging schedule. If necessary, the organization should use a collection agency to collect delinquent accounts. When cash does arrive, there should be specific procedures to safeguard it until its ultimate deposit in the bank. All these elements will now be discussed.

Preadmission Data Collection

As noted above, the process of managing accounts receivable should start before a patient is even admitted to a health care institution. Many organizations have a conference with the patient to determine the sources of payment for the patient's care. In many cases patients have Medicare, Medicaid, Blue Cross, or other insurance coverage. If that is the case, all pertinent information should be recorded so that upon discharge a bill can be expeditiously processed. All forms should be completed, signatures obtained, and insurance companies called to verify coverage and obtain all necessary preadmission approvals. Many insurers will deny coverage if the patient was admitted without prenotification to the company.

In some cases it may be determined that the patient is eligible for Medicaid but has not enrolled. Many health care organizations have specific policies regarding helping patients enroll for Medicaid. In fact, some hospitals actually have state Medicaid employees working in the hospital to enroll patients. Enrolling an eligible patient often represents the difference between a substantial payment for the care provided to that patient and receiving little payment, if any at all.

If the patient has no insurance coverage, financial planning for payment can take place at the preadmission conference. In some cases this will mean establishing a payment schedule so that patients can pay what they can afford over an extended period. In some cases it will be determined that patients have no capacity to pay, and they will be classified as indigent for medical purposes. In that case their care will be considered charity care. In some states, there is financial assistance to health care organizations to reimburse some part of the charity care provided. However, careful documentation is required so that a claim can be properly filed.

Credit Policies

Some medical care represents true emergency care, and standards in the United States require that such care be provided regardless of the patient's ability to pay. This certainly is justified on moral or ethical grounds. Other care, however, is elective. Health care providers have a greater ethical and legal latitude in deciding what nonemergency care to provide to whom. At the opposite extreme from emergency care are things such as cosmetic surgery. Few would blame a health care organization that refused to provide a cosmetic rhinoplasty to an indigent patient.

Health care organizations must establish clear rules that guide their decisions on whether to offer credit to patients. These rules must reflect both the financial condition of the patient and the medical condition. There should be a clear policy on when patients are treated regardless of their ability to pay, and when they are not. Some organizations will be more permissive than others for a variety of reasons. For example, one organization may have a better financial position than another and be able to better withstand bad debts.

To carry out the organization's credit policy, preadmission data collection is essential. In addition to providing the information needed for prompt, accurate billing, it provides the information the organization needs to make its decisions on when to provide care. While it is distasteful to have to deny any care to anyone, it is a reality of the existing health care system. Organizations have credit policies to protect the organization so it can remain in business and continue to provide essential care to all.

Ongoing Data Collection

During a patient's course of treatment, there should be a continuous collection of data. The organization must track the services that the patient is consuming so that they may properly be included in the patient's bill.

If data collection is postponed until discharge or shortly thereafter, there is the risk that some charges will be overlooked. The number of patient days, x-rays, and lab tests must all be accumulated on an ongoing basis.

Nursing has always had a responsibility to participate in this ongoing data collection in a number of ways. Inventory items used are recorded on the patient chart. Charge slips for various procedures are also often placed in the chart by the nursing staff. While it may seem cumbersome to have to place a charge slip for a catheter on the patient's chart, without that step the patient will not be billed for that item. In that case the organization will lose that money and have fewer resources available for the provision of patient care.

This role is likely to grow in the future, as variable billing for nursing services becomes more widely used. Specifically, to charge for nursing services it is necessary to have information on the patient's consumption of nursing resources. This is generally obtained from the patient classification system. While all acute care hospitals have such systems, they do not all actively use them. To charge patients for nursing, information on their daily classification level must be accumulated on an ongoing basis.

Discharge Review and Billing

Upon discharge, a number of activities must take place in short order. The original patient payment information must be reviewed to ensure that it is complete. Something as minor as a missing zip code in the patient address could lead to a payment delay of several months or more.

The diagnosis of the patient must be firmly and clearly established at discharge. Medicare DRG payments for inpatients rely on the DRG assignment. That assignment in turn relies on a number of factors recorded in the medical report, such as principal and secondary diagnoses, surgical procedures, and age. If any of those elements is missing, a DRG cannot properly be assigned, and payment will be delayed. Once a patient bill is "kicked out" of the system, a payment delay of at least several months is the rule rather than the exception.

When the record has been reviewed and found to be complete both with respect to payer information and clinical information, a bill should be promptly issued. Many large payers now accept billing on electronic media such as computer tapes rather than requiring paper bills. Some payers require electronic submission of bills. Computer information may even be electronically transmitted, eliminating the entire time that a bill would normally be in transit.

Even a savings of two or three days can have a significant impact. For any one bill it does not seem to matter if there are a few delays. However, when all bills are considered, the impact of prompt billing is significant. For example, suppose that a large hospital issues $200 million in patient billings each year. Also assume that the hospital has outstanding loans from banks at a 10% interest rate. If electronic processing of bills directly to payers means that each bill is collected three days sooner than it otherwise would be, the interest savings would be over $164,000 a year! ($200 million × 10% ÷ 365 = $54,800 interest per day. $54,800 × 3 days is approximately $164,000 per year.)

Electronic processing is only one element. Consider a hospital that processes lab charges only once a month. Bills for patients discharged in January could not be issued until lab charges are processed for January. That might not be completed until February 5. Then all the lab charges would have to be posted to the individual patient accounts. That might take another week. It is conceivable that in a totally manual system, it might well be February 15 until any bills were issued for patients discharged anytime in January. On average, it would be a month after discharge until a patient bill was issued.

Delaying billing by a month delays receipt of cash by a month. In a hospital with $200 million of charges, such a delay could cost over $1.5 million per year. It should be no surprise that most health care organizations have automated data entry and billing systems. Every day earlier that bills can be issued saves a significant amount of money.

Aging of Receivables

Once bills have been issued, it is important for the organization to monitor receivables and to follow up on unpaid bills. This is true not only for self-pay patients, who are viewed as bad-debt risks, but also for the government and insurers. Often the large third-party payers will not pay a bill if they find any problem with it. The health care organization must be on top of receivables to ensure that any problems preventing specific bills from being paid are resolved.

A tool used to keep track of potential accounts receivable problems is an *aging schedule*. An aging schedule shows how long a receivable has been outstanding since a bill was issued. For example, at the end of June a summary aging schedule might appear as the example in Table 14–3.

The aging schedule allows managers to monitor outstanding receivables. In Table 14–3, we notice that only 53.4% of the receivables outstanding are outstanding for less than one month. Almost half the receivables are outstanding more than thirty days since the date the bills were issued. On the other hand, a relatively small 3% of outstanding receivables are more than ninety days old.

If large payers constitute a significant portion of the organization's revenue, the organization should attempt to arrange for periodic interim payments (PIP). In a PIP arrangement, the payer makes payments in advance of the receipt and processing of specific bills. For instance, in the example in Table 14–3 the hospital might find that every month it bills Blue Cross for about $700,000.

❖ **TABLE 14–3**
Sample Aging Schedule—June 30 Aging Report

Payer	1–30 Days	31–60 Days	61–90 Days	>90 Days	Total
By Total Dollars					
Medicare	$ 802,054	$ 795,633	$402,330	$ 52,050	$2,052,067
Medicaid	325,020	342,943	85,346	28,345	781,654
Blue Cross	682,285	114,538	14,354	4,364	815,541
Insurers	437,899	46,722	8,563	7,773	500,957
Self-pay	174,799	103,295	67,322	43,588	389,004
Total	$2,422,057	$1,403,131	$577,915	$136,120	$4,539,223
By Percent					
Medicare	17.7%	17.5%	8.9%	1.1%	45.2%
Medicaid	7.2	7.6	1.9	.6	17.2
Blue Cross	15.0	2.5	.3	.1	18.0
Insurers	9.6	1.0	.2	.2	11.0
Self-pay	3.9	2.3	1.5	2.0	8.6
Total	53.4%	30.9%	12.7%	3.0%	100.0%

399

Rather than wait for the billings, each month Blue Cross could issue a payment of perhaps $500,000 for care to patients during the current month. The balance to be paid for each month's care would wait until the specific bills are received. This allows the health care organization to receive its revenues in cash sooner than would otherwise be the case. Unfortunately, in recent years payers, also under financial pressure, have been reluctant to make PIPs.

The over-ninety-day category in the aging is a particular concern, even though it is a small part of the total. These accounts probably reflect problems encountered in processing the bills by third-party payers or else an inability or unwillingness to pay by self-pay patients. The health care organization should have specific follow-up procedures. These procedures should include sending monthly statements and making phone calls to determine why payment has not been made.

Some of this process can be avoided if indigent patients are clearly identified in advance. While the health care organization will want to pursue those individuals who can pay for the care they receive, it is a costly waste of effort to spend resources trying to collect payment from the truly indigent.

In some cases it is necessary to use a collection agency if other efforts have failed and it is believed that the patient can afford to make payments. This is a costly approach, since collection agencies retain as much as half of all amounts that they are successful in collecting.

Cash Receipt and Lock Boxes

When cash does arrive, there should be specific procedures to safeguard it. One common approach is to direct all payments to a *lock box*. This is generally a post office box that is emptied directly by the bank. The bank removes the payments and processes them directly to the organization's account. The paperwork associated with the payment is then forwarded to the organization.

There are two key advantages to this approach. First, since the bank empties the boxes at least once a day, the receipts are deposited to interest-bearing accounts immediately rather than sitting around a business office for several days or weeks until they are deposited. Second, there is substantially decreased risk that receipts will be lost or stolen. As discussed earlier, maintaining security over cash resources is a key element of working capital management.

Inventory

The last major current asset category is inventory. This is the category that nurses are most directly involved with. Health care organizations tend to have a wide variety of inventory items. For example, there are clinical supplies, drugs, office supplies, food, and housekeeping supplies. The cost of inventory in health care organizations is generally much smaller than the level of accounts receivable. Nevertheless, careful inventory management can result in significant savings. A general rule of thumb is that inventory levels should be kept as low as possible, consistent with patient needs. The less inventory on hand, the less money tied up in inventory.

The major problem health care organizations face with respect to inventory is the unpredictability of patient flow and patient needs. If the organization runs out of an item, it could mean the difference between life and death.

However, that fact is sometimes used to justify excessive stockpiles of a wide variety of inventory items that do not have life-and-death implications. Management needs to develop a system that ensures that inventory is available when needed but also that it is used efficiently and that levels are kept as low as possible.

Inventory should be ordered and stored in a centralized fashion whenever possible. Although ready access to supplies justifies maintaining some items in a number of different areas, the amount in each area should be a bare minimum, with restocking from one central point. Otherwise, each area will have a large inventory, and resources will needlessly be tied up in inventory that may not be used for weeks or even months. This is an area that is sometimes difficult for staff nurses. Nurses do not like to run out of supplies. The nurse manager must balance the staff nurse needs for immediate access to supplies with the organization's needs to control inventory costs.

Perpetual Inventory

One approach that can be helpful is maintenance of a perpetual inventory of high-cost items. A perpetual inventory is one in which each use of an item is recorded and a running balance maintained. This allows the organization to know how much it has of each item at any point in time. Reordering can take place when inventory falls below a certain level.

Generally less inventory is required when a perpetual system is used. There is less need to hold a large safety stock, since the manager always knows how much inventory is available. Reordering can take place whenever an item runs low. Without a perpetual system it is necessary to take a physical count of inventory to determine how much is available. That is a costly, time-consuming process that is not frequently undertaken.

Perpetual inventory systems are costly and time-consuming as well. However, automated systems have reduced the cost of such perpetual systems substantially. Supermarkets, for example, use uniform price codes (bar codes) to automatically update their perpetual inventory records as each item is sold. If inventory is maintained on an automated perpetual system, managers have greater control over their stocks and therefore can get by with less of each item.

Economic Order Quantity (EOQ)

Not only does inventory require a cash outlay when it is acquired but there are also other costs related to inventory. It must be stored. That requires physical storage space. Over time inventory may become damaged or obsolete or may pass an expiration date. There are costs related to placing an order and having it shipped. As noted, there are potentially high costs of running out of an item. These many factors can be balanced using a method called the economic order quantity (EOQ).

EOQ is a quantitative technique that weighs all the pros and cons of ordering large amounts of inventory infrequently vs. ordering small amounts on a more frequent basis. The result of an EOQ calculation is the optimal number of units that should be ordered each time an item is restocked and how frequently orders should be made. The EOQ technique is presented and explained in Chapter 17, along with other quantitative techniques of management.

CURRENT LIABILITIES

Management of current liabilities often receives less attention than current asset management, but it is also important. Careful planning and management of short-term obligations can save the organization significant amounts of money.

The typical current liabilities that most organizations have and that must be managed as part of working capital are accounts payable, payroll payable, notes payable, and taxes payable. Accounts payable represent amounts that are owed to suppliers. Payroll relates to obligations to employees. Notes payable represent short-term debt, usually loans from banks. Taxes payable would include not only income taxes for proprietary organizations but also a variety of payroll taxes for all organizations.

The basic approach to management of current liabilities is deferral of payment and avoidance of borrowing to the extent possible. The longer the organization waits to make payments, the longer the cash will remain in the organization's interest-bearing accounts. This allows it to earn a return that can be used to provide more services. The less money the organization borrows and the later it borrows it, the less interest it must pay.

Accounts Payable

Accounts payable are often referred to as *trade credit*. Trade credit is generally free for a short time. After a purchase is made, the organization has several weeks or a month to pay the bill. After that time some suppliers charge interest; others do not. A more common practice than charging interest for late payments is to offer a discount for prompt payment.

Discount terms are often stated as 2/10 N/30. That means a 2% discount is given for payments received within ten days of the invoice date. Otherwise the full amount, referred to as the net amount, is due thirty days from the invoice date. Sometimes only a 1% discount is offered, in which case it would be referred to as 1/10 N/30. Some vendors use terms based on the end of the month. For example, 2/10 EOM means that the buyer can take a 2% discount for payments made by ten days after the end of the month in which the invoice is issued. In general, trade credit is only offered to trustworthy buyers. In some cases, when the supplier has not had a long-term relationship with the buyer, goods will be sold COD, which means cash on delivery.

Does it pay to take the discount when it is offered? In most cases it clearly does make sense to take the discount. A formula can be used to determine the annual interest rate implicit in trade credit discounts:

$$\text{Implicit interest rate} = \frac{\text{Discount}}{\text{Discounted price}} \times \frac{\text{365 Days}}{\text{Days sooner}} \times 100\%$$

For example, suppose that your organization purchased $1,000 worth of goods and was offered "terms" of 2/10 N/30. A 2% discount on a $1,000 purchase would be $20. This means that if the discount is taken, only $980 would have to be paid. If the discount is taken, payment is due on the tenth day rather than the thirtieth day. This means that payment is made twenty days sooner than would otherwise be the case.

$$\text{Implicit interest rate} = \frac{\$20}{\$980} \times \frac{365 \text{ Days}}{20 \text{ Days}} \times 100\% = 37.2\%$$

While the discount appears to be a very small percentage, on an annualized basis the rate is actually 37.2%! Effectively one can think of this as if the organization has an obligation of $980 due on the tenth day. If it waits an extra twenty days to make payment, the interest charge is $20. Twenty dollars of interest on a $980 loan for twenty days represents a 37% annual interest rate. Clearly, if the organization takes the discount, it is avoiding a high charge for deferring payment by a few weeks.

What if the organization does not have enough cash to take all discounts? In that case, it pays to incur short-term debt, i.e., to borrow the money from the bank to pay the bill on the tenth day as long as the bank charges a rate less than 37%.

However, that assumes that the organization will in fact pay the bill on the due date if it does not take the discount. What if a hospital is in financial difficulty and is paying its bills after 150 days? That is an undesirable position to be in, as suppliers may stop making future sales. Nevertheless, it is not uncommon to find some health care organizations paying bills 90 days, 120 days, or even 150 days late. If a hospital would normally pay a bill after 150 days, then taking the discount on the tenth day means that payment is made 140 days sooner than it otherwise would be.

$$\text{Implicit interest rate} = \frac{\$20}{\$980} \times \frac{365 \text{ Days}}{140 \text{ Days}} \times 100\% = 5.3\%$$

In this situation the implicit interest rate is much lower. Any hospital paying after 150 days probably has a cash shortage. It is unlikely that this hospital could borrow from a bank for a rate as low as 5.3%. Therefore, in that situation it is not financially advantageous to take the discount. The decision to take or not take a discount is not automatic. It depends on both the amount of the discount and the implications for how much sooner payment must be made.

Payroll Payable

Payroll payables are generally very short in duration. At the end of each payroll period, salaries and wages are paid and the obligation eliminated. This does not mean, however, that management has no ability to manage in this area.

First, there must be policy decisions regarding when and how often employees are paid. Paying some employees monthly instead of every two weeks effectively defers payment of half their salary by two weeks. Over the course of the year, that adds up to a significant amount of savings for the organization. Similar savings accrue from paying employees every two weeks instead of every week. Additionally, less frequent payments mean that there is less paperwork and other administrative costs.

Second, there is the issue of how long the delay is from the end of the payroll period until payment. If the payroll period ends on Friday and payroll is paid on the following Thursday, the organization has gained the use of the money for nearly an extra week.

On the other side of the ledger, one must consider the organization's relationship with its employees. While it will require some time to process the amounts due to employees and to print checks, a good relationship between employer and employees calls for as prompt a payment of payroll as is possible.

Short-term Debt

The most common type of short-term debt owed by health care organizations is *unsecured notes* payable to banks. Many health care organizations also borrow money from financing and factoring companies, using their accounts receivable as collateral. Additionally, some health care organizations issue commercial paper.

Unsecured notes are loans that do not have any *collateral*. Collateral is a specific asset pledged to the lender. If the borrower defaults on the loan, the lender can sell the collateral to recover its money. In the case of an unsecured note, if the organization fails to repay the money, the lender would not have any specific claim on an asset owned by the organization. Rather, it would be a general creditor and would share the assets of the organization with all the other general creditors. This makes lending money more risky and drives up the interest charged.

An alternative available to health care organizations is to put up accounts receivable as security or collateral for the loan. This is called *financing accounts receivable*. It is also possible to directly sell receivables. That is called *factoring*. The buyer of the receivables, called the factor or the factoring agent, then takes on the risk that patients or third-party payers may not pay. Factoring tends to be an expensive alternative because of that risk that the factor takes. Financing, on the other hand, is less expensive. The health care organization borrows money, and the receivables are simply back-up security in case the organization fails to repay the loan. Since much of the receivables are due from the government, they are seen as reasonably good collateral. This may make borrowing less costly than an unsecured bank loan would be.

A last alternative is *commercial paper*. This is a form of borrowing in which the borrower issues a financial security that can be traded by the lender to someone else. This is an uncommon approach for any organization other than large, for-profit chains. Although the commercial paper is referred to as a security, it is generally unsecured.

In general, short-term debt bears a higher interest rate than long-term debt. This is because short-term debt is typically unsecured, while long-term debt is generally secured by specific assets. Also, there are transactions costs related to the borrowing and repaying of loans. These costs are more substantial for short-term loans because they cannot be spread out over a long lifetime of a loan. Therefore, if an organization needs an amount of money for a long time, it usually borrows on a long-term basis. Long-term borrowing is discussed in the next chapter. Short-term debt is generally used only for short-term needs.

Taxes Payable

Even not-for-profit organizations get involved with taxes. For the most part, these relate to FICA (Social Security taxes) and employee income tax withholding. FICA is paid by both the employee and the employer. The organization must withhold an amount for FICA from its employees and then must make payments to the government for both its share and the employees' share. The organization must also withhold a portion of each employee's wages and pay it to the government for the employee's income taxes. Generally, specific rules determine when these tax payments are due. Aside from not paying the taxes before they are due, there is relatively little management can do in this area.

IMPLICATIONS FOR NURSE MANAGERS

Nurse managers may question the importance of this chapter. Except for a minority of nurse managers, readers of this book are unlikely to be in charge of decisions concerning collection of accounts receivable and payment to suppliers. However, working capital management is important for all nurse managers.

It is important because managers do not just manage their cost centers; they manage a part of an organization, and they should understand the financial workings of the organization. It is important because in many instances the actions of nurse managers impact on working capital. And it is important because decisions made about working capital impact on nurse managers and their cost centers or departments.

Nurse managers at one time were restricted primarily to clinical management. Over the last several decades this role has changed, and it continues to change. Nurse managers control the largest share of resources in most health care institutions. The financial management of the entire organization should be a concern of nurse managers. Inefficient use of working capital invariably impacts on the resources available for patient care.

The impact nurse managers can have on working capital should not be understated. The most obvious area that nurses impact on is inventory management. Efficient control of inventory resources is one working capital ingredient. Another is payroll liabilities. Nurse managers through their staffing decisions do impact on that current liability. Decisions to purchase supplies and equipment come into play as well. The timing of such purchases should be made in light of their implications for working capital.

On the other hand, while delaying purchases of equipment until the equipment is actually needed makes sense, delaying it beyond that point reduces quality of care. Understanding working capital management can help nurse managers understand why a financial manager would want an acquisition to be delayed as long as possible. That understanding should help the manager in a dialogue with financial management over the acquisition. Mutually beneficial solutions are more likely to be achieved when both parties understand the needs and concerns of their counterparts.

KEY CONCEPTS

Working capital   Organization's current assets and current liabilities.

Working capital management   Management of the current assets and current liabilities of the organization to ensure that there is adequate cash on hand to meet the organization's needs and to minimize the cost of short-term resources.

Cash requirements Cash is needed by organizations for three main purposes: transactions, safety, and investments.

Cash management Management of inflows and outflows of cash.

Cash budgets Starting cash balance, plus expected cash receipts, less expected cash payments.

Management of accounts receivable Minimization of the time between provision of care and receipt of payment. Accounts receivable earn no return for the organization. The sooner cash is collected, the sooner the organization can use that cash for its operations or else invest it.

Aging schedule Tool used to keep track of potential accounts receivable problems by showing how long each receivable has been outstanding since a bill was issued.

Inventory management Managers need to develop a system that ensures that inventory is available when needed, while keeping inventory levels as low as possible.

Management of current liabilities Process of deferring payment and avoiding borrowing to the extent possible. The longer the organization waits to pay, the longer the cash is in the organization's interest-bearing accounts, earning a return that can be used to provide more services. The less the organization borrows and the later it borrows, the less interest it must pay.

Trade credit Accounts payable. Often subject to credit terms such as 2/10 N/ 30. The implicit interest rate contained in such terms may be calculated as follows:

$$\text{Implicit interest rate} = \frac{\text{Discount}}{\text{Discounted price}} \times \frac{\text{365 Days}}{\text{Days sooner}} \times 100\%$$

Short-term debt Unsecured short-term loans.

SUGGESTED READINGS ❖

Anderson, Suzanne, "Hospitals Can Improve Cash Flow by Managing Pre-authorizations," *Healthcare Financial Management*, Vol. 42, No. 12, December 1988, pp. 56–60.

Barenbaum, Lester, and Thomas Monahan, "Developing a Planning Model to Estimate Future Cash Flows," *Healthcare Financial Management*, Vol. 42, No. 3, March 1988, pp. 50–56.

Blackmore, Alice, "How Better Cash Management Can Increase the Hospital's Income," in Gerald E. Bisbee and Robert A. Vraciu, *Managing the Finances of Health Care Organizations*, Health Administration Press, Ann Arbor, MI, 1980, pp. 302–309.

Brigham, Eugene F., *Fundamentals of Financial Management*, 5th edition, Dryden Press, Chicago, IL, 1989.

Dominiak, Geraldine F., and Joseph G. Louderback, *Managerial Accounting*, 5th edition, PWS-Kent Publishing Co., Boston, 1988.

Finkler, Steven A., *Finance & Accounting for Nonfinancial Managers*, revised edition, Prentice-Hall, Englewood Cliffs, NJ, 1992.

Mark, Barbara A., and Howard L. Smith, *Essentials of Finance in Nursing,* Aspen Publishing, Rockville, MD, 1987.

Neumann, Bruce R., James D. Suver, and William N. Zelman, *Financial Management: Concepts and Applications for Health Care Providers,* 2nd edition, National Health Publishing, USA, 1990.

Pelfrey, Sandra, "Understanding the Tools for Managing Cash," *Journal of Nursing Administration,* Vol. 20, No. 10, October 1990, pp 23–27.

Van Horne, James C., *Fundamentals of Financial Management,* 7th edition, Prentice-Hall, Englewood Cliffs, NJ, 1989.

CHAPTER

15

Long-Term Financial Resources

CHAPTER GOALS

The goals of this chapter are to:

♦ Describe the different sources of long-term financing for health care organizations

♦ Explain the relative merits of equity financing vs. debt financing

♦ Distinguish among the different equity sources of financing

♦ Consider the changing roles of equity sources of financing

♦ Explain the different types of debt financing and the trade-offs for each type

♦ Introduce bond ratings and bond insurance

♦ Explain what bond refinancing is and why it takes place

♦ Explain the purpose of and methods used for feasibility studies

♦ Consider the future of long-term financing for health care organizations

❖

INTRODUCTION

In the previous chapter we discussed a number of sources of short-term financing for health care organizations. We now turn to sources of long-term financing. Long-term financing represents sources of money that the organization can use for longer than a year. In many cases these sources are critical to the existence of the organization.

Most, if not all, buildings and equipment are financed on a long-term basis. It would probably be impossible to find a lender willing to make a ninety-day or six-month loan to acquire a building. It is unreasonable to expect that enough profits could be earned within a short period to repay the entire cost of a building. It is more likely that at the *maturity* or due date of the loan a new loan would be required to get the money to pay off the old loan. If a new loan cannot be obtained, the organization would likely have to default on its loan. The lender would consider the risk of not being repaid too high.

As a result of that problem, long-term assets are generally acquired with money that the organization knows it can keep and use for a long time. The two principal sources of long-term money are debt and equity. Debt represents borrowed money. Interest must be paid during the period of the loan, and the original amount borrowed will have to be repaid. Equity represents ownership. In some cases equity represents money that outsiders have given the organization in exchange for owning it and having a claim on its profits. In other cases equity represents money that the organization itself owns.

EQUITY SOURCES OF FINANCING

The four principal sources of equity financing for health care organizations are philanthropy, corporate stock issuance, government grants, and retained earnings.

One main advantage of equity financing is that there is no legal requirement to make annual payments. This is in contrast to debt, which generally calls for at least annual payments of interest. Even if a health care organization has a bad year, it is legally required to make interest payments on its debt. If it does not have enough cash to make those interest payments, it might have to go out of business. That risk is not associated with equity sources of financing.

If a for-profit health care organization has a bad year, it can skip dividend payments to its stockholders. The usual form of stock, called *common stock*, has no requirements that dividends of any amount be paid, even if the organization is making a profit. A special form of stock called *preferred stock* requires a specific dividend of a specific amount each year, but in hard economic times payments can be delayed.

Other forms of equity such as retained earnings and philanthropic funds do not have required payments of any type. This freedom from interest payments relates to a concept called *leverage*. The greater the extent to which an organization uses debt financing, as opposed to equity, the more highly leveraged it is said to be. The benefit of leverage is that high leverage implies a low amount of required equity investment. The detriment of leverage is that it creates risk because of the need to make interest payments.

Philanthropy

Philanthropy represents gifts to the organization. These gifts may be small, or they may come in the form of multimillion dollar endowments. There may be costs related to generating the gifts, but once received they do not require interest or dividend payments, and the amount of the gift need never be repaid to someone outside the health care organization. Philanthropy has been a declining percentage of long-term financing for health care organizations.

The decline in philanthropy is probably caused by a number of factors, most of which are outside the control of any specific health care organization. These include changes in the tax rates, the introduction of Medicare and Medicaid, the proliferation of for-profit health care organizations, increased competition from non-health-care charities, cuts in federal support of social welfare, and the rising costs of generating philanthropic donations. Additionally, the existence of other sources for financing has made health care managers less aggressive in pursuing philanthropy.

Tax changes in the 1980s made it less advantageous to donate money to charitable organizations. In the past many philanthropists were in a 70% federal income tax bracket. A donation of $1 resulted in a 70¢ tax savings. Considering the tax implications, it only cost a person in that bracket 30¢ to be able to make a $1 contribution. With state income taxes added on, the effect was even more extreme. With the current lower maximum tax rates, each dollar contributed costs the donor more on an after-tax basis. For example, a gift of $1 million in 1980 might have cost a rich benefactor only $250,000 after considering the savings in federal and state taxes. That same contribution now might cost $650,000 after considering the tax savings.

Prior to the introduction of Medicare and Medicaid, many philanthropists believed that they had a mission to help provide for the health care of the poor and aged. With the government role that was created by Medicare and Medicaid, many philanthropists no longer believe that the same degree of need still exists. While it is true that many people are still uninsured or underinsured, the mere existence of a major role for the government in payment for health care has possibly made many people believe that the need for charity has disappeared from the health care industry.

At one time hospitals were viewed as community benefit organizations whose mission was to serve the people in the community. In many cases, especially in large cities, this is no longer true. Thus people in the community do not have the same sense of responsibility to the hospital.

This is probably reinforced by the fact that health care organizations have been viewing themselves more and more as businesses rather than charities. While running health care organizations in a financially sound, business-like manner does not eliminate their charitable mission, it does change the way people perceive the industry. The proliferation of for-profit health care organizations tends to make the entire industry appear more like a business. And many people believe that the last place they would donate money is to a business.

At the same time that health care organizations were losing some of their allure as a charity, there has been tremendous growth in the not-for-profit sector. More charities are competing for dollars, and they are learning how to do it better. This increased volume of charities and improved fund-raising skills has occurred at the same time as a cutback of social services by the government. During the 1980s the federal government pushed more of its social welfare function back to localities. The result was numerous cuts. Many charitable organizations stepped in to try to restore some services. That created an additional, highly visible outlet for philanthropic giving.

Another problem with philanthropy for health care organizations has been the rising cost of generating philanthropic donations. As competition for philanthropy has grown, organizations have had to develop more sophisticated and more expensive approaches to generating gifts. Expensive advertising campaigns join the more traditional dinners as a way to raise money. Full-time personnel must be hired to work at the task of "development" (i.e., gift generation).

Most, if not all, of the above factors contributing to the decreasing role of philanthropy cannot be greatly influenced by managers of an organization.

Nevertheless, many not-for-profit health care organizations have dropped the ball with respect to raising philanthropic funds. Not only have philanthropists started to view health care as a business; many health care managers have as well. There is a need to distinguish between running the organization in a business-like manner and being a business.

Many health care managers believe that among Medicare, Medicaid, Blue Cross, private insurers, HMOs, and other payers, there should be enough revenue to run a health care business. The error in that perception is that in the case of not-for-profits, health care is not a business. The mission is not centered on making money but rather on providing service to the community. Not-for-profits inherently undertake some activities at a loss because of their mission. One way to offset those losses is to earn high profits on other services. Most health care organizations try to accomplish that. However, another way to offset those losses is to actively solicit donations from a wide variety of sources, including past patients and community leaders.

Realistically, however, while efforts to receive donations should continue and perhaps even be stepped up, philanthropy can no longer be viewed as the major source for long-term financing. The costs of the health care industry have grown too high. New buildings are so expensive that in most cases their cost has gone beyond the reach of the best philanthropic efforts.

Corporate Stock Issuance

A major growth area in health care financing during the 1970s and 1980s was the issuance of corporate stock. In direct contrast with philanthropy, this approach says that health care can in fact be a business. Individuals can give money to health care organizations in exchange for stock. The stock makes the individuals the owners of the business. As the business earns profits, it distributes part of them to the owners in the form of dividends. The owners can sell the stock to someone else as a way of getting back their original investment, perhaps with a profit. The new owner of the stock can then receive the future dividends from the business's profits.

The issuance of stock has slowed considerably in the health care industry. Maxicare, a large for-profit HMO, filed for bankruptcy during the late 1980s due to extreme financial difficulties. Large for-profit hospital chains also found difficult financial conditions that saw their stock prices plunge during the 1980s. The for-profit sector is still growing and still seen as potentially profitable. Apparently, however, the rapid growth of the health care for-profit sector, which saw it take over approximately one-third of all acute care hospital beds in the space of less than two decades, is over. Nevertheless, many small new health care organizations are still getting their start using stock issuance to get much of their initial financial resources.

Stock issuance is only available to for-profit organizations. It is unlikely that health care organizations will generally switch to being for-profit simply to access this form of financing. Such a step would likely have wide ramifications for the organization. On the other hand, organizations that are already for-profit must decide how much equity financing of this form they want. It is conceivably possible to issue enough stock to raise all the necessary long-term financing for an organization. However, that may not be an optimal strategy.

When stock is issued, the benefit to the owners who invest money in the business is the dividend flow. Dividends are a distribution of profits. They are paid after taxes have been calculated on profits. Interest, on the other hand, is a tax-deductible expense of the organization. By issuing some stock and some debt, some of the payments for financing become tax deductible, therefore lowering the taxes paid to the government. That is one reason that most for-profits have a mixture of stock and debt.

Government Grants

Government grants were a common financing mechanism at one time, especially for hospitals. Hill-Burton funds were available in the 1950s for the construction of new hospital buildings. In recent years, however, there has been a growing reluctance by the government to create more capacity in the health care system. Studies have demonstrated that increased capacity tends to create higher levels of utilization ("a bed built is a bed filled"). Further, there is an excess of capacity for health care services in many areas of the country. As a result, government grants are no longer a significant source of financing for health care organizations.

Retained Earnings

The last significant source of equity financing is retained earnings. Each year that a health care organization makes a profit that profit is either paid to owners in the form of a dividend or else retained in the organization. Money retained can be used for short-term operations or to finance long-term assets.

Retaining earnings is a critical factor in the long-term survival of health care organizations. To stay viable, it is necessary to replace plant and equipment as they become physically deteriorated or technologically obsolete. In addition, organizations must add new services and technology to remain current as medical care changes. The combination of inflation plus technological change plus expanding community needs often drives the cost of replacement buildings and equipment well above the original items' cost. It would not be surprising for an old hospital building that cost $50 million to build sixty years ago to be replaced now for $250 million. If profits have been earned, retained, and invested, the organization will have some of the money needed for the new facility.

Even on a less grand scale, retained earnings are essential. Suppose that a hospital wishes to buy a patient monitor for $25,000. If it goes to a bank to borrow the money, the bank will want the hospital to make a down payment probably of 20% or more. The reason for this will be discussed later under the heading of mortgages. If there is adequate philanthropy or cash from stock issuances, the hospital will be able to buy the equipment. If not, then it is likely that it will only be able to acquire the equipment if it has enough money for the down payment available from earnings that have been retained and have not yet been used for another purpose. Retained earnings represent a source of equity financing that is of growing importance to health care organizations.

DEBT SOURCES OF FINANCING

Relatively few health care organizations are entirely free from debt. The need to raise large amounts of long-term financing causes many, if not most, health care organizations to borrow money. There are a number of different approaches to borrowing. Depending on the specific circumstances for which money is needed, at times some approaches will be superior, while at other times other approaches will be more suitable.

The major forms of long-term debt are mortgages, long-term notes, leases, and bonds. Mortgages and long-term notes generally represent money that a bank lends to the organization. However, it is possible to have a mortgage or note with a nonbank. For instance, some equipment manufacturers will lend the buyer the money to acquire equipment. Leases are arrangements to rent equipment or facilities under a contract. Bonds are financial obligations that can be traded from one party to another.

Mortgages and Long-term Notes

Mortgages and long-term notes are referred to as *conventional debt.* A long-term note is a loan to the health care organization. It is sometimes secured by collateral and sometimes is unsecured. If secured, the collateral is often in the form of financial securities rather than physical property. The obligation to repay the loan is generally evidenced by a formal legal document, called a note, that is signed by the borrower. When a note is secured by a specific piece of physical property such as a building, piece of equipment, or land, it is referred to as a mortgage. If the borrower fails to repay a mortgage, the lender can foreclose on the property, sell it, and pay the borrower only the amount realized from the sale that exceeds the outstanding loan balance.

Mortgages and long-term notes are very common, can be issued with little delay, and require relatively little paperwork and involvement of lawyers. They tend to be more expensive than bonds but less expensive than leasing.

Mortgages are often used to finance a specific acquisition. Usually lenders require that the borrower make a down payment of anywhere from 20% to 50% of the purchase price of the asset. This protects the lender in the case there is a payment default and the asset cannot be sold for its full original cost. Mortgages generally call for monthly payments of a constant amount. The payments consist of interest on the balance of the loan that was outstanding during the previous month, plus a repayment of a portion of the original loan. Over time the amount of interest in each payment declines and the amount of loan repayment in each payment rises. At the end of the term of the mortgage, the loan has been fully repaid. In contrast, notes generally call for monthly payments of interest only. At the maturity date of the loan, the full amount of the original loan is repaid.

For example, suppose that an HMO wanted to purchase equipment for a new group practice office. The total cost of the equipment needed is $500,000. The HMO plans to invest $100,000 of its own funds and borrow $400,000. Suppose that if it borrowed on an unsecured long-term note, the interest rate would be 14%. If it took a mortgage, using the equipment as collateral, the interest rate would be 12%. The collateral lessens the lender's risk, so a lower interest rate is available. Assume for this example that payments are only made once a year. What are the annual payments under the two alternatives?

The long-term note has annual payments of $56,000, as seen in Table 15-1. This is 14% of $400,000. The loan balance of $400,000 remains constant over the 10-year life of the loan. At the end of the loan there is an interest payment, plus a payment for the full $400,000.

❖ TABLE 15–1
Payment Schedule for a Long-term Note

Year	Loan Balance Start of Year	Interest Payment	Loan Repayment	Total Payment	Loan Balance End of Year
1	$400,000	$56,000	$ 0	$ 56,000	$400,000
2	400,000	56,000	0	56,000	400,000
3	400,000	56,000	0	56,000	400,000
4	400,000	56,000	0	56,000	400,000
5	400,000	56,000	0	56,000	400,000
6	400,000	56,000	0	56,000	400,000
7	400,000	56,000	0	56,000	400,000
8	400,000	56,000	0	56,000	400,000
9	400,000	56,000	0	56,000	400,000
10	400,000	56,000	400,000	456,000	0
				$960,000	

The annual mortgage payments on a $400,000 loan would be $70,794.[1] Note that this is a higher amount than the annual $56,000 payment on the long-term note, even though the interest rate on the mortgage was only 12% while the rate on the note was 14%. This is because the mortgage payments include not only interest but also repayment of a portion of the original loan (see Table 15–2).

Note that in the early years most of each payment is interest. However, because there is some repayment of the original loan, each year a smaller amount is owed. Since less money is owed, there is less interest. The annual payments are a constant amount. If the amount of interest is dropping each year, then the amount of the annual payment available for paying off the loan is rising. Thus, in the latter years most of each payment is loan repayment rather than interest. By the end of the ten years the loan is fully paid off.

Note that in total the mortgage payments came to $707,940, while the note payments came to $960,000. The reason for this is that there is more interest on the note. This is partially because of the higher interest rate and partly because for the note the full $400,000 is owed during the entire ten years, while the mortgage obligation declined over the ten years.

Leases

Leases are rental agreements evidenced by a contract referred to as a *lease*. The *lessee* rents a building or equipment from the *lessor*. Unless otherwise agreed, at the expiration of a lease the lessor continues to own the property. It is possible, however, to design the lease to transfer the property to the lessee

---

[1] The $70,794 constant annual payment is exactly the amount of money that is needed to provide for a 12% interest payment on the outstanding balance of the loan, plus repayment of the loan so that there is no remaining balance at the end of ten years. That number can be calculated using the time-value-of-money techniques discussed in the appendix of Chapter 11. In this case the number of compounding periods is ten, the interest rate is 12%, the present value of the loan is $400,000, and the annual payment is being sought.

at the end of its term. It is also possible to design the lease to give the lessee the option to purchase the property at the end of the lease for a specified price. Leases usually call for equal payments payable at the beginning of each month.

Lease payments generally have three components, although the lessee is only told the total monthly payment. The first component pays for part of the cost of the property being leased. This is equivalent to the principal portion of a mortgage payment. The second component is an interest charge equivalent to the interest portion of a mortgage payment. The last component is a profit for the lessor.

In many ways leases are simply an alternative to mortgages. In both cases the organization wishes to have the use of an asset, but it does not have the cash to go out and buy the asset. It needs to use cash from someone else, either the mortgage lender or the lessor. Leases in effect obligate the lessee to make monthly lease payments for a number of years into the future in the same way that the user of the equipment would be obligated to make monthly mortgage payments had the property been purchased with a mortgage. It is because of the long-term obligation to make payments on a lease that accountants treat long-term noncancelable leases as long-term debt.

Other things being equal, leases are more costly than mortgages. In either case the user of the property must ultimately pay the cost of the property. In either case the user of the property must pay interest for the use of the money needed to buy the property. That interest includes a profit for the lender. In the case of a lease, however, the lessor has generally borrowed the money to buy the property. Suppose that the lessor borrows from a bank to finance the asset purchase. The bank and its depositors must receive interest, and the lessor must also earn a profit. This extra party to the transaction, the lessor,

❖ **TABLE 15–2**
Payment Schedule for a Mortgage

Year	Loan Balance Start of Year	Interest Payment	Loan Repayment	Total Payment	Loan Balance End of Year
	(A)	(B)	(C)	(D)	(E)
1	$400,000	$48,000	$22,794	$ 70,794	$377,206
2	377,206	45,265	25,529	70,794	351,677
3	351,677	42,201	28,592	70,794	323,084
4	323,085	38,770	32,023	70,794	291,060
5	291,062	34,927	35,866	70,794	255,195
6	255,195	30,623	40,170	70,794	215,025
7	215,025	25,803	44,991	70,794	170,034
8	170,034	20,404	50,390	70,794	119,645
9	119,645	14,357	56,436	70,794	63,209
10	63,209	7,585	63,209	70,794	0
				$707,940	

(A) Loan balance at the start of the year is the original loan balance in the first year. In subsequent years it is the ending balance from column E for the previous year.
(B) 12% interest rate multiplied by loan balance in column A.
(C) = (D) − (B).
(D) = Annual payment calculated using time-value-of-money techniques. See Chapter 11 appendix.
(E) = (A) − (C).

adds the need for additional profits and therefore additional costs to the lessee. The bank and its depositors *and* the lessor earn a profit. With a mortgage, only the bank and its depositors need earn a profit.

Then why would one lease rather than buying a property and taking a mortgage? For one thing, leases do not require a down payment. If the organization does not have the 20% to 50% of the asset cost needed for a down payment, then the lease may be viewed as advantageous even if it is more expensive. Another advantage of leasing is that the leasing company may be better able to sell the used property than the user of the property.

Consider a home health agency that provides cars to its nursing staff for making home visits. At the end of three or four years the agency may wish to replace the cars. The agency probably cannot get a high value for the cars when it sells them because it is not an expert in the used car market. On the other hand, if the cars are leased, the leasing company can probably sell the cars for a reasonable price because it is an expert. By sharing the extra amount received on the ultimate sale with the lessee, the lease may become attractive.

Another potential advantage of leasing is that in some leases the lessee can call for the equipment to be replaced if it becomes obsolete. This removes some risk that health care organizations take when they buy equipment. On the other hand, the leasing company will probably charge a higher monthly amount to pay it for taking that risk.

The total rate being charged to cover interest and profits on a lease can usually be estimated using the time-value-of-money techniques. Suppose that a nursing home is considering buying some equipment for $200,000 or leasing it for $5,000 per month for five years. If it purchases the equipment, there will be an immediate down payment of $50,000, plus monthly mortgage payments based on a 12% interest rate, for five years. If it leases the equipment, it will have sixty monthly payments of $5,000. If the number of months equals sixty, the payment each month is $5,000, and the present value of the equipment is $200,000, then the annual interest rate on the lease is approximately 18%.[2] This is substantially higher than the bank rate of 12%. On the other hand, the nursing home would need only $5,000 at the start for the first month, as opposed to $50,000 for a down payment.

Bonds

Bonds are formal certificates of indebtedness. The certificate indicates a promise to pay interest, usually semiannually, and the face value of the bond at a future specified maturity date. Bonds are financial obligations that can be traded from one party to another. For example, Mr. Smith can lend money to the health care organization (i.e., he can buy a bond) in exchange for a promise that interest plus the original loan will be repaid. That promise is evidenced by the bond certificate. In turn Mr. Smith can sell the bond certificate to someone else, and the borrower will then owe the money to the new owner of the bond instead of to Mr. Smith. Bonds are issued by the borrower. Sometimes it is said that the borrower sells the bonds or floats a bond.

---

[2]Using the methods from the Chapter 11 appendix, i = ?% per month, N = 60 months, the present value is $200,000, and the monthly payments = $5,000. Note that with a lease, payments are made in advance of each period rather than at the end of each period.

Bonds are an advantageous way of obtaining debt for several reasons. First of all, the borrower obtains the money directly from the ultimate lender. Second, bonds tend to disperse risk.

In the case of a bank loan, the borrower gets money from a bank, which in turn gets money from depositors. The depositors must make a profit and the bank must make a profit. With a bond, the money is borrowed directly from individuals, who might otherwise put their money in a bank. By eliminating the middleman bank, the depositors can be paid more than the bank would pay them, and the borrower can pay less than would be paid to a bank. Both the borrower and the ultimate lender are better off if they can eliminate the bank's role.

The second major advantage is that there is a dispersal of risk. If a bank were to lend $100 million for a hospital expansion, it would take on a tremendous amount of risk. If the hospital were to default, the bank would be faced with a huge potential loss. Bonds, however, are often divided into hundreds or thousands or even hundreds of thousands of relatively small loans. For a $100 million total debt, each lender may lend as little as $5,000. Thus no one single person or organization takes on the full risk of one organization's defaulting on a loan.

With mutual funds, investors may effectively disperse their risk even further. An individual could invest $5,000 in a mutual fund that has combined the investments of thousands of individuals to buy hundreds of different bonds. Thus an individual's risk from any one hospital's defaulting might be several hundred dollars or less. By lowering risk, the borrower lowers the interest rate that must be paid to adequately reimburse the lender for the risks taken.

Bonds are also advantageous because they do not require down payments for projects, and they may have extremely long maturity periods. Forty-year bonds are not uncommon. These factors can be very important to a health care organization borrowing money to construct a new building. The organization can have the full depreciation period of the building to accumulate the money needed to pay for its construction.

Usually bonds pay interest *semiannually*. Every six months a payment is made based on a stated interest rate and the face value of the bond. Bonds are generally issued in denominations of $5,000 and multiples of $5,000, such as $10,000, $25,000, and $100,000. The total amount issued by the borrower is generally quite large, often over $100 million. At the due date or maturity of the bond the original face amount must be repaid.

Although bond interest is paid at the stated rate and the face value is repaid at maturity, the bonds may actually be issued for a greater or lesser amount than the face value. That is because interest rates fluctuate in the financial marketplace. Bond certificates may be printed indicating a promise to pay a 10% interest rate. If the issuer finds that market conditions have changed and no one is willing to lend money unless it is possible to earn a 10.1% return on the money, then a discount will have to be offered to get anyone to buy the bonds.

Thus, on a $10,000, 20-year, 10% bond paying interest semiannually, the issuer might accept payment of $9,915. In exchange for getting $9,915, the borrower will make payments of $500 twice a year for twenty years (i.e., the $10,000 face multiplied by 10% a year, divided by two payments per year), plus a payment of $10,000 at the end of twenty years. The borrower received

$9,915 but repays $10,000. This converts the 10% stated interest rate to the 10.1% market interest rate.

If interest rates fall, the bond will be issued at a premium. If interest rates in the marketplace are only 9.8% and this bond offers 10% based on a face value of $10,000, then investors will be willing to pay more than $10,000 to get the bond.

A number of decisions must be made before bonds are issued. These decisions can have a dramatic impact on the interest rate that must be paid on the outstanding bond obligations. Bonds may be issued in either taxable or tax-free form. The issuer can request to have the bond rated. The issuer can also purchase insurance that guarantees the payments of bond interest and principal. Another decision concerns whether to make interest payments or let the interest accrue and pay both the interest and face value at the maturity date. That is called a zero-coupon bond. After bonds have been issued, another question that sometimes arises is whether the bonds should be refinanced. These issues are discussed below.

Taxable vs. Tax-free Bonds

A taxable bond is one on which the lender of the money (also called the buyer of the bond) must pay income tax on the interest received. Under certain conditions it is possible to offer bonds free of federal income tax and free of state and local income taxes in the state or locality issued. The advantage of a tax-free bond is that people are willing to lend money in exchange for a lower interest rate if they can avoid paying taxes.

Suppose, for example, that a hospital wanted to borrow money and found that with a taxable bond it would have to pay a 12% interest rate. However, there are a number of potential lenders from the state where the hospital is located. Many of these lenders are in a combined federal and state income tax bracket of 33%. That means that they will have to pay one-third of any interest received in taxes. If they could earn the interest free of taxes, it would save a lot of money. In fact, if the hospital paid just two-thirds as much interest, or 8% interest on a tax-free bond, the lenders would still have just as much money after taxes!

In fact, not all lenders will necessarily be in such a high tax bracket. Also, some lenders may be from another state, which will tax the bond interest. As a result, it is likely that the hospital can issue the bond for a rate somewhere between 8% and 12%. If the bond is issued at a 10% rate, that can still mean a savings of millions of dollars per year to the hospital.

One key to this savings is the ability to borrow money directly from individuals. Note from Figure 15–1 that individuals (households) lend about 40% of the money organizations receive from tax-exempt bonds, while they lend only about 7% of the money received by for-profit corporations or foreign borrowers.

To issue a tax-free bond, however, requires compliance with a number of federal and state regulations. Generally, a health care organization itself cannot issue a tax-free security. That is a privilege reserved for governmental bodies. For that reason, tax-free bonds are usually referred to as *municipal* bonds. In most states there are governmental bond-issuing authorities. They act as a link allowing not-for-profit health care organizations to issue tax-free securities. However, they usually assume no liability for repayment.

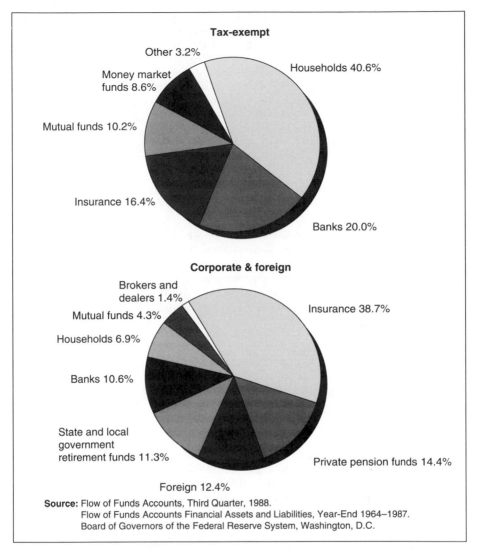

Figure 15–1. Holders of tax-exempt, corporate, and foreign debt. (Reprinted from John Aderholdt and Charles Pardue, "A Guide to Taxable Debt Financing Alternatives," *Healthcare Financial Management*, July 1989, p. 60, with permission of Healthcare Financial Management Association.)

Given the possibility of avoiding taxes, why would taxable bonds ever be issued? There are several reasons. First of all, for-profit organizations are generally not given access to the tax-free market. Second, laws govern the total amount of bonds that can be issued on a tax-free basis. If that ceiling has been exceeded, only a taxable bond offering may be possible. The most common reason for issuing taxable bonds, however, is because it is possible to have lower expenses related to the issuance of the bond.

A number of costs are related to the issuance of bonds. Legal fees are one type of cost; placement fees are another. Bonds tend to require a great deal of sophisticated legal work to properly protect all parties. There is counsel for the issuer, counsel for the investors, and counsel for the investment firm that finds the buyers. Additionally, substantial amounts of money are paid to the investment firm, called the *underwriter* of the bond. The underwriter is generally an investment banking company that places the bonds with investors. A health care organization does not typically have direct access to the thousands of potential investors necessary to issue a bond successfully. Investment bankers have that large client base and are expert at finding buyers for bonds.

Despite the high legal and placement costs, it is worthwhile to issue bonds. Even a 1% savings in the interest rate as compared with conventional debt would save $1 million per year on a $100 million bond flotation. To borrow that much money for forty years, issuance costs of $2 or $3 million may be considered quite reasonable.

However, for a smaller bond such as $5 to $20 million or a shorter-term bond such as ten years or less, the issuance costs may be too much. Taxable bonds do not require the organization to go through nearly so great a legal and regulatory process as tax-exempt bonds. Further, if the bond is issued to a small group of investors rather than to the public at large, both legal and placement costs can be reduced even further. In such a case it may be worthwhile to pay the higher interest rate on a taxable bond. Consider the fact that a 2% interest difference on a $7 million, three-year bond would only amount to about $400,000. If the costs of a tax-exempt issuance would always exceed a million dollars, then the taxable approach would make sense. Why not just borrow $7 million for three years from a bank? The bank would probably charge a higher interest rate than even a taxable bond. Recall that the bank represents an extra middleman that must make a profit.

Bond Ratings and Insurance

As has been noted, a primary reason for issuing bonds rather than using conventional debt is to get a lower interest rate. One of the most important determinants of interest rates is risk. If investors perceive an investment to be risky, they require a higher return than they otherwise would. The way they get a higher return on money they lend is by charging a higher interest rate. The purpose of bond ratings and bond insurance is to lower perceived or actual risk levels to lower the interest rate that must be paid on a bond.

The two dominant bond-rating agencies in this country are Standard and Poor's and Moody's. For a fee, they will evaluate the issuer of a bond and assign a rating to the quality of the bond. Quality is a measurement of the likelihood of the borrower to make all payments required by the bond. The highest rating is triple A. This rating is indicated by AAA or Aaa. The ratings then decline to double A, single A, triple B, double B, single B, and down into the C and D range. Anything below single B is considered a risky, speculative investment.

Triple A bond ratings are reserved for only the safest of investments. Extremely few, if any, health care organizations can merit a triple A rating on the basis of their financial condition. Even double A ratings tend to be reserved for the most elite of health care organizations. Ratings of single A and below are common in health care. The specific rating assigned to an organization's bonds will have a significant bearing on the interest rate it must pay.

There is no requirement that an organization have its bonds rated. The organization can avoid paying a fee to the rating agency and simply issue "nonrated" bonds. The fee for rating a bond is quite high, since the bond rater must continue to follow the organization's financial condition over the life of the bond so that it can change its rating if the financial circumstances of the organization change. Failure to have a bond rated is not an indication that the bonds are a safe or unsafe investment. It may simply mean that the bond offering is too small to warrant the expense of a rating. However, many investors will be reluctant to invest in such a bond.

Another alternative to rating, however, is bond insurance. The premium for such insurance is even more costly than obtaining a rating. The borrower pays a company to insure its obligations under the bond. The principal insurers of tax-free bonds are the American Municipal Bond Assurance Company (AMBAC) and the Municipal Bond Insurance Association (MBIA). Both these organizations undertake a study of the financial situation of the bond issuer to assure themselves that the chance of default is extremely low. If they are satisfied, then they issue the insurance.

Both Standard and Poor's and Moody's currently give an automatic rating of triple A to any bonds that have such insurance. We say currently because substantial defaults could affect the financial status of the insurer, in which case the ratings of the bonds could be lowered. The benefit of obtaining a triple A rating in terms of interest rates is so great that it often makes insurance a worthwhile investment for the bond issuer, if the organization's financial condition is sufficient to allow it to obtain the insurance.

Zero-coupon Bonds

Typical bonds pay interest semiannually. Another type of bond, called a *zero-coupon* bond or simply "zeroes," does not make periodic interest payments. Instead, the interest is calculated every six months and added onto the outstanding loan balance. At the maturity date the payment consists of the original loan plus all the accrued interest. Note that every six months the accumulated obligation grows, and in future periods interest accrues on prior interest as well as on the original principal amount. In other words, since interest is not paid out every six months, compound interest applies to all amounts owed to the lender.

Zero coupons are issued at deep discounts, and the interest is built into the face value of the bond. For example, a $10,000, 10%, twenty-year-maturity, zero-coupon bond might be issued for $1,420. The $10,000 payment at maturity would cover both the original $1,420 loan and also the interest from the entire life of the loan.

Zeroes have a great advantage in that they do not require any payments of interest at all until the maturity date. At the same time, there is also an increased risk. Lenders generally receive at least interest over the life of a loan. If they have to wait until the very end of a loan before they receive any payment at all, they are likely to demand a higher rate of interest to compensate them for that increased risk.

Zero-coupon bonds get their name from an era when bond certificates had a coupon attached for each interest payment. The lender would clip a coupon every six months and present it for payment. At that time bonds were often issued in bearer form. When a bond was sold from one party to another, the borrower was not informed. Whoever presented the coupons for payment was assumed to be the owner. For reasons of safety (to avoid loss or theft) and for tax purposes (to avoid people not paying taxes on taxable bonds), bonds are no longer issued in bearer form. They are all *registered*. The borrower maintains a record of the owner of the bond. The interest payments are automatically made without presentation of a coupon. Zero-coupon bonds were so called because they had no coupons attached, since there were no periodic interest payments.

Debt Refinancing

From time to time organizations review their bond obligations and consider whether it would be advantageous to *refinance* the debt. Generally, refinancing means that the organization pays off outstanding debt with high interest rates and substitutes new debt with a lower interest rate.

Interest rates in the financial markets tend to rise and fall with the economy. When there are recessions, interest rates fall. This is largely because there is not much business demand for money. When demand is low, the price of borrowed money (i.e., the interest rate) falls. When the economy is strong and there is a great demand for loans, the price rises.

Sometimes a health care organization borrows money despite relatively high interest rates because there is a pressing need for the assets that will be bought with the money. The economy's cycles take a long time. It might be five years, ten years, or even longer before interest rates decline. When the rates do decline, however, the organization must consider whether it pays to refinance the outstanding bonds.

Refinancing is not automatic for a number of reasons. First of all, there are all the costs related to a new bond issuance. These costs are expensive but make sense when spread out over a long period. If the bonds are refinanced every five years, the issuance costs could overwhelm much, if not all, of the interest rate benefit. Second, when bonds are issued, assurances are given to the lenders (i.e., the buyers of the bonds) that they will earn the stated interest rate. Often there is a penalty charged to the issuer of the bond for early re-payment of the bonds. The borrower may have to pay not only the face value of the bonds but also an extra amount.

The amount of the penalty, if any, depends on the *call provisions* of the bond. Call provisions are the conditions in the bond agreement that specify the rights the borrower has to call in the bond early and pay it off. If the call provisions are very easy on the borrower, the original interest rate will be higher. If the call provisions make it difficult to call in and pay off the bond, the interest rate is somewhat lower. When the bond is first issued, a trade-off must be made as the call provisions are established.

So far, we have considered refinancing from the point of view of calling in and paying off an outstanding bond at its face value. A related element of refinancing is the purchase of the organization's own bonds on the open financial market. However, unlike the refinancing done when interest rates fall, purchase refinancing is likely to occur when interest rates rise. If interest rates climb, the market price of bonds drops. Why would anyone want a bond that pays 10% when new bonds pay 12% or 13%?

If interest rates have risen and bond prices have fallen and if the organization has some cash available, it can buy its own bonds at the market price. The advantage of this is that the price is less than the organization will have to pay if it waits for the maturity of the bond.

In many cases organizations establish a *sinking fund* when they have an outstanding bond liability. A sinking fund is a pool of money being accumulated for a specific purpose. The purpose of a bond sinking fund is to accumulate money to eventually pay the bond face value at maturity.

If interest rates have risen and the bonds are selling below their face value, money from the sinking fund can be used to buy the bonds and retire them early. By retiring the bonds, the interest payments for those specific bonds purchased no longer have to be paid. And by buying them below face value, the organization saves the difference between the price paid and the face value that would eventually have had to be paid. On the other hand, the money is no longer in the sinking fund, earning interest at the relatively high current rate.

FEASIBILITY STUDIES

When large amounts of money are borrowed on a long-term basis, the lenders often require that the borrower undertake a feasibility study to demonstrate the organization's capacity to repay the loan. The organization will generally hire an outsider such as a certified public accounting firm to perform the study. Feasibility studies evaluate all the financial implications of the proposed investment. They show expected revenues and expenses over a long period, usually five to ten years.

A feasibility study will not only show the expected profitability of a particular investment or venture but will also project pro forma financial statements for the entire organization.[3] In addition, feasibility studies include ratio analysis showing the capacity of the organization to cover the interest charges and principal payments on its total debt, including the proposed borrowing.

One of the most telling elements of the feasibility study is the ratio that relates to interest coverage.[4] If the organization cannot make interest payments when due, it risks having to seek protection of the bankruptcy laws and possibly even closure. Therefore lenders are interested in how much of a cushion is anticipated for coverage of such payments.

Another element of feasibility studies that is considered fairly important relates to the attitude of the staff of the organization. If the bulk of the organization's people believe in a project and are committed to its success, that does not guarantee success. But when the majority of people in an organization are opposed to a project, disinterested, or not committed to it, there is a strong likelihood of failure.

If a commissioned feasibility study raises serious questions about the success

---

[3]Pro forma financial statements are discussed in the section on business plans in Chapter 10.
[4]A discussion of ratios was included in Chapter 6.

of an expansion or new venture, the organization should very seriously consider the weaknesses that have been raised. Not only will there be a question about whether financing can be obtained; there is also the more important question concerning whether the organization is making a mistake in undertaking the project.

THE FUTURE OF HEALTH CARE FINANCING

To thrive an organization must be able to maintain its major facilities. Buildings must be modernized and eventually replaced. Equipment must be kept up-to-date. This all requires major capital investments, which in turn require cash resources. For example, as Figure 15–2 indicates, capital spending by long-term care facilities over a five-year period is expected to range anywhere from $5,080 to $14,380 *per bed*.

The source of financing for health care has changed quite a bit over the last fifty years, and there is a likelihood that it will continue to change. Early in this century philanthropy was a major source of cash for long-term investments by health care organizations. Then the government became the major supplier of cash resources. Most recently, long-term debt has become the single largest element for new construction.

However, the continued availability of debt is not assured. There are movements to eliminate tax-free bonds. That would severely hurt health care organizations, hospitals in particular. Even with the continued existence of tax-

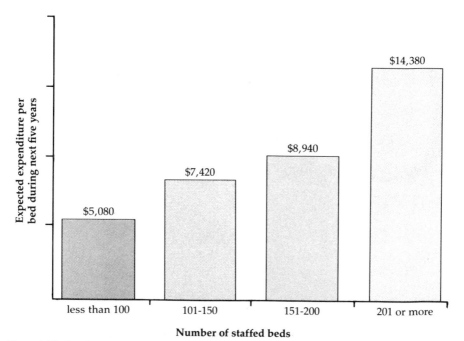

Figure 15–2. Long-term care expenditures by facility size. (Reprinted from Jimmie Hinze, "Providers Forecast 5 Year Construction Spending," *Healthcare Financial Management*, May 1990, p. 58, with permission of Healthcare Financial Management Association.)

free bonds, there is cause for concern. The introduction of DRGs in 1983 had a dramatic effect on the health care bond market. This is because the health care industry has been riskier since the shift of hospital Medicare payments from cost-based reimbursement to the DRG prospective payment system. The basic ability of the organization to issue bonds depends on its actual and perceived riskiness.

Approximately half of all hospital revenues comes from Medicare and Medicaid patients. In the pre-DRG era the bond market perceived those revenues as nearly risk free. Certainly hospitals could count on receiving their annual stream of revenues from the government. That allowed hospitals to incur large amounts of long-term debt at relatively favorable interest rates.

With the advent of DRGs, the guaranteed revenue base was affected. Payments were shifted to a fixed fee rather than cost reimbursement. Substantial losses might occur on Medicare patients. In fact, the number of hospital closures has increased dramatically since the introduction of DRGs.

To the bond market that represents increased risk. Not only are hospitals now able to lose money on Medicare patients but the change also increases the likelihood of additional regulatory changes that might hurt all health care providers. Thus, the bond market is not as welcoming to health care providers as it was a decade ago. Whether this is likely to close off a major source of financing for health care, or simply make it more expensive, cannot be determined at this time. However, the poor financial health of the health care industry makes it more likely that long-term debt will become less and less available.

Where will the resources come from in the future? Some have suggested that corporations will have to get together to generate the monies needed. In effect that proposal is a return to philanthropy but at a corporate level, since individuals do not have the vast sums necessary for modern health care facility construction.

Another view of the future is that the government will take over the health care system similar to the approaches of England or Canada. In that view, the government will decide what facilities are needed and will build them using tax dollars.

Yet another view is that many health care organizations will go out of business, reducing excess capacity. The remaining organizations will be financially healthy and will continue to have access to the major debt markets.

We have no special insight regarding a solution. We do, however, clearly see a problem. Nationwide and particularly in certain regions such as the Northeast, the severe financial distress of health care institutions such as hospitals and nursing homes has prevented them from replacing, or even adequately maintaining, their facilities. Given this state, there is clearly the potential for a health care financing crisis before the end of this century.

IMPLICATIONS FOR NURSE MANAGERS

The highest levels of nurse managers in any health care organization must be involved in the specific long-term financing decisions. Other nurse managers also have an important role in the financing process.

The decision to finance using conventional debt, tax-free bonds, or leasing will have a dramatic impact on the financial well-being of the institution. This decision should not be left solely to the financial managers because they may lack vision about the organization. They have greater financial expertise than nurse managers, but they may not have as good judgment about the clinical aspects of the organization.

This fact is evidenced by the interest that lenders, bond raters, and bond insurers all have in the attitude and thoughts of the staff of a health care institution. If the physicians are unhappy, they will not admit patients. If the nurses are unhappy, patients will not want to come to the institution. Financing should be done for investments that will make the organization as a whole work better. The nursing staff can provide critical input in this area.

It is important to bear in mind that major long-term financing such as a bond issuance is not an area of expertise of *anyone* in most health care organizations. Except for the larger academic medical centers, a bond floatation may be something that occurs just once in the career of a chief executive officer, chief financial officer, or chief nurse executive. The input of all areas of the institution can help the organization to make the correct decisions.

Some other types of long-term financing are more common. Mortgages and leases occur with great frequency. However, the choice of a mortgage or a lease is not strictly financial. Rather than having financial managers make such decisions on their own, nurse managers should provide input to the process. From a departmental or unit point of view, what are the advantages of the lease or the advantages of ownership as compared to a lease? Does the lessor provide some essential support service that is otherwise not readily available? Perhaps the equipment is subject to repeated breakdowns. A lease arrangement may provide cheaper service than ownership plus a service contract.

Nurse managers should not assume that the financing of the organization is something outside their management sphere of activity or expertise. A participatory team attitude and approach between nursing and finance is more likely to result in financing decisions that will benefit the entire organization, including nursing services.

KEY CONCEPTS _____ ❖

Long-term financing   Sources of money that the organization can use for longer than one year.

Debt   Borrowed money. Interest is generally paid on the debt as well as eventual repayment of the original loan balance.

Equity   Represents ownership sources of financing. In some case equity represents money that outsiders have given the organization in exchange for an ownership interest. In other cases equity represents money that the organization itself owns. The four principal sources of equity for health care organizations are philanthropy, corporate stock issuance, government grants, and retained earnings.

   Philanthropy   Gifts to the organization.

   Stock issuance   Sale of ownership interests in the organization; only available to for-profit organizations.

Government grants   Direct payments to health care organizations, usually to finance construction.

Retained earnings   Profits earned by the organization and retained in the organization to finance assets.

Long-term debt   Represents borrowed sources of financing. This includes mortgages, long-term notes, leases, and bonds.

Mortgages and long-term notes   Conventional loans to the organization. Notes are sometimes secured by collateral and sometimes are unsecured. When a note is secured by a specific piece of physical property such as a building, piece of equipment, or land, it is referred to as a mortgage.

Leases   Rental agreements evidenced by a contract referred to as a lease. Considered long-term debt because they obligate the organization to making payments over a period of years.

Bonds   Formal certificates of indebtedness. The certificate indicates a promise to pay interest, usually semiannually, and the face value of the bond at a future specified maturity date.

Call provisions   Elements of the loan agreement between a bond issuer and a bond purchaser indicating the rights of the bond issuer to call in and pay off the bonds early and specifying penalties that must be paid if a bond is retired early.

Bond sinking fund   Pool of money being accumulated for the eventual repayment of the face value of outstanding bonds.

Feasibility study   Analysis designed to determine the organization's capacity to repay a long-term loan.

SUGGESTED READINGS ———————————————————————

Bayless, Mark, and David Diltz, "Leasing Strategies Reduce the Cost of Financing Healthcare Equipment," *Healthcare Financial Management*, Vol. 39, No. 10, October 1985, pp. 38–49.

Brigham, Eugene F., *Fundamentals of Financial Management*, 5th edition, Dryden Press, Chicago, 1989.

Cavouras, Carol Ann, Ricki Harvey, and Pamela McGann Bordelon, "A Guide to Tax-Exempt Bonds," *Journal of Nursing Administration*, Vol. 19, No. 6, June 1989, pp. 36–38.

Dominiak, Geraldine F., and Joseph G. Louderback, *Managerial Accounting*, 5th edition, PWS-Kent Publishing Co., Boston, 1988.

Finkler, Steven A., *Finance & Accounting for Nonfinancial Managers*, revised edition, Prentice-Hall, Englewood Cliffs, NJ, 1992.

Greenfield, James, and William McGinly, "Where Does Philanthropy Fit in Fiscal Imperatives," *Healthcare Financial Management*, Vol. 42, No. 1, January 1988, pp. 66–70.

Mark, Barbara A., and Howard L. Smith, *Essentials of Finance in Nursing*, Aspen Publishing, Rockville, MD, 1987.

Neumann, Bruce R., James D. Suver, and William N. Zelman, *Financial Management: Concepts and Applications for Health Care Providers*, 2nd edition, National Health Publishing, USA, 1990.

Van Horne, James C., *Fundamentals of Financial Management*, 7th edition, Prentice-Hall, Er glewood Cliffs, NJ, 1989.

VI

ADDITIONAL
MANAGEMENT TOOLS

Most nurse managers recognize the importance of financial management. To successfully manage finances the nurse manager must understand the underlying financial concepts. The preceding chapters of this book have described these concepts. In addition to understanding the concepts, it is necessary to have sound financial information on which to base financial decisions. The first step in getting information is to know what to ask for.

Nurse managers generate some of the information they need themselves. Other information is readily available in health organizations; the nurse manager needs to ask for it. Still other information is available but not in a format that is useful for the nurse manager. Some information is not available and will need to be generated either by the nurse manager directly or by other departments in the organization.

The following chapters describe management tools that can be used both to generate information and to reconfigure it into a useful format. In addition, the chapters explore the kinds of information that are useful in making financial decisions.

The first chapter in this part of the book, Chapter 16, relates the use of information systems and computers to financial management. The chapter begins with a description of computer hardware and software. The use of both mainframe and microcomputers is reviewed. Major types of software for microcomputers are identified. The use of this software for forecasting, costing, personnel management, budgeting, and acuity systems is then described. Finally, we assess the future use of computers in financial decision making.

Chapter 17, Forecasting and Other Methods for Decision Making, focuses on quantitative and qualitative methods useful for nurse managers. The chapter begins with a discussion of probability, which forms the basis for many of the methods discussed later in the chapter. The use of specific techniques to predict future events, such as patient volume and staffing needs, is stressed. Finally, this chapter provides methodologies for inventory control and tracking a project.

The last chapter in this part of the book, Chapter 18 on Marketing, begins with a discussion of why marketing is important for nurse managers. The difference between marketing and advertising is clarified. Marketing concepts are then defined. The elements of a marketing plan and the role of these elements is discussed. ❖

16

The Role of Management Information Systems and Computers in Financial Management

CHAPTER GOALS

The goals of this chapter are to:

- Describe computer hardware and software
- Identify the use of computers for information management
- Describe the use of mainframe computers for financial management
- Discuss the use of microcomputers for financial management
- Discuss special purpose software, such as that used for forecasting, costing, personnel management, budgeting, and acuity systems
- Analyze the future use of computers in financial management
- Discuss the implications of computers for financial management for nurse managers

❖

INTRODUCTION

The purpose of this chapter is to describe the use of computers in nursing financial management. Computers are a tool to help the nurse manager summarize and organize information. Computers decide neither what information is provided nor the format in which it is displayed. Previous chapters of this book identified the types of financial information the nurse manager needs to effectively manage a unit or an organization. This chapter will focus on how the computer can be used to collect and summarize that information.

COMPUTER HARDWARE AND SOFTWARE

Computers and their related pieces of equipment such as printers, monitors, and terminals are referred to as *hardware*. The instructions that tell computer equipment what to do are referred to as *software*.

Types of Computers

The three major types of computers are mainframes, minis, and microcomputers. Mainframe computers are large (both physically and in computing capacity), fast, and expensive. Microcomputers are small, relatively slow, and inexpensive. Mini computers fall somewhere in between. Each of these types of computers has a variety of manufacturers such as IBM, Apple, and VAX. Computer manufacturers make a large variety of models. Some manufacturers make only mainframes or microcomputers. Others make all types of hardware. Within the category of microcomputers, for example, a company may make as many as fifty different models.

When health care organizations first used computers to manage financial information, they used mainframe computers. They either purchased or leased time on a mainframe. Sometimes they leased time on a mainframe and accessed the computer over telephone lines. Many hospitals and nursing homes contracted with a computer services company to provide both the time on the computer and the staff services to process financial information.

Some health care organizations purchased mini computers, hired information systems staff, and processed their own financial information. In the 1980s as the cost of microcomputers decreased and their processing speed increased, health care organizations began investing in them. As of the writing of this book, mainframe or mini computers are still required and used by most large health care organizations to perform the major financial operations such as billing. Many clinical information systems operate using terminals linked to a mainframe computer. However, an increasing number of nurse managers are using microcomputers for managerial functions.

Telling Computers What to Do

Computers require software to operate. Software is a *program* or set of instructions for the computer. All computers must use a type of software called an operating system, the basic language used to give the computer instructions about what to process. When a computer is purchased, an operating system is purchased as well. However, that only provides a starting point. Someone must program or write the instructions for the computer to follow for various specific applications. Initially, individuals (programmers) wrote specific sets of instructions for each computer and each application. It soon became clear that many organizations had common needs and could all use the same set of basic programs. Since many people want to use a computer to calculate the arithmetic sum of a set of numbers, one person wrote a program (software) to calculate sums for his or her own organization. Proprietary companies wrote more sophisticated software using the operating system to perform complex operations. Other people can then use the software (usually by purchasing it) to do sums. These programs are often called *software packages* or *packages*.

To understand the use of computers for financial management the nurse manager must know both the hardware and software capabilities available at the institution. Since hardware is often more expensive than software, once an organization owns hardware, it is less likely to purchase new equipment. Some commercially available software is available to operate on a variety of computers. Other software will only operate on one model of computer. Some software packages are sold prepackaged, and little or no tailoring is needed. Other software is designed (at much greater expense) to meet the specific needs of a particular organization.

USES OF COMPUTERS

The three principal uses of computers for nursing are for general information needs, clinical applications, and financial management.

General Information Management

Computers are tools to store and process information. In health care organizations computers are used for various types of information. These uses are quite varied, from keeping a calendar or computerized telephone directory to word processing. When information is computerized, it is often called *electronic*. Over time the number of applications continues to grow.

Clinical Care

Computer uses for clinical care fall into two general areas. The first area is for the assessment of patients. This includes computers used in laboratories to measure blood levels, in radiology for MRIs, and for physical assessment measures such as blood pressure. Each of these applications requires both hardware and software.

The second clinical care area is the storage and management of patient information. Often called the hospital information system or nursing information system, these computer systems store data such as patient demographics; admission, transfer, and discharge information; and documentation of nursing care provided.

While clinical information systems are not directly related to financial management, data produced by these systems can be used to make financial decisions. Clinical systems are being used to directly link the use of services to the billing for them. Ultimately, financial management is based on the allocation of resources; clinical information systems offer the nurse manager data about the use of resources in the organization.

Clinical information systems that combine information from a variety of sources, such as laboratory, radiology, dietary, and nursing, are called *fully integrated* systems. In these systems the data are entered once and are accessible all over the organization (with the appropriate confidentiality precautions). These integrated systems improve the flow of information.

Financial Management

Computers can greatly aid nurse managers in the area of financial management information. The first step for the nurse manager is to decide what financial information is needed for management. This includes information the manager needs from others and information the manager must report to others. Earlier chapters of this book discuss various types of information needed for financial management. Some examples are budget information and variance reports. An example of computerizing some aspects of variance analysis is provided in the article reprinted at the end of this chapter.

Later chapters also discuss financial information that could be generated by a computer, e.g., forecasting analyses. After identifying the needed information, the nurse manager should identify information currently available in the organization. Some information may already be routinely reported to managers (e.g., occupancy, average length of stay, and payroll). Next the manager should identify information that is likely available but not systematically reported. After assessing whether the required information can be obtained in a useful format, the nurse manager must decide how best to collect and analyze unavailable data.

Computerizing everything is not always the best solution. Using a computer for data management has equipment and human costs. Adding to and retrieving information from a computer requires an ongoing human resource commitment. Unless that commitment exists, the benefits of computerizing may not be worth the cost. For example, setting up a computerized checkbook system requires that all entries be entered in timely fashion. If data are not entered on an ongoing systematic basis, the computerized system is no better than the paper record with missing entries.

The key to the use of computers is that they must accomplish one of two things. One is to electronically generate information that is currently generated manually, saving human effort in doing it with a computer. The other is that information is generated that would not otherwise be available and that the value of information is worth more than the cost of obtaining it.

Mainframes and Financial Management Information

As described earlier, most hospitals and many other health care organizations have mainframe computers for patient billing and other aspects of organizational financial management. In many cases the CNE was not involved in planning for these systems. In most health care organizations the CNE receives periodic reports generated by the system, and in many organizations midlevel nurse managers also receive regular reports. Often the format of these reports was designed by the financial or information systems departments and does not give the nurse manager the type of information needed. In some cases the information is provided months after appropriate decisions based on that information should have been made.

As a nurse manager you may want to know the average length of stay by DRG for each unit for which you are responsible. Your hospital provides the CNE with the average length of stay by DRG hospital-wide. While that information as reported for the entire hospital is useful for overall hospital efforts to decrease length of stay, it may not assist you in identifying variation in length of stay by unit.

After assessing information needs, the first step is to learn what information is currently collected electronically. These data may be collected by the finance department, the management information systems department, the nursing department, or other departments. Data collected by other departments may be useful to you. By understanding how finance, personnel, or information systems departments collect and organize data, you will be able to identify the data that you can request. Most hospital finance systems can prepare special reports on request. However, you should keep in mind that such requests are often time-consuming and expensive. If you will be requesting these data on a regular basis, you should communicate that.

Computers allow for storing, processing, and reporting huge amounts of information quickly. First, the nurse manager can easily become overloaded with computer-generated reports. Second, processing and reporting data is not costless. What may appear to be a simple request may take hours of programming by the information systems department.

Clear communication with the data processing department is an essential aspect of obtaining appropriate information. The first step is to carefully determine what information is needed. Next, that specific need must be clearly communicated to data processing. The nurse manager should be sensitive to the fact that many demands are placed on the data processing department. Seemingly simple requests may in fact require substantial programming time. There should be an exchange of information concerning how hard it will be to generate the data and how valuable the data will be. In some cases the cost of obtaining the data may exceed the benefit. Finally, the nurse manager should give data processing a sufficient amount of time to generate the information. Undertaking this process of communication and consideration will make the nurse and information managers partners in meeting the needs of the organization.

Microcomputers and Financial Management Information

Many types of microcomputer software applications are useful for financial management. There are currently two standard microcomputer hardware systems, IBM and MacIntosh. *Clones*, equipment made by competitors and intended to function on a completely compatible basis, are available for both, usually substantially cheaper. Although many software applications are available for IBMs and MacIntoshes, some are available on only one or the other. Information is not readily transferable between the two types of hardware, although conversion processes do exist.

Four major types of software are especially useful for financial management:
♦ Word processing
♦ Data base
♦ Spreadsheet
♦ Statistical packages

There are both general purpose and application-specific programs available for each of these. General purpose programs require that the person using the program set up many of the parameters.

Word processing software is used to prepare correspondence and reports. While not directly related to financial management, the presentation of budget justifications, business plans, and other proposals virtually requires that the nursing department have this capability. WordPerfect, Word, and Wordstar are examples of commercially available software for word processing.[1]

It is strongly suggested that most people in the organization use the same word processing package. Because the use of computers developed gradually in most organizations, each department and even each person in a department

---

[1]WordPerfect is a trademark of WordPerfect; Word is a trademark of Microsoft; Wordstar is a trademark of Wordstar International.

initially may have selected and used different software. Unfortunately, most software is not *compatible*. In a way it is like asking a computer that only understands French to read something in Spanish. Although there are ways to "translate" files, in many cases the translation is not very good, particularly formatting such as spacing and paragraphs. While staff initially may be resistant to learning a new program, in the long run having everyone use the same program will save hours of retyping.

Related to word processing programs are graphics programs to present information in pictorial form. These programs can produce charts and graphs. Many word processing programs now include the capability to produce graphics.

Data bases are compilations of related information systematically organized. The telephone directory is a data base of names, addresses, and telephone numbers usually organized alphabetically by last name. Most nursing departments have numerous data bases. The nursing department and each nursing care unit likely have a data base of employees. The nursing department also maintains a data base of equipment inventory. These data bases may be handwritten, on 3 × 5 cards, or typed on paper. They also may be electronically stored for use on a computer.

Many data base software packages are available commercially. Paradox and dBase are examples of data base software programs.[2] The software may be for general applications and useful for a variety of tasks or designed for specific applications. General application programs tend to be more difficult to learn but are flexible and offer the advantage of integrating a variety of data bases.

Specific-application data bases such as those used for mailing labels and health records are often easier to learn to use but may limit the integration of data. Data bases allow one to store information in a systematic manner and then retrieve information according to criteria one chooses.

Once you have decided to use a computerized data base, choosing which software to use will depend on a variety of factors. The general rule is to use what everyone else in the organization is using unless there is a compelling reason not to. First, there will be people to help you use the program; second, your data bases will be compatible with theirs.

Because most nonelectronic data bases are organized in only one way (e.g., alphabetically, by date, by dollar amount), it is difficult to look for information by other than the organizing category. For example, if you received a garbled message that someone called you and his phone number was 348-8125, how would you determine who called? You might remember that this is the number of the supply salesperson who has been bothering you about buying new equipment. You could look through your phone book page by page and find out who the person is. You will likely just call the number and see who it was. With a computerized data base of phone numbers you can ask the computer to locate the name of the person with this phone number. The computer will look through your list of phone numbers and identify the name associated with that number. However, as discussed above, it is not always cost effective to computerize every data base you have.

Spreadsheets are large ledger sheets often used by accountants for financial

---

[2]Paradox and dBase are trademarks of Borland International.

calculations. A spreadsheet has columns and rows of cells. These cells contain text or numbers that can be manipulated. Electronic spreadsheets allow cells to contain formulas for mathematical manipulation. The formulas are decided by the person who develops the spreadsheet and can contain any mathematical formula. The power of an electronic spreadsheet is the speed with which a whole series of numbers can be recalculated.

Spreadsheets are often used for budgeting. For example, Figure 12–6 in Chapter 12 shows a spreadsheet for the calculation of positions needed. As you probably noted, the calculations can be tedious, particularly if someone changes one of the underlying assumptions and the entire budget must be recalculated. There are several commercially available spreadsheet packages available. LOTUS 1-2-3 is an example.[3] As with the data base programs described above, there are both general purpose and specific programs available. The same general rules apply. It is often advisable to use what the rest of the organization uses and get a generic program unless there is a compelling reason not to.

Statistical software is used to perform statistical analyses. Statistics refers to both the way in which data are organized and analyzed and the data themselves. Nurse managers frequently perform statistical analyses and use the results from these analyses. They need to know the average number of sick days, the range of sick days, the average staff salary per category of worker, or the average overtime per unit per day. An example is an estimate of the average number of sick days per month for different categories of staff. One approach is to estimate based on memory. The usual approach is to count the sick days per category of worker, add up the days, and divide by the number of workers.

All statistical calculations can be done with pencil and paper. They can be done more quickly with a calculator and often even more quickly with a statistical software program on a computer. As discussed earlier, it is not always more efficient to do tasks with a computer. For example, to calculate the average number of nurses who worked during a five-day period, it is far easier to use a calculator. Using a computer is more efficient for manipulating a large quantity of numbers, for performing complex analyses such as forecasting that are time-consuming to do by hand, and for repetitive tasks.

Again a variety of software programs are available for purchase. The most sophisticated programs were initially designed for use on mainframe computers and have been rewritten for microcomputers. SPSS – PC + (Statistical Package for the Social Sciences Personal Computer Version) is an example.[4] The versions for microcomputers do not include as many options as the mainframe versions, but they are more than adequate for most nursing departments. Additional statistical programs are available that were developed for microcomputers. Careful use of these programs is advised for those nurse managers who have not studied statistics.

Special Purpose Software

The previous section described the general types of software that will assist the nurse manager. The following section describes how these general purpose

---

[3]LOTUS 1-2-3 is a trademark of the LOTUS Development Corporation.
[4]SPSS – PC + is a trademark of SPSS, Inc.

programs can be used for specific financial management activities and discusses special applications programs.

Forecasting

Chapter 17 discusses forecasting in depth. Computers can be extremely useful in forecasting. Forecasting is used to predict the future. One of the best predictors of the future is the past. Obviously, the past is not a perfect predictor, and other factors will have to be taken into account. Statistical models can be used to predict the future based on past performance and assumptions about the future. Both spreadsheets and statistical software packages are useful for forecasting. Table 17–5 in Chapter 17 shows a computer printout of the estimated hours of nursing care needed for a nursing unit, based on historical hours.

Costing

Determining the cost of providing nursing care is discussed in Chapter 8. Goals are to determine the cost of providing care to a particular patient, to groups of similar patients, or to a group of patients on a particular unit. The more valid and reliable data collection is at the patient level, the more reliable and valid the aggregated data will be. Much of the literature on determining the cost of nursing care advocates using acuity systems. The section below on acuity discusses the use of computers for acuity measurement.

However, as discussed in Chapter 8, using acuity is not the only way to determine costs. Costs are really a dollar determination of resources used. How can computers be useful in determining resources used? In the nursing department the major resources consumed are personnel and supplies. Clinical information systems can provide an electronic data base of resources consumed. Each time a supply is used for a patient, it is noted in the electronic record and the appropriate cost is allocated. Each time the nurse notes that care is provided, that resource use can be captured by the computer and the appropriate costs determined. There are potential flaws in this system. It requires the nurse to note every care activity. Although noting activities on a computer may be easier than writing them, many nursing activities are not documented in either system.

The same activity provided for two different patients may require different amounts of time. This is obvious for something such as patient education, but it is also true for activities such as initiating a venous line. Depending on the use of the cost estimates, standard measures of resource use may be acceptable (see Chapter 8 discussion of standard costs). For example, Hospital A may assume that starting a line takes ten minutes, recognizing that there may be variation from patient to patient.

Some hospitals are experimenting with *bar coding*. Each patient's wristband contains a bar code. Each time the nurse begins care and again when care is completed the nurse uses a scanner to *scan* the patient's bar code. Data are then collected about real time spent providing care to patients. Computers then use these data to tabulate resources used. However, nursing includes both the care giver and care integrator role.[5] The care integrator role involves commu-

---

[5]M. L. McClure and J. J. Nelson, "Trends in Hospital Nursing," in L. H. Aiken, ed, *Nursing in the 1980s: Crisis, Opportunities, Challenges*, J. B. Lippincott, Philadelphia, 1982, pp. 59–73.

nication with other health providers and family members and is less easy to document with the scanner.

While using computers may decrease the time required to collect and analyze data to determine the cost of care, the expense is still not trivial. The nurse manager must make the decision about the level of detail that is necessary and cost/benefit of collecting the data.

If the nurse manager does not believe it is cost effective to document the cost of care provided to each patient on every unit, the computer can still be useful for summarizing cost data that are available. The manager can use a spreadsheet program with existing data from payroll combined with data generated from unit variance reports and acuity numbers to estimate costs on various units.

Personnel Management

Personnel management requires the systematic organization of information about employees. This includes information about staff skill levels, work preferences, health background, salary, work history, and other factors. A computerized data base is a helpful tool to organize this material. In most health care organizations payroll is computerized. In many organizations with a personnel department distinct from the nursing department, it is likely that some personnel data are computerized, although that will vary from organization to organization.

From a financial management viewpoint the nurse manager needs to have information to most efficiently use these personnel resources. One main use of data bases is for staffing. The organizational structure of the hospital will impact on the way data bases are set up. For example, a home health agency may want a data base of all RNs employed. This data base will include demographic information, health status, continuing education record, full- or part-time status, and preferred work hours. It is particularly useful to include special skills such as knowledge of foreign languages and high skill in parenteral fluid administration in the data base. The data base may also include vacation time used. If nurse managers need a nurse to work on the weekend, they can use this data base to identify a nurse in the appropriate geographic area who has the requisite skills and who is willing to work extra shifts.

Staffing is the major responsibility of the nurse manager. Special application programs are available for staffing. These programs are combinations of data bases and spreadsheets. Examples are ANSOS and RESQUE. Private computer consultants will also develop software programs to meet the specific needs of organizations. Data about available staff are stored in the data base. Staffing needs are identified by nurse managers, often using an acuity system. Exhibit 16–1 shows an example of data showing scheduled staffing produced using RESQUE.

Staffing rules are determined by the nurse manager. Rules can include: (1) no nurse can work more than seven consecutive days; (2) no nurse can work more than every other weekend; (3) each nurse must have at least two consecutive days off. Using the established rules, the computer provides staffing options. These programs can also incorporate individual preferences. For example, Nurse A prefers not to work Thursday evenings or requires Mondays off to attend school. For years nurse managers have been staffing units and taking staff preferences into account. The use of a computer greatly reduces

❖ **EXHIBIT 16-1**

The RES-Q RN System
MEDICAL MANAGEMENT PLANNING HOSPITAL
SCHEDULED STAFFING PROJECTIONS - BY UNIT WITH SCHEDULE CODES AND NOTATIONS
(AS OF 09/11/90)

THU, AUGUST 16, 1990   3 SOUTH

---------------------------------- DAY SHIFT ----------------------------------

RN	LPN	TECH	AIDES	MGMT	CLERK	ED	ORIENT
D ALDRIDG., M.	D CHAPMAN, E.	D HAZEN, H.		7 BROCKMA., R./CHG	6C PARKER, S.	E2 BEARDAL.. W./2.00/EKG	
D BAKER, A./16.00		D HYATT, L.			7 SMITH, L.	E2 COMPTON, R./2.00/EKG	
D BUTRES., B.		D MEISEL, M.				E2 LOVELAN, C./2.00	
D BUTZERF., C.						E2 MOORE, T./2.00/EKG	
7A GAAR, N./4C						E2 ST.JEOR, S./2.00/EKG	
7A HELLER, J.							
D ROTH, K.							

-------------------------------- EVENING SHIFT --------------------------------

RN	LPN	TECH	AIDES	MGMT	CLERK	ED	ORIENT
E BELLING., K.		E PESSES, K.			3 ALVORD, M.		
7P BENDER, K./4.00					6C PARKER, S./1.00		
E DEARDA., T.							
7A GAAR, N./4.00/4C							
7A HELLER, J./4.00							
7P KELLER, S./4.00							
E MONDFRA., L.							
7P TRUDEAU, C./4.00/CHG							

--------------------------------- NIGHT SHIFT ---------------------------------

RN	LPN	TECH	AIDES	MGMT	CLERK	ED	ORIENT
7P BENDER, K.					11 LEATHAM, J.		
7P KELLER, S.					6C PARKER, S./1.00		
N MCCANN, J.							
7P TRUDEAU, C./CHG							

440

From *Micro Management Systems*, Medical Management Planning, Inc., Calabasas, CA, August 1991.

the time needed to do this and can quickly adjust for changes in staff requirements. This frees the nurse manager to spend time on other elements of management.

The advantage of spreadsheets is the ability to quickly determine "what if" options. For example, "what if" the number of sick days increases or three more staff decide to go back to school and need to switch work days? The most sophisticated systems can provide staffing patterns based on acuity and patient need. While staffing is a general management function rather than a specific aspect of financial management, efficient use of available staff will likely improve the financial strength of the hospital. Exhibit 16–2 shows a productivity report generated by RESQUE.

Budgeting

Chapter 12 discusses the budgeting process. This is often seen as one of the most painful parts of a nurse manager's responsibility, but computers can dramatically decrease the frustration and tedium of budget preparation. Budget preparation involves collection of historical data, estimates of future resources and needs, and proposed allocation of resources to meet those needs.

Using the computer for forecasting, costing, and personnel will give the nurse manager many of the data needed for successful budgeting. A spreadsheet is the most common computer application for budgeting. Commonly used software packages are LOTUS 1-2-3, Excel, and Quattro Pro.[6] Exhibit 16–3 shows a simple spreadsheet for overtime hours. Overtime hours for each of five workers for five months are shown. Total overtime hours are shown in row 9. Assume the nurse manager realizes that overtime hours for Smith and Jones were erroneous. Instead of working three and two hours, respectively, they each worked ten hours. Exhibit 16–4 shows the corrected spreadsheet. The nurse manager corrects only the hours for the individuals, and the spreadsheet automatically recalculates the total shown in cell G9. This same spreadsheet can be used to calculate "what if" scenarios. For example, if overtime increased to fifteen hours per worker, what would be the implications of total overtime? These are, of course, very simple examples of the very complicated calculations the computer can do automatically.

It is becoming increasingly common for health care organizations to use flexible budgeting (discussed in Chapter 13). Spreadsheets can be particularly useful in calculating, understanding, and justifying flexible budget variances (see, for example, the article reprinted at the end of this chapter). A series of multiplications is used to identify the actual cost, the budgeted cost of actual resources used, the acuity category, the flexible budget, and the original budget. Further calculations are required to determine the price, quantity, acuity, and volume variances. In some institutions these calculations are performed by the finance department. If these data are not available, the nursing department can create a spreadsheet template to do these calculations. Secretarial staff can type in the information, and nurse managers can benefit from sophisticated variance data.

Information can be presented in a variety of formats. The appendix at the end of this chapter provides a reprinted journal article that gives examples of

---

[6]Quattro Pro is a trademark of Borland International. Excel is a trademark of Microsoft.

❖ **EXHIBIT 16–2**

The RES-Q RN System
MEDICAL MANAGEMENT PLANNING HOSPITAL
PRODUCTIVITY AND ACUITY MANAGEMENT REPORT
FOR THE PERIOD: 08/16/90 TO 08/16/90

ACTIVITY DATA

UNIT	BUDGTD DAILY CENSUS	ACTUAL DAILY CENSUS (AVG)	ACTUAL DAILY CENSUS BY CATEGORY (AVG)							TOTAL CENSUS	% OCCUP	HOURS WORKED DIRECT	TOTAL
			1	2	3	4	5	6	7				
OB/GYN	28.0	37.0	5.0	15.0	15.0	2.0	0.0	0.0	0.0	37.0	77.1	132.00	148.00
NURSERY	16.0	24.0	4.0	10.0	10.0	0.0	0.0	0.0	0.0	24.0	60.0	116.00	124.00
NICU	15.0	9.0	2.0	2.0	4.0	1.0	0.0	0.0	0.0	9.0	40.9	126.00	124.00
L&D	8.3	8.0	8.0	0.0	0.0	0.0	0.0	0.0	0.0	8.0	80.0	76.00	104.00
PEDS	12.0	24.0	5.0	10.0	8.0	1.0	0.0	0.0	0.0	24.0	85.7	100.00	132.00
3 SOUTH	20.0	24.0	4.0	5.0	15.0	0.0	0.0	0.0	0.0	24.0	100.0	164.00	207.00
4 NORTH	20.5	23.0	3.0	10.0	10.0	0.0	0.0	0.0	0.0	23.0	76.7	104.00	140.00

From *Micro Management Systems*, Medical Management Planning, Inc., Calabasas, CA, August 1991.

ways to show the information contained in a variance report generated by LOTUS 1-2-3. Note that there are a number of cells with "xxx" or "err." The "xxx" represents data not yet available and the "err" represents where the program has been unable to carry out a calculation because the needed data have not been made available. Data can be presented in a variety of graphic formats. Figure 16–1 shows variances in the form of a bar graph, and Figure 16–2 shows the same information in the form of a pie chart. Figure 16–3 shows variance data for six months in line-graph form.

Acuity Systems

It is becoming more and more common for staffing to be based on actual patient care needs. This has led to a greatly increased focus on measurement of patient acuity.

Home health agencies base the amount of care provided (usually visits per week and total number of visits per episode of care) on the patient's need for

❖ **EXHIBIT 16–3**
Example of LOTUS 1-2-3 Spreadsheet

	A	B	C	D	E	F	G	H	I	J	K
1			Nursing Hospital—4 South West: Overtime Hours								
2											
3			Jan.		Feb.		Mar.		Apr.		May
4											
5	Smith		28		30		16		12		3
6	Jones		25		25		14		8		2
7	Kovner		34		35		24		14		5
8	Finkler		15		28		20		10		2
9	Moga		40		35		18		13		2
10											
11	Totals:		142		153		92		57		14

❖ **EXHIBIT 16–2**—Continued

	PRODUCTIVITY PERFORMANCE								ACUITY PERFORMANCE			
HOURS REQUIRED		ACTUAL HPPD		GOAL HPPD			YTD		INTEN OF CARE	HOURS REQUIRED WITH ACUITY		PROD INDEX WITH	YTD PROD INDEX
DIRECT	TOTAL	DIRECT	TOTAL	DIRECT	TOTAL	PROD INDEX	PROD INDEX	RESP MANAGER	INDEX	DIRECT	TOTAL	ACUITY W/ACTY
103.23	137.23	3.57	4.00	3.72	4.48	93	91	M JACOBS	2.38	151.97	185.97	126	121
90.00	115.00	4.83	5.17	3.77	4.78	93	89	M JACOBS	2.25	93.24	109.24	95	90
117.90	136.89	14.00	14.00	13.10	15.21	109	110	T. EDWARDS	2.44	41.09	57.09	98	99
77.84	97.84	9.50	13.00	9.73	13.78	94	99	K. ZUNDEL	1.00	26.32	46.32	45	80
136.86	158.86	4.17	5.50	7.92	9.88	120	114	F. LINDQUIST	2.21	89.54	111.54	84	90
146.99	170.99	6.83	8.63	8.39	10.23	82	81	R. BROCKMAN	2.46	165.88	189.88	91	88
117.82	162.82	4.52	6.09	6.74	8.76	116	104	t. MILLER	2.90	125.50	170.50	122	125

care. This assessment of need is usually ordered by the physician, but in actuality it is determined by the nurse doing the initial assessment and on an ongoing basis by the nurse providing care. Increasingly, payers are and will be requesting more systematic determination of care required.

The Joint Commission on Accreditation of Healthcare Organizations (JCAHO) now requires that hospital staffing be based on patient needs. While hospitals have always done this, JCAHO now expects some evidence of systematic assessment of patient needs. Most hospitals are using some type of acuity system to make this determination.

Numerous articles describe approaches to determining acuity, and many hospitals have developed their own system. The usual method is for nurses to rate the patient's needs periodically (usually once per day), to sum the scores for each patient, and, based on a predetermined relationship for score to hours of care needed, determine the required staff for the following time period (often the next twenty-four hours). Usually the score sheets are sent to a centralized

❖ **EXHIBIT 16–4**
Revised Example of LOTUS 1-2-3 Spreadsheet

	A	B	C	D	E	F	G	H	I	J	K
1			Nursing Hospital—4 South West: Overtime Hours								
2											
3			Jan.		Feb.		Mar.		Apr.		May
4											
5	Smith		28		30		16		12		10
6	Jones		25		25		14		8		10
7	Kovner		34		35		24		14		5
8	Finkler		15		28		20		10		2
9	Moga		40		35		18		13		2
10											
11	Totals:		142		153		92		57		29

ABC HOSPITAL – MED/SURG 4B
VARIANCES – JUNE 1991

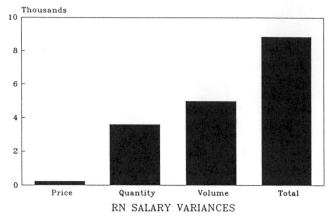

RN SALARY VARIANCES

Figure 16–1. Bar graph of price, quantity, and volume variances for June. (Reprinted from Steven A. Finkler, "Variance Analyses Part II, The Use of Computers," *Journal of Nursing Administration,* Vol. 21, No. 9, September 1991, p. 13, with permission of the publisher.)

location for tabulation. The average acuity measures over time are also reviewed for long-range planning for staffing requirements.

The entire process can be computerized. In the most sophisticated model the nursing plan of care is entered into a clinical information system. Data from the plan of care are electronically transmitted into an acuity system, patient acuity is determined, and those data are analyzed to determine future staffing needs and aid in budgeting. This totally electronic system is beyond the re-

ABC HOSPITAL – MED/SURG 4B
VARIANCES – JUNE 1991

Figure 16–2. Pie graph of June price, quantity, and volume variances. (Reprinted from Steven A. Finkler, "Variance Analysis Part II, The Use of Computers," *Journal of Nursing Administration,* Vol. 21, No. 9, September 1991, p. 14, with permission of the publisher.)

ABC HOSPITAL – MED/SURG 4B
VARIANCES – JAN. TO JUNE 1991

RN SALARY YEAR–TO–DATE PRICE VARIANCES

Figure 16–3. Line Graph for Year-to-Date Price Variances. (Reprinted from Steven A. Finkler, "Variance Analysis Part II, The Use of Computers," *Journal of Nursing Administration*, Vol. 21, No. 9, September 1991, p. 14, with permission of the publisher.)

sources of most hospitals as this book is being written. Figure 16–4 depicts a staffing system integrated with the clinical information system. Information generated by nurses about patient needs determines appropriate staffing needs.

Most acuity systems require completion of a paper form on each patient to determine acuity. This form can be a *scansheet*. Scansheets are forms with preprinted markings, usually filled out with a number 2 pencil. These forms can then be read electronically by a computerized scanner and directly entered as data. Those data can then be analyzed by the computer and printed for review by the nurse manager. This process decreases data entry time by clerical staff and dramatically decreases transcription errors. Both Medicus and GRASP have the capability to provide this service to hospitals. Hospitals using other systems, including their own, can purchase software to do this. Scanners and customized forms can be purchased from National Computer Systems and other vendors.

For those hospitals which choose not to invest in a scanner, a spreadsheet program is useful to calculate staffing requirements based on acuity. The spreadsheet program can be set up to perform routine calculations. Data on the acuity status of each patient are entered manually, and the calculations of weighing and summing are performed by the computer.

THE FUTURE

In the section on clinical information systems the fully integrated system was discussed. In an ideal future vision financial, personnel, and clinical systems will be fully integrated. In the hospital world of the future, as the nurse, physician, and other health care providers plan care for a patient, the units required to provide care will be alerted. As the care is ordered and provided, data will be electronically stored and appropriate bills generated. Reports of

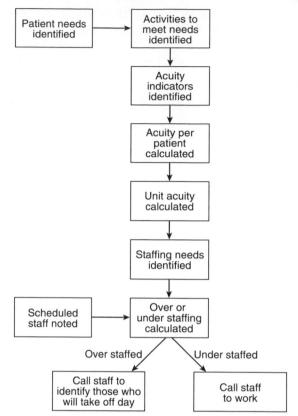

Figure 16–4. Computerized information flow worksheet.

care provided for patients will be identified as well as care provided by various categories of workers (and even individual workers). These data can then be summarized in a variety of formats so that the nurse manager can analyze the way care is provided for types of patients by type of nursing staff and by individual nurses.

Computer programs are available to simulate a health organization. The programs can be developed for a specific hospital, nursing home, or home health agency. The programs are similar to very sophisticated spreadsheets in that they allow the user to present "what if" scenarios. After analyzing the work flow in the organization, a complex computer model is developed. Using this model the nurse manager can test on the computer a variety of organizational models and estimate the impact that changes will have on the other parts of the organization.

For example, what if the admitting department assumed the responsibility for orienting the patient to the hospital? What would the implications be in terms of paper flow, personnel, and costs? Obviously, without a computer it is clear that the work level for admitting would increase. However, with the computer this could be more exactly determined. The modeling approach can handle the impact of many concurrent changes simultaneously. What if admitting handled orientation, sent an admitting staff person with the patient to the unit, and each unit had its own food preparation area and small lab for routine tests and transport workers used beepers and guaranteed less than a ten minute response time?

When organizations explore changing the way care is provided, implications for the various departments are almost always considered. However, the implications of multiple simultaneous changes are more difficult to analyze. A computerized model can assist with the assessment of multiple simultaneous changes. The options are simulated on the computer without disrupting even one pilot unit prior to implementation.

IMPLICATIONS FOR NURSE MANAGERS

One of the most difficult decisions about using computers is the determination of the set of activities that should be done by the manager and those activities which others (secretaries, clerks, nursing staff, finance, etc.) should do. The authors believe that all nurse managers should have a basic understanding of how computers are used and their capabilities. This skill level can be reached by taking a one-semester college course in information systems or some combination of one-day workshops. Some managers have the capacity to be self taught using the computer and a few books.

We also think the nurse manager should take a seminar in spreadsheets and data bases. These are essential management tools. We think that using computers and related software will greatly increase the nurse manager's ability in the area of financial management. That does not mean that the manager must learn or become proficient in all (or any) of the software used. Realizing the benefits of the software is the key; implementing the use of the software can be left to nonclinical personnel if the nurse manager prefers.

The level of skill required can be compared to the level of clinical knowledge required by a nurse manager. Managers must understand the concept of parenteral fluid administration. They must know what can be done to provide fluids and what can go wrong. Does that mean they must be proficient at working every new pump the organization uses? Probably not. Might there be times when the manager needs to set the dials? Maybe. The manager should know enough about the principles to be able to read and understand the manual or know where to get the help needed. Other managers want to know how to work every piece of equipment. They want to be able to "do the work themselves" if they expect their subordinates to do it.

Computers are like that. The nursing office may provide staff to develop computer spreadsheet programs for unit budgets. Nurse managers may be expected to hand in changes and then wait for results. Sometimes the wait may be too long. The organization may have central staff to set up the spreadsheet shell (tailored model for the application, often referred to as a template) and even enter the numbers. Perhaps you don't need to do that. With enough knowledge of the program you can change the numbers and try different options. Finally you may want to do it all yourself.

The authors' experience is that it is useful to know the basics of how to use a few software programs. Although we have staff to assist us, our experience is that the day before a research grant budget is due, our colleagues want to use that same staff. We'd rather do it ourselves. However, neither of us is a software expert, and we rely on organizational experts to help us. You may have noticed in the acknowledgement page that there was no thank you to our spouses or secretaries for typing the manuscript. We wrote this book directly using a word processing program on a microcomputer. We can't imagine having done it any other way. We believe there should be a microcomputer on every nurse manager's desk and that it should be used.

The nurse manager can use computers to assist in financial management. The manager can use the computer for data base management, financial simulations, and report generation. In addition to general programs for these uses, specialized programs are available for staffing and acuity.

KEY CONCEPTS

Hardware   Computers and their related pieces of equipment such as printers, monitors, and terminals. The three major types of hardware are mainframes, minis, and microcomputers.

Program   Set of instructions for the computer to do a task. Some programs are tailored for specific organizations. Other programs used to perform a specific task can be purchased "off the rack."

Software packages   Computer programs. All computers use a type of software called an operating system, which is the basic language used to give the computer instructions. In addition, software is available to perform a variety of functions such as word processing, budgeting, and statistical analyses.

Electronic   Computerized information.

Fully integrated   Information system in which all the components are able to communicate with each other. In health care organizations these systems integrate clinical and financial information from a variety of sources such as dietary, nursing, and radiology. The data are usually entered only once and are available all over the organization (with the appropriate confidentiality precautions).

Word processing   Electronic production and storage of documents. Word processing software is used to prepare correspondence and reports. The presentation of budget justifications, business plans, and other proposals can be improved using word processing software.

Data base   Compilation of related information systematically organized. Electronic or computerized data bases are used to organize information in the nursing department. Examples of data bases are an equipment inventory or personnel directory.

Spreadsheet   Large ledger sheets often used by accountants for financial calculations. Spreadsheets have columns and rows of cells. These cells contain text or numbers that can be manipulated. Electronic spreadsheets contain formulas in some of the cells. When a number is changed in one cell, other cells are automatically recalculated according to the formulas.

Special purpose software   Software used for a specific purpose such as budgeting, statistics, or assessing acuity.

Statistical software   Computer software used to perform statistical calculations.

Acuity systems   Systems to assess how much care is required by patients. These systems are developed for a particular hospital or can be purchased. Special purpose software is available to determine acuity.

Scansheet   Forms with preprinted markings and markings added, usually with a number 2 pencil, which can be read by an optical scanner.

SUGGESTED READINGS ———————————————————————

Adams, Rella, and Pam Duchene, "Computerization of Patient Acuity and Nursing Care Planning: New Approach to Improved Patient Care and Cost-Effective Staffing," *The Journal of Nursing Administration*, Vol. 15, No. 4, April 1985, pp. 11–17.

Behrenbeck, Julia G., Patrick Davitt, Pamela Ironside, et al., "Strategic Planning for a Nursing Information System (NIS) in the Hospital Setting: Development of a Nursing System Model," *Computers in Nursing*, Vol. 8, No. 6, November/December 1990, pp. 236–242.

Bergmann, Corinne, and JoAnn Johnson, "Managing Staffing with a Personal Computer—Part I," *Nursing Management*, Vol. 19, No. 7, July 1988, pp. 28–32.

Budd, Marjorie, Judy Blaufuss, and Susan Harada, "Nursing: A Revenue Center, Not a Cost Center," *Computers in Health Care*, Vol. 9, No. 11, November 1988, pp. 24–26.

Day, Lurana, "Automated Staff Scheduling in Long-Term Care Facilities," *Nursing Management*, Vol. 20, No. 3, March 1989, pp. 76–78.

Dick, Richard S., and Elaine B. Steen, eds., *The Computer-Based Patient Record*, National Academy Press, Washington, DC, 1991.

Finkler, Steven A., "Microcomputers in Nursing Administration," *The Journal of Nursing Administration*, Vol. 15, No. 4, April 1985, pp. 18–23.

Finkler, Steven A., "Variance Analysis Part II: The Use of Computers," *Journal of Nursing Administration*, Vol. 21, No. 9, September 1991, pp. 9–15.

Fitzpatrick, Therese, Louice Y. Farrell, and Mary Richter-Zeunik, "An Automated Staff Scheduling System That Minimizes Payroll Costs and Maximizes Nurse Satisfaction," *Computers in Nursing*, Vol. 5, No. 1, January/February 1987, pp. 10–14.

Garre, Patricia P., "A Computerized Recruitment Program," *Journal of Nursing Administration*, Vol. 20, No. 1, January 1990, pp. 24–27.

Garre, Patricia P., Linda M. Lutey, and Linda S. McElroy, "Apply Technology Today: A Computerized Nursing Recruitment Database," *Computers in Nursing*, Vol. 8, No. 1, January/February 1990, pp. 10–15.

Giovannetti, Phyllis, and Judith M. Johnson, "A New Generation Patient Classification System," *Journal of Nursing Administration*, Vol. 20, No. 5, May 1990, pp. 33–40.

Kilby, Sally A., Carolyn C. Fishel, and Ann D. Gupta, "Access to Nursing Information Resources," *IMAGE: Journal of Nursing Scholarship*, Vol. 21, No. 1, Spring 1989, pp. 26–30.

Kropf, Roger, *Service Excellence in Health Care Through the Use of Computers*, Foundation of the American College of Healthcare Executives, Ann Arbor, MI, 1990.

McClure, Margaret L., and M. Janice Nelson, "Trends in Hospital Nursing," in Linda H. Aiken, ed., *Nursing in the 1980s: Crisis, Opportunities, Challenges*, J.B. Lippincott Co., Philadelphia, 1982, pp. 59–73.

McCormick, Kathleen A., "Conceptual Considerations, Decision Criteria, and Guidelines for Development of the Nursing Minimum Data Set from a Research Perspective," in Harriet H. Werley and Norma M. Lang, eds., *Identification of the Nursing Minimum Data Set*, Springer Publishing Company, Inc., New York, 1988, pp. 34–47.

McLaughlin, Katherine, Susan Taylor, Jane Bliss-Holtz, et al., "Shaping the Future: The Marriage of Nursing Theory and Informatics," *Computers in Nursing*, Vol. 8, No. 4, July/August, 1990, pp. 174–179.

Malvey, Mari, *Simple Systems, Complex Environments: Hospital Financial Information Systems,* Sage Publications, Beverly Hills, CA, 1981.

Mills, Andrew C., Sandra L. Blaesing, and Joan H. Carter, "Preparing Nurses to Use Microcomputers for the Work of Management," *Computers in Nursing,* Vol. 9, No. 5, September/October 1991, pp. 179–183.

Mowry, Mychelle M., and Ralph A. Korpman, *Managing Health Care Costs, Quality, and Technology,* Aspen, Rockville, MD, 1986.

Patterson, Carole H., "Quality Assurance, Control, and Monitoring: The Future Role of Information Technology from the Joint Commission's Perspective," *Computers in Nursing,* Vol. 8, No. 3, May/June 1990, pp. 105–110.

Pierskalla, William P., and Deirdre Woods, "Computers in Hospital Management and Improvements in Patient Care—New Trends in the United States," *Journal of Medical Systems,* Vol. 12, No. 6, 1988, pp. 411–428.

Richards, Julie, "Implementing a Computer System: Issues for Nurse Administrators," *Computers in Nursing,* Vol. 10, No. 1, January/February 1992, pp. 9–13.

Schroder, Mary Ann, and Joann Carter, "Development of a Database Management System for an Obstetrics Unit," *Computers in Nursing,* Vol. 7, No. 3, May/June 1989, pp. 112–118.

Silva, Nettie, and Betty Aderholdt, "FTE Reports and Fiscal Management," *Nursing Management,* Vol. 20, No. 11, November 1989, pp. 46–48.

Strasen, Leann, "Implementing Salary Cost per Unit of Service Productivity Standards," *Journal of Nursing Administration,* Vol. 20, No. 3, March 1990, pp. 6–10

Tamarisk, Nancy K., "Personal Computer Databases for Middle Managers," *Nursing Management,* Vol. 21, No. 7, July 1990, pp. 49–51.

Warnock-Matheron, Ann G., and Kathryn J. Hannah, "Comparative Analysis of Computer-based Operating Room Information Systems: An Evaluation Research Study," *Computers in Nursing,* Vol. 6, No. 4, July/August 1988, pp. 147–156.

Werley, Harriet H., Elizabeth C. Devine, Cecilia R. Zorn, et al., "The Nursing Minimum Data Set: Abstraction Tool for Standardized, Comparable, Essential Data," *American Journal of Public Health,* Vol. 81, No. 4, April 1991, pp. 421–426.

Wiewandt, Jerry, "Bar Codes Help Contain Costs at Florida Hospital," *Computers in Healthcare,* Vol. 10, No. 3, March 1989, pp. 54–55.

Zinn, Tim K., "HIS Technology Trends," *Computers in Healthcare,* Vol. 11, No. 2, February 1991, pp. 46–48.

FINANCIAL MANAGEMENT SERIES

Variance Analysis
Part II, The Use of Computers

Steven A. Finkler, PhD, CPA

This is the second in a two-part series on variance analysis. In the first article (*JONA*, July/August 1991), the author discussed flexible budgeting, including the calculation of price, quantity, volume, and acuity variances. In this second article, the author focuses on the use of computers by nurse managers to aid in the process of calculating, understanding, and justifying variances.

In recent years, there have been great strides in the degree of sophistication of variance analysis in healthcare organizations. This is the second in a two-part series on variance analysis. In the first article, flexible budgeting was discussed, including the calculation of price, quantity, volume, and acuity variances. Many healthcare organizations use some form of flexible budget variance analysis, but many do not. The focus of this second article is on the use of computers by nurse managers to aid in the process of calculating, understanding, and justifying variances.

Part I concluded that, at a minimum, nurse managers should be receiving variance reports that in some way allow for the impact of changes in the workload volume. As the number of patients increases, nurses should not have to waste their time explaining that more patients consume more resources. Therefore, some type of volume variance measure is a necessity. The calculation of price, quantity, and acuity variances can also be a great aid. Such variances can help nurse managers focus their variance investigation attention on the specific areas in which the variances arose.

The calculation of flexible budget variances is a straightforward matter with a personal computer (PC). Even if variance reports provided to nursing departments do not provide such information,

nurses can readily calculate the variances on a PC. This article describes what is involved in computerizing flexible budget variance analysis. Furthermore, even in departments that receive flexible budget variance information from the finance or information systems departments, the *form* of the information is not always conducive to understanding the variances. This article also focuses on the development of graphs to aid nurses in understanding, investigating, explaining, and justifying variances.

Use of an Electronic Spreadsheet

Basics

The basic role of an electronic spreadsheet is to make repetitive, quantitative calculations less laborious. The key to the value of electronic spreadsheets is that a model is developed that uses formulas based on relationships rather than specific numbers. For example, if employee benefits are calculated in an institution as 20% of salaries, and a department's salaries are expected to be $100,000, we could expect benefits to be $20,000.

In a spreadsheet model, however, we would simply indicate that benefits are 20% of salaries. If subsequent changes in forecasts lead us to believe that salaries are going to be only $90,000, the computer can automatically update the amount of benefits because it has been programmed with the 20% relationship between salaries and benefits. A long sequence of calculations, with each calculation being affected by the result of some earlier calculation, can be linked in the spreadsheet model. One change in a beginning assumption will set off a series of recalculations by the spreadsheet program, and hours or days of manual arithmetic can take place in seconds on the computer.

To make a spreadsheet a useful tool for any specific application, it cannot be used directly from the manufacturer. Someone must program

Steven A. Finkler, PhD, CPA, Professor of Health Administration, Accounting, and Financial Management, Robert F. Wagner Graduate School of Public Service, New York University, New York City.

Reprinted from *Journal of Nursing Administration*, Vol. 21, No. 7/8, July/August 1991, pp. 19–25.

the specific relevant relationships. There is no need for nurse managers to perform the actual programming. It is quite feasible, as well as reasonable in cost, to employ a programmer to generate a specific model (or template). Once the template has been developed, the use of a spreadsheet is quite simple.

There are a large number of electronic spreadsheets for use on microcomputers. The examples used in this article are based on LOTUS 1-2-3 (Lotus Development Corp., Cambridge, Massachusetts), the most widely used spreadsheet program.

Spreadsheets and the Calculation of Variances

In Part I, flexible budget variances were calculated manually. The mathematics involved are not advanced. A series of multiplications are required to determine the actual cost, the budgeted cost of actual resources used, the acuity category, the flexible budget, and the original budget. Several subtractions are then required to determine the price, quantity, acuity, and volume variances.

For one unit, for one time, for one line item, the calculation of the variances is not unduly time-consuming or difficult. If we were to suppose, however, that a hospital had 30 different nursing units, each with a separate unit budget, it would be necessary to perform those calculations 30 times for each variable cost line item. Furthermore, we would have to perform the calculations every month in order to have the information we need to investigate variances on a timely basis. Devoting the time of 30 nurse managers on a regular basis to perform a series of repetitive mathematical tasks is not a good use of their time.

In some cases, finance or information systems will provide the variance information. If they do not, then the nursing department can have a simple spreadsheet template created, specifying the mathematical relationships in the variance calculations. The template can be used on a monthly basis by secretarial staff to generate a wealth of information promptly and efficiently for the nurse managers to use. Nursing departments can have the benefit of sophisticated variance information, relieve unit managers of numerous repetitive calculations, and in all likelihood increase accuracy as well by reducing arithmetic errors.

There are many different ways that the variance information can be reported once it has been calculated. For example, our printed report could appear as the one shown in Table 1. In this example, only one line item is shown. Typically, each

unit would have a number of line items for their flexible budget variance report. Additionally, the report would include columns for an acuity variance if the institution has a patient classification system that collects the necessary data, as discussed in Part I. The report could also show more detailed information, month by month for each specific line item, if desired.

The exact form of the report is quite flexible once the variance information has been calculated. Each manager can design a reporting form to suit their needs. Therefore, the remainder of this article will not focus on the form and content of the report. Instead, it will consider some of the tasks that are required, who is capable of performing them, some of the types of graphs that can be generated for the purposes of analysis, and the types of analysis that can be done.

Table 1 represents the portion of a spreadsheet model that would be printed out each month. The remainder of the spreadsheet appears in Table 2. This section of the spreadsheet would be updated each month, but would not necessarily be printed unless specific detailed information were desired.*

Note that there are a number of cells in Table 2 with either a dash or the letters ERR. The dashes represent data that are not yet available. The ERRs indicate areas where the program has been unable to carry out a calculation because needed data have not been made available. As each month's information is entered into the computer, those error messages automatically are replaced with variance information. Once a template is designed, it is used to calculate all flexible budget variances for that unit month after month, year after year.

At the beginning of each year, a secretary could be assigned the task of inserting all budgeted data. This task can be performed by one secretary for all units, or individually unit by unit. In this example, all that is involved is typing in the values for budgeted patient days, budgeted rate, and budgeted RN hours, for each of the 12 months. A total of 36 numbers have to be typed. For each line item, there would be a budgeted rate and budgeted amount of resource. If ABC Hospital, Med/Surg Unit 4B, also wanted variance information for LPN labor and for nurse's aides, it also

---

* A computer disk with the example template is available from the author at the Robert F. Wagner Graduate School of Public Service, New York University, 738 Tisch Hall, 40 West 4th Street, New York, NY 10003.

Flexible Budget Variance Report*: June 1991 and Year-to-Date Variances

This is Month Number _____ 6

| | This Month | | | | | | Year-to-Date | | | | | |
	Budget	Actual	Variances Price	Quantity	Volume	Total	Budget	Actual	Variances Price	Quantity	Volume	Total
RN salaries	$90,000	$98,847	$247	$5,600	$5,000	$8,847	$652,000	$684,333	$11,333	$6,000	$15,000	$32,333

*ABC Hospital Med/Surg Unit 4 B Variance Report.

❖ TABLE 2
Remaining Portion of Computer Template

	Jan	Feb	Mar	Apr	May	Jun	Jul	Aug	Sep	Oct	Nov	Dec
Workload measure												
Budgeted pt. days	1,200	1,230	1,140	1,050	1,000	900	900	850	950	1,000	1,050	1,100
Actual pt. days	1,180	1,200	1,200	1,100	1,040	950	—	—	—			
RN salary information												
Budgeted rate	$20.00	$20.00	$20.00	$20.00	$20.00	$20.00	$21.00	$21.00	$21.00	$21.00	$21.00	$21.00
Budgeted RN hours	6,000	6,150	5,700	5,250	5,000	4,500	4,500	4,250	4,750	5,000	5,250	5,500
Actual rate	$20.00	$20.50	$21.00	$20.30	$20.10	$20.05	—	—	—			
Actual RN hours	5,930	5,990	5,890	5,550	5,360	4,930	—	—	—			
RN salary variances												
This month												
Price	$0	$2,995	$5,890	$1,665	$536	$247	ERR	ERR	ERR	ERR	ERR	ERR
Quantity	$600	($200)	($2,200)	$1,000	$3,200	$3,600	ERR	ERR	ERR	ERR	ERR	ERR
Volume	($2,000)	($3,000)	$6,000	$5,000	$4,000	$5,000	ERR	ERR	ERR	ERR	ERR	ERR
Total	($1,400)	($205)	$9,690	$7,665	$7,736	$8,847	ERR	ERR	ERR	ERR	ERR	ERR
Year-to-date												
Price	$0	$2,995	$8,885	$10,550	$11,086	$11,333	ERR	ERR	ERR	ERR	ERR	ERR
Quantity	$600	$400	($1,800)	($800)	$2,400	$6,000	ERR	ERR	ERR	ERR	ERR	ERR
Volume	($2,000)	($5,000)	$1,000	$6,000	$10,000	$15,000	ERR	ERR	ERR	ERR	ERR	ERR
Total	($1,400)	($1,605)	$8,085	$15,750	$23,486	$32,333	ERR	ERR	ERR	ERR	ERR	ERR
Budget this month	$120,000	$123,000	$114,000	$105,000	$100,000	$90,000	$94,500	$89,250	$99,750	$105,000	$110,250	$115,500
Actual this month	118,600	122,795	123,690	112,665	107,736	$98,847	ERR	ERR	ERR	ERR	ERR	ERR
Budget year-to-date	120,000	243,000	357,000	462,000	562,000	652,000	746,500	835,750	935,500	1,040,500	1,150,750	1,266,250
Actual year-to-date	118,600	241,395	365,085	477,750	585,486	684,333	ERR	ERR	ERR	ERR	ERR	ERR

would be necessary to type in the budgeted average hourly rate for each of these types of employees, and the budgeted number of paid hours. It would not be necessary to type in the budgeted patient days, since the workload measure will remain constant for all line items for a given unit. It should not take a secretary much more than several days to enter the initial budget data for all 30 units at ABC hospital, for each line item for which flexible budget variance information is desired, for all 12 months.

Each month, the variances can be calculated by having the secretary enter the actual information for that month. For example, assume that the hospital's fiscal year begins in January. In July, the secretary is asked to prepare a June variance report. The secretary would start by entering 6 as the month number at the top of the template (Table 1). This monthly numerical indication is needed so that the computer program knows which set of data to show as being the variances for the current month and year-to-date. The variance numbers in Table 1 come from the June column in Table 2. However, it is not necessary to type those numbers. They are automatically transferred from the June column in Table 2 to Table 1, once the computer knows that it is Month 6.

The next step for the secretary each month is to enter the actual data for the month into the computer template. In this example, in the June column of Table 2, the secretary would type the actual values for patient days, rate, and hours: 950, $20.05, and 4,930, respectively. Once those three pieces of information are entered, the computer calculates the four variances for the month and the four variances for the year to date and transfers that information to the Table 1 portion of the template automatically. If the table also contained lines for variances for LPNs and nurse's aides, then the secretary also would have to enter actual average rates and hours for those types of employees. The Table 1 portion can then be printed out, providing a monthly flexible budget variance report. (The actual formulas used for the calculations are discussed in Part I.)

This monthly process of data entry and report production should take less than 2 days each month for one secretary for all 30 units. However, it is important to establish a system that generates the raw data (actual number of patients for each unit, etc.) each month for the secretary to input.

Different nursing units will use slightly different templates. Some units may use orderlies, while others may not. Some units may use the number of patient days as a measure of workload, while others may use emergency room treatments or hours of operations. Although the templates may vary somewhat from unit to unit, the process of entering information at the start of the year as well as each month will be basically the same for all units. If desired, a master template can be prepared, which takes the data from each of the unit templates and prepares a summary report for the nursing department as a whole.

Graphics

Once variance information has been generated and is available, it must be analyzed and investigated by nurse managers. The knowledge, judgment, and experience of the nurse manager is critical to understanding what is causing the variances. The use of flexible budget variance analysis is meant to be a time-saving aid to the nurse manager. Rather than just being faced with the total variance for any line item, the manager knows how much of the variance is due to more patients, how much to higher prices paid for a resource such as nursing labor, and how much to the amount of nursing labor per patient. This can simplify the variance investigation process substantially. Using graphics to display the variances is another step in providing the nurse manager with tools to improve variance analysis capability.

The advantage of graphs is that in many cases a visual display of relationships either highlights certain items that would otherwise go unnoted, or else makes it easier to spot certain relationships and key focal points. The discussion that follows highlights only a few of the possibilities. It should be noted that, once the spreadsheet model is constructed, LOTUS 1-2-3 or similar software can generate graphs based on a few additional instructions to the computer, with no additional input of data. All the graphs discussed below were generated from the data in Table 2. A standard set of graphs can be developed and built into the template. The same graphs can then be produced each month with automatically updated information.

One type of graph that is frequently used is a bar graph. Figure 1 is an example of a bar graph showing the price, quantity, volume, and total variances for RN salaries for the month of June 1991. This graph gives a very quick and vivid picture of the extent to which each type of variance is having

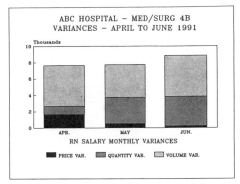

Figure 1. Bar graph of price, quantity, and volume variances for June.

Figure 3. Stacked bar graph for April through June variances.

an impact on the total variance for this line item for this month. For example, Figure 1 emphasizes the importance of investigating the quantity and volume variances. Although the volume variance is not usually under the control of the nurse manager, if it becomes significant in amount she must try to understand it, because if it persists it will have considerable significance for future staffing decisions. Figure 2 provides somewhat more information at a glance by showing not only the price, quantity, volume, and total variance for June, but the variances for the 6-month year-to-date period as well.

An alternative to a simple bar graph is a stacked bar graph. In Figure 3, one can see the

Figure 2. Bar graph with June and year-to-date variances.

price, quantity, and volume variances all in one bar for each month. In this graph, the user quickly notes that the total variance has been rising despite the fall in price variance. The main change took place in the middle segment. The quantity variance increased substantially during the 3 months. Despite some advantages, stacked bar graphs can become quite confusing if any of the variances are negative numbers. The combination of a positive and negative variance in one bar makes interpretation of the graph quite difficult. Since variances can be either favorable or unfavorable, stacked bar graphs should be used for variances only with a great deal of caution.

Another way to look at information is from the perspective of the relative size of each variance compared with all variances—in proportions rather than specific dollar amounts. A pie graph (Figs. 4–5) provides a very easy and quick assessment of which variances are large in size relative to the other variances. In some instances, displaying this information in the "exploded pie" format of Figure 5 may be preferred, although the information content is the same in both graphs. In Figure 5, the quantity variance is highlighted by the explosion of that section away from the remainder of the pie. This helps to emphasize the size of the quantity variance, which is often viewed as being the one variance most directly under the manager's control. Figures 4 and 5 show the volume and quantity variances in June to be quite significant, and substantially less effort could be spent investigating the price variance. Pie graphs are somewhat limited as the amount of data to be pre-

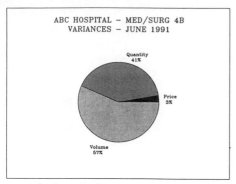

Figure 4. Pie graph of June price, quantity, and volume variances.

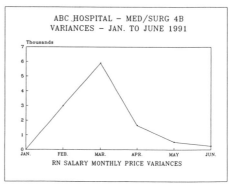

Figure 6. Line graph for year-to-date price variances.

sented increase. It would not be possible to show both the monthly values and the year-to-date values on one pie graph.

For information that reflects what is happening during a period of time, a line graph often is a helpful tool for evaluating possible problematic trends. However, even a potentially good format, such as a line graph, will not make our information useful unless we carefully decide on the appropriate information. For example, Figure 6 presents a line graph for year-to-date information on the price variance through June. Our first reaction to this graph may one of concern over the large and apparently growing variance. The year-to-date variance is substantial by the end of June. The monthly price variance information of Figure 7, however, should produce a different reaction. Although the price variance was a problem in the early months of the year, it does seem to have been brought substantially under control. The graph quickly informs the user that the price variance has been decreasing for a number of months and has now reached a quite modest level. Although this data could be obtained from the numbers in Table 2, in many cases it is hard to ferret information out of a table full of numbers; a selected graph (Fig. 7) quickly conveys what has been happening. Figure 8 shows monthly quantity variances. In contrast to the price variance, we quickly observe a problem. The quantity variance is modestly unfavorable in the first month (January) and then favorable for two months (February and March). In the last several months, however, there appears to be a serious unfavorable trend. This would warrant immediate attention.

When desired, more than one set of informa-

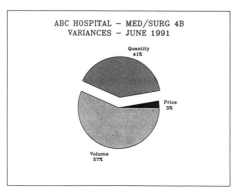

Figure 5. Pie graph with exploded section.

Figure 7. Line graph for monthly price variances.

tion can be shown on a time graph simultaneously. For example, Figure 9 shows monthly price, quantity, and volume variances. However, adding more items to a line graph may not always be desirable. In Figure 9, the price and volume lines intersect in March. Look at those two lines carefully. It is quite easy for the viewer's eye mistakenly to switch from one line to another at the intersection point. If that occurs, the use of the graph will be damaging because it will be conveying misinformation. In a case such as this, presenting the same information in three separate line graphs, or in a bar graph format, may be more informative.

Essentially, graphs do not present information that we don't already have in the form of numbers. After all, these graphs were derived directly from the information in Table 2. They can be very helpful, however, in spotting areas that need prompt attention and trends that may be early warning signals of oncoming problems.

Conclusion

Variance analysis is an area of growing attention as control of costs becomes more and more vital to the financial well-being of healthcare organizations. Adequate data for variance analysis often are not being generated by the organization's financial and information systems departments. Recent advances in terms of availability of reasonably priced PCs, however, has placed the ability to generate useful variance information within the reach of most nurse managers.

Calculations that would be an imposing task, if performed manually each month for each line

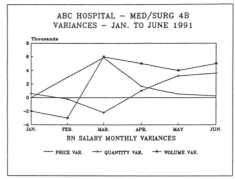

Figure 9. Line graph for monthly price, quantity, and volume variances.

item for each unit or department, can be processed by a spreadsheet program in rapid fashion. Some data will still have to be collected, but once the system is in place, the monthly effort involved in collecting actual information should be quite small for each unit. The data entry, computation, and generation of reports can be done by secretarial or other support staff and should not take an unreasonable amount of time.

In addition to yielding information on price, quantity, volume, and possibly acuity variances, as opposed to simply a total for each line item, it is also possible to use the computer to make the information much more usable through the generation of graphs. A variety of types of graphs, if thoughtfully considered, can generate supplements to variance reports, which should reduce the time needed to grasp the impact of the information and be an aid in both variance investigation and interpretation.

Suggested Readings

Austin C. Information systems for health services administration. Ann Arbor, MI: Health Administration Press, 1988.

Finkler SA. Microcomputers in nursing administration: a software introduction and overview. J Nurs Adm 1985;15(4): 18–23.

Hannah KJ, Ball MJ. Nursing and computers: past, present, and future. J Clin Comput 1984;12(6):179–84.

Spitzer R, Poate W. Effective budgeting variance reporting. In: Spitzer R, ed. Nursing productivity: the hospital's key to survival and profit. Chicago: 5-N Publications, 1986:21–25.

Tortora ML. Integrating computers into the nursing environment. Nurs Forum 1989;24(2):8–12.

Figure 8. Line graph for monthly quantity variances.

17

Forecasting and Other Methods for Decision Making

CHAPTER GOALS

The goals of this chapter are to:

♦ Describe quantitative methods useful for nurse managers in decision making

♦ Discuss probability theory

♦ Explain forecasting techniques used to predict resource use, patient volume, and income

♦ Discuss the reasons for forecasting

♦ Discuss the use of microcomputers for forecasting

♦ Explain the use of qualitative approaches to forecasting

♦ Explain the use of other quantitative methods such as linear programming and expected value for decision making

♦ Discuss quantitative methods of inventory control

♦ Describe the use of techniques for tracking projects

INTRODUCTION

Uncertainty exists when there is doubt about future events. The delivery of health care is uncertain. We do not know for certain who will need nursing care tomorrow. Yet the nurse manager must make decisions each day about the allocation of resources. Many of the resource allocation decisions are about what to do today. Others are decisions about expending resources in the near or distant future.

An example of a decision that must be made today occurs when two RNs call in sick. Should the manager replace one or both staff? Should the manager use agency nurses or try to find in-house overtime staff? The manager makes these decisions based on organizational policies, experience, and knowledge about what is currently happening on the unit. The decision making requires the exercise of managerial judgment. Many of these decisions must be made with less information than the nurse manager would like. Everything seems under control on the unit. There are four empty beds and no one waiting in the ER for admission. However, what if the unit gets three new admissions? Is that likely?

Nurse managers must also make decisions about resource allocations for the next year. What should the staffing pattern be? What will occupancy be? Which units will need new infusion pumps? These long-range decisions are often made with even less information than is available for the daily decisions. Some information is available, however. Other chapters in this book have suggested what information is needed to make financial decisions.

It should be remembered that the nurse manager along with other key managers decides the organizational and programmatic goals. These goals then form the basis for the decision-making process. The methods outlined in this chapter assume that the manager has decided what key decisions need to be made. For example, many of the methods described below can be used to determine if a decision will likely lead to increased profits. If the manager does not have increased profits as a goal, knowing how to maximize profits will not be very useful. As in many managerial issues, the first question is, "What is the question?" It is up to the manager to decide what question to ask. The focus of this chapter is the use of forecasting and other techniques to assist nurse managers in making judgments about the questions they have posed.

PROBABILITY THEORY: FOUNDATION FOR FORECASTING AND DECISION MAKING

Probability is the likelihood of an event's occurring. Managers of health organizations depend on knowing the probability of events' occurring to plan for care. We know with complete certainty where the hospital ER is today. We are very certain it will still be there tomorrow. We know with less certainty that it will be there three years from now. We know with a great deal of certainty that at least one patient will come to the ER for care in the next twenty-four hours, but what is the likelihood that someone will come into the ER in the next hour? What is the likelihood of 100 people coming into the emergency room in the next hour? The answer to these questions is unknown, yet the probability of each possible answer to these questions can be based on information that is known.

Suppose we expect to have 100 maternity patients who will deliver babies. We know from our past records that it is highly likely that forty patients will have cesarean sections and sixty patients will have normal vaginal deliveries. The type of delivery affects the unit's staffing needs. If a patient arrives at the unit, before we have any other information we know that the chance of a C-section is 40 out of 100. We could also say that if 1,000 patients arrive this year, the percentage of C-sections would be about 40 and the percentage of vaginal deliveries would be about 60.

Mathematically, if an event can happen in X ways and not happen in Y

ways, the probability of its happening is $X/(X+Y)$. The possibility of its not happening is $Y/(X+Y)$. To determine probabilities it is necessary to specify events. Each patient either has a C-section or does not. These events are mutually exclusive and are the two possible events upon the arrival of a patient who will deliver a baby. If events are mutually exclusive, the sum of the probability of each event's occurring must equal 100%.

Two general rules apply to probability. One relates to the likely occurrence of one or another mutually exclusive event. The second is the likelihood of each of two mutually exclusive events' occurring simultaneously or in succession. For example, what is the likelihood of rolling a 1 on a die on the first try or a 2 on the die on the second try? We know that the likelihood of rolling a 1 is 1/6. We also know that the likelihood of rolling a 2 is also 1/6. The likelihood of either of these events' occurring is 1/6 + 1/6 or 1/3.

The likelihood of rolling a 1 is 1/6, of rolling a 2 is 1/6, of rolling a 3 is 1/6, of rolling a 4 is 1/6, of rolling a 5 is 1/6, and of rolling a 6 is 1/6. The sum of 1/6 + 1/6 + 1/6 + 1/6 + 1/6 + 1/6 is 1. We know that if we roll a die, a 1, 2, 3, 4, 5, or 6 will result. Therefore the likelihood of one of these numbers' being rolled is the sum of each probability or 1. The *additive probability rule* states that the likelihood of either one event or another event's occurring is the sum of the likelihood of each event's occurring.

The likelihood of two specific events' *both* occurring is much less. The likelihood of rolling a 1 on the first try and a 2 on the second try is 1/6 × 1/6 or 1/36. The second rule of probability is the *multiplication rule;* the likelihood of two or more events is the product of each event.

Nurse managers implicitly use probability theory on a frequent basis. The nurse manager in the ER knows that there is a 90% probability that two people are in the ER waiting to be admitted. The nurse manager knows there is 100% probability that it will take the lab more than ten minutes to send someone up to draw blood. The nurse manager knows that one in four or 25% of the nurses who are asked to work an extra shift will say yes. These probability estimates, sometimes called "guesstimates," are based on previous experience of the nurse manager and the manager's colleagues.

The probability of events' occurring in the future can be based on historical data. The following example shows how to estimate the probability of staff's calling in sick on a weekend day shift based on historical data. The nurse manager knows that for a three-month period there were thirteen weekends each with two days or a total of twenty-six day shifts (13 × 2 = 26). There were five nurses scheduled for each of these shifts. Therefore there were a possible 130 nurse shifts scheduled (26 × 5 = 130). During this time period ten nurses called in sick. There were sick calls for ten of the possible 130 shifts or 8% of the time. Therefore the likelihood of a sick call on this unit on a weekend is about 8%, calculated as follows:

$$\text{Day shifts scheduled} = 13 \text{ weeks} \times 2 \text{ days} = 26$$
$$\text{Nurses scheduled per shift} = 5$$
$$\text{Total nurse shifts possible} = 26 \times 5 = 130$$
$$\text{Actual number of sick calls for day shift} = 10$$

$$\text{Probability} = \text{Actual number of sick calls} \div \text{Total nurse shifts}$$
$$P = 10 \div 130 = 8\%$$

In future planning for staff the manager can assume that about 8% of weekend day shifts will require coverage for sick leave. This may not turn out to be exactly correct, but it provides the manager with a reasonable estimate.

In some cases the nurse manager does not have historical data on which to base probabilities and must estimate. For example, suppose the hospital now has twelve-hour shifts. Historical data for sick time are based on eight-hour shifts. The nurse manager believes that some nurses take a sick day because they are really tired and just need a day off. The manager thinks that nurses who have four days off per week will take fewer sick days than those who have two days off and therefore estimates the sick-time probability at less than 8% — perhaps 5% or 6%. Such an estimate is referred to as *subjective probability*. It relies not only on the scientific application of the laws of chance but also on the judgment of the manager. The need for nursing units to be managed by experienced and skilled nurses exists partly because of the frequency and importance of decisions based on the managers' subjective probability estimates.

The concepts of probability are used in the following sections that describe forecasting and other quantitative approaches to decision making.

QUANTITATIVE METHODS FOR FORECASTING

The preparation of budgets and other financial decision making require a number of preliminary steps, including forecasting. A budget cannot be prepared without knowing the types of patients that the organization will likely be treating. A staffing plan to implement a new liver transplant unit cannot be developed without an estimate of the number of patients the unit will serve. Nor can financial decisions be made without being aware of who the competition is and the actions competitors are likely to take. Similarly, a budget cannot be prepared without knowing information such as *how many* patients are likely to be treated or *how sick* they are likely to be. That is where forecasting comes in.

Forecasting techniques allow for prediction of how many patients or patient days the organization or a particular unit or department will treat. Forecasting allows prediction of how sick the unit's patients will be. If a nurse manager were to attempt to prepare an operating budget without some prediction of these elements, there would be no way of determining how much staff is needed. Forecasting can help to estimate how many chest tubes the ICU will need or how many heparin locks a med/surg unit will consume. This will enable the nurse manager to plan the supplies portion of the unit's budget.

Forecasting is a tool that helps in the preparation not only of the operating budget but also of other budgets. If trends in the demographics of the community can be forecast, it is possible to prepare better long-range and program budgets. If it is forecast that a growing portion of the patient population will be Medicare patients, it can be determined what impact that will have on how quickly the organization gets paid. That will help in preparation of the cash budget.

The range of items that can be forecast is fairly unlimited. It is possible to predict patients, patient days, various supply items, the percentage of total operations performed by a specific doctor, and so on. Generally, forecasting focuses on items that the manager must respond to rather than items that can be controlled. For example, a nursing unit may forecast how sick the patients will be. It cannot control severity of illness, but its budget must be a plan that responds to how sick the patient population is expected to be.

Forecasting should be undertaken as an early step in the budget preparation and financial decision-making process. Virtually all managers forecast in some manner. Unsophisticated managers may forecast by simply using their best judgment or by assuming that the previous year's results will occur again the next year. It has been found that more formalized analysis of historical data can yield more accurate predictions than such less sophisticated approaches. These predictions in turn form a basis for many decisions in the planning process.

A formalized forecasting process can be divided into several steps. The first step is collection of historical data. The next step is graphing the data. The third step is analysis of the data to reveal trends or seasonal patterns. The fourth and final step is developing and using formulas to project the item being forecast into the future.

Before these steps are considered one point must be stressed. When a forecast is made, it is just an estimate of the future based on probabilities. Sophisticated approaches to forecasting allow the projection to be an educated estimate, but it is still an estimate. Your intuitive hunch or gut feeling should *not* be ignored. The most sophisticated methods lack the feel for the organization that a manager develops over time. Never accept forecasts on the blind faith that if it is mathematical or computerized, it must be superior.

Quantitative forecasts are merely aids or supplements that managers should take into consideration along with a number of other factors, many of which often cannot be quantified and entered into formalized predictive models. The best forecasts result from neither naive guessing nor advanced mathematics, but from an integration of quantitative methods with the experience and judgment of managers.

Data Collection

The first step in formalized forecasting is the collection of historical data. Consider several examples. If a nurse manager wishes to make the most basic of projections, workload, she will first have to decide upon a workload measure, such as patients or patient days. Then it is necessary to determine what the workload was in the past so that it can be projected into the future. This is referred to as a *time-series* approach to forecasting. Historical changes over time are used to help anticipate the likely result in a coming time period.

The methodology that will be discussed in this section is broadly applicable. If one wanted to predict diaper usage in the maternity unit, one could use historical data based on the number of diapers used. Once the number of diapers needed is predicted, it would probably be necessary to focus on the expected cost per box of diapers. If the purchasing department has a good degree of certainty about the price of diapers for next year (such as a purchase contract specifying price), this would be a pretty accurate approach. On the other hand, if it was desired to predict the total cost for diapers directly rather than focusing first on the expected number of diapers, it would be possible to gather information on what total amount was spent on diapers in the past and use that for a direct cost estimate.

In other words, it is possible to first forecast diaper usage and then calculate the projected cost or to forecast diaper cost directly. The preferred choice would depend partly on whether information about the number of diapers to be used in the coming period is considered valuable. Similarly, both the number of patient days and the patient severity of illness can be predicted. Then those data can be used to project the number of nursing hours needed, or historical information about the number of nursing hours consumed can be used to directly forecast nursing hours.

Appropriate Data Time Periods

There is often a tendency to try to make do with annual data. In fact, many operating budgets are annual budgets, specifying the total amounts to be spent on each line item for the coming year. However, when a manager is preparing an operating budget, it makes a lot of sense to use monthly rather than annual predictions of costs.

The easiest way to make monthly predictions is to take annual budget information and divide it by twelve. In many industries it would be possible to use such a simple approach; production in one month may be much the same as in any other month. In the health care sector, such an expectation is not reasonable. If for no other reason, the weather alone is likely to cause busy and slow periods. Winters are often busier periods for health care organizations than summers. Health care organizations must be prepared to have more staff available in busier periods. It is desirable to plan more vacations in slow periods and fewer during peak periods. Thus it is important to be concerned with month-to-month variations within each year as well as with the predictions for the year as a whole.

Furthermore, the number of days in a month will affect monthly costs. Many health care organizations such as clinics, labs, or radiologists' offices might only be open weekdays. Some months have as many as twenty-three weekdays, while other months have as few as twenty weekdays. A three-day difference on a twenty-day base represents a 15% difference. Clearly a difference that large would have a significant impact on the resources required for the month. Similarly, for a hospital it is quite likely that the number of weekdays will have an influence, since on certain days of the week admissions and discharges tend to be higher.

Monthly budgets are also important because they can be compared to the actual results as they occur. If there is a difference (variance) between the plan and the actual results, the cause can be investigated and perhaps a problem can be corrected immediately. Such variance analysis is the topic of Chapter 13. Without monthly subdivisions of the budget, it might be necessary to wait until the end of the year to find out if things were going according to plan. By then, of course, it would be too late to do anything about it for this year.

Thus, it is very important for most health care institutions to have their costs broken down on a monthly basis and to do so in some manner that is more sophisticated than dividing the year's expected cost or volume by twelve. Therefore, the data collected should generally be historical *monthly* data. For each type of item to be forecast (patients, chest tubes, diapers, costs) twelve individual data points are needed per year, representing values for the item being forecast for each month.

How far back should the data go? One year seems convenient, and it provides twelve data points. However, one year's worth of data provides only one piece of information about January, not twelve. If this January was unusual (either very costly or unusually low in cost), that would not be readily apparent. It is likely that next year would be predicted to be like this year. Therefore, more than one year's data is needed.

The use of ten years of data is often suggested for forecasting, although that has weaknesses as well. It is possible that so much has changed over the last ten years that the data are no longer relevant. For that reason, it would seem that five years of data (or a total of sixty months) is a reasonable rule of thumb. If a nurse manager knows that things have not changed much on the unit in a long time, using more years of data will make the estimate a better predictor. If there have been drastic changes recently, then five years might be too long. Judgment is needed. One of the most important things a manager does is to exercise judgment. Throughout the budgeting process, as in other managerial functions, a manager can never escape from the fact that thoughtful judgment is vital to the process of effective management.

What Data Should Be Collected?

The fact that it is necessary to collect historical data on the item to be forecast has already been discussed. Too often managers stop at that point because those data are sufficient to make a forecast. However, those data points are not all the data that are really needed to make a *good* forecast.

Forecasting techniques mindlessly predict the future as an extension of the past, even though many things change over time. Whenever forecasting is done, the manager should question whether factors might have changed that will make the future different from the past. Are there in fact things that are changing? For instance, are demographics shifting? When it is predicted that next January will be like the previous five Januarys, is the fact that last July there was a large influx of refugees into the community being ignored? Is a sudden shift in population caused by the closing of the town's auto plant being ignored? The forecasting formulas to be developed will not take these recent factors into consideration. Forecasting formulas are based solely on historical information. The manager should collect additional data to use as a judgmental adjustment to forecast results.

For example, availability of personnel can have a dramatic impact. For years many health care organizations suffered from a shortage of available nurses. The result was high overtime payments to staff nurses and high agency charges for per diem nurses. If there has been a noticeable increase in the number of nurses available, then a manager should realize that the average hourly cost for nursing can now be brought down by the elimination of much overtime and agency cost. A quantitative model for forecasting will not take that into account. Information about nurse availability must be collected, and the manager should give specific consideration to that information.

Note that a unit manager does not have to be a one-person information service. The personnel department can be asked about the outlook for hiring additional staff nurses. Administrators can be asked whether changes in third-party coverage are likely to have any impact. It is unreasonable to expect a home health agency's director of nursing to budget correctly for the coming year if the number of Medicare-reimbursable visits has changed and she does not know about it. Most home health agency financial officers would quickly be aware of such a change. That information should promptly be communicated to the chief nursing officer. It is vital to open communication links with other managers throughout the organization to ensure receipt of necessary information that could help in the budget process.

Some changes will not be easy to get information about. For instance, there may be no central clearing person to provide an update on changing technology that will dramatically shift the demand for nursing personnel. Nevertheless, a unit manager must try to get that information and consider its likely impact on the unit. To some extent, nurse managers may have better information on changing technology than the organization's administrators. First of all, nurse managers have clinical knowledge superior to administration's. Second, nurse managers are likely to know what kinds of changes physicians in their clinical area are planning to implement.

It is also important for nurse managers to be aware of the organization's long-range plan, program budgets, and capital budgets. Many hospitals tend to guard budget data closely with an "eyes only" attitude. Only people with an immediate need are allowed to see any budget other than their own. It is important that administrators begin to understand that managers do need to see any budget that even indirectly may impact on their unit or department. For example, if a new service winds up consuming a significant amount of nursing time that had not been planned on, much of it will likely be at overtime rates or will result in overtime elsewhere in the hospital. Had the service been planned for, overtime premiums might have been avoided. If a manager is to be held responsible for that overtime, then the manager is entitled to have the information needed to anticipate demands on the unit and to plan for adequate staffing.

Graphing Historical Data

Having collected all the relevant data that might help predict the future, the next step is to lay out the historical data on a graph. In the forecasting approach to be discussed here, time is plotted on the horizontal axis. For instance, suppose that the unit manager wants to predict next year's total nursing hours starting with Janaury 1994. Assume that it is currently October 1993 and that historical data from the past five years are going to be used. Data for October through December of 1993 are not yet available. Therefore, the horizontal axis begins in October 1988 and goes through September 1993 (Fig. 17–1).

The vertical axis provides information on the item to be forecast. This is nursing hours in Figure 17–1. The forecasting methodologies to be discussed later in this chapter will allow a manager to predict work-load estimates for the future, such as the number of patients and the number of patient days, the actual amounts of resource consumption (e.g., the number of nursing hours or the number of rolls of bandage tape), or to predict costs. Depending on the procedures of your specific institution, some of these forecasts may be made by the accounting department rather than by nurse managers.

If costs or some other financial measure expressed in dollars is being predicted directly, the impact of inflation must be considered. If inflation is ignored as forecasting is done, the forecast becomes more complicated because it must predict not only a work-load measure, such as the number of diapers for the coming year, but also the rate of inflation for the coming year. The problem of inflation and adjustments that can be made to allow for it are discussed in Chapter 7.

If a prediction is being made for next year's nursing hours (Fig. 17–1), the

Figure 17–1. Basic graph for nursing hours forecast.

first point graphed would be the number of nursing hours worked in October 1988. The next point would be the number of nursing hours in November 1988, and so on. It is important to keep in mind that this forecasting approach is a time-series analysis—that is, the variable on the horizontal axis is always time. In time-series analysis, whether the manager is trying to predict workload, resources, or cost, the basic process is to look at how much of that item there was in the past and project that into the future. To make such predictions, the manager will need to be able to analyze the underlying cause of the variations in the data that have been graphed.

Analysis of Graphed Data

Before any predictions can be made, it is necessary to assess the basic characteristics of the data that have been graphed. For instance, do the data exhibit *seasonality?* Is there a particular *trend?* Do variations from month to month and year to year appear to be simply random fluctuations? There may be patterns related to the passage of time that can be uncovered.

A visual inspection can usually give a good picture of the type of pattern that exists. Here it is quite important to focus on a reasonably long period, at least several years, as opposed to several months. By just looking at the past few months, it is possible to get a very distorted impression of what is occurring. For instance, see Figure 17–2. (Note: These are not the same data as shown in Fig. 17–1.) It appears that the number of nursing hours has a definite downward trend, but this graph covers a period of only six months.

Figure 17–3 shows the pattern for the full year. Now the graph gives a totally different impression. The number of nursing hours has not been steadily de-creasing over time. For the first half of the year it was decreasing, and for the second half it was increasing. The pattern being observed is not likely to be indicative of a long-term decline. It is still not possible to tell, however, if some basic change has occurred that caused a downward trend to reverse or if the pattern is seasonal behavior. Next year will the number of nursing hours con-tinue to rise, as it appears to be doing near the end of the year, or will it turn downward, as it did at the beginning of the graphed year? To answer that question it is vital that data for at least several years be graphed.

Now look at Figure 17–4, which covers a period of five years. A pattern of falling and then rising hours occurs each year. This is clearly a seasonal pattern rather than a trend. Each year the same pattern repeats itself.

When data for a sufficient number of years are graphed, the pattern that becomes apparent will generally fall into one of four categories: random fluc-tuations, trend, seasonality, and seasonality and trend together. Each of these patterns will be discussed.

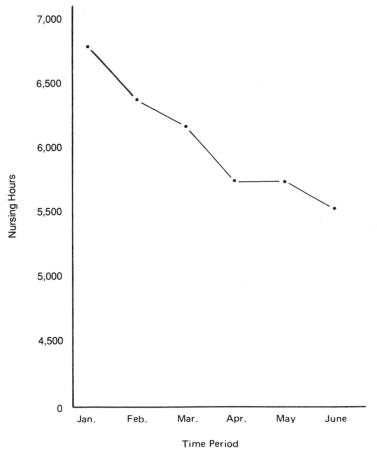

Figure 17–2. Six months' data for nursing hours forecast.

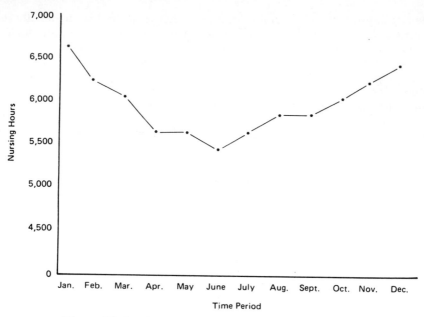

Figure 17–3. One year's data for nursing hours forecast.

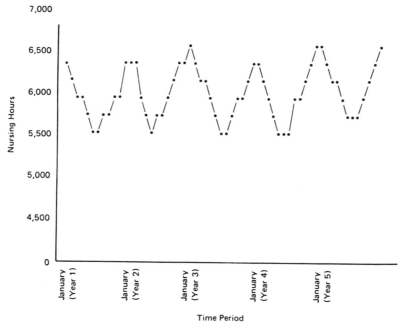

Figure 17–4. Five years' data for nursing hours forecast: seasonality.

Random Fluctuation

It would be quite surprising if a unit or department consumed exactly the same amount of any resource two months or two years in a row. One year the winter will be a little colder than another, and more people will get pneumonia. Another year prices will rise a little faster. One year some staff members will take more sick days than another. Yet these events are not likely to be trends—it does not get colder and colder year after year. Nor are they seasonal. They are just random, unpredictable events.

When a graph exhibiting random patterns only is viewed, it should look something like Figure 17–5. As can be seen, there is no clear upward or downward trend. You may also notice that each year there is no discernible seasonal pattern. May is not usually particularly busy nor particularly slow. May is a low month in the first year and a high month in the next year, relative to the values for the other months in those years.

Trend

In Figure 17–6, it should be noted that although the graph has its ups and downs, there is a clear upward trend. Because nursing hours rather than dollars are being considered here, this is not caused by inflation. Rather, it is probably caused either by an increased number of patient days or else by an increase in the amount of nursing time provided per patient day.

The underlying causes of observed patterns will not be determined in the

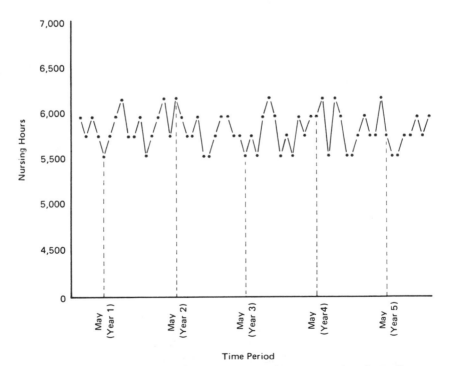

Figure 17–5.   Five years' data for nursing hours forecast: random fluctuations.

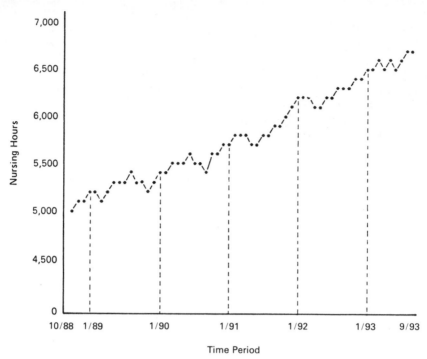

Figure 17–6. Five years' data for nursing hours forecast: trend.

forecasting process described here. The focus is strictly on projections of past items into the future. Whatever the cause, it appears that a definite trend exists. Unless there is information about expected patient days or a new policy regarding the relative ratio of nurses to patients, it would have to be assumed that this trend will continue. However, managers should try to understand the underlying causes of patterns such as trends. This will better enable them to forecast correctly if something does change the underlying cause of the pattern.

Note further in Figure 17–6 that although the overall trend is upward, there is no discernible seasonal pattern. For example, January does not appear to be consistently high or low each year relative to the other months of those years.

Seasonality

Seasonal patterns are sometimes quite visible to the eye, as was the case in Figure 17–4. In health care, one is especially likely to see seasonal patterns because of seasonal disease patterns and as a result of the weather. Winter months bring different ailments than summer months do. For hospitals and home health agencies, this will affect overall patient volume. On the other hand, nursing homes may be running at full occupancy all year round. Therefore the number of patient days at a nursing home might not show any seasonality, although the specific care needs of the patients in a nursing home are likely to vary with the different seasons of the year.

Seasonality may not always be easy to spot. Therefore, it might be a worthwhile exercise to examine certain months that are known as peak or slow periods. Suppose that Janaury is compared to June for each of the last five years and it is found that January almost always has higher levels of the item being forecast than June does. In that case seasonality does exist, even if it is not readily apparent when the graph is visually inspected.

Seasonality and Trend

It is quite common for health care organizations to experience at least some seasonality. At the same time, due to increasing patient volume or the effects of inflation, upward trends are quite common as well. Downward trends may also occur. It is not at all unusual therefore for the organization to experience both seasonal influences and trends at the same time. Figure 17–7 shows an example of a historical pattern exhibiting both seasonality and trend.

Often the trend is more obvious than the seasonality in patterns that contain both. In these cases, it becomes especially useful to make several comparisons to see if certain months are always higher or lower than other months. Valid forecasts require an awareness of seasonal patterns if they exist.

Forecasting Formulas

At this point historical data have been gathered and graphed, and there has been a visual inspection of the graphs for apparent trend or seasonal patterns. It is finally time to begin using the information to make forecasts for the coming year. The approach taken for forecasting depends to a great degree on whether seasonal patterns, trends, both, or neither are present.

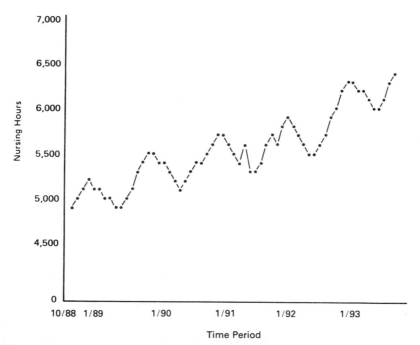

Figure 17–7. Five years' data for nursing hours forecast: seasonality with trend.

An approach to forecasting each of these patterns will be discussed below. First, however, it should be noted that the formulas below assume very limited use of computer technology in performing the forecasting function. The most sophisticated element of the formula approach is the use of a calculator or computer for simple linear regression. Much of the tedium and difficulty of the forecasting process is avoided if a sophisticated computer forecasting program is used. Although the formulas discussed below are valuable in situations in which a computer approach is unavailable, a computer solution is preferred. It takes less management time and can produce superior results. The costs of appropriate software are readily offset by the saved managerial time. A computer approach to forecasting is presented later in this chapter.

Random Fluctuations

The easiest forecasting occurs when there is no seasonal pattern or trend. For example, consider the budget for office supplies for the office of the chief nurse executive. The need for these supplies may not vary much over time or with the particular work-load level faced by the clinical nurses.

The most obvious approach in this case would be to simply add up the sixty monthly data points for the past five years and divide by sixty. That will give a monthly average. If every month is like every other month in terms of the item being forecast, this would be a reasonable approximation.

Caution must be exercised, however. Different months have different numbers of days. Even if there is no strong seasonal influence or trend, longer months may consume more of a resource. Months that have more weekdays may consume more of a resource. It may be necessary to adjust for factors such as days in a month or weekdays in a month. For example, if weekdays use much more of a resource than weekends, rather than dividing the total for the last sixty months by sixty, the total could be divided by the number of weekdays in the past sixty months. The result would be a predicted value per weekday. That value would be multiplied by the specific number of weekdays in each month in the coming year to get the appropriate forecast for each month.

Seasonality

If seasonality exists in the item being forecast, it means that some months are typically low and other months are typically high. If all sixty months for the last five years are averaged together, the seasonality becomes lost in the broad average. An approach is needed that is more sensitive to fluctuations within each year. The most obvious approach is to add together the values for a given month for several years and divide to get an average just for that month. For example, the last five February values can be totaled and then divided by five. That provides a February average for the last five years that can be used as a prediction of next February.

This approach is not always acceptable. Suppose that seasonal variations do not repeat in the exact same month each year. For instance, suppose that February is usually the coldest month, causing patient days to peak because of many flu cases. Sometimes, however, January or March will be colder. Because of this variation in seasonality from year to year, a better prediction may result from adding January plus February plus March for the last five years. Thus, February is being based on January, February, and March. This total should be divided by fifteen to get a prediction of February of next year. Then March is estimated by adding February plus March plus April for each of the last five years and dividing by fifteen.

The key to this *moving-average* approach is to add up not only the month in question for the last five years but also the month preceding and the month following the month being predicted. This formula will often give a good prediction. However, there are also problems with this approach. Peaks and valleys in activity will be understated. For instance, what if January were typically the busiest month of the year, with both December and February being less busy? Then, by averaging December and February with January, the slower December and February will cause the busier January to be understated in the forecast.

How can a nurse manager determine whether predictions will be improved by using calculations such as this one? Should the manager simply take an average of five Februarys or use January, February, and March information for five years to predict next February? One good way to make that determination is to try to use historical data (excluding data from the most recent past year) to predict the results of the past year. For instance, if 1993 has just ended, take data from 1988 through 1992 and use them to predict 1993. Since the actual results for 1993 are already known, the prediction can immediately be compared to the actual results. This is a good way to test any formula to see if it is a reasonable predictor.

Keep in mind two things, however. First, no forecast will predict the future perfectly. The future is uncertain, and all the specific events that will occur can never be fully anticipated. Therefore, the prediction should not be expected to match the actual results precisely. Second, the predictions or forecasts using formulas must be adjusted based on the manager's own knowledge about the future. The formulas just use information about the past. If managers have some information about the future that leads them to believe that the future will not follow the patterns of the past, that information must be used to adjust the predictions of the formulas. The role of an intelligent manager should never be relinquished to the mathematical precision of a formula.

When a formula is tested by seeing how well it can predict what actually happened last year, there should be a determination of whether the predictions based on the formula are closer to what actually happened than the predictions that would have been used in the absence of the formula. If so, then it is a useful tool. Otherwise, the formula should be either modified or discarded.

Trend

If a trend is observed, it is desirable to project that trend into the future. Trends are usually represented by a straight line. However, trends tend to have some random elements within them. If one were to draw a straight line, it would not generally go through each historical point. Some points would be above the line and some would be below the line. A manager could just eyeball the points on the graph and try to draw a line that is as close as possible to all the points and that extends into the future. However, such manual attempts are likely to be fairly inaccurate.

If the line is drawn too high or too low, the estimates for the future will also be too high or too low. Even worse, if the slope of the line is too high or too low, the error will be magnified, as seen in Figure 17–8. In this figure the

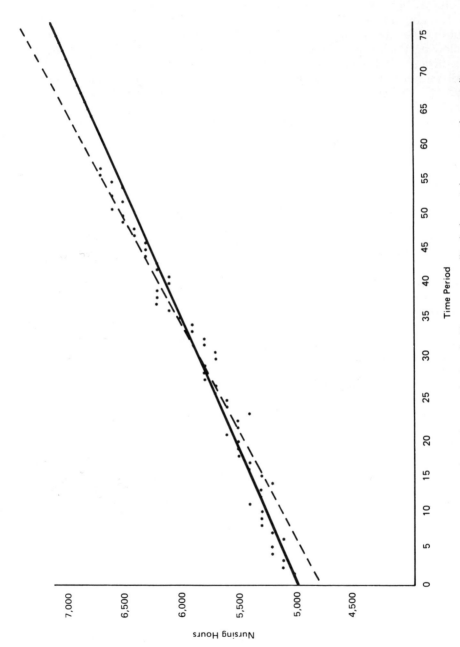

Figure 17–8. Nursing hours forecast for trend with no seasonality: judgmental vs. regression results.

solid line represents the best straight line that uses the known data to forecast the future. The dashed line represents a judgmental, eyeball estimate. Note that near the center of the graph, the two lines are relatively close. However, in the area of the forecast for the coming year, the two lines have diverged to the point that the number of nursing hours predicted differs a great deal depending on which line is used.

One solution to this problem is to use a statistical technique called *regression analysis*. The goal of regression analysis is to find the unique straight line that comes closest to all the historical data points. Regression analysis can be readily performed by a nurse manager using many types of hand-held calculators or on a computer using statistical software packages such as the Statistical Package for Social Sciences (SPSS), spreadsheet packages such as LOTUS 1-2-3, or forecasting packages such as SmartForecasts II.

Regression analysis is a technique that applies mathematical precision to a scatter diagram. The scatter diagram used in regression analysis is a graph that plots points of information. Each data point represents a dependent variable and one or more independent variables. The independent variable is sometimes referred to as the causal variable. It is responsible for causing variations in the dependent variable.

When making forecasts, time is considered an independent variable, and a second variable is considered a dependent variable. For example, the dependent variable could be the number of patients treated by the organization. As time passes, the organization may have more or fewer patients. The change in the number of patients over time may reflect a random pattern, seasonal effect, trend, or seasonality and trend, as discussed in this chapter. If a trend exists, regression analysis will generate a line that is a good predictor of the future.

Regression is a tool that can help managers to manage better. The major difficulty in using regression is simply a fear of the process (and this relates not only to nurse managers but to all managers). However, when using a computer program, regression analysis does not require the user to do extensive mathematical computation. The computer carries out all the calculations.[1]

Since regression analysis requires the manager to provide numerical values, months and years cannot be used by their names for the independent variable. An independent variable cannot be referred to as January 1988. Instead the month names can be replaced by assigned numerical values. The historical months used for the analysis can be identified as one through sixty instead of October 1988, November 1988, and so forth to September 1993. Table 17–1 presents the data. After feeding the information into a calculator or computer (e.g., in month 1, there were 5,000 nursing hours; in month 2, there were 5,100 nursing hours; and so on through month 60, with 6,700 nursing hours), the calculator or computer is instructed to "run" (compute) the regression. When the computation is complete, it is possible to determine how many nursing hours would be expected in months 64 through 75, which represent the twelve months of next year. Note that months 61 through 63 have been intentionally skipped over. There are neither historical data points nor forecast points plotted

---

[1]Although regression is easy to perform using a computer, the user should have some familiarity with regression to interpret the regression results and their significance. See the regression discussion in Chapter 7 and/or a statistics text.

❖ TABLE 17–1
Nursing Hours—Historical Data for Trend with No Seasonality

Data Point	Date		Nursing Hours
1	October	1988	5,000
2	November		5,100
3	December		5,100
4	January	1989	5,200
5	February		5,200
6	March		5,100
7	April		5,200
8	May		5,300
9	June		5,300
10	July		5,300
11	August		5,400
12	September		5,300
13	October		5,300
14	November		5,200
15	December		5,300
16	January	1990	5,400
17	February		5,400
18	March		5,500
19	April		5,500
20	May		5,500
21	June		5,600
22	July		5,500
23	August		5,500
24	September		5,400
25	October		5,600
26	November		5,600
27	December		5,700
28	January	1991	5,700
29	February		5,800
30	March		5,800

for those three months. That is because those months represent the remaining months of the current year for which data are not yet available. The goal is to develop predictions for the months in the coming year.

The results are shown in the scatter diagram in Figure 17–9. The regression results are plotted as a solid line for 1994 and are extended back from 1993 to 1988 with a dashed line. The specific predictions of nursing-hour requirements for 1994, by month, are as follows:

January	6,772	May	6,884	September	6,995
February	6,800	June	6,911	October	7,023
March	6,828	July	6,939	November	7,051
April	6,856	August	6,967	December	7,079

Note in Figure 17–9 that the projections for next year all fall on the trend line, even though in the past many points are not on the extended (dashed) trend

❖ **TABLE 17–1**
Nursing Hours—Historical Data for Trend with No Seasonality—*Continued*

Data Point	Date		Nursing Hours
31	April		5,800
32	May		5,700
33	June		5,700
34	July		5,800
35	August		5,800
36	September		5,900
37	October		5,900
38	November		6,000
39	December		6,100
40	January	1992	6,200
41	February		6,200
42	March		6,200
43	April		6,100
44	May		6,100
45	June		6,200
46	July		6,200
47	August		6,300
48	September		6,300
49	October		6,300
50	November		6,400
51	December		6,400
52	January	1993	6,500
53	February		6,500
54	March		6,600
55	April		6,500
56	May		6,600
57	June		6,500
58	July		6,600
59	August		6,700
60	September		6,700

line. Actual results are not expected to fall right on the line; however, in the absence of any other information, the points on the trend line are the best prediction that can be made for the actual uncertain outcome. To guess higher than the trend-line value would probably be too high. To guess lower than the trend-line value would probably be too low.

Seasonality and Trend

Seasonality together with trend poses a more complex problem; yet it is likely to be a common occurrence, so the reader should pay special attention to the approach discussed here. This example will use the data provided in Table 17–2. The first step is to use a regression to predict a trend line for the coming year. Once a set of results for the regression is plotted for each month in the coming year (January 1994 through December 1994) it should be noted that there is no seasonal appearance to the line predicting next year. It is simply an upward-trending line (see Fig. 17–10 for 1994).

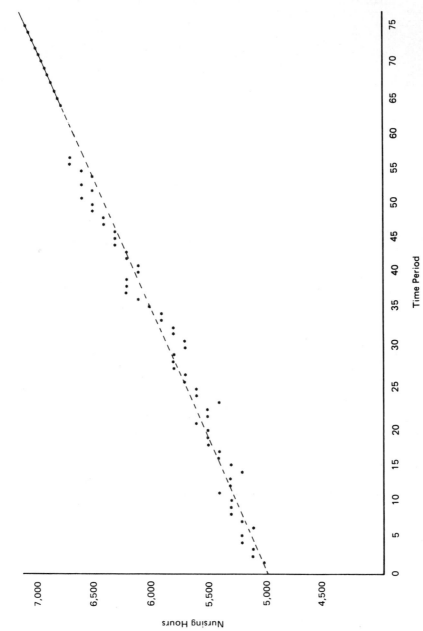

Figure 17-9. Nursing hours forecast for trend with no seasonality: regression results.

The next step is to extend the trend backwards into the five years for which there are historical data. This is fairly straightforward, since it simply requires extending backwards a straight line that has been already located for the coming year (see the dashed line on Fig. 17–11).

Once the line has been extended backwards, the manager must calculate how much above or below the line the actual value was each month for the last five years. Those amounts must then be converted into a percentage. For example, in January 1989 on Figure 17–11, there were 5,200 nursing hours, but the trend line was at a vertical height of 5,000. The actual value was 200 hours above the trend. Because it is a trend, however, it is necessary to convert this to a percentage. In this case, it is a positive 4%, because 5,200 is 4% above the trend-line point of 5,000.

Now simply revert to the seasonal approach. Add together the percentages that December, January, and February are over and under the trend line for the last five years and divide by fifteen. The result is a prediction of what percent above or below the trend line January will be next year. Find the point on the trend line next year for January and multiply it by the moving-average percent to find how much above or below the trend line the predicted point is. This process can be repeated for each month of the coming year. For example, Table 17–3 shows the actual number of nursing hours incurred and the extended trend-line information for December, January, and February for five years.

The trend-line prediction for January 1994 from Figure 17–11 is 6,204. This is before adjustment for seasonality. In the calculation shown in Table 17–3, it was determined that for January the moving-average percentage is a positive 3.2% of 6,204. By adding 3.2% of 6,204 to the trend-line value of 6,204, the resulting prediction adjusted for seasonality is 6,403. That point has been plotted for January 1994 on Figure 17–11. Similarly, to get the 1994 forecast for the entire year, this process should be repeated on a moving-average basis for each month in turn.

Using Computers for Forecasting

The previous section on forecasting formulas demonstrates how complicated forecasting can become when historical data are influenced by both trend and seasonality. However, health care organizations frequently do have at least seasonality; both trend and seasonality are not uncommon. In recent years, nurse managers' ability to deal with such patterns has improved dramatically as a result of personal computers and specially designed computer software. These computer programs make the work of forecasting easier and the results more accurate.

A number of forecasting programs are available. This section will discuss some of the capabilities of one such program, SmartForecasts II.[2] This program

[2]SmartForecasts II is a trademark of Smart Software, Inc., 4 Hill Road, Belmont, MA 02178; telephone (617) 489-2743. Version 2.15 for IBM PC/XT/AT, PS/2, and compatible personal computers was used for Exhibits 17–1 to 17–4, Figures 17–12 and 17–13, and Tables 17–4 and 17–5 in this chapter. This chapter does not attempt to demonstrate all the capabilities of this software. The software program is used simply as an example of the use of computer forecasting.

Permission has been obtained from the vendor for the use of these examples. The use of the example in this chapter does not represent a formal endorsement of the product.

❖ TABLE 17–2
Nursing Hours—Historical Data for Trend with Seasonality

Data Point	Date		Nursing Hours
1	October	1988	4,900
2	November		5,000
3	December		5,100
4	January	1989	5,200
5	February		5,100
6	March		5,100
7	April		5,000
8	May		5,000
9	June		4,900
10	July		4,900
11	August		5,000
12	September		5,100
13	October		5,300
14	November		5,400
15	December		5,500
16	January	1990	5,500
17	February		5,400
18	March		5,400
19	April		5,300
20	May		5,200
21	June		5,100
22	July		5,200
23	August		5,300
24	September		5,400
25	October		5,400
26	November		5,500
27	December		5,600
28	January	1991	5,700
29	February		5,700
30	March		5,600

is an example of personal computer forecasting software that is not limited to linear forecasting. Regression analysis produces a straight-line forecast. When there is seasonality, certain months are always above the regression line and others are always below it. Software such as SmartForecasts II can generate *curvilinear* (curved line) forecasts. That means that the forecast line generated will come closer to the historical points, and therefore its projections are likely to be closer to the results that will actually occur.

Additional advantages of this particular software package are that it does not require the user to have a strong statistical background, and it is particularly easy to use. Although it is always advisable to use tutorials and user manuals, there is sufficient information on the SmartForecasts screen to help users move through the various steps to get the type of analysis they desire. The basic screen display when one enters SmartForecasts II is shown in Exhibit 17–1.

The dots on the left-hand side of the display become replaced by the relevant historical dates for up to 150 periods. The top row becomes replaced with the

❖ **TABLE 17–2**
Nursing Hours—Historical Data for Trend with Seasonality—*Continued*

Data Point	Date		Nursing Hours
31	April		5,500
32	May		5,400
33	June		5,600
34	July		5,300
35	August		5,300
36	September		5,400
37	October		5,600
38	November		5,700
39	December		5,600
40	January	1992	5,800
41	February		5,900
42	March		5,800
43	April		5,700
44	May		5,600
45	June		5,500
46	July		5,500
47	August		5,600
48	September		5,700
49	October		5,900
50	November		6,000
51	December		6,200
52	January	1993	6,300
53	February		6,300
54	March		6,200
55	April		6,200
56	May		6,100
57	June		6,000
58	July		6,000
59	August		6,100
60	September		6,300

names of variables being examined. The column for V1 (i.e., variable one) could be used for a prediction of the number of patients, V2 for patient days, V3 for nursing hours, and so on, up to sixty different variables. Each column is used to record the historical information on the variables that are going to be forecast.

Notice that the display lets the user know how to get further information about any possible command by telling the user how to access the on-screen help function. The bottom two rows also tell the different commands that can be given at that point in the program, such as clearing the screen, for which one would type CLE, exploring the data (EXP), entering or replacing data in the table (REP), or forecasting (FOR). Working with a computer allows managers to use advanced mathematics to produce forecasts. But it should always be kept in mind that the computer knows only what it is told. To the extent that the manager is aware of information that has not been given the computer, it will be necessary to adjust the resulting forecast.

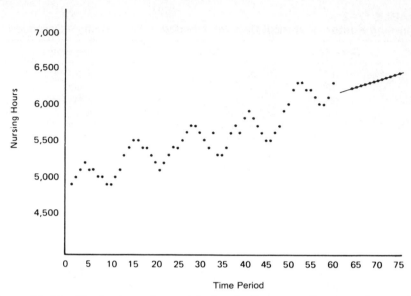

Figure 17–10. Nursing hours forecast for trend with seasonality: regression results.

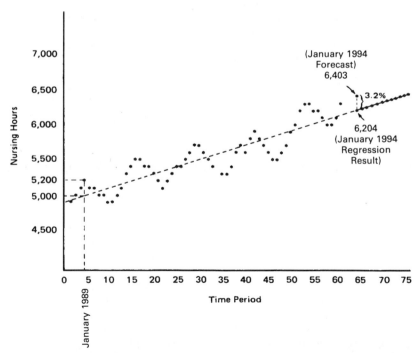

Figure 17–11. Nursing hours forecast for trend with seasonality: regression results extended back into historical data.

❖ **TABLE 17–3**
Calculation of Moving-Average Percent for January 1994

Month		Actual	Trend Line	Difference	Difference as a Percentage of Trend Line
December	1988	5,100	4,980	120	2.4%
January	1989	5,200	5,000	200	4.0
February	1989	5,100	5,020	80	1.6
December	1989	5,500	5,221	279	5.3
January	1990	5,500	5,241	259	4.9
February	1990	5,400	5,261	139	2.6
December	1990	5,600	5,461	139	2.5
January	1991	5,700	5,482	218	4.0
February	1991	5,700	5,502	198	3.6
December	1991	5,600	5,702	(102)*	(1.8)*
January	1992	5,800	5,723	77	1.3
February	1992	5,900	5,743	157	2.7
December	1992	6,200	5,943	257	4.3
January	1993	6,300	5,963	337	5.7
February	1993	6,300	5,983	317	5.3
Total					48.4%
Divided by 15 =					3.2%

*Negative amounts.

❖ **EXHIBIT 17–1**
SmartForecasts II Beginning Screen Display

```
SmartForecasts II      (C) 1986, 1987, 1988, 1989  Smart Software, Inc.

             ..............  ..............  ..............
                  V1              V2              V3
             ----------------------------------------------
.............. C1    |      *               *               *
.............. C2    |      *               *               *
.............. C3    |      *               *               *
.............. C4    |      *               *               *
.............. C5    |      *               *               *
.............. C6    |      *               *               *
.............. C7    |      *               *               *
.............. C8    |      *               *               *
.............. C9    |      *               *               *
.............. C10   |      *               *               *
.............. C11   |      *               *               *
.............. C12   |      *               *               *
             ----------------------------------------------

EDIT MODE :

For help, type  HELP EDIT  or  HELP  followed by one of these commands:

CLEar  DEFine  DELete  EXPlore  FORecast HELp   INSert   LABel  LISt  OOPs
PAGe   QUIt    REAd    REPlace  SAVe     SEE    SEQuence SPAce  TITle VARiables
```

Exhibit 17–2 shows the software display with historical information in place. The left-hand column shows that October 1988 is the starting point. Although the display only has room to show through September 1989, on the computer one could move the "window" of the display down farther to reveal historical information through September 1993.[3] Variable 1 represents the historical number of nursing hours each month. The data used in Exhibit 17–2 have been taken from Table 17–2.

As discussed earlier in the chapter, it is useful to graph historical data as part of the forecasting process. In SmartForecasts II the user would type EXP to enter the explore mode. A new display would then appear on the screen, presenting options for the user within the explore mode. Exhibit 17–3 presents the *menu* section from the bottom of the new display.

By typing TIM V1 on the computer keyboard one can get a time plot showing the historical points connected, with months on the horizontal axis going from October 1988 through September 1993 and nursing hours on the vertical axis going from 4,000 to 7,000. Examination of the time plot in Figure 17–12 quickly alerts the user to the seasonal nature of the data; a closer inspection reveals the upward trend.

Next the user can type FOR to move to the forecasting mode. The commands available for forecasting can be seen in Exhibit 17–4.

Quite a few different forecasting models are available. For example, REG is a command to do regression analysis. With SmartForecasts II it is possible to

---

[3]When using a computer one can only see a portion of a large data table on the screen at one time. It is as if a wall is in front of the table and the user looks through a window in the wall. By moving the window to different spots on the wall, different parts of the table can be viewed.

❖ **EXHIBIT 17–2**
SmartForecasts II Display with Data

```
        SmartForecasts II      (C) 1986, 1987, 1988, 1989  Smart Software, Inc.

                            NURSING.HOURS..  ..............  ..............
                                  V1              V2              V3
                            -------------------------------------------------
    OCT1988........ C1           4900.00            *               *
    NOV1988........ C2           5000.00            *               *
    DEC1988........ C3           5100.00            *               *
    JAN1989........ C4           5200.00            *               *
    FEB1989........ C5           5100.00            *               *
    MAR1989........ C6           5100.00            *               *
    APR1989........ C7           5000.00            *               *
    MAY1989........ C8           5000.00            *               *
    JUN1989........ C9           4900.00            *               *
    JUL1989........ C10          4900.00            *               *
    AUG1989........ C11          5000.00            *               *
    SEP1989........ C12          5100.00            *               *
                            -------------------------------------------------

    EDIT MODE :

    For help, type  HELP EDIT   or   HELP   followed by one of these commands:

    CLEar  DEFine  DELete  EXPlore  FORecast HELp  INSert    LABel  LISt  OOPs
    PAGe   QUIt    REAd    REPlace  SAVe     SEE   SEQuence  SPAce  TITle VARiables
```

❖ **EXHIBIT 17–3**
SmartForecasts II Explore Mode Screen Display

```
-------------------------------------------------------------------
EXPLORE MODE :

For help, type HELP EXPLORE or HELP followed by one of these commands:

CORrelate  DECompose  DEScribe   EDIt   FORecast   HELp
PAGe       QUIt       SCAtter    SPAce  TIMeplot   VARiables
```

forecast nursing hours using a regression analysis technique. However, if that is done, given the seasonality that has been observed in the time plot, the same problem will occur as existed in Figure 17–10, requiring the same manual adjustments shown in Figure 17–11 and Table 17–3.

The key advantage of this software is that it allows for use of a curved line for forecasting. This should remove the necessity to adjust the trend line for seasonality. However, which forecasting approach should be used? Available methods shown in Exhibit 17–4 include DOU for double exponential smoothing, LIN for linear moving average, SIM for simple moving average, SIN for single exponential smoothing, WIN or Winters' exponential smoothing, and so on.

Moving-average approaches were used in the earlier section on forecasting formulas in this chapter. However, will that approach give the best result if other advanced statistical techniques are available? The best approach until one is very familiar with forecasting is to use the AUT command. This stands for automatic forecasting and will let the computer choose the best approach. Under the automatic approach, the computer will calculate the forecast by using a number of different methods to see which predicts the best.

After the AUT command is entered, the program will ask how far ahead you wish to forecast. In this case, to get all of next year, it is necessary to predict fifteen months into the future. That will provide three months of fore-

Figure 17–12. SmartForecasts II timeplot graph of historical data.

❖ **EXHIBIT 17–4**
SmartForecasts II Forecast Mode Screen Display

```
-------------------------------------------------------------------------
FORECAST MODE :

For help, type HELP FORECAST or HELP followed by one of these commands:

AUTomatic  DOUble  EDIt     EXPlore  EYEball  HELp   LINear     MULtiseries
PAGe       QUIt    REGress  SIMple   SINgle   SPAce  VARiables  WINters
```

cast data to complete the current year, plus twelve months of data for next year. The computer will indicate whether sufficient historical information has been provided to project out as far as is desired. With sixty data points, one can reasonably predict as far as thirty months into the future. The computer will also inquire as to whether the data being used are monthly, quarterly, or annual. Once these questions are answered, the computer will generate a forecast. Figure 17–13 will appear on the computer screen.

What does this graph consist of? The historical data points are connected by a solid line. The forecast line is dotted. Compare this dotted line to the regression line shown in Figure 17–11. During the first five years in Figure 17–11 the actual points are usually substantially above or below the regression line. Therefore it is reasonable to assume that as the line is used to project next year, each month's actual result is likely to be substantially above or below the forecast trend line.

Although the statistical theory is complex, effectively, the closer the forecast line comes to the actual results in the past, the more likely the forecast line is to come close to the actual results in the future. When the computer performs forecasting automatically, it examines how close the forecast line is to the historical actual points for each of a series of different forecasting methods. The computer can be given a command to examine the relative accuracy of the different forecasting methods examined. Table 17–4 shows the results of the

Figure 17–13. SmartForecasts II forecast of nursing hours.

❖ **TABLE 17–4**
Tournament Rankings for AUTOMATIC Forecasts of V1 Nursing Hours

Rank	Method	% Worse than Winner
1	WINTERS' exponential smoothing with weights = 10%	(winner)
2	DOUBLE exponential smoothing with weight = 10%	49
3	LINEAR moving average of twelve periods	57
4	SINGLE exponential smoothing with weight = 50%	107
5	SIMPLE moving average of two periods	111

competition among forecasting methods for this example. The best technique is Winters' exponential smoothing method. Winters' is a curvilinear approach that works extremely well for seasonal data. The data points were 49% further away from the forecast line for the next best method.

Looking at Figure 17–13, it is evident that the dotted forecast line during the first five years followed extremely closely the actual results. In some cases the solid and dotted lines are so close that they cannot be distinguished from each other. Therefore, the dotted line projected through 1992 is likely to give a fairly accurate estimate.

In the graph shown in Figure 17–13 there are solid lines above and below (bracketing) the forecast line projected into the future. These lines represent a margin-of-error interval. Forecasts can never be expected to be exactly correct. It is possible, however, to use statistics to get some idea of how large the difference might be between the forecast and the actual result. In this case, based on the statistical analysis there is a 90% likelihood that the actual result will fall somewhere between these solid lines. But graphs, while visually very informative, are hard to read when it is time to write down the actual forecast. Another computer command provides a numerical table of the forecast results. See Table 17–5 for the forecast results.

In this table not only the forecast is seen but also the margin of error or confidence interval above and below the forecast. If desired, that interval could easily be changed so that there would be a 95% or 99% confidence that the actual result would fall within the range of values between the lower-limit and upper-limit estimates. If the percentage is raised to a higher confidence level, the interval around the forecast line becomes wider. For example, for January 1994, the prediction is 6,619.98 nursing hours and there is 90% confidence that the actual nursing hours would not be less than 6,420.80 or more than 6,819.17. If a manager wanted to be 99% confident that the actual results would not exceed the boundaries of the projection, the lower-limit value would become 6,307.67 and the upper limit would be 6,932.29.

In practice it is rarely necessary to be so precise. While 95% or 99% confidence may be important for academics' research studies, in practice managers tend to have a greater degree of latitude. In fact, the SmartForecasts software program is preset by the manufacturer to give a 90% confidence. While it is simple for the user to change that confidence level given the way the software is set up, one must question whether it is desirable. Essentially, a 90% confidence interval implies that nine times out of ten, the actual result will fall within the

❖ **TABLE 17–5**
**Forecasts of V1 NURSING HOURS Using Multiplicative WINTERS'
METHOD**

Time Period	Approximate 90% Forecast Interval		
	Lower Limit	FORECAST	Upper Limit
OCT 1993	6101.21	6265.37	6429.53
NOV 1993	6213.73	6391.15	6568.56
DEC 1993	6305.24	6494.07	6682.90
JAN 1994	6420.80	6619.98	6819.17
FEB 1994	6396.38	6605.52	6814.67
MAR 1994	6322.39	6544.84	6767.28
APR 1994	6225.13	6460.03	6694.93
MAY 1994	6126.02	6375.28	6624.54
JUN 1994	6075.40	6336.45	6597.50
JUL 1994	6020.32	6298.44	6576.56
AUG 1994	6110.48	6400.92	6691.37
SEP 1994	6249.74	6550.19	6850.64
OCT 1994	6365.76	6666.64	6967.51
NOV 1994	6501.27	6798.30	7095.33
DEC 1994	6612.58	6905.59	7198.60

bounds of the interval. That is an extremely good result for most managers' forecasts.

Compare the result from Winters' exponential smoothing method (Table 17–5, Fig. 17–13) with the earlier result obtained by the combined regression analysis–moving-average approach (see January 1994 in Fig. 17–11). As can be seen, the results differ. This is because the approach used earlier is less accurate than Winters' method. Earlier the January 1994 number of nursing hours was projected to be 6,403, while Winters' predicts it to be approximately 6,620. In fact the earlier estimate is below the lower-limit value of the 90% confidence interval. It is clear that using more sophisticated techniques can generate results that differ markedly from the manual approaches used before computer software was readily available. It is probable that the manual moving-average calculation would be more accurate than simply a judgmental guess. However, the computer-based Winters' solution is likely to be even more accurate.

It is also possible to refine Winters' method even further. The computer makes some general assumptions when it performs forecasts under the automatic approach. If Winters' method was immediately selected as the forecasting method instead of selecting automatic, some additional options would be provided to improve the forecast further. Specifically, the SmartForecasts II software can be informed of the relative importance of the most recent level, trend, and seasonal factors. If the user knows that the trend is changing due to shifts in the underlying demographics of the community population, it is possible to give more weight to the most recent trend, as compared to the trend in the earlier years.

Not only can information be supplied to enable the computer to be more accurate, such as the relative importance of the recent trend, but it is also possible to modify the results of the computer analysis. SmartForecasts II provides a feature called "eyeball" forecasting, which allows the user to take the results and modify the graph (and simultaneously the numbers in the forecast table) based on some judgment or knowledge the user has that is not reflected in the historical information.

Most managers would initially only use a forecasting program to forecast one item at a time. However, as one becomes more adept at using computer-based forecasting, the program would probably be used to generate forecasts on a number of different variables. The user will also want to be able to save the data file to avoid having to reenter data each time an analysis is to be performed. The SmartForecasts II program has its own data files, and the data can also be stored in a wide variety of formats for future use, including LOTUS 1-2-3 worksheet files, ASCII (generic) files, or DIF files. By the same token, data in another format such as LOTUS, ASCII, or DIF can be read into SmartForecasts.

SmartForecasts is one of a number of forecasting programs that can be used on a microcomputer. The most significant aspect of using sophisticated software programs is that they can generate a substantially improved result. The ability of the forecast line to curve in synchronization with the actual historical seasonal pattern decreases the required effort by the manager substantially, while enhancing the result.

QUALITATIVE METHODS FOR FORECASTING

The discussion of this chapter has assumed that reasonably reliable historical data are available. However, there will be many instances, especially in the case of new ventures, where a forecast will be needed for a budget even though there are no reliable historical data. Subjective estimates will be required. In such cases regression analysis or even computerized curvilinear forecasting will be inadequate to provide a solution. Two approaches commonly used to aid in making reasonable subjective forecasts are the Delphi and Nominal Group techniques.

In both approaches a team or panel must be selected who are likely to have reasoned insights with respect to the item being forecast. Although no one may have direct knowledge or experience, an attempt should be made to select a qualified group. Industrial experience has shown that by arriving at a consensus among a team of experts, subjective forecasts can be reasonably accurate.

Nominal Group Technique

The *Nominal Group Technique* is one in which the group of individuals is brought together in a structured meeting. Members write down their forecasts. Then all the written forecasts are presented to the group by a group leader without discussion. Once all the forecasts have been revealed, the reasoning behind each one is discussed. After the discussions, each member again makes a forecast in writing. Through a repetitive process, eventually a group decision is made.

Obviously there are weaknesses to the Nominal Group Technique. One problem concerns lack of information. If different forecasts are made based on different assumptions, it may be impossible to reach consensus. Another problem concerns politics and personalities. As members of the group defend their forecasts, extraneous issues having to do with whose idea it is may bias the group decision.

Delphi Technique

With the *Delphi technique* the group never meets. All forecasts are presented in writing to a group leader who provides summaries to all group members. For those forecasts which differ substantially from the majority—either high or low—a request is made for the reasoning behind the forecast. That information is also shared with group members. Then a new round of forecasts is made. This process is repeated several times, and then a decision is made based on the collective responses.

Delphi has several particular advantages. By eliminating a face-to-face meeting, confrontation is avoided. Decisions are based more on logic than on personality or position. The dissemination of the respondents' underlying reasoning allows erroneous facts or assumptions to be eliminated.

These two methods both make use of the fact that individual managers cannot be expected to think of everything. Different individuals, bringing different expertise and different points of view to bear on the same problem, can create an outcome superior to what any one of them could do individually. It is a cliche to say that two minds are better than one. Nevertheless, it is true that in many forecasting instances, the Delphi and Nominal Group approaches can substantially improve results.

OTHER DECISION-MAKING TOOLS

A number of other tools can aid managers in making decisions. In particular, the remainder of this chapter will focus on the following techniques:
- Expected value
- Linear programming
- Inventory control
- Gantt
- Critical Path Method and PERT

Expected Value

One approach to making decisions in the uncertain world of health care is to estimate the probability of events' occurring. An *expected value* is a weighted average using the probabilities as weights. For example, assume that the nurse manager of a home health agency is considering two possible approaches to providing nursing care to the elderly. On the basis of previous experience, reading the literature, and talking with managers of other similar agencies, the manager makes the predictions of cash receipts for care provided under each approach, as shown in Table 17–6. The expected value for each project in Table 17–6 is the weighted average of the possible cash flow outcomes. Each cash flow is weighted by its probability. Therefore the expected value of Project A, denoted as E(A), is as follows:

$$
\begin{aligned}
E(A) = \ & 0.3 \times 5{,}000 = \$1{,}500 \\
+\ & 0.5 \times 8{,}000 = 4{,}000 \\
+\ & \underline{0.2} \times 10{,}000 = \underline{2{,}000} \\
& \underline{\underline{1.0}} \phantom{\times 10{,}000 =} \underline{\underline{\$7{,}500}}
\end{aligned}
$$

The expected value of Project B is:

$$
\begin{aligned}
E(B) &= 0.1 \times \$3{,}000 = \$\ \ 300 \\
&+ 0.8 \times \ \ 6{,}000 = \ \ 4{,}800 \\
&+ \underline{0.1} \times 11{,}000 = \underline{\ \ 1{,}100} \\
&\ \ \underline{\underline{1.0}} \qquad\qquad = \underline{\underline{\$6{,}200}}
\end{aligned}
$$

Thus if the goal of the agency were to choose the option that maximized revenue, option A offers the greatest likelihood of achieving that goal. Such an option is probably desirable if it has no negative impact on quality.

When using the expected value approach it is essential to bear in mind that the expected value provides information on the *average* outcome. Sometimes the results will be better. Sometimes they will be worse. Over a large number of decisions they should average out to the expected value.

For the example above, Table 17–6 indicates that the possible outcomes for Project A are $5,000, $8,000, or $10,000. The expected value of the project is $7,500. However, $7,500 is not one of the possible outcomes. When we say that the expected value is $7,500, we recognize that we really expect the outcome to be $5,000, or $8,000, or $10,000. Sometimes the result might turn out to be the low $5,000, sometimes the high $10,000, and sometimes $8,000. Over time, however, we would expect the average cash flow from many projects with similar possible outcomes to be $7,500.

The nurse manager should also remember that expected value is based on the assumed probabilities. The manager should get the best estimate of the probabilities of the events' occurring, but this information is not perfect. Often it will be based on subjective estimates by managers. Even with the best information poor outcomes can occur. All decisions must be made on the basis of information available at the time the decision is made. As the probability data indicate, by choosing option A there is still a .30 chance that cash flow will be only $5,000. That may occur, but that does not mean that it was a poor decision. Even further, the actual result might be lower than $5,000. It is possible that an unanticipated event may cause actual results to be lower or higher than the manager even believed was probable. However, use of techniques such as expected value should still improve a manager's ability to assess information and make correct decisions.

Linear Programming

Linear programming (LP) is a technique to determine how best to allocate scarce resources to achieve a certain goal. It is based on solving simultaneous

❖ TABLE 17–6
Projected Cash Receipts for Two Different Projects

Project A		Project B	
Probability	Cash Flow	Probability	Cash Flow
.30	$ 5,000	.10	$ 3,000
.50	8,000	.80	6,000
.20	10,000	.10	11,000

equations. Given that two or more resources are available, the linear programming model helps determine the best combination to achieve a desired goal. The goal is usually to maximize an outcome such as revenues or sales, or minimize an outcome such as personnel costs. The equations developed for these models can be solved for a specific value either graphically or mathematically.

Efforts to achieve goals are often limited by a number of constraints. Most nurses do not want to work weekends or nights. Yet some nurses must work those shifts to maintain a desired level of quality. The nurse manager of the OR wants to increase the hours of OR time, yet most surgeons do not want to operate on Saturday. In complex organizations balancing the various constraints in achieving goals is complicated.

Linear programming can assist the nurse manager in making complex decisions that are constrained by a variety of factors. The first step is to develop the objective function. This equation states the relationship between the objective and other organizational factors. Developing the objective is not as simple as it would appear. Is the objective of the nursing unit to maximize revenue, maximize patients served, maximize quality, minimize errors? One advantage of LP is that any objective can be tempered by constraints established by the manager. Therefore an objective could be to maximize profits but not let quality fall below 3 on a nursing quality scale.

For example, suppose that the OR has been told that it should maximize its profits. The objective function would be

$$\text{Profits} = \text{Revenues} - \text{Expenses}$$

where revenues are the sum of revenues from all operations and expenses are the costs of all operations. For simplicity, assume that there are three types of operation: hernia, heart, and gallbladder surgery. The average price charged for a hernia operation is $1,000. The average price charged for heart surgery is $10,000. The average price for a gallbladder procedure is $5,000. At first glance, one would not think it would be complicated to determine which mix of operations would be most profitable. Clearly, devoting all OR space to heart surgery will yield the largest total revenue.

However, it will not necessarily yield the maximum profit. Suppose that heart surgery takes five hours, while gallbladder cases take only two hours on average and hernias only one hour. One could do five gallbladders (total revenue $25,000) in the time it would take to do two heart cases (total revenue $20,000). Therefore, in preparing an analysis one would want to consider the length of each procedure as well as the revenue, assuming that the total hours of procedures is limited.

Thus, we have an objective function: maximize profits. We also have a constraint: the total number of hours of operating room time available. We also have several existing conditions: total revenue is the sum of the revenue of each case; total cost is the sum of the cost of each case; hernia operations take one hour; gallbladder operations take two hours; heart operations take five hours.

It seems to be getting complicated, but we have only begun to establish all the conditions. Dr. Smith does hernias; Dr. Jones does gallbladders; Dr. Brown does heart procedures. Dr. Brown will only operate from 6 AM to 4 PM on Tuesdays through Fridays. Dr. Jones will operate anytime from 6 AM to 8 PM on Mondays through Saturdays. Dr. Smith will operate from 6 AM to 10 PM on any day except Tuesdays, when she has office hours until 1 PM in the afternoon. On Tuesdays she will operate from 2 PM to 10 PM. However, Dr. Smith will not perform surgery more than five days per week. Anytime that the surgeons cannot operate at this hospital, they will operate at the hospital across town. Therefore, if the patients cannot be done within the OR schedule, the revenue will be lost. The problem is growing in complexity.

The OR contains six suites. However, because of difficulties in recruiting nurses it has been determined that we will probably only staff one room for one shift on Sundays and two rooms for two shifts on Saturdays. On weekdays, three rooms will be staffed for one shift and three rooms for two shifts, if necessary. Nurses working on the second shift get a $3 per hour premium. The complexity grows.

Hernia operations, although low priced, are relatively simple and require only one nurse during the procedure. The nurse may be experienced ($27/ hour) or inexperienced ($20/hour). Gallbladders require one nurse for the procedure, and the nurse may be experienced or inexperienced. Heart surgery requires two nurses, and they must both be experienced.

Note that not only is the problem growing in complexity, but the number of constraints is growing as well. Even if we wanted to provide only heart surgery, we probably could not because we would be constrained by both Dr. Brown's operating schedule and by the need for experienced nurses only for that procedure. The equations would have to include the possible supply of shifts by inexperienced nurses and the supply of shifts by experienced nurses.

How can all the various factors be simultaneously taken into account to ensure that the OR time is preferentially given to the correct surgeon to maximize the OR's profit? Linear programming establishes an approach that solves multiple equations simultaneously to arrive at the optimal result. Human beings are not nearly so adept at taking all the factors into account and balancing them to determine the actual profit-maximizing solution. Note that in the real world the OR might have hundreds of different types of procedures and dozens of nurses and surgeons to balance.

Computer programs are now available that perform linear programming. Therefore it is not necessary to be able to work out the mathematics (which involve inversion of a linear algebra matrix). The nurse manager needs to be able to specify the relationships and constraints. Using computer software, the manager can spend less effort on trying to solve the problem and more effort on trying to correctly specify the relationships. Only the unit's or department's manager usually has adequate knowledge about such relationships to accurately specify them.

Will the organization schedule staff in the manner LP deems is most profitable? Will it keep the number of ORs open the optimal number of shifts as determined by the mathematical solution? Will it create the specific patient mix that generates the most profit? Very possibly not. Hospitals and other health care organizations tend to be very political places to work. As was discussed in Chapter 3, managers must learn to understand and take into account the various unofficial lines of authority. Sometimes it is better to give in a bit to a demanding surgeon than to fight that surgeon and possibly lose the surgeon and all the surgeon's patients.

The LP solution to each problem generates not only the optimal solution but also an ability to determine the cost of giving in to politics. The profits can be calculated at the optimal-mix solution. The profits can then be calculated at a solution that would appease either all the surgeons or perhaps just the most vocal surgeon. In either case, the manager can now determine how much profits would decline from the optimal because of the accommodations being made. A rational decision can then be made concerning whether it is worth the reduced profit in the short run to keep the surgeon(s) happy.

For small sacrifices in profit it probably pays to keep the surgeons happy. For large sacrifices in profit the organization may want to find some other way to appease the surgeon (a fancier office or title) rather than foregoing the extra profits. The key is that the manager who uses linear programming can easily determine how much profit it will cost the organization to keep the surgeon happy.

The LP model also has the capability to determine (automatically) the impact on the objective function of the relaxation in certain constraints. For example, how much extra profit would be earned if Dr. Smith were willing to start her surgery hours one hour earlier on Tuesdays? It may be that the optimal mix and scheduling of patients result in the nurses on Tuesdays being paid for a full shift, even though they have no surgical duties during one hour of the shift. If Dr. Smith performed one more hernia operation on each Tuesday, it would allow the unit to eliminate one Saturday shift a month. This would generate much more efficient use of staff, lowering the average cost per operation. Once the impact on profits of such a change is known, it can be determined how hard we should work to induce Dr. Smith to make that change.

The key to LP is that it helps managers to obtain information to make improved decisions. Using LP the nurse manager will be able to assimilate a huge amount of information and provide guidance to make decisions and achieve the organization's goal.

The following example is presented so the reader can understand how LP works. The goal of the nurse manager is to provide care at the lowest cost per patient. Most decisions have some inherent constraints. In this case the manager has determined that to maintain an adequate level of quality when the census is thirty, at least six staff must work on the day shift. The unit has a "partners" or "dyad" nursing model. Therefore, there must always be a number of RNs equal to or greater than the number of aides. RNs are paid $200 per shift and aides are paid $80. What is the best combination of RNs and aides that will achieve the desired goal?

OBJECTIVE FUNCTION: MINIMIZE AVERAGE COST PER PATIENT

Minimum cost = [$200 × (Number of RNs) + $80 × (Number of aides)]
Average patient census

Let R = number of RNs; A = number of aides

Minimum cost = $(200R + 80A)/30$

The manager identified two constraints that can be mathematically depicted as:

1. The number of RNs *(R)* plus the number of aides *(A)* must be at least 6:

$$R + A \geq 6$$

2. The number of RNs must be at least equal to the number of aides:

$$R \geq A$$

Although the nurse manager's constraints indicate that the number of RNs must be equal to or greater than the number of aides, to simplify the calculation in this example, assume that the number of RNs must equal the number of aides. In addition, to simplify the calculation assume that the number of aides plus the number of RNs must be equal to 6. Therefore we remove the greater than signs and have the following equations:

$$R + A = 6$$
$$R = A$$

Using algebra, these equations are solved simultaneously. The second equation states that $R = A$. In the first equation if we substitute A for R we get the following:

$$A + A = 6$$
$$2A = 6$$

By dividing both sides by 2 we get:

$$\frac{2A}{2} = \frac{6}{2}$$
$$A = 3$$

Thus if the unit is staffed with three RNs and three aides, costs will be minimized. Minimum cost = [($200 × 3 RNs) + ($80 × 3 aides)]/30 = $28 per patient per shift.

We recognize that this trivial example is intuitive. In the more complex situations of the real world, all the known constraints would be depicted and the many equations would be solved simultaneously using a computer.

Inventory Control

Operations management is that area of management which analyzes the use of resources to produce the desired product. Most of this book has focused on nursing personnel as the major resource used in providing nursing care. Although nursing personnel are the costliest resource in providing nursing care, nurse managers are often also responsible for management of clinical and other supplies. In areas such as the OR, supplies are a major expense. On other nursing units and for outpatient programs supply costs can be considerable. One aspect of the management of supplies is the appropriate use of supplies.

Another aspect of management of supplies is *inventory management*. Inventory management refers to the appropriate ordering and storage of supplies. This section will focus on inventory management.

Horngren and Foster describe five categories of costs associated with supplies: (a) *cost of the product,* (b) *ordering costs,* (c) *carrying costs,* (d) *stockout costs,* and (e) *quality costs.*[4] Cost of the product is what the organization must pay for the product and can be affected by quantity discounts and timing of payment. Ordering costs include those costs associated with the order such as clerk time for preparation of a purchase order. Carrying costs are often called *opportunity costs* or those costs of having money tied up in inventory rather than in a revenue-producing endeavor such as an interest-bearing bank account. Stockout costs are the costs incurred when the supply is not available but is needed. If this is a supply item that the nurse must have for patient care, often the supply must be purchased at a higher price from a local vendor. Finally, quality costs are those costs incurred to ensure that the product is of the required quality. This may include costs such as inspection or replacement or the patient harm done by using a low-quality item.

Nurse managers are most often concerned with stockouts. Because many of the supplies used have a direct impact on the quality of patient care provided, nurse managers are particularly sensitive to this issue. In some cases supplies are not readily available from other sources. Patient care will suffer, or a patient may need to be transferred to another institution and revenues lost. Although the manager cannot predict with certainty what supplies will be needed, previous experience and expectations about future patient care needs can be used to estimate supply needs.

At the unit level the nurse manager is usually concerned with balancing the space required to store supplies with the goal of avoiding a stockout. The following example shows how to calculate the reorder point for catheter kits. Suppose that the nurse manager knows that the unit usually uses about .2 catheter kits per patient day.

Identify the average daily census on the unit = 25
Identify average catheter kits used per patient day = .2

Calculate daily usage = Census × Usage per patient day
= 25 × .2
= 5 kits needed per day

Identify safe level of supply on unit = 10
Identify lead time to order supplies = 2 days

Reorder point = (Lead time × Average daily use) + Safe level
= (2 × 5) + 10 = 20

---

[4]Charles T. Horngren and George Foster, *Cost Accounting A Managerial Emphasis,* 7th ed., Prentice-Hall, Inc., Englewood Cliffs, NJ, 1990, p. 741.

Therefore assuming that the census remains at about twenty-five, catheter kits should be reordered when there are twenty remaining.

This simple approach to determine inventory supplies, however, does not take into account either the carrying costs or the ordering costs. Often the unit-based nurse manager is concerned with the reorder costs. Many decide that supplies will be ordered weekly, unless there is an emergency. This may not be the most efficient system for the entire organization. Although the unit-based nurse manager is not usually directly concerned with carrying cost, it does affect the financial health of the organization and is therefore relevant for all managers having responsibility for inventory.

Economic order quantity (EOQ) is an approach to determine the balance between ordering costs and carrying costs. The goal of inventory control is to minimize costs while not encountering a stockout. The manager estimates the optimal quantity of supplies to order and lead time necessary to place that order. For example, suppose that based on historical use the nurse manager on a med/surg unit knows that when the unit has twenty-five patients the staff uses 5,000 syringes per year. It takes two days from the time the request is made to the time the supplies reach the floor. Preparing a central supply request costs $5 of a clerk's time. The central accounting office has determined that the organization currently borrows money at a rate of 10% to pay some of its bill and that it costs the organization $.50 per unit for insurance, storage, and other carrying costs per year. This $.50 includes 10% interest on the average inventory level.

Table 17–7 shows an example of the calculations that can be used to estimate the balance between ordering costs and carrying costs. *A* is defined as the demand for the supply for the year. *E* is the size of each order. The average inventory on hand will therefore be $E \div 2$. There will be one purchase order for each order, so the total number of purchase orders per year will be $A \div E$. The cost of planning orders will be the cost per purchase order (*P*) multiplied by the number of orders ($A \div E$). The total cost of carrying inventory is the cost to carry one unit for one year (*S*) multiplied by the average inventory level ($E \div 2$). The total inventory costs, *C*, in addition to the purchase price of the units will be the order cost $P \times (A \div E)$ plus the carrying costs $S \times (E \div 2)$. The nurse manager has estimated that the demand (*A*) for syringes is about 5,000 per year (or about fourteen per day). In the example shown three possible order sizes (*E*) are identified: 50, 316, and 5,000.

The easiest approach might appear to be the third alternative—order once

❖ **TABLE 17–7**
Economic-Order-Quantity for Purchase of Syringes

A	Demand	5,000	5,000	5,000
E	Order size	50	316	5,000
E ÷ 2	Average inventory	25	158	2,500
A ÷ *E*	Number of purchase orders	100	16	1
P(A ÷ *E)*	Annual ordering costs @ $5.00	$ 500	$ 80	$ 5
S(E ÷ 2)	Annual carrying costs @ $0.50	13	79	1,250
C	Total annual relevant cash	$ 513	$ 159	$1,255

per year. In that case there would be just one order, at a cost of $5. However, the average inventory on hand would be 2,500 syringes. That would result in high carrying costs of $1,250. The total cost would be $1,255. At the other extreme, an order size of fifty is sufficient stock for the unit. The costs to the organization of that alternative are $513.

Both the first and third alternatives are substantially more expensive than the economic order quantity (EOQ). The EOQ is 316 (cost = $159). Ordering a little more than once per month (sixteen times per year) will minimize costs of inventory. The EOQ is calculated using the following formula:

$$EOQ = \sqrt{2AP/S}$$

$$= \sqrt{2 \times 5,000 \times \$5/\$.50}$$

$$= 316$$

This formula approach does not take into account the fact that there are sometimes discounts for quantity. The manager should consider what discounts are available and calculate the higher carrying costs associated with larger orders to determine if it is worth taking the discount.

For example, suppose in this problem that there was a $250 discount in purchase price for five orders of 1,000 units each as opposed to sixteen smaller orders. To order 1,000 units at a time, there would be five orders at a cost of $5 each. Therefore the order cost would be $25. The carrying cost would be $S \times (E \div 2)$, or $.50 \times (1,000 \div 2) = \$250$. The total costs would be $275. This is $116 higher than the EOQ cost of $159. If we can reduce the purchase cost of the inventory units by $250, the savings would more than offset the $116 increase in inventory management costs. Five orders per year instead of sixteen would be justified.

Even if the nurse manager is not responsible for inventory control, an appreciation of the costs incurred in inventory may make the manager and the staff more sensitive to the issues. It is common for nurse managers to stockpile supplies. Because nurses believe that they cannot provide care without certain supplies and because they have run out of supplies in the past, often extra supplies are hidden for future use. Organizations incur costs associated with inventory. The use of organizational resources can be optimized by efficient inventory control.

PLANNING AND TRACKING A PROJECT

Organizations often face the opportunity to pursue new ventures or programs. Careful analysis of the steps involved in the planning and implementation of such projects will lead to smoother implementation.

Successful implementation of a project requires the completion of many activities in a timely fashion. A variety of specific techniques can be used to aid the planning and implementation of a project. Examples of these approaches are Gantt, PERT, and the Critical Path Method. Each of these methods provides an approach for laying out the specific steps to be taken and when each activity must be accomplished.

A major benefit of these techniques is that they force the manager to think through all the steps necessary to complete a project. To use them successfully the manager must outline the timing of the necessary steps. In addition they serve as a map of how the project is proceeding. In many cases certain steps must be completed before other steps can occur. If a necessary step is not completed, further work on the project cannot proceed. These methods highlight such "bottleneck" points.

For example, if a hospital plans to open a hospital-based home care agency, the nurse manager may be responsible for the successful implementation of the project. Planning for the project may include activities such as obtaining a certificate of need, hiring staff, renovating space, and developing a marketing strategy. Some of these steps cannot be completed until a prerequisite step is completed. Some may be done concurrently.

The initial step in using any of these techniques is to identify the activities that must be completed. Next the manager estimates the amount of time required to complete the activity and finally the sequence of tasks in relation to other activities.

Gantt

A *Gantt chart* depicts necessary activities or goals in a matrix format with the horizontal axis indicating the time frame and the vertical axis the activities in the project. Exhibit 17–5 shows a Gantt chart for the implementation of a skin risk assessment program on two units of a hospital.

The vertical axis shows the activities that must be completed. The horizontal axis shows when the various activities will occur and the expected date of completion. For example, item 5 states "collect baseline data." Collection of baseline data is expected to take two months. Prior to this period, the nursing staff will need to develop a consensus for a skin assessment protocol to use to collect baseline data. Item 5 will occur during April and May. However, item 6 "implement education program" will not occur until June, or after the baseline data are collected. Note that data analysis begins during October, even though some data are being collected during that month.

Critical Path Method and PERT

The *Critical Path Method* is a diagram or model of the sequencing of events that must be completed for successful implementation of the project. The first step is to identify all activities that must be completed. The second step is to identify approximately how long it will take to complete the activities. With this information the work flow is diagramed. See Figure 17–14 for an example of a critical path to conduct a comprehensive zero-based budget review. Various methods of depicting the activities (often identified by a number) and the time required to complete the activity are noted. Those points which must be completed prior to the next step are identified and highlighted. In many projects only a few of the steps are critical. An activity may take a month to complete, but the time line may show several months to complete the activity. However, some steps in a project are critical, and subsequent steps cannot be done until these steps are completed. These are the critical steps that must be very carefully monitored. The critical path is generally shown as a bold line on the diagram.

❖ EXHIBIT 17–5
Example of a GANTT Chart

Project Timeline	1993											
	JAN	FEB	MAR	APR	MAY	JUN	JUL	AUG	SEP	OCT	NOV	DEC
1. Hire projector director	X											
2. Review literature	X											
3. Train data collectors	X	X										
4. Develop consensus on skin assessment			X									
5. Collect baseline data				X	X							
6. Implement education program on two units						X	X	X				
7. Collect post data												
8. Analyze data									X	X		
9. Prepare report for QA committee										X		
10. Place for further implementation or options											X	X

Figure 17–14. Critical path method. (Reprinted from Hospital Cost Management and Accounting, Vol. 3, No. 6, p. 3, with permission of Aspen Publishers, Inc., © 1991.)

In Figure 17–14 the days needed to complete an activity are noted under the activity. It can be seen that developing audit guidelines will take thirty-one days. The top path shows that auditing departments B, C, and D will take fifteen, thirteen, and nine days, respectively, for a total of thirty-seven days. The bottom path indicates that auditing departments A and E will take twenty-two and nineteen days, respectively, for a total of forty-one days. This path is part of the critical path and is shown in bold. Activity 6, review audits, cannot be completed until this path is completed.

Steps 2-4-6 are critical because a delay of even one day in that path will delay the entire project by a day. By contrast, a delay in path 2-3-5-6 will not delay the project at all. Since this latter path takes thirty-seven days as compared to forty-one days for the critical path, it has four days of slack. It is not worthwhile to push to shorten work in departments B, C, or D. However, any savings in time in the work in departments A and E could speed up the entire project.

PERT (program evaluation and review technique) is a more sophisticated version of the critical path method.[5] All activities are noted in a network format with events and activities identified. Time estimates are made for optimistic, likely, and pessimistic outcomes. Figure 17–15 shows a PERT chart for a simple project.

The development of a PERT network often begins at the end and works backward to identify those activities which must be completed. The project depicted must be completed in sixteen weeks. Three sets of activities must be completed. The numbers in triangles indicate the earliest week that an activity can start, and the squares indicate the latest week that an activity can start and still have the project completed on time. The circles indicate the likely time frames. The activities on the top and bottom rows can be completed in four weeks (two weeks plus two weeks) and three weeks, respectively. The middle set of activities will take at least eleven weeks to complete, but twelve weeks are allowed. This path is shown in bold because the entire project cannot be completed until activities on this path are completed, and these activities must be done in sequence. Sophisticated tables may be prepared in addition to the

---

[5] See, for example, D. M. Warner, D. C. Holloway, and K. L. Grazier, *Decision Making and Control for Health Administration*, 2nd edition, Health Administration Press, Ann Arbor, MI, 1984, for a detailed description of PERT and other quantitative methods for decision making.

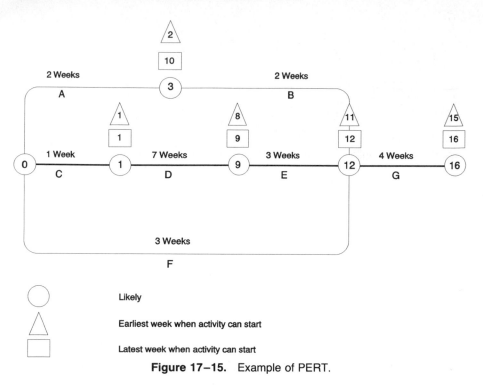

Figure 17–15. Example of PERT.

graphic depiction outlining the slack time and the probabilities of events' occurring.

For some projects it is necessary to complete the activities as quickly as possible. It may be possible to complete the project sooner, but that will require additional expenditures. For example, it may be possible to complete activity D in five weeks if extra resources are devoted to that activity. The project manager can estimate the time savings and related costs and estimate whether these costs are justified. In the example above it is unlikely that the costs could be justified. However, the additional revenues generated by opening a new transplant unit two months earlier may justify incurring additional expenses to complete the project more quickly.

In all these methods the person responsible for each activity is usually identified. This identification then offers the manager in charge of the project an opportunity to hold someone accountable for the completion of the various components. That tends to create an environment in which there is increased likelihood of completion of the various phases of the project on a timely basis.

IMPLICATIONS FOR NURSE MANAGERS

Forecasting is an essential part of the budgeting process. A number of items such as patients, length of stay, and acuity are essential ingredients of an operating budget. Preparation of an operating budget cannot begin without some prediction of the values for these variables. The same holds true for other types of budgets.

Most forecasting is based on the theories of probability. Probability is the likelihood of an event's occurring and is usually based on historical data.

Managers have great flexibility in selecting the variables that they choose to forecast. They can forecast the number of patients, patient days, the quantity of a resource that will be consumed (e.g., the number of chest tubes needed or the number of nursing care hours), the amount that will be spent on supplies or personnel, or the acuity level of patients. Any variable for which historical data are available can be forecast using the methods of this chapter.

The forecasting process consists of collecting data, graphing the data, analyzing the graphed data, and preparing prediction formulas. Care must be exercised regarding consideration of things that are changing and that will prevent the future from being like the past. For example, a change in federal regulations concerning types of treatments covered by Medicare might have a dramatic impact on volume. While managers are aware of such changes, computerized formulas are unlikely to take discrete, recent changes into account. The human role in the forecasting process is critical to generating accurate forecasts.

Analysis of the graphed data will help a manager determine whether the item to be forecast has been exhibiting seasonal or trend behavior, both, or neither. Formulas can then be used to make predictions of the future.

It is important for managers not only to use common techniques of management but also to be prepared to be leaders in the development of new uses. The 1990s will likely see a rapid increase in the use of computers by health care managers. The first wave of microcomputer use in the late 1970s and early 1980s saw widespread introduction of personal computers in positions where the same rote function was performed over and over. Computers clearly increase productivity by being faster at performing a calculation currently done many times. The next wave of computer use in the mid to late 1980s often represented a novelty. Computers were widely introduced, but in many cases they were used only as sophisticated typewriters (word processors).

In the 1990s, however, the average manager will start to use personal computers to manage better—not just to do an existing calculation faster and not just to type nice-looking letters, but to manage better. Forecasting is one area where the results of a manager's efforts will be superior because the use of a computer can allow a greater degree of sophistication to be merged with the already existing judgment and experience of the manager.

Specific decision-making tools such as expected value, linear programming, and economic order quantity can be used by the nurse manager to make better decisions. In addition, approaches such as Gantt and PERT can be used by the nurse manager to plan and manage new programs or projects.

At the same time, one must always bear in mind that the sophisticated quantitative techniques for decision making lack the judgment and experience of managers. Therefore, whether one is using a subjective Delphi technique or a high-powered computer program, the role of the manager in making the final forecast should never be understated.

KEY CONCEPTS

Probability   Likelihood of an event's occurring. The probability of future events can be estimated based on data from historical events.

Additive rule   States that likelihood of either one event or another event's occurring is the sum of the likelihood of each event's occurring.

Multiplication rule   Likelihood of two or more events' occurring simultaneously or in sequence is the product of each event.

Subjective probability   Relies not only on the scientific application of the laws of chance but also on the judgment of the manager.

Forecasting   Making a prediction of some future outcome. A great number of management decisions are based on forecasts.

Trend   Patterns related to the passage of time. A trend may be generally upward, constant, or downward over time.

Time series   Approach to forecasting in which historical changes over time are used to help anticipate the likely result in a coming time period.

Seasonality   Variations related to seasons of the year. For example, there may be more communicable diseases in the winter when people are indoors more.

Regression analysis   Mathematical technique to find the unique straight line that comes closest to all the historical data points. This regression line is then used to predict future events.

Curvilinear   Curved line. Most of the methods described assume that there is a straight-line relationship between changes in the variables. Sometimes the relationship is curved. A curvilinear approach to forecasting is especially useful when seasonal patterns exist.

Expected value   Method used to estimate the likely value of undertaking an activity that has alternative possible outcomes. It is the weighted average of the value of each possible outcome using probabilities as weights.

Nominal Group Technique   Method for qualitative forecasting in which the group of individuals is brought together in a structured meeting. A consensus forecast is developed.

Delphi technique   Method for qualitative forecasting in which the group never meets. A consensus forecast is developed that is less biased by personalities of group members than with the Nominal Group Technique.

Linear programming (LP)   Technique to determine how best to allocate scarce resources to achieve a certain goal, which is subject to a number of constraints.

Inventory management   Refers to the appropriate ordering and storage of supplies, considering the product cost, ordering costs, stockout costs, and carrying costs.

Economic order quantity (EOQ)   Approach to determine the optimal quantity for each order. It is based on creating a balance between ordering costs and carrying costs.

Gantt chart   Depicts necessary activities or goals in a matrix format with the horizontal axis indicating the time frame and the vertical access the activities in the project.

Critical Path Method (CPM)   Diagram or model of the sequencing of events that must be completed for successful completion of the project. Those points which must be completed prior to the next step are identified and highlighted.

PERT (program evaluation and review technique)   More sophisticated version of the critical path method. All activities are noted in a network format with events and activities identified. Estimates are made for optimistic, likely, and pessimistic actual times to complete each step.

SUGGESTED READINGS

Barenbaum, Lester, and Thomas Monahan, "Developing a Planning Model to Estimate Future Cash Flows," *Healthcare Financial Management*, Vol. 42, No. 3, March 1988, pp. 50–56.

Broyles, R.W., and M.L. Colin, *Statistics in Health Administration*, Vol. I, 1979, Aspen Systems Corp., Rockville, MD, pp. 145–146.

Finkler, Steven A., "Regression-based Cost Estimation and Variance Analysis: Resolving the Impact of Outliers," *Hospital Cost Accounting Advisor*, Vol. 3, No. 4, September 1987, pp. 1–5.

Hicks, Lanis L., Kenneth Bopp, and Richard Speck, "Forecasting Demand for Hospital Services in an Unstable Environment," *Nursing Economics*, Vol. 5, No. 6, November/December 1987, pp. 304–310.

Marsh, John J., and James A. Hoover, "Management Engineering," in *Handbook of Health Care Accounting and Finance*, William O. Cleverley, ed., Aspen Publishers, Rockville, MD, 1982, pp. 909–931.

Romano, Carol A., "Innovation: The Promise and Perils for Nursing and Information Technology," *Computers in Nursing*, Vol. 8, No. 3, May/June 1990, pp. 99–104.

SmartForecasts II, Smart Software, Inc., Belmont, MA.

Synowiez, Barbara B., and Peter M. Synowiez, "Delphi Forecasting as a Planning Tool," *Nursing Management*, Vol. 21, No. 4, April 1990, pp. 18–19.

CHAPTER
18

Marketing

CHAPTER GOALS

The goals of this chapter are to:

- Explain the essential elements of marketing management
- Relate the roles of nursing and marketing
- Discuss the importance of understanding the needs of customers
- Define basic marketing concepts, including the market, market segmentation, customer behavior, market measurement, market share, market research, determinant attributes, and advertising
- Define the elements of a marketing plan and discuss the role of each element
- Discuss the roles of the BCG matrix and life-cycle analysis in the development of marketing strategy
- Explain the difference between strategy and tactics and discuss the importance of tactics for carrying out strategy
- Introduce the four Ps of marketing: product, price, place, and promotion
- Discuss the implementation and control of marketing plans

❖

INTRODUCTION

Virtually every organization desires to provide a high volume of services. Health care *marketing* is a management science that attempts to maintain and increase the organization's patient volume. High volume is desirable because of its financial implications, which are related to the concepts of fixed and variable costs (discussed in Chapter 7). If any costs of the organization are fixed, then increasing volume will inherently spread those costs more widely. Each unit of service will bear a smaller share of the fixed costs. The average cost per unit declines as volume increases because of the sharing of fixed costs.

For example, the costs per patient in a half-full hospital are much higher than in a full hospital because certain costs must be incurred to operate the hospital, regardless of how full it is. These include administration, heat, light, depreciation, and a wide variety of other fixed items. With fewer patients, each must cover a larger share of those costs. If the prices at which services are provided are maintained at a fairly constant level, then rising volume and declining average costs will lead to a higher profit margin per unit of service. This is turn leads to greater financial stability.

Organizations with higher volume can use their improved financial stability in a variety of ways. They can offer a wider range of services, improving health care in the community. They can offer services without an internal environment of perpetual financial crisis. This means that adequate levels of staff and improved quality of care are more likely to exist. Financial remuneration of employees can be determined based on factors other than what an austerity situation allows.

Many people in health care believe that the key to a successful organization is to provide high-quality care and to let potential patients know that your care is high quality. Surprisingly, quality is not necessarily a key determining factor in the demand for an organization's health care services. To many consumers, when it comes to health care, quality goes without saying. They would not expect the government to allow any organization to offer health care services that are not high quality. This perception may well be incorrect. However, it is a common belief.

Factors other than quality often make the difference in where a patient goes for health care services. Convenience, amenities, price, and a wide variety of other factors come into play.

Marketing is an area of management that tries to ensure that the organization achieves and maintains a high volume level. However, to the surprise of many people not familiar with marketing, the essence of marketing is not selling the organization's product. Attaining the high revenues and the profits that result from the provision of a high volume of service is more complicated than simply going out and finding customers to buy the organization's goods and services.

The concept of marketing may be counterintuitive to many nurses. Clinical education focuses on a perspective that people come for care when they are ill or want preventive services such as immunizations. Nurses are not selling patient monitoring in the same way that a department store sells blouses. However, health care organizations are selling their services, and there is nothing inherently unethical about that. If you believe that your facility provides the best care, you want potential patients to be aware of that. If your care is as good as that provided by other facilities in your area, encouraging patients to use your facility will result in higher volume, economies of scale, and ultimately lower costs and/or better services for all your organization's patients.

THE ESSENCE OF MARKETING: ASSESSING CUSTOMER NEEDS

The short-run focus of marketing efforts is on finding customers for the organization's goods and services. However, that effort is really not the main theme of marketing. Rather, the goal of marketing efforts is to enable the organization to determine what customers want or need and to develop and offer those goods or services. Selling is a minor focus of marketing, while determining what to sell is the essence of marketing.

Most nonmarketing specialists mistakenly assume that marketing consists primarily of determining what type of advertising to use and then implementing an ad campaign. The major efforts of marketing managers, however, are directed toward assessing customer needs.

Too often, organizations formed to respond to an unfilled need remain the same over time, even though they exist in a changing environment. The marketplace faced by each organization tends to be dynamic, in a constant state of flux. Successful organizations respond to changes in the marketplace. The sooner a health care organization can identify changing customer needs, the more promptly it can respond and the more successful it is likely to be.

Prior to the 1950s there were few if any supermarkets. Shoppers went to a variety of different stores to purchase meat, dairy products, fruits, and other groceries. The food suppliers who anticipated the notion of one-stop shopping and developed supermarkets flourished, while other food stores went out of business. The same process was true in the development of department stores.

In the 1990s, however, supermarkets and department stores have come under financial pressure in the marketplace. Many affluent shoppers want better service than they get from large department stores, and they are willing to pay for it. Boutiques and other specialty stores are on the increase, reversing the one-stop shopping trend. Supermarkets in wealthy neighborhoods are upscaling their stores, particularly in the area of service and quality. Fresh-baked breads, salad bars, and other amenities are appearing in many supermarkets. The trend we observe is recognition by the companies of the changing needs and desires of their customers.

Health care organizations are similarly in a constantly changing environment. The desires of the customers change. Most health care organizations would be quick to state that they are well aware of the constant change in the technologies and methodologies for providing health care. Many health care organizations are on the technological edge in providing care. However, simply deciding on what is a good health care product and then setting about providing it may not be enough. Designing a better mousetrap will make you rich only if potential customers are interested in catching mice.

Focusing on customer needs often leads to the development of new products, services, and other innovations sooner than they would otherwise be adopted. This in turn makes it easier to market the organization's services. Marketing becomes more oriented to informing potential customers of what is available, rather than trying to sell what you have, whether it is what they want or not. Ultimately, such a focus on customer needs means that the organization provides more service to the community rather than simply using the community to serve the needs of the organization.

UNDERSTANDING CUSTOMERS

For health care organizations, marketing represents an unusually great challenge because it is not always clear who the customer is. It is a well-known concept in health care that the physician is often viewed as the true customer, particularly by hospitals. In recent years, it has become more and more apparent that to some extent the insurance company is a customer of health care providers. And in some cases a relative of the patient, rather than the patient, has the decision-making power commonly associated with the ultimate customer.

If you were to buy a gift, would you consider yourself or the ultimate recipient of the gift the customer of the store selling the gift? Clearly, you are the customer. The same thing could be said in the case of mental health or long-term care. Often the patient lacks the capacity to make choices about the selection of a provider of health care services. For a mental health provider or nursing home, the customer often may be a relative of the patient.

In marketing such services it is essential to consider the needs of the relative. Certainly, it is likely that the relative wants the patient to receive high-quality care. Beyond that, however, it may be necessary to provide additional features that make the relative feel the organization is the right one. Perhaps the organization could offer written monthly progress reports to the significant relative. Or perhaps the visiting hours could be made particularly convenient for working relatives. A simple change in visiting hours from 2 to 4 PM to 6 to 8 PM could make a significant difference in ultimate patient volume. The key for the organization is to know who the customer is and then to focus on the needs or desires of the customer. For most health care organizations there is more than one category of customer.

If the key customer is the insurer, that must be taken into account in the organization's decisions. Sometimes health care organizations try to respond to the needs of their potential patients, incorrectly viewing them as the decision-making customer. New buildings are built with substantial amenities that the patients want. However, patients often want more than they (or the insurers) are willing to pay for. They request amenities knowing that they have insurance that will pay for their care.

Insurance companies are starting to find ways to prevent such "moral hazard" behavior. *Moral hazard* refers to the fact that people behave differently if they are insured than if they are not. For example, a homeowner is less likely to have fire extinguishers in the house if there is fire insurance on the house than if there is no insurance. A car owner is more likely to leave an expensive camera on the car seat if there is theft insurance than if there is not. Similarly, patients are more likely to consume more health care services if they have health insurance. They are more likely to see their doctor for minor complaints, and they are more likely to allow the doctor to order a wide range of tests than they would if they did not have insurance.

As a result of widespread health insurance, many people have become used to receiving health care services without direct cost to themselves. Insurance companies, however, have started to encourage patients to use preferred providers (discussed in Chapter 2). They sometimes offer patients full reimbursement for care from preferred provider organizations and only partial reimbursement for care from other providers. In such cases the insurer may not be willing to pay for the high costs of fancy amenities. And often, given a choice of paying 20% of a hospital bill and having the amenities or going to a preferred provider with fewer amenities but no coinsurance, the patients choose the latter. The insurance companies have so much power to steer patients to providers they prefer that it would be foolish for a marketing effort not to consider the needs and desires of the insurer as well as the patient.

The physician still has a dominant role in health care and cannot be ignored in any discussion of health care customers. Physicians can steer patients to hospitals and other providers of health care services in an even more direct way than insurers. Some patients may have a preference for one hospital over another. On the other hand, very few patients will have a preference for a particular home health agency. If their physician refers them to a particular agency for after-hospital home care, they are likely to use that recommended agency. The marketing efforts of home health agencies would have to be based on the realization that a significant segment of their customers consists of physicians.

Even though the services are primarily provided by nurses directly to patients, without physician recommendations business may be lost. Marketing efforts would therefore have to focus to a great extent on physicians. Alternatively, a home health agency might attempt to generate referrals from hospital discharge-planning nurses. In that case the nurse becomes a key customer of the agency, along with physicians and patients.

WHY IS MARKETING IMPORTANT FOR NURSE MANAGERS?
Keeping the Organization Current

In light of the above discussion of the main goal of marketing efforts, it should become easier to understand why marketing is an important topic for nurse managers to comprehend. Organizations that succeed learn the lesson of marketing—that customer needs must be determined. In health care it is virtually impossible for the organization to fully understand the needs of its customers without input from the nursing staff.

The nursing staff has the pulse of the organization's customers in its hands (both literally and figuratively). Nurses constantly hear from the patients what is good and bad about the organization. They have the most frequent patient contact, and the contact is of substantial duration. They are most likely to hear from the patients about what the organization should be doing better or differently. They are likely to hear from the patients about all the good things some other organization does that this one does not do.

From the marketing manager's perspective, the nursing staff can serve a significant market research role. They can listen to the patient comments and pass the information along to the marketing department. Marketing in turn can use the information to assess the changes that the organization should be making to meet the desires of the patients.

Customer needs should be a focal point of the organization. Nurses should be considering whether their activities are focused on responding to those needs. Clearly, specific activities may be required that have little direct impact on making the patient feel better. And in no case can all customer needs be satisfied regardless of cost. Nevertheless, there should be an evaluation of whether the work of a nursing unit is communicated to the patients so that the patients realize that their needs are being addressed.

A recent study indicated that the single factor most often cited by patients as related to their satisfaction is "staff sensitivity to inconvenience of sickness and hospitalization." As one can quickly see looking at the results of that study, reprinted in Table 18–1, the three most important indicators of patient satisfaction have a direct bearing on nurse treatment of patients. However, it is not strictly *clinical* treatment that is involved but rather the extent to which nurses relate to the patients' psychological needs. Based on this, it would appear that

Importance of Individual Satisfaction Indicators

Indicator	Correlation	Indicator	Correlation
Staff sensitivity to inconvenience of sickness and hospitalization	.94	Volunteers	.80
Staff concern for patient's privacy	.93	Information regarding diet	.79
Extent to which nurses take patient's problem seriously	.92	Likelihood of receiving food checked on the menu	.79
Time physician spends with patient	.91	Respiratory care	.79
Overall cheerfulness of hospital	.91	Speed of admissions	.79
Nurses' attention to personal and special needs	.90	Courtesy of intravenous care starter	.79
Nurses' attitude toward patient calling them	.90	Courtesy of transportation staff members	.79
Technicians' explanations of tests and treatments	.89	Length of wait for X-ray	.78
Nurses' information about tests and treatments	.88	Physical therapy	.77
Hospital's concern not to discharge patient too soon	.87	How well television worked	.75
Nurses' friendliness	.87	Skill of intravenous care starter	.75
Technical skill of nurses	.87	Social services	.73
Likelihood of recommending hospital to others	.87	Adequacy of advice for home care	.73
Courtesy of business office	.86	Nurses' attitude toward visitors	.73
Adequacy of information given to family about patient's condition and treatment	.86	Discharge waiting time	.70
Skill of technician taking blood	.85	Daily cleaning of room	.69
Courtesy of technician taking blood	.85	Adequacy of visiting hours	.69
X-ray technicians' concern for patient's comfort	.84	Noise level in and around room	.68
Nurses' promptness in responding to call button	.84	Physicians' information to family	.67
Cheerfulness of room	.82	Physicians' information to patient regarding treatments	.66
Accommodations and comfort for visitors	.81	Courtesy of information desk personnel	.64
Cafeteria or coffee shop rating	.81	Quality of food	.64
Courtesy of cleaning personnel	.81	Temperature of food	.61
Courtesy of admissions personnel	.80	Temperature of room	.59
		Physicians' concern regarding questions	.53

a. The higher the correlation coefficient, the greater its importance to patients. Correlation coefficients can range from −1.0 to +1.0.
Reprinted from Irwin Press, Rodney Ganey, and Mary Malone, "Satisfied Patients Can Spell Financial Well-Being," *Healthcare Financial Management*, February 1991, p. 40, with permission of Healthcare Financial Management Association.

the key to marketing success in health care organizations rests not so much on spending money as on having a very nurturing and supportive staff attitude toward patients.

The issue of patient satisfaction is essential to every health care organization. A dissatisfied patient is not likely to return to a health care provider. That potential lost future revenue is readily apparent. However, since people talk to each other, the effects of dissatisfaction are multiplied. An article several years ago hypothesized that *each* dissatisfied patient might cost a hospital $400,000. The calculation is reprinted in Table 18–2.

Marketing the Importance of Nursing

Nurses do many things for patients that the patients are never aware of. One aspect of marketing should be to create a greater level of patient education concerning some of the many things nurses do for the patient behind the scenes. This can result in a more satisfied customer, and that in turn leads to additional customers later on. For example, even though in many cases patients do not pick their hospital, there are probably many cases in which patients do become aware of the reputation of a hospital and affiliate specifically with a physician who uses that hospital. In other cases physicians may be affiliated

❖ **TABLE 18–2**
Costs of Dissatisfied Patients

Hard Costs	
Dissatisfied patient	1
Assumed revenue associated with a typical hospitalization	× $5,000
	$5,000
Assumed average number of hospitalizations in the patient's remaining lifetime	× 5
	$25,000
Soft Costs	
Dissatisfied patient	1
Additional patients who have a significant complaint but do not register the complaint	+ 6
Significant patient complaints	7
A dissatisfied customer typically tells nine to 10 people of their dissatisfaction	× 9
People eventually receiving negative word-of-mouth information pertaining to the hospital	63
Assuming that one-fourth of the 63 people are influenced by the negative word-of-mouth to the degree that they seek hospitalization elsewhere, apply the "hard" cost assumptions from the analysis above to develop an indication of the potential opportunity cost:	
People receiving negative word-of-mouth information	63
Assumed level of influence	×.25
People choosing to be hospitalized elsewhere	16
Previously determined "hard" costs	× $25,000
Potential lost revenue	$400,000

Reprinted from Virginia Regan Rosselli, Jody Moss, and Randall Luecke, "Improved Customer Service Boosts Bottom Line," *Healthcare Financial Management,* December 1989, p. 22, with permission of Healthcare Financial Management Association.

with several hospitals, and patients will specify a preference when they need an elective procedure.

A vital role played by marketing is the provision of information. Customers may know what they want, but they may not understand the best way to get it. People know that when they are sick, they want to obtain the care needed to get well. The nursing profession should respond to that desire by informing the public of its role in helping them to get well.

If patients were informed of the essential role of high-quality nursing care, they would be likely to consider nursing care in their choices of health care providers. The financial remuneration of nurses has been shown to be related to the demand for nurses. When demand is high and there is a shortage of nurses, salaries tend to rise. This is in line with the principles of basic economics (see Chapter 4). Therefore, it is in the interest of the nursing profession to keep the demand for nursing services high.

The demand for nursing care would be higher if people demanded that health care organizations provide high-quality nursing care. Therefore, there is likely to be a direct return to all nurses from efforts made by the profession to inform the public about what nurses do and why it is important to their health. Marketing should not simply be something that health care organizations do as a way to compete with each other.

MARKETING CONCEPTS
Understanding the Market

To make any assessment of the desires and needs of a group of customers, it is first necessary to understand as much as possible about the set of customers that constitutes the relevant *market*. The market is defined as the potential customers for a product or organization. Information about the market will affect not only the mix of services that should be offered but also the advertising message, price, and other critical factors.

The information about the market that is needed represents primarily demographic information. The age, race, religion, ethnic background, and mobility of the population should be assessed. The likelihood of change in the existing demographics should also be considered. The marketing efforts of the organization should also include collection of data that will help the organization assess the income and assets of the market, the educational level, and the density of the population.

Understanding the market additionally requires understanding various factors that impact on the types of services that can be offered and the prices that can be charged. For example, it is crucial that the organization consider available technologies as well as the wide variety of regulations that impact on the organization.

In attempting to understand the market, many organizations also identify key success factors, sometimes called *determinant attributes*. Determinant attributes are factors that ultimately impact on a consumer's purchase decision. Generally these factors can be divided into two major types: *decision variables* and *environmental variables*. Decision variables are factors controllable by the organization that can affect volume. Environmental variables are also factors that can affect volume. However, they are not controllable by the organization.

Data must be collected for both types of variable. Such data, for either decision or environmental variables, may require action by the organization. In the case of decision variables the organization may take steps to impact directly on the variable. For example, price, the amount of advertising, and the hours that a service is offered are all decision variables. Suppose that a health care organization found that patients who do not use its services would not only use them but would also be willing to pay a higher price than is currently being charged if the service were offered at more suitable hours. The organization can take a set of definite actions. It can adjust its hours of service, advertise the new hours, and raise the price to cover any higher costs associated with the new hours.

On the other hand, the general economy is not a factor within the control of the organization. However, the organization can respond to the economy. High unemployment during a recession will lead to many psychological problems. Rather than focusing as much on services for stress caused by overwork, the organization can emphasize services available for problems such as depression that result from being laid off. And it can offer to defer payment until the patient is re-employed. Although the organization can do little about the general economy, it can find a way to serve its community and at the same time increase its patient volume.

Market Segmentation

One essential tool of marketing is to *segment* the overall market. Segmentation means division of the market into several specific subsections. Some health care organizations have done this already to a great extent. Charging a low price to Blue Cross, perhaps an even lower price to an HMO, and yet a higher price to private insurers represents a segmentation of the market based on the payer for the services.

By dividing the overall market a number of different objectives can be achieved. Not only is it possible to charge different prices to different buyers but it is also possible to target preferred customers. For example, suppose that private insurance patients are the most profitable. The organization can target its advertising to media that primarily reach individuals who have private insurance. Advertisements can be placed in magazines read primarily by affluent individuals.

Markets can be segmented in a variety of ways. They can be divided by socioeconomic factors such as age, sex, occupation, and income; by geography; by personality traits; or by buyer behavior. For example, some customers are price sensitive, others are quality sensitive, and some consider amenities important. If elderly individuals are most likely to need a service, then that service can be advertised in a magazine read by the elderly. The impact of the advertisement is not dispersed over a general public, most of whom do not need the service. The result is that advertisements become more cost effective. It is not only how many people an ad reaches per dollar of cost; it also matters which people the ad reaches.

In general, segmentation is based on three factors. First, one attempts to divide the customer base into groups that have distinct and measurable needs. Second, it is vital that one can assess the specific segments. Finally, the segment must be big enough to merit a distinct effort.

Customer Behavior

Understanding how consumers behave is vital to fashioning the proper mix of services. Not only customer desires and needs but also attitudes and behavior are critical to developing a marketing plan that will create the volume of patients needed by the organization.

Consider a hospital that was losing maternity patients. The hospital was a prestigious research center, known for excellent-quality care. Yet over time its maternity volume was declining. The problem was potentially easily solvable, but the hospital was unaware of buyer behavior and therefore not tuned in to the problem. Unlike other diagnoses, for which patients are unexpectedly rushed to the hospital, maternity provides plenty of advance notice. In fact, many expectant women toured the maternity area as part of their prepared childbirth classes. However, the maternity area was not very presentable. It gave an old appearance. One expectant mother called it "dirty" and said that she refused to deliver her baby at that hospital regardless of its reputation. A coat of paint and perhaps some minor remodeling would probably have easily paid for itself from increased patient volume. The hospital, however, failed to tune in to the effect that the condition of the facilities had on preadmission visitors.

Many things affect the behavior of customers. Price, image, or an advertising message are just a few examples. Organizations need to perform market research to ascertain which factors affect consumer behavior, and how. The buying process consists of perceiving a need, getting ready to make a purchase, purchasing, consuming, and after-the-fact reacting. Lavidge and Steiner have described the process of getting ready to make a purchase as:

Awareness → Knowledge → Liking → Preference → Conviction → and Purchase[1]

A buyer must first perceive a need for health care services. The perceived need is not the marketer's domain. Marketing does not create needs; it satisfies them. Then there must be awareness that the provider exists and knowledge that the provider can meet the need. The buyer must like the provider enough to consider it among other possible choices. The buyer must decide that the provider is the preferred way to go. The preference must be reinforced until it becomes a conviction, and finally a purchase will take place. At any point in the process, the customer may decide to purchase a competitor's services.

Making sure that the potential buyer is aware of the health care organization as a possible source for satisfying needs is an essential role of marketing. Marketing must also put forth information that is likely to cause the buyer to like the organization's product, to prefer it, and to become convinced that the organization is the appropriate source for care. The organization must make sure that its actual production process does in fact fill the perceived need. The after-the-fact reaction of customers will influence future purchase decisions by the patient and the patient's friends and family.

[1]Robert J. Lavidge and Gary A. Steiner, "A Model for Predictive Measurements of Advertising Effectiveness," *Journal of Marketing*, Vol. 25, October 1961, p. 59.

Market Measurement

An important aspect of marketing is the conversion of qualitative information into quantitative estimates of demand. This is referred to as market measurement. Such measurement is made for analysis, planning, and control. Analysis is made of what services to offer. Planning is undertaken to develop the services. Control is conducted to keep performance on target.

The central aspect of market measurement is estimation of market demand. How much will be the total volume purchased by all patients in a defined market area. This measurement requires a thorough definition of the specific product or service whose demand is being estimated. It also requires a clear understanding of the time period for which the estimate is being made, such as a week, month, or year into the future. The longer the time period for the estimate, the less reliable the data obtained.

Environmental factors must be considered in making an estimate for market demand. Since the demand for any service is affected by various factors outside the organization's control, the assumptions leading to a specific forecast of demand must be understood. For instance, a home health agency might plan a geographical expansion into an elderly community under the assumption that Medicare will continue to reimburse for a certain number of home visits. If legislation were to change Medicare reimbursement, the demand estimates might prove faulty. To know how much to rely on demand predictions, one must be able to assess the reasonableness of the underlying assumptions about the environment faced by the organization.

Market demand will also depend, at least to some extent, on the actions taken by the organization itself. The price charged, the advertising campaign undertaken, and other controllable factors can impact on the market demand and should be considered in attempting to determine it. Finding the demand for a hospital-based product may not tell the actual demand that would exist if care could be delivered to patients' homes. Estimating demand must be based on the approaches to providing the product or service that the organization is considering or intends to undertake.

Market measurement requires that demand be forecast. Forecasting demand can be done by a variety of methods ranging from crude to sophisticated. The most common of these approaches are surveys, acquisition of expert opinion, and statistical analyses.

Potential patients can be surveyed as to what they would be inclined to do under a given set of circumstances. Insurance companies and physicians should also be included in the survey process if they have a significant role in steering patients. It should be noted that surveying potential customers is a time-consuming and expensive process.

Another approach would be to obtain expert opinion. For example, the organization could survey members of the nursing staff. In many instances, nurses have the closest experience with what typically happens after the introduction of new services. They may have an insight about the process that occurs after the introduction of new services and the length of time before services typically reach certain levels of patient volume. They may also have an insight about the attitudes of patients. For example, if one were considering how accepting patients would be of endoscopic removal of gall bladders, OR nurses who have had years of experience with endoscopic gynecological procedures would be in a good position to provide an important perspective on what the likely acceptance of the new procedure would be. An alternative to the survey technique would be to develop focus groups and have them discuss the issue under consideration.

Other approaches to market forecasting include time-series analysis (discussed in Chapter 17) and regression analysis (discussed in Chapter 7). These are both sophisticated forecasting tools. However, both these techniques require historical information about the items being forecast. When such data are unavailable, the time-consuming survey approach is generally used.

Market Share

Related to the concept of market measurement is *market share*. Market share represents the portion or percentage of the overall market that a specific organization controls. If half of all broken-leg patients in your area come to your ER, then you have a 50% share of the broken-leg market.

Market share is important because rather than being an absolute number, such as the number of broken legs you treat, it shows your status relative to the competition. If your total number of hospital inpatients is rising 4% per year, that may seem good. However, if the number of inpatients in your city is rising at a rate of 15% per year, then each year your hospital has a smaller share of the total market. This can be a direct warning sign that your competitors are passing you by. It can tell you about your long-term prospects, if you remain as you are.

Market Research

Related to market measurement is the broader question of *market research*. This includes gathering, recording, and analyzing information to improve decisions made by the organization. Market research is needed to determine what the customer really wants and is willing to buy. The major areas for market research are advertising, business economics, products, and sales.

Advertising research focuses on issues such as the appropriate copy to use and the appropriate media for advertisements for a product or service. Business economics research considers forecasting general trends in the environment. Product research considers potential acceptance of new products, analysis of competitors' products, and other factors related to the delivery of services. Sales research focuses on issues such as market characteristics and market share.

The market research process consists of defining the problem to be investigated, constructing the model, collecting data, and interpreting data. The statement of the problem must be carefully framed and the intended use of the research understood to avoid wasting substantial effort. The result of the research should be to produce not just interesting information but rather information that is useful for making a particular decision.

A model must be constructed to ensure a full understanding of all the possibilities. For instance, the research might focus on the outcomes of a decision by a hospital to increase advertising to raise the hospital's profile in the community. The market research model would consider each possible ramification of the campaign. One element of the model would cover possible competitive responses. The competing hospitals might not react to the campaign, might react modestly, or might react strongly. Based on the competitive reaction, consumers might react in a variety of ways. Each possible outcome and its likelihood must be evaluated.

To evaluate the outcome of each possibility, data must be collected. They can be collected from primary sources, such as observations, experiments, or surveys, or from secondary sources, such as existing files, service organizations that collect and sell data, or available publications. Secondary data are much easier to obtain and less costly, but they may not be relevant to the particular problem at hand. Primary data, in addition to being costly, have other inherent problems. Surveys, whether by mail, telephone, or in person, have a nonresponse rate. Are nonresponses randomly distributed? Those who feel strongly, either positively or negatively, may be more or less likely to respond. Failure to get data from that group may bias the results. Surveyors themselves may bias the results by the way they ask questions.

It is important that data collected be valid and reliable. Ensuring quality of data requires a high level of expertise. While nurse managers can help their organizations by having a basic knowledge of the field of marketing, many elements of marketing such as market research should be conducted by experts in the field.

It is incumbent on the organization to employ market research to determine which factors are really important to the ultimate purchase decision. Therefore market research should always include analysis of the product or service's determinant attributes (discussed earlier). Depending on the product or service, this may mean considering the impact of convenience, price, special services, or any of a number of other characteristics.

Advertising

Advertising makes people aware of an organization and its products, provides knowledge about the product, and hopefully creates a preference for and loyalty to the organization's services. Advertising can come in the form of paid advertisements, personal selling, sales promotions, and other forms of publicity. The level of expenditures on advertising should be established so that the extra benefits from extra advertising always exceed or are at least equal to the extra cost of the extra advertising. This is based on the concepts of marginal costs and marginal benefits discussed in Chapter 4.

In advertising there are many critical questions to be addressed. How many people are reached by a campaign? Are they the right people? Is the message making the desired impact? It is not sufficient to have a slick presentation. The message must be designed and presented based on what is likely to work with the desired audience. The presentation and timing of the message are as important as simply reaching a large number of people.

MARKETING PLANS

Marketing is based on a strategic planning approach. Plans are made to achieve a goal. An unusual aspect of marketing plans is that they often tend to be disruptive. The plan is often aimed at making change occur. At a minimum, marketing may take patients away from competitors. Often, marketing plans call for changes in the current operations of the organization. Change generally meets resistance. For the marketing plan to be effective in an environment in which reactions to the plan both internally and by competitors are likely, the plan must be carefully established.

Marketing plans should first consider the organizational mission and goals. Then internal/external analyses must be performed, a strategic marketing plan developed, and specific tactics developed. Plans must then be revised, integrated, and implemented. Finally, control and feedback are essential to an effective plan.[2]

Organizational Mission/Goals

The marketing plan should support the organizational mission. Most health care organizations have realized the importance of having a basic mission statement to guide the organization. Based on the mission statement, organizational goals can be set and strategic plans made to carry out those goals. Strategic planning was discussed in Chapter 10.

It is inappropriate to develop a marketing plan without referring back to the organization's mission and strategic plan. Marketing plans often encompass major changes in product offerings, not simply the sale of existing services. Therefore, the organization can very easily find itself working at cross-purposes unless there is a mesh between the overall direction that the organization wants to take and the direction in which the marketing plan takes it.

Internal/External Analyses

The internal/external analysis consists of an analysis of the environment, including the competition, and the organization's internal capabilities in light of the needs and desires of the consumer. There must always be a continuing focus first and foremost on what the organization's customers need. The ability of the organization to satisfy those needs, in light of the competition, is the basis for an internal/external analysis. The opportunities and threats disclosed by this analysis must be carefully considered before any strategies can be developed. The analysis itself makes use of tools such as market measurement and market research, discussed above.

The organization's environment is a critical piece of the puzzle of trying to determine how to successfully provide services to the community. Questions about the environment that should be addressed in a marketing plan include the size of the market, the growth rate of the market, stability of prices, and the degree of competition. Factors such as social attitudes and reimbursement rules must also be considered.

The next element of the internal/external assessment is identification of the market and its needs. This assessment should include both internal and external markets. For example, if physicians are considered crucial to generating patients, they should be assessed along with patients. An example of a data collection form for identifying markets and needs is given in Exhibit 18–1.

Knowing the basic markets is a critical first step. Next, the markets must be fully understood. What factors result in changes in the marketplace? Are the key factors that cause the market to change related to demographics (e.g.,

---

[2]Steven G. Hillestad and Eric N. Berkowitz, *Health Care Marketing Plans: From Strategy to Action*, 2nd edition, Aspen Publishers, Gaithersburg, MD, 1991, p. 54.

❖ **EXHIBIT 18–1**
Identification of Major Markets and Needs

Part I—Identifying markets. A market or market segment consists of a group of people who have common demographic, specialty, or social characteristics that represent a size large enough for the organization to concentrate resources around.

Potential Markets	Importance of Market (check one column for current and future)						Current Attitude Toward You (circle one number)				
	Current			Future			Very Favorable				Very Unfavorable
	High	Med	Low	High	Med	Low	1	2	3	4	5
Gen. medicine M.D.'s							1	2	3	4	5
Surgeons							1	2	3	4	5
OB/gyn							1	2	3	4	5
Peds							1	2	3	4	5
Other M.D.'s							1	2	3	4	5
Inpatients (by specialty)							1	2	3	4	5
Outpatients							1	2	3	4	5
Community at large							1	2	3	4	5
Donors							1	2	3	4	5
Board of directors							1	2	3	4	5
Insurance companies							1	2	3	4	5
Regulators							1	2	3	4	5
Business/ industry (specify)							1	2	3	4	5
Have no doctor market							1	2	3	4	5
HMO patients							1	2	3	4	5
Over-65 market							1	2	3	4	5
Nonuser market							1	2	3	4	5
Females							1	2	3	4	5
Males							1	2	3	4	5
Others _____							1	2	3	4	5
_____							1	2	3	4	5
_____							1	2	3	4	5

Part II—Based on the mix of actual and potential markets listed in Part I, indicate the size and future potential.

Key Market Segments from Part I	Size Today	Future Size— Three Years	Your Current Market Share
25 thru 34-year-old males - athletics	*9% of metro area*	*14%*	*32% of medical care needs in sports medicine programs*

Part III—Based on completion of Parts I and II, indicate the needs major market segments are likely to exhibit.

Key Market Segments	Needs
25 thru 34-year-old males in sports medicine program	*Greater emphasis on strength, training, cardiovascular fitness*

Reprinted from *Health Care Marketing Plans*, 2nd ed., by S. Hillestad and E. Berkowitz, with permission of Aspen Publishers, Inc., © 1991.

population aging), regulatory changes (e.g., in reimbursement), or available medical services (e.g., as a result of technology)? Can the market be segmented and, if so, how attractive a market is each segment? The organization must make every effort to know not just what the markets are but why they are. What influences them and causes them to change, or to remain the same, over time?

Having gained some insight to the markets that are relevant for the organization and the needs of the market, the analysis must thoroughly examine the competition. Strengths and weaknesses of the organization vis-à-vis its competition are crucial foundations for the development of any market strategy. Exhibit 18–2 presents an example of a form that can be used to collect and record data concerning competition.

Organizations should attempt to understand any *differential advantages* they have. A differential advantage is some characteristic that provides the organization with a distinct advantage over a competitor. Such advantages might include location, cost, services offered, or other factors. For example, a women's care center may have a distinct advantage over a general care center for treating particular problems. Organizations should constantly be attempting to develop differential advantages for themselves and trying to find ways to overcome differential advantages held by the competition. One can think of a differential advantage as creating a barrier that keeps out competition.

Just as the strengths and weaknesses of the competition must be known, so also must the organization assess its own relative merits. Being aware of the external environment is only helpful to the extent that the organization can take advantage of that information. Unless the organization conducts a thorough internal analysis of what it can and cannot do, it will be unable to take advantage of such information.

Strategic Marketing Plan

According to Hillestad and Berkowitz, many managers "call the marketing staff with the following question: 'I would like to involve you in a strategy to help our orthopedics program; could you help us put together a brochure that we can send out to doctors about the program?'"[3] The problem with this approach is that it implies that the previous two steps—evaluating the mission and goals and performing an internal/external review—probably have not been undertaken. Furthermore, the brochure represents not a strategy but a tactic.

Strategies are broader frameworks by which goals can be attained. *Tactics* represent the specific activities that must be undertaken to carry out a strategy. There are many strategic approaches that organizations can adopt. An organization can choose to charge lower prices than the competition to achieve a high market share. Or it can adopt a strategy of high prices with the expectation of a highly profitable low market share. Organizations can decide to push their product, going to the customer, or use a pull strategy, making the customer come to them.

Organizations can develop strategies to create barriers to prevent other potential providers from competing. One approach is to charge low prices to gain a large market share. Competitors are likely to be reluctant to enter a market

---

[3]Ibid., p. 107.

❖ **EXHIBIT 18–2**
Relative Competitor Assessment Form

Competitor (specify): _____

	Much Worse	Somewhat Worse		About the Same			Somewhat Better		Much Better
	−4	−3	−2	−1	0	+1	+2	+3	+4
1. Medical care									
A. Emergency									
B. Surgery									
C. Gen. medical									
D. Special care									
2. Nursing care									
3. Housekeeping (hospital)									
4. Food service (hospital)									
5. Staff morale									
6. Facility: Capacity/attractiveness									
7. Public relations									
8. Reputation									
9. Image (overall)									
10. Management									
11. Lab services									
12. Convenience									
13. Staff education									
14. Equipment: Capability/technology									
15 Range of services									
16. Marketing plan									
17. Ad/promo budget									

Competitive Assessment: For each competitor on which you have a Competitor Assessment form, indicate the level of competitive intensity, your share of the market, and the basis for competition.

Competitor	Market Share	Level of Competitive Intensity						Basis for Competition			
		Very Intense				Not Competi- tive at All		Product	Price	Promotion	Distri- bution
1.	_____	1	2	3	4	5		_____	_____	_____	_____
2.	_____	1	2	3	4	5		_____	_____	_____	_____
3.	_____	1	2	3	4	5		_____	_____	_____	_____
4.	_____	1	2	3	4	5		_____	_____	_____	_____
5.	_____	1	2	3	4	5		_____	_____	_____	_____
6.	_____	1	2	3	4	5		_____	_____	_____	_____
7.	_____	1	2	3	4	5		_____	_____	_____	_____
8.	_____	1	2	3	4	5		_____	_____	_____	_____

Conclusion:

where there is already a dominant force. Another approach to the creation of barriers would be to make it costly for consumers to shift to another care provider. Yet another strategy is to offer a product that only this one organization can provide.

Sometimes strategies involve creating a high profile for quality leadership or focusing efforts on the development of one new product. A strategy can be to become known for patient service or for convenience. One key element in setting strategies relates to the nature of the specific product or service being considered. Several techniques have been developed that can help an organization develop appropriate strategies for different products. In particular, the BCG matrix and life-cycle analysis have proven to provide excellent information for use in strategy development.

The BCG Matrix

To help organizations with strategic planning for products, the Boston Consulting Group (BCG) developed a product matrix that has become widely used in developing product strategy. The matrix considers growth potential and market share for different products or services an organization offers. The matrix is somewhat simplistic, assuming that each product or service has either a high or low market share and either a high or low potential for growth. The BCG framework is presented in Figure 18–1.

If a product has a high market share and a high potential for growth, it is considered a "star" performer in the BCG approach. It is clearly worthy of continued attention and efforts on the part of management. Just the reverse is true for a service with low current market share and low potential for growth. Management would not be using its time wisely to put substantial efforts into trying to market that product. BCG refers to such products as "dogs."

The other two cells in the matrix are less clear-cut. A product or service for which the organization has high market share but that has low growth potential is generally referred to as a "cash cow." Since there is a high market share, it is likely that the organization can charge a high price, generating substantial profits. Even if prices are not high, the high market share should mean that the organization has a cost advantage. It can spread the fixed costs over a larger

Figure 18–1. BCG matrix.

number of patients, generating a lower cost per patient than is possible for competitors with smaller market share. Therefore profits should still be high for cash cows.

Cash cows not only are profitable but also throw off cash dividends. A star is profitable, but its growth may require that much of the profit be reinvested in additional capacity. Since the growth potential is low for a cash cow, it often does not require reinvestment of the cash it generates. That cash is available for providing other services.

The last cell is referred to as a "problem child." Will its high growth potential be enough to offset the disadvantage of low market share? Over time this type of service may become either a dog or a star. Careful assessment is needed before investing resources in marketing this product.

Life-cycle Analysis

An alternative to the matrix developed by BCG is an approach called life-cycle analysis. Such analysis argues that early in the life of a new product or service, the organization will have a low market share in a product that has high growth potential (BCG's problem child). This is the new-product stage of the life cycle.

If the product's introduction is successful, it will become what BCG calls a star. That will represent a period when the organization has a significant market share in a growing market. The product will be profitable and growing. This is therefore considered the growth stage of the life cycle.

At some point, the growth potential will diminish; most of the pent-up demand for the new product will have been satisfied. There will have been a spurt of growth by competitors to the point that market demand is stable and is supplied by an existing set of organizations. Each will have its own market share, but no one will be having much growth. Although BCG terms this stage a cash cow, it is not at all clear that at this mature stage in the life cycle there will be substantial profits. BCG's model simplistically assumes high or low market share. It is possible to have a number of major competitors, which basically split the market and which compete to a point at which there are few if any profits.

When the product or service starts to be replaced by a new alternative, volume starts to drop. Since fixed costs cannot decline in the short term, profits drop sharply. It is this declining point in the life cycle of the product that BCG refers to as a dog. Figure 18–2 shows the volume potential likely at each stage in the life cycle of a product.

Strategically it is very important to remain aware of the stage of each of an organization's services. When a product reaches the dog or declining period, the organization should already have focused on the replacement product that consumers will need instead of the declining product and should have made substantial progress on introducing a new replacement product. Organizations that persist in simply stepping up their marketing efforts to keep selling an existing service often miss the boat. Marketing wisdom is not to sell the product you have but to provide the products and services that customers need and want. This means that marketing requires most organizations to constantly revise their thinking about what their product is and how it can best be provided to the customer.

As new innovations enter the health care marketplace, they impact on ex-

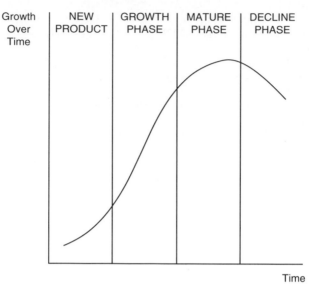

Figure 18–2. Product life cycle.

isting services. Figure 18–3 shows the history of diagnostic imaging. As nuclear imaging and ultrasound have become more widely used, the growth of x-rays has leveled off. PET scanning, on the other hand, is still in its early, new-product growth stages.

Choices of Strategy

The determination of where a product or service is in its life cycle has a direct bearing on the type of strategies that should be employed. Early in a product's life cycle the organization's strategy should be aggressive. Introduction of the product should be rapid, with an attempt to gain dominant market share before competitors can react. However, that does not require low price. Prices can be set high if there is little competition. However, it should be realized that the higher prices are set, the more competitors are encouraged that the potential benefits make it worthwhile to enter the market for that service or product. New products require an aggressive advertising campaign to inform the public about the product.

During the growth stage for the product it becomes important to differentiate the organization's product or service from that of any competitors. There needs to be some feature that would make the customers prefer the product offered by this organization. Obviously a unique superiority of the product is preferable. Failing that, the organization must decide if price, convenience, or some other factor can be affected to result in customer preference.

At a mature stage in a product's life cycle, most services are well established. The focus of marketing efforts is primarily on maintaining market share. Aggressive behavior will often not be rewarded—competitors with a major stake in the same service will not likely allow significant shifts in market share. Aggressiveness may well lead to a costly battle with competitors, with little gain if any in volume. Marketing becomes a maintenance operation. Slight modifications are made to the product to keep it current if possible, advertising efforts are made to reinforce customer awareness, and responses are made to repel the effects of any moves by competitors.

In the declining period of a product's life cycle the organization has a difficult choice. Should the organization try to establish its own special place in the declining market; should it gradually phase out a product; or should it drop the product completely? This question can only be answered by looking at each individual case.

Sometimes, even if a product is declining on an industry-wide basis, there is room for one provider. To be that provider it must be decided whether the key characteristic of the surviving provider will be price, service, convenience, or some other factor. Before it becomes too late, the organization must build a reputation in line with that characteristic. An advertising campaign late in a product's life may be worthwhile if it can convey the fact that the organization has that special feature that the ultimate survivor in the industry must have to attract sufficient volume. Loyalty among the base of customers who are likely to still be consuming the service in five years must be developed before it becomes too late in the decline of volume for the product or service.

Tactics

Strategies define the overall desired approach to marketing products and services. To carry out the strategy a set of tactics must be employed. Tactics represent the specific actions taken. The types of tactics generally considered have often been referred to as the four Ps of marketing: *product, price, place,* and *promotion.*

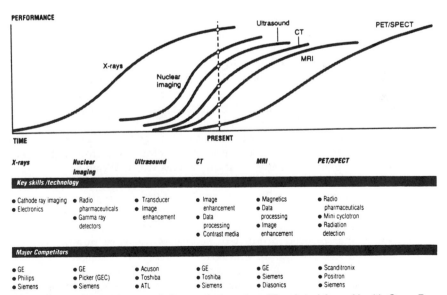

Figure 18–3. Development of diagnostic imaging. (Reprinted from *Health Care Forum Journal*, Vol. 32, No. 5, p. 25, with permission of the publisher, © 1989, Association of Western Hospitals.)

Product

The product is the essential element that the marketing plan is attempting to sell. The product has been selected and developed based on prior analysis of customer needs, the organization's mission, internal/external analysis, and finally strategy. However, several tactical issues must still be addressed about the product.

First of all, the organization must make a decision concerning the specific characteristics of the product, such as its quality. Will quality be the least the organization can get away with, average, or noteworthy? The actual decision relating to the level of quality is a strategic one. Carrying out the decision is tactical. How does one go about attaining a noteworthy level of quality? One approach is to attract famous surgeons to the staff and then let the public know. An alternative tactic would be to increase nursing care hours per patient day and inform the public of that fact and its positive implications. An alternative approach would be to beef up the quality assurance team. The choices of how to go about quality attainment are tactical.

Another feature is service. Again, it is a strategic question whether the organization is willing to incur the costs associated with high levels of service. But it is a matter of tactics whether service should consist of free taxi service to and from the organization. It might be worthwhile to have a host or hostess greeting patients upon arrival at the front door and taking them to admitting. Perhaps service should be provided in the form of follow-up phone calls several days after the service has been provided to ask about how the patient is doing and whether any further service can be provided. In some cases a basket of fruit awaiting the patient in the room might be appropriate. The key to service is to do more than expected, to go the one extra step to make the customer take note.

Nurse managers should consider their tactics carefully, since they often come into direct contact with two different classes of customers—the patients themselves and physicians. The marketing motto, "the customer is always right," can be irritating to anyone who actually must try to deal with a rude or irrational customer. Nurses, however, cope well with the irrationalities of patients, understanding how miserable it is to be sick. Nurses have on occasion shown a higher level of resentment of the other customer—the physician.

One hears many anecdotes about physicians who mess up and need nurses to save the day. There is no question that nurses serve a vital role and that physicians could not get along without them. However, from a marketing perspective, that result is exactly what one would want. When physicians feel that they receive no direct benefit from a hospital, they start providing a greater range of patient services, including surgery, out of their own offices. The reason that physicians rely on hospitals, even for outpatient surgery, is that the hospital provides some desired product or service to the physician as a customer. In many cases that desired product or service is the very nursing care that many physicians *seem* to take for granted.

As long as the physician is a key element in bringing the ultimate paying customer into a health care organization such as a hospital, the physician remains a customer, and the organization must respond by developing a set of tactics to keep the customer coming to this organization. One reason many hospitals provide unequal treatment to doctors and nurses is not a question of professionalism; it stems to a much greater extent from the fact that doctors are viewed as customers, while nurses are viewed as employees.

Viewing doctors as customers results in attempts by organizations to determine their needs. A strategy might be to increase efforts to make the organization accessible to affiliated physicians. If a particular physician wants OR time at 7 AM on Tuesdays, then a tactic to carry out the strategy is development of a specific incentive for other surgeons to use the OR on days other than Tuesday. That incentive might be a special effort to assign specific OR nurses requested by surgeons on days other than Tuesday.

Price

Price matters. Many people assume that with most of the population insured by Medicare, Medicaid, Blue Cross, or other private insurers, price does not matter. However, a growing portion of the buyers of health care services are becoming sensitive to price variations. HMOs and PPOs negotiate aggressively for the best prices they can obtain. Each organization must determine how sensitive its customers are to price and base a policy accordingly.

There are a number of different approaches to setting prices. Some organizations like to simply use a *markup*. That is, they determine the cost of providing care and raise, or mark up, their price a certain percentage over the cost. The problem with this policy is that the low-volume producer will have the highest cost (because fixed costs are not shared over a large volume of patients) and therefore the highest price. It will be difficult to increase volume and therefore reduce costs and reduce prices if you start out as a high-priced producer.

Another alternative is to charge a particularly low price, perhaps even lower than cost, to gain a substantial increase in market share. The philosophy is that even though you may lose money on each patient, as volume increases, average cost will decrease and patients will eventually become profitable at the price being charged. Further, capturing a substantial share of the market may force other providers to discontinue offering the product or service. When there are fewer providers, it may be possible to raise prices to increase the profit margin. Legal input is required to ensure that price is not set so low that it would violate antitrust laws.

Another tactic is to charge a high price, knowing that market share will be low, but planning to make a high profit on the volume achieved. This is sometimes referred to as *skimming*.

There are many other tactical approaches to price setting. The organization can charge different prices depending on the time of the day or the day of the week. For example, if an HMO wants a discounted price, a hospital that is running near capacity can offer the discount only if most patients are admitted during slower periods. For example, the HMO can agree that operations on its patients will take place on weekends or other slow days or during the slower parts of the day. In this way the organization can continue to take all full-price patients at the time most convenient for the patients and their physicians. The patients with the price break will give up some convenience for the lower price.

Place

In real estate the three most important factors that establish the value of property are location, location, and location. In marketing health care services much the same is true. Traditional health care services generally expect the patient to come to the service. If the service is in an inconvenient location, it will be difficult to attract patients. While home health agencies generally visit patients, many other health care services have lagged in coming to the patient. However, more innovative approaches to health care services do make attempts to bring the services closer to the patients. For example, there are now national mail-order pharmacies. Many disabled patients can avoid the high cost of a taxi to go to and from the pharmacy.

The issue of "place" is closely tied to the concept of *distribution channels*. The concept of distribution channels relates to moving the product from the producer to the consumer. How does the product get from the provider of the service to the ultimate consumer? In the case of a home care agency, the provider brings the product directly to the patient. In the case of a hospital, the patient comes to the provider. Clearly, if the distribution channel can be modified to bring the product closer to the consumer, there is a better chance of being the provider of choice.

Distribution channels are referred to as being direct or indirect, depending on whether the consumer and the provider have a direct relationship or whether there is some intermediary. When a patient is admitted to a hospital on the advice of a personal physician, there is an indirect channel between the patient and the hospital. The hospital is at risk if the intermediary—the physician—decides to use a different hospital. If the hospital opens a series of clinics around the community staffed with full-time physician employees of the hospital, then the distribution channel is direct.

Clearly, it is to the advantage of a health care provider to have a direct channel to the patient. However, this arrangement creates its own costs and risks. In the above example the hospital must take on the burden of operating a series of clinics. The clinics may be unprofitable, more than offsetting the advantage of the direct linkage. They may also alienate the other physicians in the community who resent the hospital's competition. A hospital must adopt a strategy concerning whether it wants to establish direct channels of distribution or is willing to accept indirect channels.

One potential solution to this problem is to arrange a confederation with one or more physician group practices. Figure 18–4 presents a possible form for such an arrangement. The group practice and the hospital each provide half the members of a management committee. The committee gives the physicians a greater amount of input in running the hospital. The hospital gains a direct distribution channel.

Once the strategic decision regarding the use of direct or indirect channels is made, tactics must be developed. If the strategy is to employ direct channels, then the tactics concern the exact location of clinics and their size, staffing pattern, and hours. If the strategy is acceptance of indirect channels, then the tactics concern the actions the hospital could take to keep the referring physicians happy and ensure that they do not start referring patients elsewhere. The tactics are less certain here, and a great deal of effort must go into determining what factors influence where a physician refers patients. If the key issue is attending to physician needs, then someone should call the physician periodically to ask whether the hospital is doing all it can for the physician. If the key issue is available beds when needed, then the hospital must develop

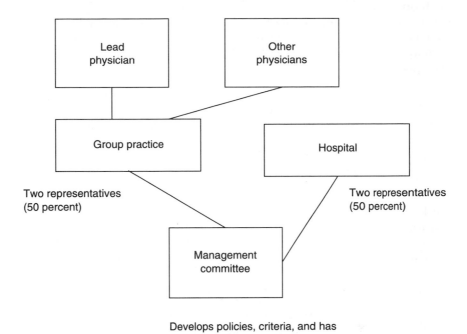

Develops policies, criteria, and has
decision making authority

Figure 18–4. Direct distribution channel. (Reprinted from Deborah Arbitman and Paul King, "Affiliated Practices Can Boost Patient Referrals," *Healthcare Financial Management,* August 1990, p. 34, with permission of Healthcare Financial Management Association.)

an admission process that ensures that certain physicians always get a bed when they need it.

Which physician should always get a bed? Should it be the one with the largest number of admissions? Or should it be a marginal physician? That is a difficult tactical issue. The physician with the largest number of admissions may not be in a position to move from this hospital, while a marginal physician may be quite likely to move. Health care providers must carefully consider the long-run implications of their tactics. Then they can make a reasoned decision about what approach is likely to be in the best interests of the organization.

Promotion

The last of the four tactical concerns is the one most people associate with marketing—promotion. Promotion consists of advertising, public relations, sales promotion, and personal selling, as was discussed earlier. The strategy of the organization will determine which products or services will receive significant promotion in a given period. The tactical questions revolve around what combination of the four promotion approaches to use and how to go about each one.

Tactics determine whether to use print media or radio or television. Tactics focus on which newspapers or magazines; on which radio or television programs; on what day of the week; on what time of the day. Should nurse managers be encouraged to teach in local nursing schools as a means of public relations? Should they be paid by the health care provider while they are teaching? How much money should be spent on mass advertising and how much on a personal sales force?

For a home care agency, advertising creates a general public awareness. However, most patients arrive as referrals by physicians, social workers, or discharge-planning nurses. One full-time sales person will likely reach only 1,000 people per year. The advertisements that could be bought for the same money might reach hundreds of thousands. Tactically, however, one must decide which is a better buy for the money and whether the money is wisely spent on either alternative.

• • •

While the four Ps of marketing are widely discussed, it is a mistake to view marketing as a subject that can be mastered through simple tools such as a BCG matrix or memorizing that tactics often fall under the rubric of the classic four Ps. Hillestad and Berkowitz note that every detail can have an impact on a customer, either positive or negative. Things as small as the little alligator on a sport shirt, a 30-minute pizza delivery guarantee, a call-back from a nurse, or a handwritten note to a referral physician—all examples of marketing tactics—can all have an impact. The depth and breadth of marketing decisions are enormous, as are the opportunities to make mistakes. Service, design, packaging of the service, promotion, location, and pricing are all interwoven to make for hundreds of possible combinations for any given service.[4]

Revision, Integration, and Implementation

Once the marketing plan is developed, it must be reviewed by top management and accepted, revised, or rejected. Management must review the plan with several key factors in mind. First of all, does the plan make sense given the mission of the organization? There may be huge potential profits from selling unproven cancer cures. It may fill a customer desire, and it may be easy to price and promote. However, if it goes against the principles of the organization, it will have to be rejected. The focus on organizational mission as the basis for the marketing plan should result in a plan that will likely call for products and services that are within the mission of the organization.

Does the internal/external analysis seem to be thorough? The plan relies upon the quality of that analysis to determine the relative position of the organization and the ultimate needs of the customers.

Do the strategies proposed respond to customer needs? Generally, a marketing plan will require the organization to make significant commitments of resources and in many cases significant changes in operations. This should not happen unless the strategies are reasoned responses to the needs of the customers in light of the relative positions of the organization and its competition. Are the tactics designed to ensure that the strategies are implemented efficiently?

If the marketing plan is accepted or sent back for revisions and then accepted after revision, it becomes critical to implement the plan not only via promotion

---

[4]Ibid., p. 149.

but also operationally throughout the organization. Marketing plans do not stand alone in an organization. The marketing plan must be integrated. It makes little sense to find out what people need and develop a plan to market that product or service without the organization's taking the various necessary actions to produce that service. Often the key to such integration is communication. The plan should not be a secret. Major strategies and individual tactics are not carried out by the marketing department but by the line staff of the organization. Nurse managers and the nursing staff are often the key to implementing many of the strategies and tactics required for the success of a marketing plan.

It does little good to advertise a health care organization as one with an extra degree of attention for the patient while changing nothing about day-to-day operations. If a strategy is adopted to provide extra attention, then the resources must be provided and the specific tactics implemented. Perhaps that means hiring a host or hostess for each unit.

Essentially, it is necessary for the marketing plan to be shared so that each cost center of the organization can evaluate its impact on the operational activities. Then the cost centers can determine the impact in terms of personnel changes and other costs. Those impacts can then be factored into the budget for the coming year. In this way the marketing plan does not stand alone but provides the resources needed to implement the changes that the plan calls for.

It should become clear that marketing does play a more substantial role than simply advertising the organization's products. Marketing is integral to deciding what products or services should be offered. When the plan is adopted, it creates change in what products and services are offered. In light of that, nursing managers should not treat informational requests from marketing as a peripheral annoyance to be handled quickly and without much thought. Six months later the decisions based on that information will come back in specific operational changes. Marketing has a significant and growing role in health care organizations, and interactions between nursing and marketing warrant careful thought and attention.

Control and Feedback

Once a marketing plan has been accepted and implemented, it is necessary to control the various aspects of the plan to ensure that it is being carried out. Generally, this means that information must be collected on how the tactics are being implemented and whether the implementation is appropriate to carry out the strategies decided upon and to achieve the goals of the plan.

For example, many nursing units around the country are hiring hosts or hostesses for each unit to relieve nurses of a number of time-consuming burdens that could be handled by a less trained individual. Many of these tasks are of a nonclinical educational nature. Showing families of patients where the waiting rooms and telephones are is an example. Other examples are explaining to the families how strict or lenient visiting hour regulations are or informing families how to inquire as to patient status.

When the marketing plan was envisioned, the intention may have been that this person would also greet arriving patients at the front door and take them to admitting, or that the host or hostess would bring a fruit basket to the patient shortly after admission. If that tactic is not being carried out, then the plan loses a minor but significant element—providing the unexpected benefit or service.

There should be a formal process by which there is reporting on which tactics have been implemented. The reporting must be specific; it is inadequate to simply indicate that a host or hostess has been hired for each unit. Furthermore, there must be feedback directly from the customers. Physicians and patients should be polled, asking their satisfaction levels at various points in time to see if the changes are having any attitudinal impact. And of course there should be quantitative measures in terms of patient volume to allow for tracking the success of the plan.

MARKETING FAILURES

It would be nice to believe that any organization that realizes the potential benefits of marketing will succeed in its marketing efforts. Unfortunately, that is not always the case. History has shown that many marketing campaigns do fail. Learning from those failures should help others to avoid them.

It is true that sometimes everything will be done right and marketing efforts will still fail. However, avoiding certain common shortcomings can reduce the likelihood of that result. Specifically, common failures are often due to several specific factors.

One major problem is failure to collect data prior to making decisions. Decisions based solely on intuition may fail after substantial financial investment, when a modest amount of market research data collection could have indicated that the financial investment was unwise.

Another problem relates to errors of analysis. Data may be collected but not carefully interpreted. One key concern that managers should have is that new products and services often have strong advocates. Such people may not neutrally evaluate information, since they have a vested interest in its interpretation.

A third key element common to failure is a lack of clear objectives. Marketing should not be rushed without careful consideration of exactly what needs to be accomplished. Focusing the marketing plan carefully on a specific set of objectives increases the likelihood of achieving them.

Finally, many organizations use incorrect tactics. It is important that carrying out the objectives of a plan be done in light of the specific clearly stated objectives. The tactics must fully and directly support the accomplishment of the goals that have been set.

THE ROLE OF MARKETING IN NURSE RECRUITMENT

There have been nursing shortages periodically throughout this century. When a health care provider is attempting to hire nurses, those nurses effectively become customers from a marketing perspective. In attempting to minimize the impact of a nursing shortage on an organization, a variety of marketing techniques can be employed. For example, advertising is often used to attract new nurse employees, and advertising is one element of marketing.

However, as was noted a number of times above, marketing does not start with advertising. It starts with the identification of the need or desire and the filling of that need or desire. These elements must precede the advertising.

Only then can a specific plan be developed regarding the communication of the strengths that the organization has to offer. The role of marketing in nurse recruitment was discussed in Chapter 9.

IMPLICATIONS FOR NURSE MANAGERS

Marketing activities are much more highly related to nursing management than most nurses realize. The first and most vital aspect of marketing is assessing the needs and desires of the customers of the organization. Nurses are in a position to be very attuned to those needs and desires, both in the case of patients and in the case of physicians.

Another major aspect of marketing is assessing the capabilities of the organization. Here again, the input of nurses is vital to gaining a clear understanding of the strengths and limitations of the organization.

The strategic and tactical issues of marketing also warrant close cooperation between nursing and marketing. Nurses are unlikely to enthusiastically work to carry out organizational strategies that they cannot support. Therefore, there should be substantive discussions between nursing and marketing as strategies are developed. Nurses should give direct input on what strategies they think are good, which ones are bad, and why. Similarly, since nursing units will be operationalizing many of the specific tactics to implement the strategies, they must have some say in the establishment of what those tactics will be.

Cost is also an important factor in marketing. The marketing department will proudly point out gains in patient volume. The nursing department will incur additional costs to implement new products, services, strategies, and tactics. There must be a clear relationship between the expectations of a marketing plan and the additional resources provided to nursing units to carry out their aspect of the plan.

Marketing plans are generally prepared by marketing experts. There will likely be times that nurses are called upon to develop a business plan for a new product or service, including the marketing plan aspects. In such cases an understanding of the marketing concepts discussed in this chapter is essential for the nurse manager. However, it would be wise for the nurse manager to employ consultants who are experts at marketing. Conducting an internal/ external analysis and developing marketing strategies and marketing tactics are tasks that require a great deal of marketing experience and in-depth expertise about marketing techniques. A poor marketing plan is not necessarily better than nothing. It can mistakenly lead to the commitment of resources in a doomed venture. Working together, nurse managers and marketing managers can provide a health care organization with significant benefits from the use of marketing techniques.

Nursing departments should consider having their own marketing plan for internal marketing. The nurse's customers include other nurses, physicians, patients, and other hospital staff. Determining the needs of each customer group can improve outcomes for both the customers and nursing.

Marketing is also important as nurses become more and more entrepreneurial in their focus. There has been a growing trend of nurses starting health care businesses. These range from home care agencies through drug treatment clinics. Nurses venturing out in innovative ways will need to concern themselves with the concepts of marketing.

KEY CONCEPTS _____

Marketing Management science that attempts to maintain and increase the organization's patient volume. High volume is desirable because of its favorable financial implications.

Essence of marketing To enable the organization to determine what customers want or need and to develop and offer those goods or services.

Market Potential customers for a product or organization. Information about the market will affect not only the mix of services that should be offered but also the advertising message, price, and other critical factors.

Determinant attributes Factors that ultimately impact on a consumer's purchase decision. There are two major types: decision variables and environmental variables. Decision variables are factors controllable by the organization that can affect volume. Environmental variables are factors that can affect volume but that are not controllable by the organization.

Market segmentation Division of the market into several specific subsections. In general, segmentation is based on three factors: each group must have distinct and measurable needs; it is vital that one can access the specific segments; and each segment must be big enough to merit a distinct effort.

Customer behavior Customers perceive a need; become aware of a provider's existence; become knowledgeable about the provider and the provider's service; develop a liking for a service and then a preference for the service, followed by a conviction to acquire that provider's service, followed by the acquisition of that provider's service; and finally have an after-the-fact reaction to the purchase. At any point up until the purchase, a customer may decide to purchase a competitor's product instead.

Market measurement Conversion of qualitative information into quantitative estimates of demand.

Market share Portion or percentage of the overall market that a specific organization controls.

Market research Gathering, recording, and analyzing information to improve decisions made by the organization. Market research is needed to determine what the customer really wants and is willing to buy. The major areas for market research are advertising, business economics, products, and sales.

Marketing plan Plan that first considers the organizational mission and goals and then, based on the results of an internal/external analysis, develops a set of strategies and tactics designed to increase the organization's volume of patients. Plans must then be revised, integrated, and implemented. Control and feedback are also essential to an effective plan.

Strategies Broad plans for the attainment of goals. Marketing strategies define the overall desired approach to marketing products and services.

Tactics Specific activities that are undertaken to carry out a strategy. The four Ps of marketing—product, price, place, and promotion—relate to tactics aimed at implementing marketing strategies.

Implementation of marketing plan   Marketing plays a more substantial role than simply advertising the organization's products. When the marketing plan is adopted, it creates change in what products and services are offered. It creates changes in the way services are produced through the strategies and specific tactics it contains. It also results in changes in the allocation of resources throughout the organization.

SUGGESTED READINGS ————————————————————

Barigar, Denise L., and Marian L. Sheafor, "Recruiting Staff Nurses: A Marketing Approach," *Nursing Management*, Vol. 21, No. 1, January 1990, pp. 27–29.

Duro, Robert, and Bjorn Sandstrom, *The Basic Principles of Marketing Warfare*, John Wiley & Sons, New York, 1987.

Frand, Erwin A., *The Art of Product Development: From Concept to Market*, Dow Jones–Irwin, Homewood, IL, 1989.

Johnson, Joyce E., Alicia C. Arvidson, Linda L. Costa, et al., "Marketing Your Nursing Product Line," *Journal of Nursing Administration*, Vol. 17, No. 11, November 1987, pp. 29–33.

Hillestad, Steven G., and Eric N. Berkowitz, *Health Care Marketing Plans: From Strategy to Action*, 2nd edition, Aspen Publishers, Gaithersburg, MD, 1991.

Ireson, Carol, and Diana Weaver, "Marketing Nursing Beyond the Walls," *Journal of Nursing Administration*, Vol. 22, No. 1, January 1992, pp. 57–60.

Kiener, M.E., "Market Segmentation and Positioning: Matching Creativity with Fiscal Responsibility," *Journal of Continuing Education in the Health Professions*, Vol. 9, No. 2, 1989, pp. 77–86.

Kotler, Philip, *Marketing Management, Analysis, Planning and Control*, 3rd edition, Prentice-Hall, Englewood Cliffs, NJ, 1976.

Magrath, Allan J., *Market Smarts: Proven Strategies to Outfox and Outflank Your Competition*, John Wiley & Sons, New York, 1988.

Porter, Rosemary T., Michael J. Porter, and Mary S. Lower, "Enhancing the Image of Nursing," *Journal of Nursing Administration*, Vol. 19, No. 2, February 1989, pp. 36–42.

Rados, David L., *Marketing for Non-Profit Organizations*, Auburn House Publishing Company, Boston, 1981.

Ries, Al, and Jack Trout, *Bottom-Up Marketing*, McGraw-Hill, New York, 1989.

Sonnenberg, Frank K., *Marketing to Win: Strategies for Building Competitive Advantage in Service Industries*, Harper Business, Division of Harper & Row, New York, 1990.

Stefflre, Volney, *Developing and Implementing Marketing Strategies*, Praeger, New York, 1986.

Strasen, Leann, *Key Business Skills for Nurse Managers*, J.B. Lippincott, New York, 1987.

Taylor, Tucker, "Healthcare Marketing and the Nurse Manager," *Nursing Management*, Vol. 21, No. 5, May 1990, pp. 84–85.

Washburn, Stewart A., *Managing the Marketing Functions: The Challenge of the Customer-Centered Enterprise*, McGraw-Hill, New York, 1988.

Weitz, Barton A., and Robin Wensley, *Strategic Marketing: Planning, Implementation, and Control*, Kent Publishing Co., Boston, 1984.

THE FUTURE

19

Nursing and Financial Management: Current Issues and Future Directions

CHAPTER GOALS

The goals of this chapter are to:

- Review the current nursing literature on financial management
- Discuss the skills that will be required of nurse managers to assume an expanded role in financial management
- Discuss the pros and cons of nurses' assuming more responsibility for financial management
- Discuss the differences in responsibility for varying levels of nurse managers
- Discuss the nurse entrepreneur role
- Discuss the role of the nurse as policy manager

❖

INTRODUCTION

In the role of manager, nurses perform a variety of functions related to financial management. To perform these functions as efficiently as possible, nurse managers must be aware of current issues in the field of financial management in nursing. This chapter will review current issues identified in the nursing literature. Discussion of the future of the nurses' role in financial management follows. By having a sense of the current issues and future directions in nursing as it relates to financial management, nurse managers will be in a better position to "work smarter, not harder." The most important thing for managers to avoid is complacency. The role of a manager includes innovation. Innovation, however, is only occasionally the result of inspiration. Often it is the product of careful attention to the changing world and what others have done in an attempt to cope with changing realities.

There is some disagreement among nurses about whether nursing financial management is nursing or financial management. We believe nursing financial management is a blend of both fields and as such is also a subset of nursing. Many nursing leaders argue that only studies about patients (clients) and the nursing interventions associated with these clients are the purview of nursing. We believe that nursing includes the organization and delivery of nursing care. Nursing financial management is a part of that general area of nursing.

NURSING FINANCIAL MANAGEMENT RESEARCH

The nurse researcher can serve as a key player in both financial management of organizations and the development of public policy that impacts on financial management of organizations. If we believe that research can give us a greater understanding of the way the world works, research can be used to impact on nursing financial management. Studies about the costs of care can influence the way care is delivered and also government policy.

Review of a profession's research and literature can provide insight into the current issues in the field. Research can be described as a continuum from theoretical to applied. Most people would agree that research is the development or testing of theory. Nursing financial management research includes studies such as those which look at market behavior (how nurses respond to recruitment and retention efforts might be based on this theory), management science (how CEOs respond to first-line nurse managers having authority and responsibility for unit finances), or nursing science (how power relates to the allocation of resources in a hospital). The applied result of research in areas such as these has been included in our discussion throughout the book.

Research Taxonomies for Nursing Financial Management

There are two major taxonomies for nursing research. One was developed by Sigma Theta Tau International. The other is the Classification of Nursing-Related Dissertations (DISSER).[1] The Sigma taxonomy uses the category "systems research," while the DISSER schema uses "nurses and nursing profession." Nursing financial management falls into both these categories. In addition, the National Center for Nursing Research has a Division of Nursing Systems, under which nursing financial management falls.

---

[1]Elaine Larson, Margaret Dear, and Margaret Keitkemper, "Comparison of Two Schema for Classifying Nursing Research," *Image*, Vol. 23, No. 3, Fall 1991, pp. 167–170.

In reviewing these taxonomies, one finds that there is little research toward the theoretical end of the spectrum in the area of nursing financial management. Most financial management theoretical research takes place within the strict disciplines of accounting and finance. The research in the area of nursing financial management tends to apply theoretical developments in accounting or finance to nursing or health administration in general.

There is a body of literature in applied nursing financial management research. One major element falls under the general rubric of policy and evaluation research. These studies describe how resources are allocated and explore relationships about the cost and financing of nursing care. Many of these studies look at the cost-benefit ratio of various approaches to providing nursing care, study the impact of various innovations on nursing costs, and develop instruments to measure the cost of providing care. Many of the cost studies use economic and/or organizational theory as the theoretical framework to answer questions. Others use no theoretical framework but rather describe the relationships among variables. The health services research in nursing literature from 1980 to 1989 was reviewed, and it was found that 22.1% of the articles were on the cost of health care and 12.4% were on productivity.[2]

In addition to the policy and evaluation research literature, increasing numbers of articles in nursing journals are about the application of financial techniques. This is another form of applied research. Almost every issue of the major nursing management journals has at least one article on the financial aspects of nursing. Likely future trends in nursing financial management can be assessed from this applied research. From a review of nursing journals for the period 1988 to 1991, several general areas related to nursing financial management emerged.

CURRENT ISSUES IN FINANCIAL MANAGEMENT IN NURSING

The broad categories of nursing financial management that recent literature focused on are (1) allocation of nursing resources[3]; (2) financial incentives and

---

[2]Gail Ingersoll, Nancy Hoffart, and Alison W. Schultz, "Health Services Research in Nursing: Current Status and Future Directions," *Nursing Economics*, Vol. 8, No. 4, 1990, pp. 229–238.
[3]For example, Kathleen G. Behner, Louis F. Fogg, Linda C. Fournier, et al., "Nursing Resource Management: Analyzing the Relationship Between Costs and Quality in Staffing Decisions," *Health Care Management Review*, Vol. 15, No. 4, Fall 1990, pp. 63–71; Janet Bostrom and Malinda Mitchel, "Relationship of Direct Nursing Care Hours to DRG and Severity of Illness," *Nursing Economics*, Vol. 9, No. 2, 1991, pp. 105–111; Sandra Edwardson and Patricia Nardone, "Resource Use in Home Care Agencies," *Applied Nursing Research*, Vol. 4, No. 1, February 1991, pp. 25–30; Gerry Hendrickson, Theresa M. Doddato, and Christine T. Kovner, "How Do Nurses Use Their Time?" *Journal of Nursing Administration*, Vol. 20, No. 3, March 1990, pp. 31–37; T. R. Misener, A. J. Frelin, and P. A. Twoist, "Sampling Nursing Time Pinpoints Staffing Need," *Nursing and Health Care*, Vol. 8, No. 4, April 1987, pp. 233–237; and Sharon Holcombe Servais, "Nursing Resource Applications Through Outcome Based Nursing Practice," *Nursing Economics*, Vol. 9, No. 3, 1991, p. 171.

compensation[4]; (3) the cost impact of various models of nursing care[5]; (4) measuring the cost of nursing care[6]; and (5) system-wide approaches to decreasing the cost of care.[7] Other articles covered a wide variety of financial management issues.[8]

A major concern in nursing is how to allocate scarce nursing resources efficiently and effectively.[9] Questions remain. What level of management should make the decisions about staffing? Who decides how much of the organization's resources should go to staffing and/or how many nursing care hours patients should receive? Can nursing decide patient care hours but not control the resources to buy those hours? Does shared governance mean control over fiscal resources as well as clinical practice? Can they be sepa-

---

[4]For example, Eunice A. Bell and Barbara D. Bart, "Pay for Performance: Motivating the Chief Nurse Executive," *Nursing Economics*, Vol. 9, No. 2, 1991, p. 92; Janice Faulkner, "Salary Equals Performance for Community Health Nurses," *Nursing Management*, Vol. 22, No. 6, 1991, pp. 28–32; Charlene Harrington, "Wages & Benefits of Nursing Personnel in Nursing Homes: Correcting the Inequities," *Nursing Economics*, Vol. 8, No. 6, November/December 1990, pp. 378–385; Sharon E. Hoffman and Marsha E. Fonteyn, "Third Party Reimbursement for CNS Consultation," *Nursing Economics*, Vol. 6, No. 5, 1988, p. 245; Joanne C. McCloskey, "Implications of Costing Out Nursing Services for Reimbursement," *Nursing Management*, Vol. 20, No. 1, January 1989, pp. 44–49; Elizabeth Manco, Kathleen Russel-Babin, and Sheryl Stevens, "An Incentive Program . . . More than Just R & R," *Nursing Management*, Vol. 22, No. 1, 1991, pp. 49–53; Mary Etta Mills, "Nursing Compensation: The Realities of Seeking Equity," *Nursing Economics*, Vol. 7, No. 5, 1989, pp. 270–272; Gaye W. Porter, Linda C. Hodges, and Nannette Goddard, "Financial Responsibilities and Preparation of Chief Nurse Executives," *Nursing Economics*, Vol. 9, No. 5, September 1991, pp. 305–309; and Helen K. Sullivan, "Developing an Incentive Program for Home Health Nurses," *Nursing Economics*, Vol. 7, No. 6, 1989, pp. 310–313.

[5]For example, Judy L. Brett and Mary C. Tonges, "Restructured Patient Care Delivery: Evaluation of the ProACT TM Model," *Nursing Economics*, Vol. 8, No. 1, January/February 1990, pp. 36–44; Gerald L. Glandon, Kenneth W. Colbert, and Mary Thomasa, "Nursing Delivery Models and RN Mix; Cost Implications," *Nursing Management*, Vol. 20, No. 5, May 1989, pp. 30–33; Phyllis Ethridge, "A Nursing HMO: Carondelet St. Mary's Experience," *Nursing Management*, Vol. 22, No. 7, 1991, pp. 22–27; Kathryn G. Gardner and Mary Tilbury, " A Longitudinal Cost Analysis of Primary and Team Nursing," *Nursing Economics*, Vol. 9, No. 2, 1991, pp. 97–104; and Michael Rogers, Jan Riordan, and Donna Swindle, "Community-Based Nursing Case Management Pays Off," *Nursing Management*, Vol. 22, No. 3, March 1991, pp. 30–34.

[6]For example, Marjorie C. Budd and Toni Proptnik, "A Computerized System for Staffing, Billing, and Productivity Measurement," *Journal of Nursing Administration*, Vol. 19, No. 7, July/August 1989, pp. 17–22; Diane Hamm-Vida, "Cost of Non-Nursing Tasks," *Nursing Management*, Vol. 21, No. 4, April 1990, pp. 46–52; and Phyllis M. Watson, Mary S. Lower, Susan M. Wells, et al., "Discovering What Nurses Do and What It Costs," *Nursing Management*, Vol. 22, No. 5, 1991, pp. 38–45.

[7]For example, Patricia A. Prescott, "Forecasting Requirements for Health Care Personnel," *Nursing Economics*, Vol. 9, No. 1, January/February 1991, pp. 18–24.

[8]For example, Hurdis Griffith, Gail Tumulty, and Barbara Nelson, "Participation of Nurse Executives in Product Decisions," *Nursing Economics*, Vol. 8, No. 2, 1990, pp. 90–93.

[9]See note 3.

rated? There continues to be discussion about the use of acuity systems for staffing.[10]

Financial compensation is an emerging issue.[11] How should nurses be compensated? Can productivity be improved by altering the way nurses are compensated? Should the CNE's compensation be based on a bonus system? Should an organization contract with nurses to provide care on a capitation basis?

When one thinks about issues in financial management, one usually thinks about the cost impact of various models of nursing care.[12] Does the use of technology change the cost of providing care? Are nurse/nurse-extender partnerships more cost effective than modular nursing? What are the pricing levels at which is it more cost effective to recruit new nurses than to retain current staff?

Measuring the cost of nursing care continues to be an issue in the 1990s. Although most CNEs agree that they must measure the cost of nursing care, discussion continues about the level of that measurement and how to do it in the least costly way.[13] Does the CNE need to measure cost of providing nursing care to each patient? To similar patients? By unit? By nurse? Is it acceptable to use acuity systems developed for staffing to estimate the costs of care already provided? How should indirect costs be allocated? Do patients requiring more direct care also require more indirect care? Does it matter how accurately this is measured?

Finally there were many articles on the financial aspects of the health care system that affect nursing. These included articles about financial management techniques. There were of course many articles on the nursing shortage of the late 1980s. Many of these articles dealt with financial issues, such as scholarships for nursing education. Other articles dealt with broader health care issues such as whether we should have a national health insurance system. How should it be structured? Should there be direct third-party reimbursement for nursing services? Is rationing health care the solution to controlling costs?

THE DEVELOPING ROLE OF THE CHIEF NURSE EXECUTIVE (CNE) IN FINANCIAL MANAGEMENT

Health care organizations are dynamic. They are in a constant state of flux. To maximize opportunities in such a situation, managers must be flexible in defining their role. A decade ago nurse managers might have been astonished to be asked to participate in the development of a business plan. Yet today CNEs have become key players in business plan development at many hospitals and other health care organizations. The role of CNEs and other nurse managers clearly has been changing and likely will continue to change. Specifically, the CNE's role in the area of financial management is likely to continue to expand.

---

[10]Ann Van Slyck, "A Systems Approach to the Management of Nursing Services, Part IV: Costing System," *Nursing Management*, Vol. 22, No. 6, August 1991, pp. 14–16.
[11]See note 4.
[12]See note 5.
[13]See note 6.

Andrica reported on a national sample of CNEs of hospitals that indicated that CNEs are responsible for operating budgets of from $5 to $333 million. The same study reports that 79% of CNEs were responsible for the OR and 71% had the ER within their realm of authority.[14] Although in the past the CNE went to the CEO and asked for a budget of $20 million for "her" department, more often than not the CNE now attends board of trustees meeting, sits on the executive committee of the organization, and is an active voice in the decision-making process for the allocation of all the organization's resources to all departments, not just nursing. In home health agencies the management team may consist almost entirely of nurses.

A more recent study surveyed a sample of members of the American Organization of Nurse Executives. Of survey respondents, 82% reported working in decentralized organizations (see the Chapter 3 discussion of centralization vs. decentralization).[15] Sixty-two percent reported decentralization to the unit level. However, only 24.8% reported using zero-based budgeting, and 35.4% reported using flexible budgeting. Most respondents reported that they used a computer printout from a mainframe to monitor nursing budgets. For those hospitals with decentralized budgeting, 55% used microcomputer-based generic spreadsheet-generated data for budgeting. Only 19% reported employing a financial person in the nursing department.

In the future the responsibility and authority for financial management by nurses is likely to expand at all levels of the organization. It does not require extraordinary imagination to realize that the CNE role will expand to participating in decisions to issue bonds for financing new buildings or for merging with competitors. Topics in this book such as financial statement analysis (Chapter 6) may reflect tools needed on a frequent basis by the typical CNE before the end of this decade. As the role expands for top management, the role of midlevel nurse managers will also likely expand. Midlevel and first-line managers will have increasing responsibility for financial management.

Setting Organizational Policy

The CNE's role will likely expand to include a greater role in setting organizational policy about financial matters.[16] As more CNEs participate in trustee meetings, trustees may look to the CNE for explanations about rising costs and, more important, options for restraining costs and increasing revenues. Often tactics require reorganization of the way services are provided. The CNE can play a key role in developing and proposing such strategies. It is likely that in more organizations nurses will become part of the top management team that makes policy decisions about finances.

A generation of CNEs is emerging who are academically prepared to more actively participate in financial management. Courses in budgeting and finance are now required in many graduate programs in nursing management. Some nurse managers are choosing joint MBA-MSN programs, and others are choos-

---

[14]Diane C. Andrica, "Changing Profiles of Nurse Executives," *Nursing Economics*, Vol. 6, No. 3, May/June 1988, pp. 112–115.
[15]Gaye W. Porter, Linda C. Hodges, and Nannette Goddard, "Financial Responsibilities and Preparation of Chief Nurse Executives," *Nursing Economics*, Vol. 9, No. 5, September 1991, pp. 305–309.
[16]Ibid.

ing graduate study in health management. As these educated nurses seek information on the financial operation of the organization and make informed observations, many senior financial managers will embrace their new colleagues as members of the executive team. Others will be threatened by the nurse manager's newfound knowledge and will put up subtle barriers to the nurse manager's full involvement in financial decision making.

The 1990s will continue the cost restraints seen in the 1980s. In an effort at fiscal solvency, it is likely that CEOs and boards will hold the CNE accountable for high-quality care at a cost the organization can survive with. The informed CNE must know enough about the financial condition of the organization to know with what costs it can in fact survive.

As information generation improves, partly through the use of computers, the CNE will have the information necessary to look at the financial management of specific units and even specific staff in the organization. The CNE will likely ask the midlevel managers to assume greater accountability and responsibility for fiscal matters, although the amount of accountability at the unit level will likely continue to vary by organization.

Intraorganizational Responsibility for Expenses

The CNE in virtually all health care organizations is currently responsible for the direct operating expense budget of the nursing department. In almost all organizations the CNE has a high degree of control of this budget. The CNE may be told to cut 3% off the budget, but in most organizations how that is done is a department decision. In some organizations the CEO may say to cut 3% but not to cut any positions. In many organizations salary increases are set by top management, with the CNE being intimately involved in these decisions, whether the raise is part of an organized labor settlement or not.

In most organizations the CNE has less control over indirect expenses and the allocation of those expenses to the nursing department. The CNE also has less control over the capital budget than over the direct department expenses. The CEO and the CFO control the expenses of the other departments and the allocation of these expenses to nursing. Various departments and the key members of the medical staff in hospitals compete for capital. Often the capital decisions are made by the CEO and the board. Since few nurses are members of the board and only slightly more are on board committees, the voice of nursing is less strong in hospital capital expenditure decision making. As more nurse executives understand capital financing, they will be in a position to lobby more forcefully for capital expenditures. As more CNEs understand supply-and-demand laws of economics, they will be able to argue regarding the likely positive organizational effects of investment in the area of nursing. As more nurses understand the allocation of indirect expenses and begin to question the allocation, the CNE's voice in these decisions may be heard.

Intraorganizational Responsibility for Revenues

Accountability for revenue is the likeliest growth area in expectations for nurse managers. The focus in the past has been to maintain costs with no reduction or improvement in quality. Many hospitals are already focusing marketing efforts at product lines. Survival has been linked to the ability to attract a sufficient volume of patients. With the wider adoption of formal structured nursing or interdisciplinary plans of patient care (used in some hospitals already), the CNE will identify those patients the hospital wants to attract and the nurse's role in that revenue generation.

As patients seek more "caring" in the services provided in hospitals and as patients recognize that nursing is a key service provided by the hospital, it is possible that the quality of nursing care will be identified in a marketing strategy. This will enhance the power of the CNE as a key manager of highly regarded service.

Intraorganizational Role in New Ventures

As hospitals seek alternatives to balancing expenses and revenues, the CNE will likely be more involved in new ventures. While in the past the CNE was told that the hospital was opening a transplant unit and that adequate staff would need to be provided, in the future the financially adept CNE will participate in the decision making about new ventures. The CNE who is familiar with business plan development and skilled at financial projections will be seen by some as a valuable asset in the decision-making process.

Extraorganizational Changes

Along with financial responsibilities within the organization, the CNE will increasingly be involved with extraorganizational financial issues, particularly those related to reimbursement. Nurse managers will be faced with the conflict among what is of professional benefit to nursing, what is in the best interest of the nursing department, and what is in the best interest of the organization.

Cross-training of health workers and use of assistive staff are two areas where the manager faces potential conflict. Nurse managers with their roots in the profession of nursing will share the professional values associated with professional licensure. The nurse manager facing increasing salaries for professional nurses and seeing that less educated workers can be trained to perform activities formerly the purview of professional nurses will be faced with a dilemma. What does the proposed government-sponsored health care plan mean for nursing at the hospital? Is it in the nursing department's best interest to have direct third-party reimbursement for nurses? Should the state develop an episode-based reimbursement plan for home health agencies?

Government Relations

Although professional associations such as the American Nurses Association and many nurse leaders have a long history of involvement with government, many CNEs in mid-size health organizations do not. Most reimbursement decisions are now regulated by government. The CNE of the 1990s must be able to interact with government officials in the executive branch as well as with legislators to influence how these reimbursement decisions are made. To do so, the CNE must understand the payment system and the financial implications of reimbursement and regulatory decisions for the health organizations with which the CNE is involved. This interaction can occur in letters, during in-person meetings with government officials, and informally at a variety of social and professional meetings.

Payer Relations

Although much of the reimbursement system is regulated by government, reimbursement decisions for individual patients are made by private insurers or by a fiscal intermediary for the government. Bills denied payment or for which payment is delayed cost health organizations a substantial amount of money.

In hospitals the responsibility for collections is usually in the finance office. Clearly nurse managers do not want to become financial analysts. However, unless they understand issues of cash flow, they will not be able to assume a role in helping the hospital solve cash-flow problems. The promptness and completeness with which records are generated impact on the cash flow of the organization. The sophisticated nurse manager who understands cash flow will realize the benefit to the organization of working with the nursing staff to document care so as to diminish the claims that are denied or delayed. In home health care denied claims and delayed payment are major issues threatening the fiscal viability of many agencies.

In all these areas there is a trade-off between the nurse manager's involvement in financial management and having others in the organization provide those services. We believe the days of the CNE "getting a budget" from the CEO are over. However, each CNE must decide the amount of information needed to effectively manage the nursing department.

THE FUTURE ROLE OF THE MIDLEVEL NURSE MANAGER IN FINANCIAL MANAGEMENT

As the CNE assumes greater responsibility for financial matters in both the nursing department and the organization, the midlevel manager will also be expected to have expanded responsibilities. In most health organizations the midlevel managers and above are responsible for more than one unit. In hospitals this responsibility includes several patient care units. In a home health agency it might include responsibility for a geographic area where care is provided by ten or more nurses. Although first-line managers in most hospitals are responsible for the staffing costs on their units, the accountability of the first-line manager likely will expand also.

In decentralizing fiscal accountability the CNE must balance the cost of having a nurse manager devote time to fiscal management against the potential benefits of increased control of unit and department resources. It is likely that midlevel nurse managers and first-line managers will have more authority for staffing allocations. Units will be run more like small businesses rather than parts of large bureaucratic organizations. Some nurse managers may elect to hire more support staff, while others may think that an all-RN staff not only provides the highest quality of care but is also more cost effective. At the same time these managers will have a greater responsibility for controlling their expenditures.

Hospitals are developing new approaches for paying nurses. For example, one approach is to pay nurses a salary rather than an hourly wage. Issues of productivity and accountability in such a payment system will challenge the nurse managers. Other hospitals are considering contracting with entrepreneurial groups of nurses to provide all the nursing care on the unit, similar to how HMOs contract with physicians to provide medical care. Many home care agencies are paying nurses on a per visit basis rather than a salary. Managers who use these approaches believe that financial incentives increase the productivity of nurses. Nurse managers from the CNE to the first-line manager will need to address the financial implications of such changes. It is not enough to know whether the staff would prefer to be salaried. Nurse managers will also have to calculate or at least understand the financial impact of such a change on their area.

The midlevel and first-line manager will have increased accountability for revenue as well. Historically nurse managers were held accountable for the fixed nursing personnel cost per year or, more progressively, the nursing personnel costs per patient day of care. As reimbursement moves to an episode basis, nurse managers are now being held accountable for the episode of care. The nurse managers will be held accountable for both the nursing cost associated with an episode and for providing an acceptable level of quality nursing care.

THE NURSE ENTREPRENEUR

The nursing literature has shown a growing focus on the nurse entrepreneur.[17] Entrepreneurs include the independent practitioner in private practice seeing clients on a *fee-for-service* basis and the small business person providing home health care services or selling durable medical equipment to Medicare patients. As health care moves in the "managed" direction, we see the fee-for-service options decreasing in prominence. However, the opportunity for nurses to contract for the provision of services will likely expand. Payers are interested in paying a predictable amount for a certain level of care for a specific population. Entrepreneurial nurses with sufficient financial management skills will be in an advantageous position for seeking such opportunities and creatively taking full advantage of them.

Herron and Herron suggest that entrepreneurial nursing can serve as a conceptual basis for in-hospital nursing practice models.[18] They suggest that models where nurses as a group contract to provide care on a unit are an example of an in-hospital entrepreneurial approach.

Business Plan

The creation of a business plan is essential to the development of any entrepreneurial endeavor whether for a new health services business or a new venture within an established organization such as a hospital. These plans were discussed in Chapter 10. Understanding the actual costs of doing business is essential to assessing the likelihood of success of any new venture. Even those nurse managers who most strongly abhor the notion that providing health care is a *business* recognize that no new services can be provided to improve the health of the community unless adequate attention has been paid to determining how those services will be paid for. A "business plan" doesn't require a "business motive."

Many nurses have ventured into providing services without a firm under-

---

[17]Dorothy G. Herron and Lanny Herron, "Entrepreneurial Nursing as a Conceptual Basis for In-Hospital Nursing Practice Models," *Nursing Economics*, Vol. 9, No. 5, September/October 1991, pp. 310–316; Brenda Wolfson and Susan H. Neidlinger, "Nurse Entrepreneurship: Opportunities in Acute Care Hospitals," *Nursing Economics*, Vol. 9, No. 1, 1991, pp. 40–43.
[18]Ibid.

standing of the regulatory environment (this is especially true in home care) and without a solid base in financial management. Starting programs that fail because of inadequate planning does not serve the health care needs of society. It is more sensible to understand if a proposed new venture has financial flaws and work to correct them. If business planning shows a service can only be provided with a subsidy, then the sources of subsidies should be determined before a significant amount of time, effort, and money has been invested.

THE NURSE AS A POLICYMAKER FOR FINANCING HEALTH CARE

The focus of this book has been on financial management in a health care organization. Although this is the role most nurses will assume in financial management, there is a role for nurses in developing the external financing and regulatory systems that impact on organizations.[19] Nurses can work in a variety of nonprovider settings that have a dramatic impact on people's health.

Lobbyist

Nurses serve as lobbyists to both the legislative and executive branches of all levels of government. Lobbyists often work for professional organizations, such as state nurses' associations or for special interest groups such as those concerned with a particular disease or cause. Many of the decisions about the provision of care are directly related to the payment for that care. Many of the payment decisions are now made by government. The nurse who understands financial management can be an informed lobbyist. For example, if the state is planning to require that all Medicaid patients be part of managed care programs, what implications does this have for the nurse?

Many policy decisions affecting the financial management of health care organizations are made in industry. Pharmaceutical companies set pricing levels. Insurance companies set reimbursement policy. Major industries such as the auto industry decide which benefits will be covered. Financial consulting organizations such as the largest accounting firms employ nurses to help their clients improve operations. Nurses, possessing finance skills combined with their understanding of clinical care, are viewed as invaluable employees in these organizations.

Policymaker

Finally, nurses can work in government and help develop the government policy for financing health care. There is a small but growing group of nurses who are knowledgeable about financial matters who work for government in financial policy development. Perhaps the best known is Carolyn Davis, former director of the federal government's Health Care Financing Administration. Others work in all levels of government developing and implementing the financial policies that impact the provision of patient care. Rather than continuing to complain about the decisions government makes about financing care,

---

[19]Camille T. Barry, "Profiles of Nurses Professionally Involved in Public Policy," *Nursing Economics*, Vol. 8, No. 3, 1990, p. 174.

the profession needs nurses who are knowledgeable about financing to make those decisions for and with us.

Many nurses say about colleagues who work in industry or government, "They've left nursing" or "They are no longer nurses." While working in industry or for government may not be providing direct patient care to an individual, we believe that nursing encompasses caring for the community as well as an individual. Nurse theorists debate what nursing is and the role of the nurse in the health of people. Is nursing caring, repatterning, and/or meeting clients' needs? However nursing is defined, it cannot be done without the provision of the resources to do so. Providing resources cannot be done without a firm understanding of financial management.

IMPLICATIONS FOR NURSE MANAGERS

As the functions of both the CNE and midlevel nurse manager expand, additional financial skills will likely be necessary. Some suggest that there is a tendency for nurse executives to obtain financial knowledge through on-the-job training.[20] As a result, many CNEs never acquire principles and conceptual foundations of financial management and budgeting.

Others propose that CEOs expect CNEs to have business skills similar to those of other health care executives. They suggest that decentralization and pressure to control costs have led to the unit-based nurse manager's being responsible for twenty-five to fifty full-time employees and budgets in excess of $1 million.[21]

As this book is being written, approximately seventy-five master's programs in nursing management exist. Some programs prepare CNEs, while others prepare first-line nurse managers. Based on a survey of nurse executives in a variety of health care settings to determine how they spend their time and on an analysis of the responses by nurse managers, nursing administration faculty, and management faculty, Scaizi and Wilson discuss content that should be required in graduate programs preparing nurse administrators.[22] Finance ranked fourth in time spent in practice setting after (1) law and health care policy, (2) organizational behavior, and (3) organizational strategy. They propose that finance should be a fundamental nursing administration content area.

The trend in the late 1970s was toward graduate programs in nursing focusing on clinical theory. As nurse managers recognized that management skills, including financial management, were necessary to be an effective manager, schools of nursing began to again include this content in their programs. Although budgeting and financial management are not required in all programs, we believe this is changing. The newly educated generation of nurse managers will obtain the conceptual foundations and principles to develop these skills. However, many managers currently working in health organiza-

[20]Porter, Hodges, and Goddard, op. cit.

[21]Barbara A. Mark, Jean T. Turner, and Sheila Englebardt, "Knowledge and Skills for Nurse Administrators," *Nursing & Health Care*, Vol. 11, No. 4, April 1990, pp. 185–189.

[22]Cynthia Scaizi and David L. Wilson, "Empirically Based Recommendations for Content of Graduate Nursing Administration Programs," *Nursing & Health Care*, Vol. 11, No. 10, December 1991, pp. 522–525.

tions do not have these skills and will be expected to obtain them either through formal academic programs or through workshops.

We hope that this book will serve as just the beginning of your efforts to learn about financial management. We have provided the foundations. A nurse manager who has studied this book need not fear embarrassment in conversations with financial managers and other administrators. A nurse manager who has studied this book is prepared to apply the concepts of financial management to health care organizations. We hope, however, that you will continue to read, study, and learn about nursing financial management. This is a field still in its infancy. You have the opportunity to participate in the innovations still to come.

KEY CONCEPTS

Nursing financial management research   Research can be described as a continuum from theoretical to applied. Research in this area is primarily applied and focuses on nursing resource use, costing nursing care, and cost-benefit analysis.

Role of CNE in financial management   This role is expanding to include participation in the major financial decisions of health organizations and setting organizational policy.

Government relations   Interaction with government officials in the executive as well as the legislative branch. The CNE must understand the payment system and the financial implications for reimbursement and regulatory decisions.

Payer relations   Relationship with payers is critical for the fiscal health of the organization. Nurse managers must understand payer policies about reimbursement, particularly those which affect denial of claims.

Nurse entrepreneur   Nurse who seeks opportunities for independent practice including fee-for-service payment and other payment mechanisms such as group contracts.

Policymaker   Nurse manager can impact health care delivery as a lobbyist or financial policymaker in government.

SUGGESTED READINGS

Andrica, Diane C., "Changing Profiles of Nurse Executives," *Nursing Economics*, Vol. 6, No. 3, May/June 1988, pp. 112–115.

Barry, Camille T., "Profiles of Nurses Professionally Involved in Public Policy," *Nursing Economics*, Vol. 8, No. 3, May/June 1990, pp. 174–176.

Behner, Kathleen G., Louis F. Fogg, Linda C. Fournier, et al., "Nursing Resource Management: Analyzing the Relationship Between Costs and Quality in Staffing Decisions," *Health Care Management Review*, Vol. 15, No. 4, Fall 1990, pp. 63–71.

Bell, Eunice A., and Barbara D. Bart, "Pay for Performance: Motivating the Chief Nurse Executive," *Nursing Economics*, Vol. 9, No. 2, March/April 1991, pp. 92–96.

Bostrom, Janet, and Malinda Mitchel, "Relationship of Direct Nursing Care Hours to DRG and Severity of Illness," *Nursing Economics*, Vol. 9, No. 2, March/April 1991, pp. 105–111.

Brett, Judy L., and Mary C. Tonges, "Restructured Patient Care Delivery: Evaluation of the ProACT TM Model," *Nursing Economics*, Vol. 8, No. 1, January/February 1990, pp. 36–44.

Budd, Marjorie C., and Toni Proptnik, "A Computerized System for Staffing, Billing and Productivity Measurement," *Journal of Nursing Administration*, Vol. 19, No. 7, July/August 1989, pp. 17–22.

Edwardson, Sandra, and Patricia Nardone, "Resource Use in Home Care Agencies," *Applied Nursing Research*, Vol. 4, No. 1, February 1991, pp. 25–30.

Ethridge, Phyllis, "A Nursing HMO: Carondelet St. Mary's Experience," *Nursing Management*, Vol. 22, No. 7, July 1991, pp. 22–27.

Faulkner, Janice, "Salary Equals Performance for Community Health Nurses," *Nursing Management*, Vol. 22, No. 6, June 1991, pp. 28–32.

Gardner, Kathryn G., and Mary Tilbury, "A Longitudinal Cost Analysis of Primary and Team Nursing," *Nursing Economics*, Vol. 9, No. 2, March/April 1991, pp. 97–104.

Glandon, Gerald L., Kenneth W. Colbert, and Mary Thomasa, "Nursing Delivery Models and RN Mix: Cost Implications," *Nursing Management*, Vol. 20, No. 5, May 1989, pp. 30–33.

Griffith, Hurdis, Gail Tumulty, and Barbara Nelson, "Participation of Nurse Executives in Product Decisions," *Nursing Economics*, Vol. 8, No. 2, March/April 1990, pp. 90–93.

Hamm-Vida, Diane, "Cost of Non-Nursing Tasks," *Nursing Management*, Vol. 21, No. 4, April 1990, pp. 46–52.

Harrington, Charlene, "Wages and Benefits of Nursing Personnel in Nursing Homes: Correcting the Inequities," *Nursing Economics*, Vol. 8, No. 6, November/December 1990, pp. 378–385.

Hendrickson, Gerry, Theresa M. Doddato, and Christine T. Kovner, "How Do Nurses Use Their Time?" *Journal of Nursing Administration*, Vol. 20, No. 3, March 1990, pp. 31–37.

Herron, Dorothy G., and Lanny Herron, "Entrepreneurial Nursing as a Conceptual Basis for In-Hospital Nursing Practice Models," *Nursing Economics*, Vol. 9, No. 5, September/October 1991, pp. 310–316.

Hoffman, Sharon E., and Marsha E. Fonteyn, "Third Party Reimbursement for CNS Consultation," *Nursing Economics*, Vol. 6, No. 5, September/October 1988, pp. 245–247.

Ingersoll, Gail L., Nancy Hoffart, and Alison W. Schultz, "Health Services Research in Nursing: Current Status and Future Directions," *Nursing Economics*, Vol. 8, No. 4, July/August 1990, pp. 229–238.

Larson, Elaine, Margaret Dear, and Margaret Keitkemper, "Comparison of Two Schema for Classifying Nursing Research," *IMAGE*, Vol. 23, No. 3, Fall 1991, pp. 167–170.

Manco, Elizabeth, Kathleen Russel-Babin, and Sheryl Stevens, "An Incentive Program . . . More Than Just R & R," *Nursing Management*, Vol. 22, No. 1, January 1991, pp. 49–53.

Mark, Barbara A., Jean T. Turner, and Sheila Englebardt, "Knowledge and Skills for Nurse Administrators," *Nursing & Health Care*, Vol. 11, No. 4, April 1990, pp. 185–189.

McCloskey, Joanne C., "Implications of Costing Out Nursing Services for Reimbursement," *Nursing Management*, Vol. 20, No. 1, January 1989, pp. 44–49.

Mills, Mary Etta, "Nursing Compensation: The Realities of Seeking Equity," *Nursing Economics*, Vol. 7, No. 5, September/October 1989, pp. 270–272.

Misener, T. R., A. J. Frelin, and P. A. Twoist, "Sampling Nursing Time Pinpoints Staffing Need," *Nursing and Health Care*, Vol. 8, No. 4, April 1987, pp. 233–237.

Porter, Gaye W., Linda C. Hodges, and Nannette Goddard, "Financial Responsibilities and Preparation of Chief Nurse Executives," *Nursing Economics*, Vol. 9, No. 5, September/October 1991, pp. 305–309.

Porter-O'Grady, Tim, "Newer Compensation Practices for the Nurse Executive," *Nursing Economics*, Vol. 8, No. 6, November/December 1990, p. 393.

Prescott, Patricia A., "Forecasting Requirements for Health Care Personnel," *Nursing Economics*, Vol. 9, No. 1, January/February 1991, pp. 18–24.

Rogers, Michael, Jan Riordan, and Donna Swindle, "Community-Based Nursing Case Management Pays Off," *Nursing Management*, Vol. 22, No. 3, March 1991, pp. 30–34.

Scaizi, Cynthia, and David L. Wilson, "Empirically Based Recommendations for Content of Graduate Nursing Administration Programs," *Nursing & Health Care*, Vol. 11, No. 10, December 1991, pp. 522–525.

Servais, Sharon Holcombe, "Nursing Resource Applications Through Outcome Based Nursing Practice," *Nursing Economics*, Vol. 9, No. 3, May/June 1991, pp. 171–180.

Starck, Patricia, "Health Care Under Siege: Challenge for Change," *Nursing and Health Care*, Vol. 12, No. 1, January 1991, pp. 26–30.

Sullivan, Helen K., "Developing an Incentive Program for Home Health Nurses," *Nursing Economics*, Vol. 7, No. 6, November/December 1989, pp. 310–313.

Van Slyck, Ann, "A Systems Approach to the Management of Nursing Services, Part IV: Costing System," *Nursing Management*, Vol. 22, No. 6, August 1991, pp. 14–16.

Watson, Phyllis M., Mary S. Lower, Susan M. Wells, et al., "Discovering What Nurses Do and What It Costs," *Nursing Management*, Vol. 22, No. 5, May 1991, pp. 38–45.

Wolfson, Brenda, and Susan H. Neidlinger, "Nurse Entrepreneurship: Opportunities in Acute Care Hospitals," *Nursing Economics*, Vol. 9, No. 1, January/February 1991, pp. 40–43.

Wood, Chris, "Health Care Rationing: The Oregon Experiment," *Nursing Economics*, Vol. 9, No. 4, July/August 1991, pp. 239–243.

GLOSSARY

accounting   system for keeping track of the financial status of an organization and the financial results of its activities.

accounting control   methods and procedures for the authorization of transactions, safeguarding of assets, and accuracy of accounting records.

accounting cycle   period of time from when cash is spent to acquire resources to provide care until cash is received in payment for the services provided.

accounts receivable   money owed to the organization or individual in exchange for goods and services provided.

accounts payable   amounts owed to suppliers (such as pharmaceutical or medical supply companies).

accrual accounting   accounting system that matches revenues and related expenses in the same fiscal year by recording revenues in the year in which they become earned (whether received or not) and the expenses related to generating those revenues in the same year.

accrue   to increase or accumulate in advance.

accumulated depreciation   total amount of depreciation related to a fixed asset that has been taken over the years the organization has owned that asset.

acuity   measurement of patient severity of illness related to the amount of nursing care resources required to care for the patient.

acuity subcategory   represents the amount that would have been budgeted for the actual output level if the actual acuity level had been correctly forecast.

acuity variance   variance resulting from the difference between the actual acuity level and the budgeted level; the difference between the flexible budget and the value of the acuity subcategory.

ADC   see **average daily census.**

additive rule   states that the likelihood of either one event or another event's occurring is the sum of the likelihood of each event's occurring.

administration   management; sometimes the term administration is used to refer to top-level policy development, i.e., charting the course of the organization, while management is used to refer to the process of supervising the accomplishment of the organizational objectives through use of resources. In recent years there has been movement away from this latter usage.

administrative control   plan of organization (for example, the formal organization chart concerning who reports to whom) and all methods and procedures that help management planning and control of operations.

age-of-plant ratio   see **plant-age ratio.**

aging schedule   management report that shows how long receivables have been outstanding since a bill was issued.

algebraic distribution   cost-allocation approach that uses simultaneous equations to allocate nonrevenue cost center costs to both nonrevenue and revenue cost centers in a manner that does not create distortions.

all-payer system   system of payment where all payers use the same payment method for paying for health care services.

allowance for bad debts   see **allowance for uncollectible accounts.**

allowance for uncollectible accounts   estimated portion of total accounts receivable that is expected not to be collected because of bad debts; sometimes called allowance for bad debts.

allowances   discounts from the amount normally charged for patient care services. These discounts are sometimes negotiated (e.g., with Blue Cross) and other times mandated by law (e.g., Medicare and Medicaid).

ALOS   see **average length of stay.**

alternative workers   use of workers not traditionally used to provide care. This includes workers who are less skilled than professional nurses but who may be able to assume some activities traditionally performed by RNs.

amortization   allocation of the cost of an intangible asset over its lifetime.

annuity   series of payments or receipts each in the same amount and spaced at even time periods. For example, $127.48 paid monthly for three years.

assets   valuable resources. They may be either physical, having substance and form such as a table or building, or intangible, such as the reputation the organization has gained for providing high-quality health care services.

audit   examination of the financial records of the organization to discover material errors, to evaluate the internal control system, and to determine if financial statements have been prepared in accordance with generally accepted accounting principles.

auditor   person who performs an audit.

average cost   full cost divided by the volume of service units.

average daily census   average number of inpatients on any given day; patient days in a given time period divided by the number of days in the time period.

average length of stay   average number of patient days for each patient discharged; the number of patient days in a given time period divided by the number of discharges in that time period.

axiom   unproven but accepted assertion that is either self-evident or is a mutually accepted principle.

bad debts   operating expense related to the care provided to patients who ultimately do not pay the organization, although they were expected to pay. Amounts included in revenues, but never paid, are balanced by the charge to bad debts.

balance sheet   financial report that indicates the financial position of the organization at a specific point in time; officially referred to as the statement of financial position.

Blue Cross   major provider of hospitalization insurance to both individuals and groups. For most hospitals one of the largest sources of revenue.

board-designated   portion of the fund balance that the board has identified and a corresponding amount of assets that the board has restricted for a specific purpose; sometimes called board-restricted.

board of directors   see **board of trustees.**

board of trustees   governing body that has the ultimate responsibility for the decisions made by the organization.

board-restricted   see **board-designated.**

bond payable   formal borrowing arrangement where a transferable certificate represents the debt. The holder of the bond may sell it, in which case the liability is owed to the new owner.

bondholder   creditor of the organization who owns one of the organization's outstanding bonds payable.

break-even analysis   technique for determining the minimum volume of output (e.g., patient days of care) necessary for a program or service to be financially self-sufficient.

budget   plan that provides a formal, quantitative expression of management's plans and intentions or expectations.

budgeting   process whereby plans are made and then an effort is made to meet or exceed the goals of the plans.

building fund   restricted fund containing assets that can be used only to acquire buildings and equipment.

business plan   detailed plan for a proposed program, project, or service, including information to be used to assess the venture's financial feasibility.

cafeteria plan   method of providing fringe benefits in which the employee chooses from a variety of options those fringe benefits which the employee wants.

capital acquisitions   see **capital assets.**

capital assets   buildings or equipment with useful lives extending beyond the year in which they are purchased or put into service; also referred to as long-term investments, capital items, capital investments, or capital acquisitions.

capital budget   plan for the acquisition of buildings and equipment that will be used by the organization for one or more years beyond the year of acquisition. Often a minimum dollar cutoff must be exceeded for an item to be included in the capital budget.

capital budgeting   process of proposing the purchase of capital assets, analyzing the proposed purchases for economic or other justification, and encompassing the financial implications of accepted capital items into the master budget.

capital equipment   equipment with an expected life beyond the year of purchase. Such equipment must generally be included in the capital budget.

capital investments   see **capital assets.**

capital items   see **capital assets.**

capitalism   see **market economy.**

career ladders   approach to promotion and compensation that allows a worker to progress in an organization or a field.

cash   money on hand, plus **cash equivalents,** such as savings and checking accounts and short-term certificates of deposit.

cash basis   accounting system under which revenues are recorded when cash is received and expenses are recorded when cash is paid. This system is not generally allowed because it does not adequately match revenues and related expenses in the same year.

cash budget   plan for the cash receipts and cash disbursements of the organization.

cash budgeting   process of planning the cash budget.

cash disbursement   outflow of cash from the organization.

cash equivalents   savings and checking accounts and short-term certificates of deposit; items that are quickly and easily convertible into cash.

cash flow measure of the amount of cash received or disbursed at a given point in time, as opposed to revenues or income, which frequently are recorded at a time other than when the actual cash receipt or payment occurs.

cash management active process of planning for borrowing and repayment of cash or investing excess cash on hand.

case mix mix of different types of patients treated by a health care organization.

case-mix index measurement of the average complexity or severity of illness of patients treated by a health care organization.

cash payment see **cash disbursement.**

cash receipt inflow of cash into the organization.

causal variable independent variable that is responsible for changes in the dependent variable.

census number of patients occupying beds at a specific time of day (usually midnight).

charge master list of the organization's prices for each of its services.

charity care care provided to individuals who are not expected to be able to pay because of limited personal financial resources.

chart of accounts accounting document that assigns an identifying number to each cost center and each type of revenue or expense. These code numbers are assigned to all financial transactions. By looking at any code number and referring to the chart of accounts, one would know exactly which cost center was involved and the specific type of revenue or expense.

chief financial officer (CFO) manager responsible for all the financial functions in the organization.

chief nurse executive (CNE) top-level nurse manager responsible for all nursing functions in the organization. This includes all nursing care provided to clients.

clone computer that is compatible with one of the major brands (IBM or Apple) and that functions almost identically to the original but is less expensive.

coinsurance percentage of a patient's health services charge that must be paid by the patient.

co-payment dollar amount that must be paid each time a health service is used.

collateral specific asset pledged to a lender as security for a loan.

collection period amount of time from when a patient bill is issued until cash is collected.

commercial paper form of short-term borrowing in which the borrower issues a financial security that can be traded by the lender to someone else.

common-size ratio class of ratios that allows one to evaluate each number on a financial statement relative to the size of the organization. This is accomplished by dividing each financial statement number by a key number from that statement such as total assets or total revenues.

competitive strategy organization's plan for achieving its goals, specifically, what will be sold and to whom.

compound interest method of calculating interest that accrues not only on the amount of the original investment but also on the interest earned in interim periods

conservatism principle   financial statements must give adequate consideration to the risks faced by the organization.

constant dollars   dollar amounts that have been adjusted for the impact of inflation.

consumer   person who receives services from a health care provider; this includes not only patients but also health workers.

contingency   event that may or may not occur.

continuous budgeting   system in which a budget is prepared each month for a month one year in the future. For example, once the actual results for this January are known, a budget for January of the next year is prepared.

contractual allowances   discounts from full charges, available to governments and some other third-party payers.

contribution from operations   contribution margin from the routine annual operations of the organization.

contribution margin   amount by which the price exceeds the variable cost. If the contribution margin is positive, it means that each extra unit of activity makes the organization better off by that amount.

control   attempt to ensure that actual results come as close to planned results as possible.

controllable   those items over which a manager can exercise a degree of control.

corporation   business owned by a group of individuals (shareholders or stockholders) that has limited liability; the owners are not liable for more than the amount invested in the firm.

cost   amount spent on something. Costs have two stages: acquisition cost and expired cost. When some asset or service is purchased, it has an *acquisition cost*. If the item is an asset, it will appear on the balance sheet at its cost, until it is used up. Once the asset is used up, it becomes an *expired cost,* or an expense.

cost behavior   way that costs change in reaction to events within the organization.

cost center   unit or department in an organization for which a manager is assigned responsibility for costs.

cost-effective   approach that provides care as good as any other approach but at a lower cost, or an approach that provides the best possible care for a given level of cost.

cost estimation   process of using historical cost information to segregate mixed costs into their fixed and variable components and then using that information to estimate future costs.

cost finding   process that finds the costs of units of service—such as lab tests, x-rays, or routine patient days—based on an allocation of nonrevenue cost center costs to revenue centers.

cost of the product   what the organization must pay for the product; can be affected by quantity discounts and timing of payment.

cost reimbursement   revenue based on paying the organization for the costs incurred in providing care to the patient.

cost pass-through   payment by a third party, which reimburses the health care organization for the amount of costs it incurred in providing care to patients.

CPM   see **critical path method.**

cr.   abbreviation for credit.

credit   bookkeeping term for an increase in an item on the right side of the fundamental equation of accounting or a decrease in an item on the left side.

creditors   people or organizations to whom the organization owes money.

critical path method (CPM)   program technique that indicates the cost and time for each element of a complex project and indicates cost/time trade-offs where applicable.

current assets   resources the organization has that either are cash or can be converted to cash within one year or that will be used up within one year. Current assets are often referred to as short-term or near-term assets.

current liabilities   those obligations which are expected to be paid within one year.

current ratio   current assets divided by current liabilities.

curvilinear   curved line. Most of the statistical methods described assume that there is a straight-line relationship between changes in the variables. Sometimes the relationship is curved.

data base   compilation of related information systematically organized.

days receivable ratio   accounts receivable divided by patient revenue per day; a measure of how long it takes on average until revenues are collected.

debit   bookkeeping term for an increase in an item on the left side of the fundamental equation of accounting or a decrease in an item on the right side.

debt   liability.

debt service   required interest and principal payments on money owed.

debt service coverage ratio   cash available to pay interest and principal payments divided by required interest and principal payments; a measure of the ability of the organization to meet required debt service.

debt-to-equity ratio   see **total debt-to-equity ratio.**

decision package   zero-based budgeting term referring to a package of all the information to be used in ranking alternatives and making a final decision.

decision variables   factors controllable by the organization that can affect volume.

decreasing returns to scale   extremely large volume may lead to increasing cost per unit produced due to capacity constraints or shortages of labor or supplies.

deductible   amount that must first be paid by an insured individual before the insurance covers any costs; usually the first $100 or $200 or $500 per year for health insurance.

deferred revenues   items that will become revenue in the future when the organization provides goods or services. These are liabilities until the goods or services are provided.

deficit   excess of expenses over revenues. This term sometimes is used to refer to the current year or budgeted year and sometimes to refer to the deficit accumulated over a period of years.

Delphi technique   technique sometimes employed for forecasting that uses an expert group, which never meets, to generate written information as the basis for making a decision. When used in forecasting, each member's written forecast is distributed to all members of the group, along with the reasoning behind it. This process is repeated several times, and eventually a group decision is made.

demand   amount of the good or service that consumers would be willing to acquire at any given price.

demand curve   quantity (horizontal axis) that would be desired by consumers for any given price (vertical axis).

demographics   characteristics of the human population, including age, sex, growth, density, distribution, and other vital statistics.

dependent variable   item whose value is being predicted.

depreciate   decline in value or productive capability.

depreciation   allocation of a portion of the cost of a capital asset into each of the years of the item's expected useful life.

depreciation expense   amount of the original cost of a fixed asset allocated as an expense each year.

determinant attributes   factors that ultimately impact on a consumer's purchase decision. There are two major types: **decision variables** and **environmental variables.**

diagnosis related groups (DRGs)   system that categorizes patients into specific groups based on their medical diagnosis and other characteristics such as age and type of surgery, if any; currently used by Medicare and some other hospital payers as a basis for payment.

differential advantage   characteristic that provides the organization with a distinct advantage over a competitor. Such advantages might include location, cost, services offered, or other factors.

direct costs   (a) costs incurred within the organizational unit for which the manager has responsibility are referred to as direct costs of the unit; (b) costs of resources used for direct care of the patient are referred to as the direct costs of patient care.

direct distribution   allocation of nonrevenue center costs directly and only to revenue centers.

direct expenses   those expenses which can be specifically and exclusively related to the activity within the cost center; see also **direct costs.**

disbursement   cash payment.

discount rate   interest rate used in discounting.

discounted cash flow   method that allows comparisons of amounts of money paid at different points of time by discounting all amounts to the present.

discounting   reverse of compound interest; a process in which interest that could be earned over time is deducted from a future payment to determine how much the future payment is worth at the present time.

discretionary costs   costs for which there is no clear-cut relationship between inputs and outputs. The treatment of more patients would not necessarily require more of this input; use of more of this input would not necessarily allow for treatment of more patients.

disequilibrium   situation where the quantity demanded at the current price is not the same as the quantity suppliers want to provide at that price. In such a situation there is pressure to either raise or lower the price until an equilibrium is achieved.

distribution channels   way a product moves from the producer to the consumer.

distributional efficiency ability of the market to allocate resources to different individuals in an efficient manner.

dividend distribution of profits to owners of the organization.

double distribution allocation approach in which all nonrevenue centers allocate their costs to all other cost centers once, and then a second allocation takes place using either step-down or direct distribution.

double-entry accounting refers to the fact that whenever a change is made to the accounting equation, at least one other change must be made as well to keep the equation in balance.

dr. abbreviation for debit.

DRGs see **diagnosis related groups.**

economic goods goods or services acquired by consumers to provide physical or psychic benefit.

economic order quantity (EOQ) approach to determine the balance between ordering costs and carrying costs.

economics study of how scarce resources are allocated among their possible uses.

economies of scale cost of providing a good or service falls as quantity increases because fixed costs are shared by the larger volume.

efficiency ratios class of ratios that examines the efficiency with which the organization uses its resources in providing care and generating revenues.

elasticity of demand degree to which demand increases in response to a price decrease or decreases in response to a price increase.

electronic data data that are computerized.

employee benefits compensation provided to employees in addition to their base salary, for example, health insurance, life insurance, vacation, and holidays.

employees per occupied bed total number of paid FTEs divided by the average daily census.

endowment fund restricted fund that contains the endowment assets that belong to the organization; only earnings may be removed from this fund under normal conditions.

entity specific individual, organization, or part of an organization that is the focus of attention; accounting must be done from the perspective of the relevant entity.

environmental variables factors that can affect an organization but that are not controllable by the organization.

EPOB see **employees per occupied bed.**

equilibrium situation in which the quantity of a good or service offered at the stated price is the same as the quantity that buyers want to purchase at that price.

equity (a) fairness; (b) ownership, e.g., the share of a house that is owned by the homeowner free and clear of any mortgage obligations is the homeowner's equity in the house.

exception report list of only those individual variances which exceed a specified limit.

expected value method used to estimate the value to be gained from various alternatives. It is the weighted average of the possible outcomes, using probabilities as weights.

expenditure payment; often used interchangeably with expense.

expenses costs of services provided; expired cost; see **cost.**

external accountant accountant who is hired by the organization to perform an audit of the organization's financial records.

externalities secondary impacts of an action by an individual or organization that present additional costs or benefits to those affected.

factoring selling the organization's accounts receivable, usually for less than their face value.

favorable variance variance in which less was spent than the budgeted amount.

feedback using information about actual results to avoid past mistakes and improve future plans.

fee-for-service system in which there is an additional charge for each additional service provided (as opposed to a prepaid system, in which all services are included in exchange for one flat payment).

fiduciary relating to holding something in trust; a fiduciary is a trustee maintaining assets in trust.

financial accounting system that records historical financial information, summarizes it, and provides reports of what financial events have occurred and of what the financial impact of those events has been.

financial statements reports that convey information about the organization's financial position and the results of its activities.

financing accounts receivable borrowing money and using the organization's accounts receivable as security or collateral for a loan.

first-dollar coverage insurance coverage that has no deductible or co-payment. The insurance company pays the "first dollar."

first-line manager person responsible for one patient care unit, area, or group of nursing staff.

fiscal financial.

fiscal year one-year period defined for financial purposes. A fiscal year may start at any point during the calendar year and finishes one year later. For example, "fiscal year 1993 with a June 30 year end" refers to the period from July 1, 1992, through June 30, 1993.

fixed assets those assets which will not be used up or converted to cash within one year; sometimes referred to as long-term assets.

fixed costs costs that do not change in total as volume changes.

flexible budget variance difference between actual results and the flexible budget.

flexible budgeting process of developing a budget based on different work-load levels. Often used after the fact to calculate the amount that would have been budgeted for the actual work-load levels attained. Depends heavily on the existence of variable costs.

float interim period from when a check is written until the check is cashed and clears the bank.

forecast prediction of some future value such as patient days, chest tubes used, or nursing care hours per patient day.

forecasting process of making forecasts.

for-profit organization whose mission includes earning a profit that may be distributed to its owners.

free enterprise   see **market economy.**
fringe benefits   see **employee benefits.**
FTE   see **full-time equivalent.**
full cost   total of all costs associated with an organizational unit or activity. This includes direct and indirect costs.
full-time equivalent (FTE)   equivalent of one full-time employee working for one year. This is generally calculated as forty hours per week for fifty-two weeks, or a total of 2,080 paid hours. This includes both productive and nonproductive (vacation, sick, holiday, education, etc.) time. Two employees each working half-time for one year would be the same as one FTE.
fully integrated   hospital information system in which all the components are able to communicate with each other.
fund accounting   system of separate financial records and controls; the assets of the organization are divided into distinct funds with separate bank accounts and a complete separate set of financial records.
fund balance   owner's equity in a not-for-profit organization.
fundamental equation of accounting   assets equal liabilities plus fund balance.

GAAP   abbreviation for generally accepted accounting principles.
Gantt chart   depicts necessary activities or goals in a matrix format with the horizontal axis indicating the time frame and the vertical axis the activities in the project.
general journal   first place that financial transactions are entered into the accounting records; chronological listing of all financial transactions.
general operating fund   unrestricted fund used for the day-in and day-out operations of the organization.
generally accepted accounting principles   set of rules that must be followed for the organization's financial statements to be deemed a fair presentation of the organization's financial position and results of operations.
goal congruence   bringing together the goals, desires, and wants of the organization with those of its employees.
goal divergence   natural differences between the goals, desires, and needs of the organization and those of its employees.
goals   broad, timeless ends of the organization meant to aid the organization in accomplishing its mission.
going-concern principle   it is assumed that the numbers reported on a financial statement are those of an organization that will continue in business for the foreseeable future. If the organization is not a going concern, that fact must be noted on the financial statements or the accompanying notes.
goodwill   intangible asset that represents a measure of the value of the organization that goes beyond its specific physical assets.
government   citizens' direction of the affairs of state.
gross patient revenues   charges for health care services provided.
group-rated   price charged for insurance based on the experience of the group.

hardware   computers and related equipment.
Hawthorne effect   psychological effect that causes productivity of workers to improve when they receive attention.
health maintenance organization (HMO)   organization that provides health care services to individuals or groups in exchange for a monthly payment.

hierarchy structure that establishes the authority and responsibility that different individuals have within the organization.

HMO see **health maintenance organization.**

hours per patient day paid hours divided by patient days.

HPPD see **hours per patient day.**

incentives activities, rewards, or punishments used to make it be in the individual's interest to act in a desired manner.

income excess of revenues over expenses for a specific period.

increasing returns to scale see **economies of scale.**

incremental costs additional costs that will be incurred if a decision is made that would not otherwise be incurred by the organization.

indemnity compensation for losses incurred, usually a dollar amount.

independent variable variable used to predict the dependent variable.

indirect costs (a) costs assigned to an organizational unit from elsewhere in the organization are indirect costs for the unit; (b) costs within a unit that are not incurred for direct patient care are indirect costs of patient care.

indirect expenses expenses such as administration or heating and lighting that are shared by all departments. These expenses are not incurred within the cost center; see also **indirect costs.**

inputs resources used for treating patients or otherwise producing output. Examples of inputs include paid nursing hours, chest tubes, and IV solutions.

intangible asset asset without physical substance or form.

interest coverage ratio cash available to pay interest divided by interest; a measure of the organization's ability to meet its required interest payments.

internal accountant accountant who works for the organization recording financial information throughout the year.

internal control system of accounting checks and balances designed to minimize both clerical errors and the possibility of fraud or embezzlement; the process and systems that ensure that decisions made in the organization are appropriate and receive appropriate authorization. This requires a system of accounting and administrative controls.

internal rate of return (IRR) discounted cash-flow technique that calculates the rate of return earned on a specific project or program.

inventory management refers to the appropriate ordering and storage of supplies.

investments stocks and bonds that the organization does not intend to sell within one year.

IRR see **internal rate of return.**

journal entry entry into the general journal or a subsidiary journal.

justification explanation used in defending a proposed budget or in explaining variances that have occurred.

key participants major groups involved in the organization and delivery of health care.

key players see **key participants.**

lease agreement providing for the use of an asset in exchange for rental payments.

ledger accounting book that keeps track of increases, decreases, and the balance in each asset, liability, revenue, expense, and fund balance account.

length of stay (LOS) number of days a patient is an inpatient. This is generally measured by the number of times the patient is an inpatient at midnight; see also **average length of stay.**

liabilities legal financial obligations the organization has to outsiders. Essentially it is money that the organization owes to someone.

linear programming (LP) technique to determine how best to allocate scarce resources subject to constraints to optimize a certain goal.

line function element of running an organization that implies direct authority, in contrast with the staff function, which is consultative and without direct authority. Nursing is a line department.

line item any resource that is listed separately on a budget. For example, all nursing labor for a unit may appear in aggregate (one line item), or head nurse costs may appear separately from RN costs and from LPN costs (resulting in three line items). Further subdivisions of nursing cost would create additional line items.

line manager manager of a line department or unit of the organization; see **line function.**

lines of authority formal lines of authority may be either direct (full authority), such as the associate director of nursing reporting to the CNE, or indirect (limited authority), such as the director of dietary reporting to the chief of the medical staff.

liquid assets cash or other assets that can quickly be converted to cash to meet the short-term liabilities of the organization.

liquidate convert into cash.

liquidity ratios class of ratio that examines the ability of the organization to meet its obligations in the coming year.

lock box post office box that is emptied directly by the bank. The bank removes the receipts and credits them directly to the organization's account.

long-range budget plan that covers a period of time longer than one year, typically three, five, or ten years.

long-range planning planning process that focuses on general objectives to be achieved by the organization over a period of typically three to five years; often referred to as strategic planning.

long-term period longer than one year.

long-term assets see **capital assets.**

long-term investment see **capital assets.**

long-term liabilities obligations that are not expected to be paid for more than one year.

LOS see **length of stay.**

lower of cost or market marketable securities and investments are recorded on financial statements at their cost or the market value, whichever is lower. This treatment results from the principle of conservatism.

managed care system for organizing the delivery of care in which someone who is not the provider of care arranges for the services that the patient uses.

management by objectives (MBO)   technique in which a supervising manager and the subordinate manager agree upon a common set of objectives upon which performance will be measured.

management control system   complete set of policies and procedures designed to keep operations going according to plan.

management letter   letter from the CPA to the management of the organization discussing weaknesses in the internal control system that were revealed as part of an audit.

management's role   three of the most essential elements are planning, control, and decision making.

managerial hierarchy   structure that establishes the authority and responsibility of different individuals within the organization.

margin   at the edge; usually refers to the impact of adding one more patient.

marginal benefit   see **marginal utility.**

marginal cost   price paid for a good or service; the additional amount that must be spent to acquire or produce one more unit.

marginal cost analysis   process for making decisions about changes should be based on the marginal costs of the change rather than on the full or average costs.

marginal utility   additional benefit or utility gained from a purchase of one more unit of a particular item.

market   potential customers for a product or organization.

market economy   system where individuals can choose whether to invest their wealth or capital in a business venture, workers can choose whether to work for that venture at the wages offered, and consumers can choose whether to buy the products of the venture at the seller's price.

market failure   situations in which the free market does not operate efficiently.

market measurement   conversion of qualitative information into quantitative estimates of demand.

market segmentation   division of the market into several specific subsections.

market share   portion or percentage of the overall market that a specific organization controls. If half of all broken-leg patients come to your ER, then you have a 50% share of the broken-leg market.

marketable investments   investments that are bought and sold in financial markets, making them readily convertible to cash.

marketable securities   investments in stocks and bonds that the organization intends to sell within one year.

marketing   management science that attempts to maintain and increase the organization's sales volume.

markup   certain percentage that is added to a product or service's cost to establish its selling price.

master budget   set of all the major budgets in the organization; generally includes the operating budget, long-range budget, program budgets, capital budget, and cash budget.

material   amount of money substantial enough that an error of that magnitude in the financial statements would cause a user of the statements to make a different decision than would be made if the user had known the correct information.

matrix distribution   see **algebraic distribution.**

matrix management   system in which a manager has responsibility that cuts across department lines.

MBO   see **management by objectives.**

Medicaid   program funded jointly by the federal and state (and sometimes local) governments that pay for medical care for eligible low-income people.

Medicare   federal program under the Social Security Administration that pays for medical care for the aged and permanently disabled.

menu   list of the options from which one can choose.

mid-level nurse manager   person responsible for nursing functions on more than one nursing unit or area.

mission   organization's set of primary goals that justify its existence, such as providing high-quality hospital care to the surrounding community or providing research and education.

mission statement   statement of the purpose or reason for existence of an organization, department, or unit. This statement provides direction regarding the types of activities that the organization should undertake.

mixed costs   costs that contain an element of fixed costs and an element of variable costs, such as electricity. A unit or department budget as a whole represents a mixed cost.

monopoly   sole seller who therefore has the power to set prices at a higher-than-equilibrium level.

monopsony   market in which there is only one buyer.

moral hazard   fact that people behave differently if they are insured than if they are not. Patients are more likely to consume more health care services if they have health insurance.

mortgage payable   represents a loan that is secured by a specific asset.

moving average   method of averaging out the roughness caused by random variation in a historical series of data points.

multiple regression analysis   form of regression analysis that uses more than one independent, or causal, variable. This can result in a better result than using only one variable.

multiplication rule   likelihood of two or more events' occurring simultaneously or in sequence is the product of probability of each event.

near term   see **current assets.**

net cash flow   net difference between cash receipts and cash payments.

net income   revenue less expense; profit.

net patient revenues   gross revenues less contractual allowances, bad debts, and charity care.

net present cost   aggregate present value of a series of payments to be made in the future.

net present value (NPV)   present value of a series of receipts less the present value of a series of payments.

net working capital   current assets less current liabilities.

nominal group technique   forecasting technique in which a group of individuals is brought together in a structured meeting and arrives at a group consensus forecast.

noncontrollable   those items which a manager does not have the authority or ability to control.

nonoperating revenue   categorization that no longer appears on the statement of revenues and expenses. All revenues are operating, unless they are incidental and peripheral to the organization, in which case they are shown as gains.

nonproductive time   sick, vacation, holiday, and other paid nonworked time.

nonrevenue cost center   cost center that does not charge directly for its services. Its costs must be allocated to a revenue center to be included in the organization's rates.

not-for-profit   organization whose mission does not include earning a profit for distribution to owners. A not-for-profit organization may earn a profit, but such profit must be reinvested for replacement of facilities and equipment or for expansion of services offered.

notes payable   written document representing a loan.

NPV   see **net present value.**

NRGs   see **nursing resource groupings.**

nurse executive   senior nurse responsible for managing the nursing services in the entire organization; see also **chief nurse executive.**

nurse manager   person responsible for organizational unit, program, or department.

nursing resource groupings (NRGs)   classifications of patients into homogeneous groups based on nursing care consumed. Any patient in one NRG would consume a similar set of nursing resources as any other patient in that NRG.

objectives   specific targets to be achieved to attain goals.

one-shot   budget that is prepared only once rather than on a regular periodic basis such as monthly or annually.

operating   related to the normal routine activities of the organization in providing its goods or services.

operating budget   plan for the day-in and day-out operating revenues and expenses of the organization. It is generally prepared for one year.

operating expenses   costs of the organization related to its general operations.

operating margin   operating income (revenues less expenses, before other gains or losses) divided by revenue; a profitability measure.

operating revenues   revenues earned in the normal course of providing the organization's goods or services.

operations   routine activities of the organization related to its mission and the provision of goods or services.

opinion letter   letter from the CPA to users of the organization's audited financial statements providing the CPA's expert opinion as to whether the financial statements are a fair presentation of the financial position and results of operations of the organization, in accordance with generally accepted accounting principles.

opportunity costs of inventory   carrying costs or costs of having money tied up in inventory rather than in a revenue-producing endeavor such as an interest-bearing bank account.

ordering costs   includes those costs associated with an order of inventory such as clerk time for preparation of a purchase order.

out-of-pocket costs   see **incremental costs.**

outputs   product being produced, for example, patients, patient days, visits, operations.

overhead   indirect costs allocated to a unit or department from elsewhere in the organization.

owner's equity   residual value after the liabilities of an organization are subtracted from the assets. This represents the portion of the assets owned by the organization itself or its owners.

partnership   business owned by a group of people (partners) who have unlimited liability; the partners may be sued for all liabilities of the firm; see also **corporation.**

pass-through costs   see **cost pass-through.**

patient classification   system for distinguishing among different patients based on their functional ability and resource needs.

patient day   one patient occupying one bed for one day.

patient revenue per day   total patient revenue divided by the number of days in the year.

patient revenues   see **gross patient revenues** and/or **net patient revenues.**

payback   capital budgeting approach that calculates how many years it takes for a project's cash inflows to equal or exceed its cash outflows.

payer   individual or organization that provides money to pay for healthcare.

per diem   (a) daily; (b) the charge per day for routine care; (c) agency nurses who work day-to-day.

performance budget   plan that relates the various objectives of a cost center with the planned costs of accomplishing those activities.

personnel   persons employed in the organization.

PERT   see **program evaluation and review technique.**

plant   building.

plant-age ratio   accumulated depreciation of buildings and equipment divided by annual depreciation expense; an approximation for the average age of physical facilities.

position   one person working one job, regardless of the number of hours the person works.

posting   process of transferring all parts of a journal entry to the specific ledger accounts that are affected by the entry.

PPO   see **preferred provider organization.**

preferred provider organization (PPO)   health care provider organization that is recommended by an insurer or employer as being a preferred provider of services. PPOs generally offer the insurer or employer discounts. Employees or insured individuals who use the PPO generally pay lower coinsurance for their medical care than if they do not use the PPO.

premium   payment to an insurance company for a set period.

prepaid assets   represents assets that have been paid for and have not yet been used but that will be used within one year. This includes items such as fire insurance premiums or rent paid in advance.

prepaid group plan   see **health maintenance organization.**

present costs   see **net present costs.**

present value   value of future receipts or payments discounted to the present.

price variance   portion of the total variance for any line item that is caused by spending a different amount per unit of resource than had been anticipated, e.g., higher or lower salary rates or higher or lower supply prices.

principal   amount of money borrowed on a loan.

private insurers   insurance companies that are not related to the government.

pro forma financial statements   financial statements that present a prediction of what the financial statements for a project, program, or organization will look like at some point in the future.

probability   likelihood of an event's occurring. The probability of future events can be estimated based on data from historical events.

product line   group of patients who have some commonality that allows them to be grouped together, such as a common diagnosis.

product-line costing   determination of the cost of providing care to specific types of patients. This approach is sometimes aided by the use of standard cost techniques, such as Cleverley's model of standard treatment protocols.

production function   financial implications of making and distributing the product.

productive time   straight time and overtime worked.

productivity   ratio of outputs to inputs.

profit   amount by which an organization's revenues exceed its expenses.

profit margin   excess of revenue over expense divided by total revenue; an indication of the amount of profits generated by each dollar of revenue.

profitability ratio   class of ratios that evaluates the profitability of the organization.

program   sequence of instructions for a computer to do a task; a project or service that cuts across departments.

program budget   plan that looks at all aspects of a program across departments and over the long term.

program evaluation and review technique (PERT)   multibranch programming technique designed to predict total project completion time for large-scale projects and to identify paths that have available slack.

programming   total organizational review with a focus on where the organization is headed.

property, plant, and equipment   land, buildings, and pieces of equipment owned by the organization.

proprietary   see **for-profit.**

proprietorship   business owned by one individual.

prospective payment   payment based on a predetermined price for any particular category of patient (such as a particular DRG) as opposed to reimbursement based on the costs of care provided to the patient.

provider   health worker or health care organization that dispenses health care to people.

quality costs   those costs incurred to ensure that the product is of the required quality. This may include costs such as inspection or replacement or harm to the patient created by using a low-quality item.

quantity variance   portion of the total variance for any line item that is caused by using more input per unit of output (e.g., patient day) than had been budgeted.

quick ratio   cash plus marketable securities plus accounts receivable, all divided by current liabilities.

R-squared (R^2)   regression analysis statistic that can range from a low of zero to a high of 1.0. The closer it is to 1.0, the more of the variability in the dependent variable has been explained by the independent variable.

rate setting   process of assigning prices to the units of service of the revenue centers. Prices must be set high enough to recover the organization's total financial requirements.

rate variance   price variance that relates to labor resources. In such cases it is typically the hourly rate that has varied from expectations; see also **price variance.**

ratio   one number divided by another.

ratio of cost to charges (RCC)   method used to convert a patient's bill to that patient's costs by applying the ratio of the organization's costs to its charges.

reciprocal distribution   see **algebraic distribution.**

recruitment   effort directed at getting potential employees to become employees.

regression analysis   statistical model that measures the average change in a dependent variable associated with a one-unit change in one or more independent variables.

regulation   government rule that has the force of law.

relative value unit (RVU) scale   arbitrary unit scale in which each patient is assigned a number of relative value units based on the relative costs of different types of patients. For example, if nursing care costs twice as much for Type A patient as for Type B patient, then Type A patients will be assigned a number of relative value units twice as high as that assigned to Type B patients.

relevant costs   only those costs which are subject to change as a result of a decision.

relevant range   that range of activity which might reasonably be expected to occur in the budget period.

reliability of patient classification system   measure of the consistency of rating across different observers.

repurchase agreements   flexible bank-related financial investment instrument. They can be for periods as short as one day.

residual   portion left over; when liabilities are subtracted from assets, the leftover or residual value is the fund balance or owner's equity.

responsibility accounting   attempt to measure financial outcomes and assign those outcomes to the individual or department responsible for them.

responsibility center   part of the organization, such as a department or a unit, for which a manager is assigned responsibility. Health care organizations generally have cost centers and revenue centers.

restricted funds   funds whose assets are limited as to their use; if the restriction is placed by the donor, it can only be removed by the donor. However, if the assets were restricted by the board, then the restriction may be removed by the board.

retention   continued employment. This is often measured as the converse of turnover or staff leaving an organization.

retrospective patient classification categorization of patients into a patient classification based on the nursing care needs that were met.

return-on-fund-balance ratio profitability ratio that measures the percentage profit earned on fund balance; excess of revenues over expenses divided by fund balance.

revenue amounts of money that the organization has received or is entitled to receive in exchange for goods and/or services that it has provided.

revenue center unit or department that is responsible and accountable not only for costs of providing services but also for the revenues generated by those services.

revenue-to-assets ratio total revenues divided by total assets; a measure of the amount of revenue generated per dollar of assets used by the organization.

RVU see **relative value unit scale.**

scansheet forms with preprinted markings and markings added, usually with a number 2 pencil, that can be read by an optical scanner.

seasonality predictable pattern of monthly, quarterly, or other periodic variation in historical data within each year.

seasonalization adjustment of the annual budget for month-to-month seasonality.

segment see **market segmentation.**

segmentation see **market segmentation.**

self-pay patients patients who are responsible for the payment of their own health care bills because they do not have private insurance and are not covered by either Medicare or Medicaid.

sensitivity analysis process whereby the financial results are recalculated under a series of varying assumptions and predictions. This is often referred to as "what if" analysis.

service unit basic measure of the item being produced by the organization, such as patient days, home care visits, or hours of operations.

short-term assets see **current assets.**

simple linear regression regression analysis that uses one dependent and one independent variable and that produces predictions along a straight line.

sinking fund segregated assets to be used for replacement of plant and equipment.

skimming charging a high price knowing that market share will be low but planning to make a high profit on the volume achieved.

software computer program or programs that instruct the computer what to do and how to do it.

software package program to direct the computer. May be purchased or developed internally.

solvency ability to meet current and future obligations.

solvency ratios class of ratios that evaluates the organization's ability to meet its obligations as they come due over a time frame longer than one year.

special purpose funds funds whose assets are restricted to a particular purpose, such as government grant research projects, student loans, or establishment of a new burn care unit.

spreadsheet large ledger sheets often used by accountants for financial calculations.

staff function provision of auxiliary assistance or service to the line managers and their departments. Finance is a staff function. Units designated to provide staff functions do not provide direct patient care.

staff manager manager with no direct line responsibility for running the organization. Most nurse managers are line managers; the director of nursing education and the director of nursing recruitment are examples of staff positions.

standard cost expectation of what it should cost to produce a good or service, usually on a per unit basis. They are targets, often established based on industrial engineering studies.

standard cost profile costs, fixed and variable, direct and indirect, of producing each service unit (SU); see also **standard treatment protocol.**

standard treatment protocol set of intermediate products or service units (SUs) consumed by a patient in each product line.

statement of financial position financial report that indicates the financial position of the organization at a specific point in time; often referred to as the balance sheet.

statistical software computer programs used to perform statistical calculations.

step-down method of cost allocation in which nonrevenue centers allocate their costs to all cost centers, both revenue and nonrevenue, that have not yet allocated. Once a nonrevenue center allocates its costs, no costs can be allocated to it.

step-fixed cost that is fixed over short ranges of volume but varies within the relevant range (sometimes referred to as step-variable).

step-variable see **step-fixed.**

stockout costs costs incurred when the supply is not available but is needed. If the supply is needed for patient care, it often must be purchased at a higher price from a local vendor.

strategic management process of setting the goals and objectives of the organization, determining the resources to be allocated to achieving those goals and objectives, and establishing policies concerning getting and using those resources.

strategic planning process of setting long-term goals and designing a plan to achieve those goals; often referred to as long-term planning.

strategies broad plans for the attainment of goals. Marketing strategies define the overall desired approach to marketing products and services.

subcategory device to allow separation of the flexible budget variance into the price variance and the quantity variance. The actual quantity of input per unit of output, multiplied by the budgeted price of the input, times the actual output level.

subjective probability relies not only on the scientific application of the laws of chance but also on the judgment of the manager.

subsidiary journal detailed journals where original entries are first made, with only a summary total entry being made to the general journal; for example, a sales journal would list each patient bill, with only a summary of total of revenue recorded in the general journal.

subsidiary ledger   ledgers where detailed information is recorded, with only a summary being posted to the general ledger; for example, a subsidiary accounts receivable ledger would keep track of each patient's receivable separately, while the general ledger would only show the total increase or decrease in receivables.

substitute   economic good that can be used as an alternative to another economic good.

supply   amount of a good or service that all suppliers in aggregate would like to provide for any given price.

supply curve   quantity that would be offered by suppliers at any given price.

surplus   see **profit.**

tactics   specific activities that are undertaken to carry out a strategy.

taxes payable   taxes owed to a local, state, or federal government.

third-party payer   someone other than the patient who pays the health care provider for the patient's care. The most common third-party payers are Medicare, Medicaid, Blue Cross, and other private insurance companies.

time-series analysis   use of historical values of a variable to predict future values for that variable without the use of any other variable other than the passage of time.

time value of money   recognition of the fact that money can earn compound interest, and therefore a given amount of money paid at different points in time has a different value—the further into the future an amount is paid, the less valuable it is.

total debt-to-equity ratio   total liabilities divided by fund balance. The higher this ratio, the less borrowing capacity the organization has left.

total financial requirements (TFR)   financial resources needed to provide for the present and future health care needs of the population served by the organization.

total variance   sum of the price, quantity, and volume variances; the difference between the actual results and the original budgeted amount.

trade credit   accounts payable. These are generally interest free for a period of time.

trend   patterns related to the passage of time. For example, although there are daily fluctuations in the census, the pattern of the census is relatively stable.

turnover   those employees who leave employment in an organization.

uncontrollable   see **noncontrollable.**

unfavorable variance   variance in which more was spent than the budgeted amount.

uniform reporting   approaches to have health care organizations improve comparability of financial information from organization to organization by completing uniform accounting reports.

unit of service   see **service unit.**

unrestricted funds   funds whose assets may be used for any normal purpose; usually only the general operating fund is unrestricted.

unsecured notes   loans that do not have any collateral.

use variance another name for the quantity variance; so called because the quantity variance focuses on how much of a resource has been used; see also **quantity variance.**

utility physical or psychic benefit one receives from goods or services.

validity of patient classification measure of the degree to which the system actually measures what it intends to measure.

variable billing system in which the amount billed to each patient for nursing care per patient day varies based on the differing resource consumption of different patients.

variable costs costs that vary in direct proportion with volume.

variance difference between the budget and the actual results.

variance analysis comparison of actual results as compared with the budget, followed by investigation to determine why the variance(s) occurred.

vendor supplier, such as a pharmaceutical company or hospital supply company.

volume variance amount of the variance in any line item that is caused simply by the fact that the work-load level has changed.

wages payable amounts owed to employees.

wealth value of all the resources the consumer currently owns.

word processing electronic production and storage of documents.

working capital organization's current assets and current liabilities.

working capital management management of the current assets and current liabilities of the organization.

workload volume of work for a unit or department; note that there should be a direct relationship between the workload and the amount of resources needed. Therefore a work-load measure such as patient days is inferior to one such as patient days adjusted for average patient acuity.

year-to-date sum of the budget and/or actual values for all months from the beginning of the year through the most recent period for which data are available.

ZBB see **zero-base budgeting.**

zero-base budgeting (ZBB) program budgeting approach that requires an examination and justification of all costs rather than just the incremental costs and that requires examination of alternatives rather than just one approach.

Index

Note: Page numbers in *italics* refer to illustrations, page numbers followed by t refer to tables.